www.harcourt-international.com

Bringing you products from all Harcourt Health Sciences companies including Baillière Tindall, Churchill Livingstone, Mosby and W.B. Saunders

- ▶ **Browse** for latest information on new books, journals and electronic products

- ▶ **Search** for information on over 20 000 published titles with full product information including tables of contents and sample chapters

- ▶ **Keep up to date** with our extensive publishing programme in your field by registering with eAlert or requesting postal updates

- ▶ **Secure online ordering** with prompt delivery, as well as full contact details to order by phone, fax or post

- ▶ **News** of special features and promotions

If you are based in the following countries, please visit the country-specific site to receive full details of product availability and local ordering information

USA: www.harcourthealth.com

Canada: www.harcourtcanada.com

Australia: www.harcourt.com.au

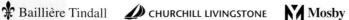 Baillière Tindall   CHURCHILL LIVINGSTONE   Mosby   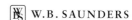 W.B. SAUNDERS

Sports Medicine for Specific Ages and Abilities

For Churchill Livingstone

Editorial Director, Health Professions: Mary Law
Project Manager: Dinah Thom
Designer: George Ajayi

Sports Medicine for Specific Ages and Abilities

Edited by

Nicola Maffulli MD MS PhD FRCS(Orth)

Professor and Chair in Traumatology and Orthopaedics, Keele University Medical School,
Stoke-on-Trent, North Staffordshire, UK

Kai Ming Chan MBBS MCh(Orth) FRCS(G) FRCS(Ed) FRCSEd(Orth) FACS FHKCOS FHKAM(OrthoSurg)

Chair Professor and Chief of Service, Department of Orthopaedics and Traumatology, Prince of Wales Hospital,
Chinese University of Hong Kong, Hong Kong, China

Rose Macdonald BA MCSP MCPA SRP

Former Director of the Sports Injury Centre, Crystal Palace National Sports Centre, London, UK

Robert M. Malina PhD FACSM

Professor of Kinesiology, Adjunct Professor of Anthropology, Michigan State University, East Lansing, Michigan, USA

Anthony W. Parker PhD FASMF

Professor and Head of School of Movement Studies, Faculty of Health, Queensland University of Technology,
Brisbane, Australia

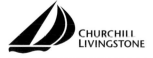
CHURCHILL
LIVINGSTONE

EDINBURGH LONDON NEW YORK PHILADELPHIA ST LOUIS SYDNEY TORONTO 2001

CHURCHILL LIVINGSTONE
An imprint of Harcourt Publishers Limited

© Harcourt Publishers Limited 2001

 is a registered trademark of Harcourt Publishers Limited.

First published 2001

ISBN 0 443 06128 9

British Library Cataloguing in Publication Data
A catalogue record for this book is available from the British Library.

Library of Congress Cataloging in Publication Data
A catalog record for this book is available from the Library of Congress.

Note
Medical knowledge is constantly changing. As new information becomes available, changes in treatment, procedures, equipment and the use of drugs become necessary. The editors, contributors and publishers have taken care to ensure that the information given in this text is accurate and up to date. However, readers are strongly advised to confirm that the information, especially with regard to drug usage, complies with the latest legislation and standards of practice.

The publisher's policy is to use paper manufactured from sustainable forests

Printed in China

Contents

Contributors

Rebecca A. Abbott BScNutrition(Hons) DipDietetics
Postgraduate, School of Human Movement Studies,
Faculty of Health, Queensland University of
Technology, Brisbane, Australia

Bruno Arena MD
Consultant, Servizio Materno Infantile, Azienda
Sanitaria Locale di Piacenza, Piacenza, Italy

Neil Armstrong PhD
Professor of Paediatric Physiology, Head of the School
of Postgraduate Medicine and Health Sciences, and
Director of the Children's Health and Exercise
Research Centre, University of Exeter, Exeter, UK

Christopher Askew BAppSci(Hons)
Research Officer, Department of Surgery, The
University of Queensland, Royal Brisbane Hospital,
Brisbane, Queensland, Australia

Simon J. Bartold BSc FASMF FAAPSM
Private Practitioner, Simon Bartold Podiatry,
Marryatville, South Australia; Consultant Podiatrist
to the Australian Institute of Sport Cycling Unit and
Cricket Academy, Australia

Adam D. G. Baxter-Jones BSc PhD
Associate Professor, College of Kinesiology,
University of Saskatchewan, Saskatchewan, Canada

Colin Boreham BA MA PhD
Professor of Sport and Exercise Sciences, University
of Ulster, Jordanstown, Northern Ireland

Treg D. Brown MD
Assistant Professor of Orthopaedics, Tulane
University, Division of Sports Medicine, New
Orleans, Louisiana, USA

Wolfgang Bruns MS DrMed
Orthopaedische Klinik und Poliklinik,
Universitaetsklinikum Leipzig, Leipzig, Germany

Kai Ming Chan MB BS MCh(Orth) FRCS(G) FRCS(Ed)
FRCSEd(Orth) FACS FHKCOS FHKAM(OrthoSurg)
Chair Professor and Chief of Service, Department of
Orthopaedics and Traumatology, Prince of Wales
Hospital, The Chinese University of Hong Kong,
Hong Kong, China

Peter S. W. Davies BSc(Hons) MPhil PhD
Director, Children's Nutrition Research Centre,
Department of Paediatrics and Child Health,
University of Queensland, Royal Children's Hospital,
Brisbane, Queensland, Australia

Maria A. Fiatarone Singh MD FRACP
John Sutton Chair of Exercise and Sport Science,
Professor of Medicine, University of Sydney,
Australia; Scientist I, Jean Mayer USDA Human
Nutrition Research Center on Aging at Tufts
University, Boston, Massachusetts, USA

David D. Fitzgerald DipEng GradDipPhys
GradDipManipTher
Private Practitioner and Lecturer, Dublin
Physiotherapy Clinic, Dublin, Ireland

Jonathan P. Folland BSc PhD
Lecturer, Chelsea School, University of Brighton,
UK

Freddie H. Fu MD
Chairman, Department of Orthopaedic Surgery,
David Silver Professor, Head Team Physician,
University of Pittsburgh, Pittsburgh, Pennsylvania,
USA

Marc T. Galloway MD
Associate Professor, Department of Orthopaedics and
Rehabilitation, Yale School of Medicine; Chief of
Orthopaedics, Associate Director for Musculoskeletal
Sports Medicine, Yale University Health Service,
New Haven, Connecticut, USA

Mike Greaves MD FRCP FRCPath
Professor of Haematology, Head of Department of
Medicine and Therapeutics, University of Aberdeen,
Aberdeen, Scotland, UK

Simon Green BAppSc MA
Lecturer, School of Human Movement Studies,
Queensland University of Technology, Kelvin Grove,
Brisbane, Queensland, Australia

Henry Ching Lun Ho MB ChB FRCS(Eng) FRCS(Ed)
Medical Officer, Department of Orthopaedics and
Traumatology, Prince of Wales Hospital, Shatin,
Hong Kong, China

Glenn Hunter CertEdFE MSc MCSP SRP
Senior Lecturer, School of Physiotherapy and
Occupational Therapy, Faculty of Health & Social
Care, University of the West of England, Bristol,
UK

David A. Jones BSc PhD
Professor of Sport and Exercise Sciences, The
University of Birmingham, Birmingham, UK

Bryan Jones BSc(Hons)
Lecturer in Sport Psychology, Department of Exercise
and Sport Science, The Manchester Metropolitan
University, Alsager, Stoke-on-Trent, UK

Toshihito Katsumura MD PhD
Professor, Department of Preventive Medicine and
Public Health, Tokyo Medical University, Tokyo,
Japan

Aileen Kelly MSc MCSP MMACP SRP
Chartered Physiotherapist, Physiotherapy
Department, The Whittington Hospital, London;
Former Head Physiotherapist to the Royal Ballet
Company, London, UK

Graham K. Kerr PhD
Senior Lecturer, School of Human Movement Studies,
Queensland University of Technology, Brisbane,
Queensland, Australia

Matthew Kiln MB BS DRCOG FRSH
Principal in General Practice and School Medical
Officer, The Rosendale Surgery, West Dulwich,
London, UK

John King FRCS
Director of Sports Medicine, Queen Mary and
Westfield College, London, UK

Arnold Koller PhD
Head of the Exercise Physiology Laboratory,
Department of Sports and Circulatory Medicine,
University of Innsbruck Medical School, Innsbruck,
Austria

Pirkko Korkia BA(Hons) MSc
Senior Lecturer, Department of Sport and Exercise
Science, University of Luton, Luton, Bedfordshire, UK

Yiannis Koutedakis BSc MA PhD
Professor, Department of Sport Sciences, Thessaly
University, Trikala, Greece; School of Sport,
Performing Arts and Leisure, Wolverhampton
University, Wolverhampton, UK

Masahiro Kurosaka MD
Professor, Department of Orthopaedic Surgery, Kobe
University Hospital, Kobe, Japan

Constance M. Lebrun MDCM MPE CCFP DipSportMed
Director, Primary Care Sport Medicine, Fowler
Kennedy Sport Medicine Clinic, 3M Centre,
University of Western Ontario, London, Ontario,
Canada

C. Terence Lee MD
Fertility Care of Orange County, Brea, California, USA

Guo Ping Li MD
Professor of Sports Medicine, Director, Department of
Sports Medicine, National Institute of Sports Science,
Beijing, China

Scott A. Lynch MD
Assistant Professor, Department of Orthopaedics and
Rehabilitation, Pennsylvania State University,
Hershey, Pennsylvania, USA

Domhnall MacAuley MD FRCGP FFPHM FISM
Professor of Primary Health Care (Research), Institute
of Postgraduate Medical and Health Science,
University of Ulster, Jordanstown, Northern Ireland

Nicola Maffulli MD MS PhD MIBiol FRCS(Orth)
Professor and Chair in Traumatology and
Orthopaedics, Keele University Medical School,
Stoke-on-Trent, North Staffordshire, UK

Robert M. Malina PhD FACSM
Professor of Kinesiology, Adjunct Professor of
Anthropology, Michigan State University, East
Lansing, Michigan, USA

William J. Mallon MD
Triangle Orthopaedic Associates, Durham, North
Carolina; Associative Consulting Professor, Duke
University Medical Center, Durham, North Carolina,
USA

Vladimir Martinek MD
Sports Medicine Fellow, Department of Orthopaedic
Surgery, University of Pittsburgh, Pittsburgh,
Pennsylvania, USA

Jenny McConnell BAppSci(Phty) GradDipManTher
MBiomedE
Director, McConnell & Clements Physiotherapy,
Northbridge, New South Wales, Australia

Jarrod D. Meerkin BAppSc MSc PhD
Australian Paralympic Committee, National Sports
Science Research Coordinator, Queensland
University of Technology, Brisbane, Queensland,
Australia

Lyle J Micheli MD
Associate Professor of Orthopaedics, Harvard
University, and Director of Sports Medicine,
Children's Hospital, Boston, Massachusetts, USA

Gabe Mirkin MD
Associate Clinical Professor, Georgetown University,
School of Medicine, Kensington, MD, USA

Kosaku Mizuno
Professor, Department of Orthopaedics, Kobe, Japan

Yuji Nabeshima MD
Chief, Department of Orthopedic Surgery, Himeji
St Mary's Hospital, Himeji, Japan

Susan A. New BA MSc PhD RPHNutr
Lecturer in Nutrition, Centre for Nutrition and Food
Safety, School of Biological Sciences, University of
Surrey, Guildford, Surrey, UK

Carolyn C. O'Brien BHMS(Hons) MHMS PhD
DipPhysEd TchCert
Lecturer, School of Human Movement Studies,
Faculty of Health, Queensland University of
Technology, Brisbane, Queensland, Australia

Anthony W. Parker PhD FASMF
Professor and Head of School of Human
Movement Studies, Faculty of Health, Queensland
University of Technology, Brisbane, Queensland,
Australia

Pasquale Patrizio MD
Assistant Professor of Obstetrics and Gynecology,
University of Pennsylvania Health System, Hospital
of the University of Pennsylvania, Philadelphia,
Pennsylvania, USA

David Perry FRCP
Consultant Rheumatologist, Department of
Rheumatology and Sports Medicine, Bart's and the
London Trust, London, UK

Ling Qin PhD
Associate Professor, Director of Research,
Department of Orthopaedics and Traumatology,
The Chinese University of Hong Kong,
Hong Kong, China

David M. Reid MD FRCP(Edin)
Professor of Rheumatology and Honorary Consultant
Rheumatologist, Department of Medicine &
Therapeutics, University of Aberdeen, Aberdeen,
Scotland, UK

Per A. F. H. Renström MD PhD
Professor, Section Sports Medicine, Tipskliniken,
Karolinska Institute, Stockholm, Sweden

Neil K. Roach BSc(Hons) MSc
Senior Lecturer, Department of Exercise and Sport
Science, Crewe & Alsager Faculty of Manchester
Metropolitan University, Alsager, Stoke-on-Trent,
UK

Christer Rolf MD PhD
Professor of Sports Medicine, Sheffield Centre of
Sports Medicine, Sheffield, UK

Marisa Z. Rose MD
House Officer, Hospital of the University of
Pennsylvania, Philadelphia, Pennsylvania, USA

L. Schlebusch MA(ClinPsych) MMedSc(Psychiat)
PhD(Natal) CPsychol(UK)
Professor and Head of Medical Psychology,
Department of Medically Applied Psychology, Nelson
R. Mandela School of Medicine, University of Natal,
Durban, South Africa

G. Schweitzer MB BS(Melb) FRACS
Orthopaedic Surgeon in Private Practice, Durban,
South Africa

Nickolas C. Smith MSc
Principal Lecturer, Department of Exercise and Sport
Science, Manchester Metropolitan University, Stoke-
on-Trent, UK

Julie Sparrow MSc MCSP SRP GradDipManip CertEd
Occupational Health Services Manager, South Lodge
Occupational Health Services, South Cleveland
Hospital, Middlesborough, UK

William Wing Kee To MB BS MRCOG
FHKAM(Obs/Gyn)
Consultant, Department of Obstetrics and
Gynaecology, United Christian Hospital,
Hong Kong, China

Thomas Parker Vail MD
Associate Professor, Division of Orthopaedic Surgery,
Duke University, Durham, North Carolina, USA

Henry G. Watson MD MRCPath FRCP(Ed)
Consultant Haematologist, Director of Haemophilia,
Department of Haematology, Aberdeen Royal
Infirmary, Aberdeen, Scotland, UK

A. D. J. Webborn MB BS MRCGP DipSportsMed
Sports Physician, Esperance Private Hospital,
Eastbourne, East Sussex, UK

Joanne R. Welsman PhD FACSM
Senior Research Fellow and Deputy Director of the
Children's Health and Exercise Research Centre,
University of Exeter, Exeter, UK

Margaret Wan Nar Wong MB BS FRCS(Ed) FCSHK
FHKCOS FHKAM(OrthoSurgery)
Honorary Consultant Orthopaedic Surgeon, Dance
Clinic, Academy of Performing Arts, Hong Kong;
Assistant Professor, Department of Orthopaedics and
Traumatology, The Chinese University of Hong Kong,
Hong Kong, China

Charles J. Worringham PhD
Senior Lecturer, School of Human Movement Studies,
Queensland University of Technology, Brisbane,
Queensland, Australia

Shinichi Yoshiya MD
Department of Orthopaedic Surgery, Meiwa Hospital,
Nishinomiya, Hyogo, Japan

Preface

Sports medicine is a relatively new speciality. It has a sound clinical grounding and its remit extends beyond traditional medical boundaries. Modern sports medicine physicians face intense demands from competitive athletes at all levels, from top sport to local youth programmes, and increasing demands from individuals who wish to exercise for health purposes. In this book we recognize the necessity of a multidisciplinary approach to the problems and ailments that physically active individuals may experience, and have therefore gathered contributors from a wide range of the health care professions.

Sports medicine has recently undergone a revolution. It started as a traditional clinically based speciality with relatively little input from the basic sciences and experimental clinical work. It has now come of age, and many recent advances represent the integration of ideas nurtured in the clinic with results obtained in the laboratory. This is major progress for the speciality and we are sure that this book fits well in this progressive, integrated environment.

There are a large number of textbooks dealing with different aspects of sports and exercise medicine, but there are still many areas that have not been adequately covered. In compiling this text, we have enlisted the help of a multinational team of experts to present their views and to share their expertise in the hope that this will lead to further discussions and a cross-fertilisation of ideas. We advised our authors not to be too didactic and to give practical advice, and we believe that their work has been exemplary. We recognize that there are some conditions which may be specific to a given sport, or to a given geographic area, and that not all of these have been included. However, we realized when planning the book that it would be impossible to cover every aspect of every condition.

Sports Medicine for Specific Ages and Abilities is aimed at those involved in the health care of athletes, both competitive and recreational. It is specifically aimed at health care professionals with a major interest in children, women, older individuals and the disabled in the context of sport and physical activity. However, it is not limited to these groups, and many of the concepts presented can be applied to other athletes and athletic activities.

This book is the first of its kind to address in one volume the specific problems of different categories of individuals in sport, and should be of major interest to the team physician, physiotherapist and athletic trainer, as well as other professionals allied to medicine in sport.

Stoke-on-Trent, Hong Kong, London, East Lansing and Brisbane, 2001

Nicola Maffulli
Kai Ming Chan
Rose Macdonald
Robert M. Malina
Anthony Parker

Children and adolescent athletes

1

Training and injuries in young athletes

Nicola Maffulli   Wolfgang Bruns

KEY POINTS

1. Although sports injuries in children and adolescents are mainly mild contusions, sprains and strains, the media often only reports the more severe skeletal injuries sustained, causing much of the concern expressed with regards to the safety of youth sport.
2. A deep knowledge of the different aspects of training, including duration, intensity, frequency and recovery, is needed to avoid serious damage to the skeletal system of athletic children.
3. Coaches and parents can minimize the risk of injury by ensuring the proper selection of sports events, using appropriate equipment, enforcing rules, using safe playing conditions and providing adequate supervision.
4. It is important to balance the negative effects of sports injuries with the many social, psychological and health benefits that a serious commitment to sport brings.

INTRODUCTION

In Britain, approximately three-quarters of all healthy youngsters between 5 and 15 years old participate in organized sport. However, only 11% of these are involved in intensive training (Rowley 1989). In the USA, up to 50% of boys and 25% of girls aged between 8 and 16 years take part in organized competitive sport (Metcalfe & Roberts 1993).

The skeletal system of children is extremely plastic (Maffulli & Baxter-Jones 1995) and shows pronounced adaptive changes to intensive sports training. As sports injuries affect bone and soft tissues, they can damage the growth mechanisms with subsequent life-long damage (Castiglia 1995, Maffulli 1992, Maffulli & Helms 1988, Williams 1981).

Around the period of peak linear growth, adolescents are vulnerable to injuries because of imbalance in strength and flexibility and changes in the biomechanical properties of bone. In immature athletes, as bone stiffness increases and resistance to impact diminishes, sudden overload may cause bones to bow or buckle. Physiological loading has been shown to be beneficial to the young skeleton, but excessive strains may result in serious injury to weight-bearing joint surfaces (Booth & Gould 1975).

INCIDENCE OF SPORTS INJURIES

The actual incidence of injury in children's sports is very difficult, if not impossible, to determine. Because of the different criteria used to define an injury, comparisons between reports are difficult, and any such comparisons should be interpreted with caution.

Between 3 and 11% of school-aged children are injured each year participating in sport. Although boys may sustain twice as many injuries as girls (Crompton & Tubbs 1977, Maffulli & Baxter-Jones 1995, Schmidt & Höllwarth 1989, Zaricznyj et al 1980), some authors report a similar incidence between genders (Castiglia 1995, Sahlin 1990). Boys, however, still sustain more severe injuries, possibly because they are more aggressive. In general, the incidence of sports injuries seems to increase with age, approaching the incidence rate of senior players in older children. Recently, using a mixed longitudinal study design, we found an incidence rate of less than one injury per 1000 h of training in 453 elite young British athletes (Maffulli et al 1994). Children also seek treatment for injuries that were previously seen almost exclusively in adults. These 'unique' injuries may represent approximately 15% of all clinically significant sports injuries in children (Maffulli et al 1996).

Injury patterns are influenced by children's physical characteristics. Joint laxity is associated with ligamentous injury, such as recurrent sprains and dislocations (Lysens et al 1984). Tightness is strongly correlated with meniscal injuries and ankle, shoulder and wrist sprains (O'Neill & Micheli 1988).

In this chapter, we shall discuss some general points relating to sports injuries in children and adolescent athletes, giving some specific examples of such injuries in the upper limb and the spine.

EPIPHYSEAL INJURIES

These injuries, with no counterpart in adult life, occur at the epiphyseal growth plates. Shearing and avulsion forces are generally responsible, but compression plays a significant role. The cartilaginous cells of the epiphysis may be damaged, producing premature closure of the epiphyseal plate and growth disturbance bone growth, with subsequent deformity.

Growth plate injuries are classified into five types (Salter & Harris 1963):

- In *types 1 and 2*, the epiphyseal plate is intact, the prognosis is excellent and, after appropriate reduction and immobilization, growth continues undisturbed (Fig. 1.1).
- In *types 3 and 4*, the fracture runs through the joint surface and through the epiphyseal plate. Through accurate closed or surgical reduction, the epiphyseal plate and the articular surface are correctly aligned. Growth can then continue, and restoration of the joint anatomy to congruity prevents secondary osteoarthritis.
- *Type 5 injuries* are often difficult to detect radiographically at the time of injury, as they are a compression injury of the growth plate. Some time after the injury, growth may cease, and deformity or growth disturbance can follow.

UPPER LIMB INJURIES

Fractures of the clavicle

These are common injuries in contact sports and in sports involving falls onto the outstretched hand or a direct fall onto the shoulder. Reduction is generally not necessary, and the child simply needs a sling to immobilize the arm for 2–3 weeks. Recovery is excellent.

Glenohumeral dislocation

Glenohumeral dislocations are rare in youngsters.

Fractures of the humerus

The mechanism of injury is usually indirect. Metaphyseal fractures are seen particularly in older children. It is rarely necessary to correct the deformity, given the great adaptability of the shoulder joint, and the good post-healing remodelling.

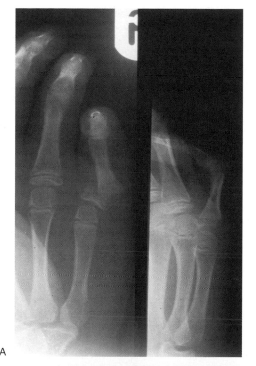

A

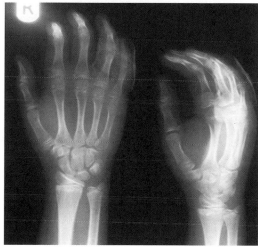

B

Figure 1.1 A: Type 2 Salter–Harris injury of the proximal phalanx of the little finger in a 10-year-old judo player whose little finger had become trapped in the judo suit of the opponent. B: After manipulation under local anaesthesia and splinting.

Elbow injuries

Elbow injuries are common. Plain radiographs in children are often difficult to interpret, damage to major vessels or nerves may occur, and some children require operative treatment. The elbow is liable to develop post-traumatic stiffness, but in this age group vigorous physical therapy is generally not needed. Damage to the growth plate can result in subsequent deformity.

Supracondylar fractures

The distal part of the humerus commonly displaces posteriorly and can involve the growth plate. The arm should be manipulated, correcting all the components of the fracture, and held either in flexion or in extension, depending on the type of fracture, in a well moulded cast. If there is an associated brachial artery injury, surgical exploration with open reduction is mandatory. If the closed reduction is acceptable but unstable, we use percutaneous wiring to maintain reduction.

Dislocation of the elbow

Common in gymnastics, this can be associated with fractures of the medial epicondyle of the humerus, fractures of the neck of the radius, or injury to the median or ulnar nerve. Most of the dislocations in youngsters are posterior or posterolateral. At all ages, they require prompt reduction. Rehabilitation should be gradual, and return to sporting activities before 8–12 weeks discouraged. The child should have regained a full range of movement before resuming full sporting activity (Fig. 1.2).

Forearm and wrist fractures

These fractures are generally due to indirect trauma from a fall onto the outstretched hand. Most fractures occur over the distal third (Fig. 1.3).

Some angulation is acceptable in young children, but angular deformity should be corrected if the child is older than 12 years. Rotational deformity should always be avoided. If manipulation under anaesthesia is unsuccessful, open reduction and internal fixation should be undertaken (Fig. 1.4).

Injuries to the distal radial growth epiphysis

Extremely common, this fracture is usually a Salter type 2 injury. Closed reduction and immobilization are generally sufficient, and results are excellent. A slight dorsal angulation can be accepted, but the young patients must be closely monitored as, in some children, the position is lost and further manipulation is necessary.

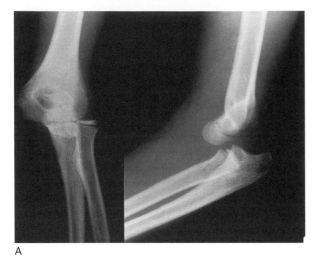

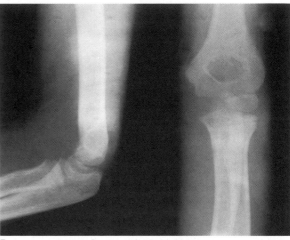

A

B

Figure 1.2 A: Posterior elbow dislocation in a 6-year-old gymnast. B: After manipulation under anaesthesia.

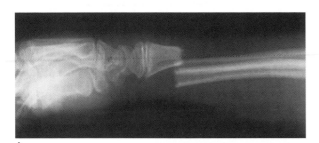

A

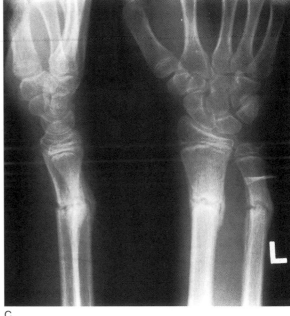

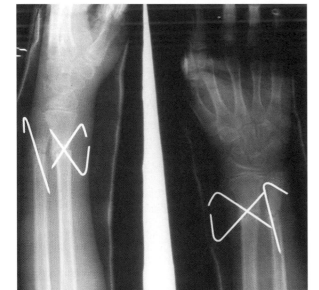

B

C

Figure 1.3 A: Fracture of the distal end of the radius and ulna with complete displacement in a 12-year-old footballer. B: After closed reduction and single percutaneous Kirschner wiring. C: Five weeks after the fracture, abundant callus can be seen despite partial loss of reduction after removal of the wires at three weeks. Full range of motion was possible.

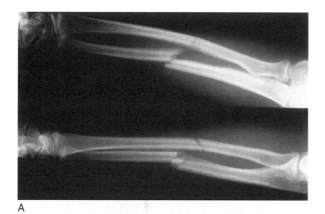

A

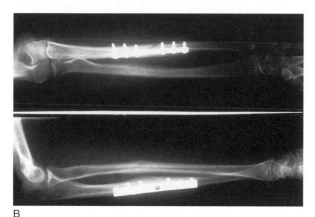

B

Figure 1.4 A: This 13.5-year-old rugby player was stamped upon by a competitor, suffering from a fracture of the radius and ulna. As the ulnar fracture was undisplaced, it was decided to plate only the radius. B: Eight weeks after the injury, there is evidence of callus formation over the ulna. The patient had started mobilization at 6 weeks.

Overuse injuries

Traction apophysilis

This condition occurs at the insertion of the triceps into the olecranon epiphysis in gymnastics, diving, wrestling and hockey, presenting with local pain and tenderness around the insertion of the triceps tendon, exacerbated by supporting the body weight with the arms. Radiographs are difficult to interpret because of normal variants in this region, and may show marked epiphyseal fragmentation. Treatment consists of a period of rest from upper limb activities, and symptoms usually settle over a few months, with no long-term problems.

Osteochondritis dissecans

Osteochondritis dissecans (OCD) of the humeral capitellum is well documented. The dominant arm is affected in little league baseball pitchers, due to valgus loading of the elbow during pitching, so that the lateral side of the joint is repeatedly compressed. In gymnasts, compression and rotation during weight-bearing through the arm, and loading of the lateral side of the elbow increased by the physiological valgus of the elbow, affect the joint surface. The youngsters present with elbow pain and some swelling, and are often unable to fully extend the elbow, which is tender over the lateral aspect. Initial signs and symptoms are often minimal. Radiographs are often diagnostic, but early diagnosis may require magnetic resonance imaging (MRI) or computed tomography (CT). The damaged area of the articular epiphysis can break away to form an intra-articular loose body.

In the early phases, conservative measures may be successful, with proscription of weight-bearing on the upper limbs or of stressing the elbow. Loose bodies should be removed surgically or arthroscopically. As the articular surface is damaged and the joint is not congruous, early osteoarthrosis can ensue. OCD of the radial head is rarer.

Panner's disease

There is impairment of blood supply of the entire epiphysis of the humeral capitellum, with pain, swelling and limitation of motion of the elbow. Diagnosis is radiological. If healing results in a deformity, there will be incongruity of the joint with the risk of later osteoarthrosis.

Epiphyseal growth plate overuse injuries

The epiphyseal growth plate may fail due to repeated microtraumas. Stress fractures through the olecranon epiphysis have been reported in adolescent baseball players, gymnasts and wrestlers. There is pain in the posterior aspect of the elbow with local tenderness over the olecranon and decreased elbow extension. The growth plate is widened. Healing usually takes place with conservative treatment. Occasionally, the epiphyseal plate fails to fuse, and internal fixation is necessary.

Stress-induced changes in the distal radial epiphysis are well recognized in gymnasts, who present with wrist pain associated with some swelling and local pain on weight-bearing and rotation of the wrist.

Radiographs show widening of the growth plate with failure of the zone of calcification. With rest, the epiphysis recovers. The prognosis is good, although growth can be interrupted. At the end of growth, the child may present a slight shortening of the radius compared with the ulna.

SPINAL LESIONS

Chronic back pain in children is rare, except in cases of Scheuermann's disease and spondylolysis or spondylolisthesis. More serious conditions, such as fractures, infections and tumours, should therefore be considered. Adolescent athletes are more prone to disc prolapse, which is best diagnosed by MRI. The high-risk sports for acute spinal injuries are American football, diving, gymnastics and trampolining. Sports injuries account for 18% of paediatric cervical spine fractures.

Although the development of scoliosis (curvature in the coronal plane greater than 10°) is not related to sport, in the sagittal plane excessive physical stress can be a factor in the development of structural kyphosis or Scheuermann's disease. This is distinct from the functional correctable kyphosis of poor posture known as functional round back. Scheuermann's disease can be diagnosed by a lateral spine radiograph showing three consecutive vertebrae with anterior wedging of 5° or more. In addition, the end-plates of the growing vertebra adjacent to the discs are often markedly irregular, and intraosseous herniation of cartilaginous disc material (Schmorl's nodes) may be a predominant feature.

Following trauma, fractures of the cervical spine are less common in children than in adults. Most spinal injuries in children below the age of 12 years involve the atlantoaxial or atlantooccipital joints, although all levels are encountered. Prevertebral soft tissue swelling greatly assists diagnosis on lateral films. Slight anterior vertebral wedging is normal in children due to incomplete ossification, and up to 2 mm of spondylolysis is acceptable in the upper cervical levels. The normally lax ligaments of children result in a greater prevalence of displacements than fractures. Down's syndrome children have such lax atlantoaxial ligaments that it is recommended that sporting activity be restricted if a lateral radiograph shows greater than 4.5 mm arch–dens separation. This laxity predisposes to atlantoaxial rotary subluxation, with abnormal displacement between the facet joints, presenting as torticollis. If this is suspected on plain radiographs, CT scanning with the head turned in both directions is required to assess whether this is fixed (a facet joint does not reduce with the head turned towards the direction of C2) or mobile. This is often seen in ballet due to rapid head rotation whilst pirouetting.

Gymnastics, dance, football, weight-lifting and running are associated with spondylolysis and spondylolisthesis (Micheli 1983). Spondylolysis is an osseous defect of the pars interarticularis between the superior and inferior facets of the vertebral body. Spondylolisthesis is the slippage of the superior vertebra on the inferior. Both can be related to hyperextension and axial loading, since there is an increased incidence in gymnasts (11%), ballet, fast cricket bowlers, and interior linemen in American football. Although spondylolisthesis can be due to a congenitally inadequate superior facet, it is usually acquired. Its frequency increases with age through childhood, especially between 5 and 7 years, to reach 6% in adults. It is thought to be a stress fatigue fracture, although occasionally it is an acute injury. Approximately 70% of spondylolistheses occur at the L5–S1 level, and only rarely above L3. They are usually bilateral. When unilateral, compensatory hypertrophy of the contralateral pedicle may be seen as increased density on plain radiograph. CT clearly shows the defect in the posterior arch, and also delineates any foraminal encroachment by bone fragments.

A much less frequent factor of low back pain in adolescent athletes is lumbar disc protrusion. The true incidence of the lesion in sporting youngsters is unknown, and no conclusion can be made. The role of acute trauma as an aetiological factor in the development of disc herniation in young and very young patients has been stressed, but degenerative changes may play a leading role, with trauma acting solely as a precipitating factor. A single traumatic episode is not sufficient to produce a disc prolapse unless a degenerative condition is present. This could explain the infrequency of the lesion in young athletes.

CONCLUSIONS

1. In general, sports injuries in children and adolescents are limited to mild contusions, sprains and strains.
2. Any sport can cause skeletal injuries, and the specific pattern and location of injuries of each sport should be known by health professionals.
3. Training programmes and performance standards should take into account the biological age of the participants, and their physical and psychological immaturity, more so than their chronological age.
4. Considerable time is needed for growing athletes to incorporate their own body changes, and it is probably difficult for the young athlete to develop speed, strength, endurance and resistance at the same time.
5. Physical injury is an inherent risk in sports participation and, to a certain extent, must be considered an inevitable cost of athletic training and competition.
6. Coaches and parents can minimize the risk of injury by ensuring the proper selection of sports events, using appropriate equipment, enforcing rules, using safe playing conditions and providing adequate supervision.

REFERENCES

Booth F W, Gould E W 1975 Effects of training and disuse on connective tissue. Exercise and Sports Sciences Review 3: 83–112

Castiglia P T 1995 Sports injuries in children. Journal of Paediatric Health Care 9: 32–33

Crompton B, Tubbs N 1977 A survey of sports injuries in Birmingham. British Journal of Sports Medicine 11: 12–15

Lysens R, Steverlynck A, van den Auweele Y et al 1984 The predictability of sports injuries. Sports Medicine 1: 6–10

Maffulli N, Baxter-Jones A D G 1995 Common skeletal injuries in young athletes. Sports Medicine 19(2): 137–149

Maffulli N, Bundoc R C, Chan K M, Cheng J C Y 1996 Paediatric sports injuries in Hong Kong: a seven year survey. British Journal of Sports Medicine 30: 218–221

Maffulli N 1992 The growing child in sport. British Medical Bulletin 48: 561–568

Maffulli N, Helms P 1988 Controversies about intensive training in young athletes. Archives of Diseases in Childhood 63: 1405–1407

Maffulli N, King J B, Helms P 1994 Training in elite young athletes (the training of young athletes (TOYA) study): injuries, flexibility and isometric strength. British Journal of Sports Medicine 28: 123–136

Metcalfe J A, Roberts S O 1993 Strength training and the immature athlete: an overview. Pediatric Nursing 19: 325–332

Micheli L J 1983 Overuse injuries in children's sport: the growth factor. Orthopaedic Clinics of North America 14: 337–360

O'Neill D B, Micheli L J 1988 Overuse injuries in the young athlete. Clinics in Sports Medicine 7(3): 591–610

Rowley S 1989 The effect of intensive training on young athletes. Sports Council, London. p 6–7

Sahlin Y 1990 Sport accidents in childhood. British Journal of Sports Medicine 24(1): 40–44

Salter R B, Harris W R 1963 Injuries involving the epiphyseal plate. Journal of Bone and Joint Surgery (Am) 45: 587–622

Schmidt B, Höllwarth M E 1989 Sportunfälle im Kindes- und Jugendalter. Zeitschrift für Kinderchirurgie 44: 357–362

Williams J G P 1981 Sports injuries in children. Medisport 3: 122–126

Zaricznyj B, Shattuck L J M, Mast T A, Robertson R V, D'Elia G 1980 Sports-related injuries in school aged children. American Journal of Sports Medicine 8(5): 3318–3324

2

The knee in children's sports

Vladimir Martinek   Freddie H. Fu

KEY POINTS

1. The knee is the most common location of sports-related injuries in children.
2. There is an increasing incidence of knee trauma in children, due to an increasing emphasis on competition in children's sports, and a greater involvement by children in passive indoor activities.
3. The growing musculoskeletal system has specific characteristics which distinguish injury patterns in children and adolescents from those in adults.
4. Increasing knowledge of joint biomechanics and the biology of healing, in addition to the availability of new diagnostic tools and techniques, has led to changes in the management of knee injuries in children during the last decade.

INTRODUCTION

The knee is the most common location of sports-related injuries in children. Increasing emphasis on competition in children's sports and improving diagnostic tools, e.g. magnetic resonance imaging (MRI) and arthroscopy, have resulted in an increasing incidence of knee trauma (DeHaven & Lintner 1986). Raising susceptibility to injury in children is also seen as a consequence of declining activity in our society. Children are more involved in passive indoor activities such as playing computer games or watching television and do not develop basic fitness and strength. As a result when they begin to participate in organized sports, they are more prone to injuries (Maffulli 1992).

The growing musculoskeletal system has specific characteristics which distinguish injury patterns and healing processes in children and adolescents from those in adults. The skeleton of a child is generally more elastic and allows more flexibility and deformation in response to external forces. The growth cartilage in the physeal plates and apophyses, however, is susceptible to injuries usually not seen in adults. Ligament laxity and muscle imbalance developing during the growth process represent an additional risk for specific injuries and overuse syndromes in children (Smith & Tao 1995, Webber 1988).

Due to increasing knowledge of joint biomechanics and the biology of healing, as well as the availability of new diagnostic tools and minimally invasive techniques, the management of knee injuries in children has changed throughout the last decade (Steiner & Grana 1988). This chapter provides an overview or etiology, diagnostic procedures and treatment of common sports-related acute and chronic injuries in the child's knee joint.

CLINICAL ASSESSMENT OF KNEE DISORDERS

The evaluation of injury history and the clinical examination of a painful, swollen knee can be difficult in children. Patients under 6 years of age are usually unable to localize the pain, and the only manifestation of a knee disorder might be a subtle limping. Physical examination contains typical knee tests and maneuvers used in adults. Special attention should be directed towards tenderness of the epiphyses. Additionally, congenital conditions, such as constitutional laxity or absence of the anterior cruciate ligament (ACL) and pain referred from the hip joint (Perthes' disease, slipped capital femoral epiphysis), should be considered. Also, systemic causes of knee pain and effusion such as hemophilia, rheumatoid arthritis or hyperparathyroidism should be included in the differential diagnosis (Smith & Tao 1995, Steiner & Grana 1988).

In cases of equivocal clinical findings, MRI may yield useful information along with the standard roentgenograms (Stanitski 1998). Views of the contralateral knee may be helpful to assess radiological abnormalities and to distinguish between normal and pathologic findings. For special considerations, computed tomography (CT) (osteochondritis dissecans, patellofemoral malalignment) and bone scans (stress fractures, osteochondritis dissecans) are recommended.

An acute hemarthrosis following trauma in the young athlete is predictive for an ACL injury in about 50% of the patients (Binfield et al 2000). Using MRI, ACL tears can be detected with a higher level of accuracy (Stanitski 1998). MRI examinations have also increased in sensitivity and specificity for the diagnosis of associated injuries such as meniscal ruptures, lesions of the articular cartilage, and injuries of the physeal plates.

KNEE LIGAMENT INJURIES
Anterior cruciate ligament injuries

Anterior cruciate ligament injuries in skeletally immature athletes are reported with increasing frequency (McCarroll et al 1988, Nottage & Matsuura 1994). This situation is attributed to increased involvement of children and adolescents in competitive sports such as soccer, football, basketball, and alpine skiing. There are two common injury mechanisms causing an ACL tear: valgus force to a flexed, externally rotated knee, and hyperextension with an internally rotated knee. The symptoms and clinical findings of ACL injuries in children do not differ from those in adults. The clinical tests for abnormal ACL laxity should substantiate the diagnosis. MRI examination can be a helpful tool in cases with equivocal physical examinations (Fig. 2.1A).

Conservative treatment

Conservative treatment of ACL injuries in skeletally immature athletes shows poor prognosis with respect to return to sport activities, functional instability, secondary articular cartilage or meniscal injuries (McCarroll et al 1994). Conservative management with rehabilitation and bracing until skeletal maturity, followed by a standard anatomical ACL reconstruction, is recommended by some clinicians because of a possible growth disturbance following operative treatment.

Operative treatment

An operative treatment approach has to evaluate and consider the risk of growth disturbance in children with open growth plates. Results of primary ACL repair in children are not better than those in adults (Grontvedt et al 1996), and primary suture cannot be recommended as a treatment for torn ACL in skeletally immature persons. Extra-articular ACL reconstruction techniques which are non-anatomical and non-isometrical have also been abandoned because of discouraging results (McCarroll et al 1994).

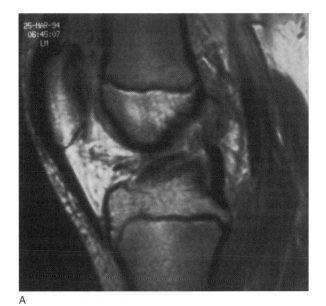

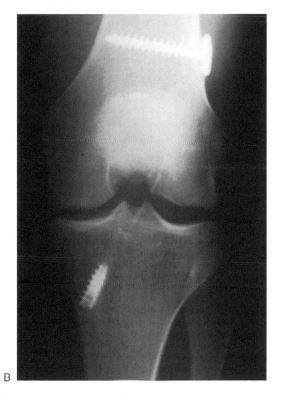

Figure 2.1 A: MRI of an ACL rupture in a 13-year-old female athlete. B: Anteroposterior radiograph 5 years after ACL reconstruction in the same patient. A semitendinosus/gracilis graft was placed through an 8 mm transphyseal tibial tunnel and over-the-top position on the lateral femur. No growth disturbance can be detected.

One of the major considerations in an ACL replacement in a child is the disturbance of the growth plate due to the transphyseal drill holes which are required by modern ACL replacement techniques. In an attempt to reduce the risk for physeal damage, an ACL reconstruction technique without the use of transphyseal drill holes has been described (Brief 1991), but the clinical result in a small group of patients was not convincing.

Intra-articular ACL reconstruction with transphyseal drill holes gives the most anatomical and isometric placement of the ACL graft in adults. Despite considerations regarding the disturbance of the growth plates around the knee, successful techniques using transphyseal drill holes for ACL placement in skeletally immature persons have been described. Using soft tissue grafts and small drill holes (up to 6 mm in diameter), this technique seems to confer only a small risk of damage to the physeal plates, even in patients with wide open physes. Our preferred technique, therefore, is to use a soft tissue graft (semitendinosus/gracilis) placed through a small transphyseal tibial tunnel and over-the-top position on the lateral femur. With this technique, no early physeal closure, limb-length discrepancy or angular deformity has been detected in our series (Fig. 2.1B).

Fractures of the tibial spine

Tibial spine fractures represent a unique variant of ACL ruptures in children which are strongly related to the level of skeletal immaturity (Fig. 2.2). In 80% of patients younger than 12 years, tibial spine avulsion is diagnosed, whereas in 90% of those over 12 years, a mid-substance disruption of the ACL is diagnosed (Kellenberger & von Laer 1990).

Meyers & McKeever (1959) classified these injuries according to the position of the avulsed tibial fragment. For non-displaced or minimally avulsed tibial spine fractures, immobilization is recommended in a long leg cast near the extension position for 6–8 weeks. Essential for adequate healing is a reduction of the fracture, which can usually be performed closed under general anesthesia using fluoroscopy or arthroscopy. For initial significantly displaced and reduced avulsions of the tibial spine, fixation of the fragment is strongly recommended. The fixation can be performed arthroscopically using pins and cannulated screws in retrograde fashion or heavy sutures passed proximally to the tibial physis.

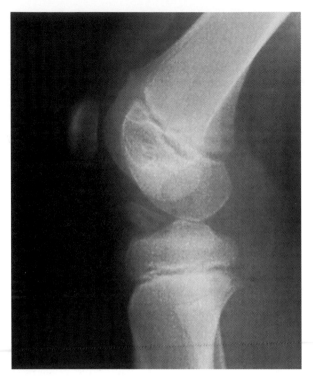

Figure 2.2 Tibial spine avulsion.

Collateral ligament injuries

Medial collateral ligament (MCL) injuries

MCL injuries are commonly caused by valgus stress to the knee in contact sports such as football or soccer. Conservative management is effective in the majority of the cases. Operative treatment will, however, be necessary for grossly displaced bony avulsions of the MCL or for associated injuries. A hinged brace should be applied for 2–4 weeks according to the severity of the injury. Return to sports activity is usually allowed as soon as free range of motion and pain-free exercise are achieved.

Lateral collateral ligament (LCL) injuries

Isolated LCL injuries are extremely rare in children and occur as a consequence of a varus stress or hyperextension of the knee. In these rare injuries, an MRI should always be performed to rule out more severe injury patterns. The management of these injuries is challenging. Isolated lesions of the posterolateral ligament complex are treated conservatively with a hinged brace and physiotherapy. Operative treatment, which should avoid drilling holes through the fibular physis, is necessary for displaced avulsions of the LCL or popliteus tendon.

Posterior cruciate ligament injuries

Posterior cruciate ligament (PCL) tears are rare in children. Clinical experience of these injuries is limited (Ringer & Fay 1990). The majority of PCL injuries in children involve avulsions from the tibial and femoral insertions. Based on biomechanical experiments, tibial avulsions occur with forceful posterior displacement in flexion, and femoral avulsions through a hyperextension of the knee joint.

The diagnosis of acute PCL injuries can be difficult. The clinical examination (posterior drawer) may reveal signs which often do not reflect the true extent of the injury. Radiographic evaluation which includes standard plain X-rays can be non-diagnostic. Usually, definitive diagnosis of the PCL tear and of the associated injuries is obtained by MRI, which is highly sensitive for the diagnosis of all ligamentous injuries in children (Stamitski 1998).

Treatment

Acute avulsions of the PCL are treated with primary intraphyseal sutures or screws. The trauma is evaluated arthroscopically to confirm the location of the PCL injury, to visualize the chondral surfaces and to repair associated meniscal tears. The reduction and fixation of the avulsed PCL can be managed in arthroscopic fashion, but in some cases an open procedure will be necessary (Ringer & Fay 1990).

For midsubstance tears of the PCL, conservative treatment with restoration of full range of motion and muscular strength is the therapy of choice. If functional instability remains a problem, PCL reconstruction should be performed at the time of skeletal maturity.

MENISCUS LESIONS

Meniscal tears

Meniscal lesions are rare in children in comparison to adults, but an increase in meniscal tears has been documented toward adulthood (DeHaven & Lintner 1986). Due to a greater vascularity, an injured meniscus has a higher healing potential in children than in adults. Therefore, more meniscal lesions, especially small stable peripheral tears, can heal without surgical intervention.

The mechanism of injury is similar to that in adults. The most common reason for meniscal tears is a non-contact twisting force to a flexed knee. The diagnosis of acute meniscal lesions can be difficult, especially in younger children. Commonly, the symptoms, such as joint line tenderness, positive McMurray test and decreased range of motion, are less specific. Plain radiographs are usually non-diagnostic but are necessary to rule out other knee disorders. MRI has become increasingly popular, because of the improved diagnostic accuracy for ligamentous knee injuries. However, the diagnostic value of MRI for meniscal lesions in children is still low. Three-dimensional MRI reconstructions have been shown to be more valuable in the diagnosis of meniscal disorders.

Treatment

The management of meniscal lesions has changed significantly during the past three decades as the biomechanical and biological importance of the menisci for the fate of the knee joint has become more and more obvious (Arnoczky & Warren 1982, Walker & Erkman 1975). Long-term follow-up studies have shown that total and partial meniscectomies lead to osteoarthritis (Abdon et al 1990). The goal of the treatment of meniscal tears is the preservation of the meniscus as much as possible. The damaged meniscus should be repaired whenever possible using arthroscopic techniques similar to those used in adults. Small stable peripheral meniscal tears (<5 mm) usually heal spontaneously. Unstable tears are repaired with sutures or with bioabsorbable staples and arrows.

Discoid meniscus

Discoid meniscus is an uncommon anomaly which can present as a 'snapping knee syndrome' in children (Raber et al 1998). It was first discovered on cadavers more than 100 years ago, and later differentiated into three types: I, stable, complete; II, stable, incomplete; III, unstable due to lack of meniscotibial attachment. Discoid meniscus is more common laterally than medially, and manifests bilaterally in 10% of patients. The frequency of this anomaly varies worldwide from 5% in Anglo-Saxons to nearly 20% in Asians (Maffulli et al 1996).

The most consistent physical findings in children with a symptomatic discoid meniscus are similar to symptoms accompanying an acute meniscal tear: restricted range of motion, lateral joint line tenderness and palpable clicking. Standard radiographs are often

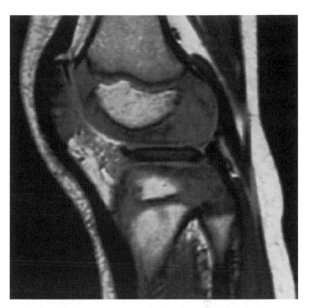

Figure 2.3 MRI showing a lateral discoid meniscus.

normal, and the preoperative diagnosis is frequently made by MRI (Fig. 2.3). Sometimes, discoid meniscus is diagnosed at arthroscopy performed for another reason.

Treatment

The existence of the discoid meniscus alone is not an indication for treatment. The treatment of symptomatic discoid meniscus is performed arthroscopically. Usually a central tear can be found. For the stable forms (types I and II), sculpting of the torn meniscus to a stable rim should be preferred to a total meniscectomy. Therapy for the unstable type III consists of stabilization of the posterior meniscal horn.

PHYSEAL AND EPIPHYSEAL INJURIES

Femoral and tibial physeal fractures

Physeal fractures around the knee are uncommon, representing only about 3% of all physeal fractures in children. The two major physeal plates of the knee, the distal femoral and the proximal tibial physes, are responsible for 70% of the longitudinal growth of the lower extremity. Consequently, injuries to these physeal plates are highly associated with growth disturbance such as leg shortening or angulation. Most of the physeal fractures occur during the adolescent

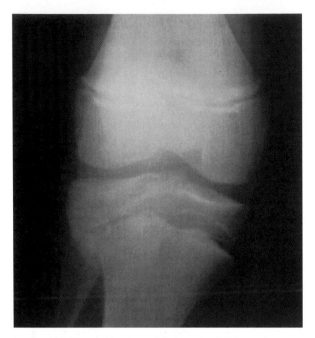

Figure 2.4 Physeal fracture of the proximal tibia.

growth spurt (males, 12–16 years) as the physeal plate becomes relatively weak in comparison to the adjacent ligaments and the bone. The main injury mechanism is a valgus or varus trauma of the knee joint, but repetitive microtrauma causing an overuse injury of the physeal plate has also been described in young gymnasts.

Among various classification systems for physeal injuries, the Salter–Harris classification is the most commonly used (I, transphyseal separation; II, transphyseal separation + metaphyseal fracture; III, transphyseal separation + epiphyseal fracture; IV, transphyseal separation + metaphyseal + epiphyseal fracture; V, crush injury of the epiphyseal plate).

Clinically, physeal fractures are difficult to distinguish from ligament injuries of the knee. Very often, excruciating pain makes a complete examination of the injured athlete impossible. Roentgenograms may not reveal the type I of this injury immediately, but they will 2 weeks following injury after periosteal new bone formation is visible (Fig. 2.4). MRI studies can again be helpful to detect physeal fractures immediately after the trauma (Jaramillo et al 1990).

Treatment

The exact anatomic reduction of displaced physeal fractures is necessary to obtain acceptable clinical results. Type I and II physeal fractures can be treated by closed reduction and casting. Occasionally, open reduction is necessary to remove the interposed soft tissue. For fractures which are unstable after reduction, or which become displaced, fixation with a smooth pin across the physeal plate is necessary. Type III and IV intra-articular injuries are treated with open reduction and internal fixation (Kirschner wires, cannulated screws), while arthroscopy is used to confirm the anatomic reduction of the articular surfaces.

Despite correct treatment, physeal injuries around the knee, especially those at the distal femur, have a high incidence of angulatory deformity and leg shortening compared with physeal injuries at other locations. About one-third of children with type I and II distal femoral physeal fractures develop angulation >5° and leg shortening >2 cm. The involved physician should always warn the parents about the risk of a growth disturbance.

Osteochondral fractures

Osteochondral injuries are frequently sports-related and are seen most commonly after patella dislocation or direct blow to the knee joint. Acute fractures are often not detectable on plain radiographic films. MRI studies are not as accurate as arthroscopic examination, but they are helpful in ruling out other injuries.

Treatment

The treatment of osteochondral fractures can be performed arthroscopically. Small fragments are removed, and the remaining crater is drilled to induce fibrocartilage healing. All larger fragments should be fixed whenever possible to reduce the risk of premature arthritis. The fixation techniques vary from Kirschner wires, pins or cortical screws to (more recently) use of Herbert screws, cortical bone plugs or bioabsorbable pins.

Tibial tubercle avulsion fractures

Avulsion of the tibial tubercle usually results from a forceful jump typically occurring in adolescent basketball or volleyball players. Patients with pre-existing Osgood–Schlatter disease and muscular athletic males near skeletal maturity are at particular risk for this injury (Steiner & Grana 1988).

These fractures have been classified into three types based on the degree of involvement of the tibial apophysis: I, fracture of tibial tubercle; II, fracture extends to tibial epiphysis; III, fracture extends into the articular surface. Patients present with marked tenderness and swelling around the tibial tubercle and are unable to fully extend the knee. Diagnosis is usually confirmed by standard roentgenograms.

Treatment

Undisplaced or minimally displaced fractures are treated conservatively with cylinder cast immobilization for 3–4 weeks. In displaced fractures, types II and III, reduction of the fragment and internal fixation with screws, sutures or Kirschner wires across the epiphysis are required to restore the articular alignment and the isometry of the extensor mechanism.

PATELLOFEMORAL DISORDERS

Disorders of the patellofemoral joint and the adjacent tendons represent a large number of congenital, developmental and traumatic conditions (Merchant 1988). For clinicians, anterior knee pain in children and adolescents very often represents a diagnostic as well as a treatment dilemma. In sports, patellofemoral disorders may originate from acute traumatic conditions (patellar dislocation, fracture, extensor tendon ruptures) or from anatomical and developmental abnormalities (patellar instability, multipartite patella, medial patellar plica, Osgood–Schlatter and Sinding–Larsen–Johansson disease, OCD of the patella, or chondromalacia patellae). In many cases of anterior knee pain, the importance of the patellofemoral dysplasia resulting in overuse problems is emphasized in children.

Osgood–Schlatter lesion

Osgood–Schlatter lesion, or tibial apophysitis, is one of the most common sources of sports disability in children (Kujala et al 1985). It is caused by failure at the chondro-osseous junction of the developing tibial tubercle. Although various theories regarding the etiology of Osgood–Schlatter lesion have been propagated, traumatic origin, especially repeated microtrauma, seems to be the most plausible. Children developing this knee disorder are usually in the midst of the adolescent growth spurt between the ages 11 and 15 (girls 2 years earlier than boys).

The affected children present commonly with antalgic gait and complain of tenderness and swelling of the tibial tubercle related to sports activities. Plain

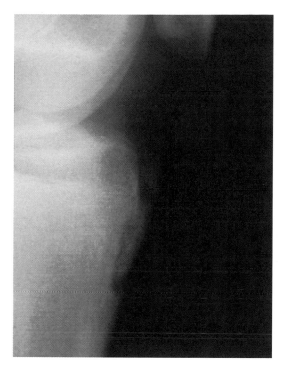

Figure 2.5 Osgood–Schlatter disease.

radiographs are sufficient to diagnose this disorder and are employed to exclude other more severe pathologic conditions such as neoplasm or infection (Fig. 2.5).

Treatment

The therapy of this self-limited condition is non-invasive (Kujala et al 1985). Restriction of activity, non-steroidal anti-inflammatory medication or ice massage is effective in the majority of the cases. After the period of acute pain, stretching programs for the lower extremity and non-aggravating activities such as swimming or cycling can be initiated. For children with severe symptoms, immobilization in a cylinder cast can be applied for 6 weeks.

Sinding–Larsen–Johansson lesion

Sinding–Larsen–Johansson lesion is another disorder of the pediatric extensor mechanism caused by the failure of the bone–tendon junction at the inferior pole of the patella. It results in calcification and ossification of the immature inferior patellar pole. Similar to Osgood–Schlatter lesion, it appears to be the sequel of repetitive traction injury to the insertion of the patella tendon. The condition is most common in prepubescent athletically active boys at 10–12 years of age who present with tenderness and swelling at the inferior patellar pole. Less frequently, the overuse problem is located at the quadriceps–patella junction. In older, skeletally mature adolescents, patella tendinopathy or jumper's knee is the presenting overuse syndrome at the lower patellar pole. Other patellar disorders causing anterior knee pain such as patella stress fractures or bipartite patella should be considered as differential diagnosis. For this reason, roentgenograms should be obtained routinely.

Therapy

The treatment of Sinding–Larsen–Johansson lesion is non-invasive. Restriction of aggravating sports activities, stretching exercise programs and applications of ice massages and non-steroidal anti-inflammatory drugs are adequate. A 4–6 week period of cast immobilization is necessary in patients with severe acute or chronic pain.

Patella instability

Patella dislocations may occur as a single traumatic event (acute dislocation), from minor trauma following previous dislocation (recurrent dislocation) or due to underlying developmental abnormality.

Acute patella dislocation

Acute dislocations of the patella occur with either a direct medial or lateral blow to the patella. Internal rotation of the femur relative to the tibia while the knee is extended or slightly flexed can also lead to an acute patella dislocation. Usually, the patella is forced laterally, the medial retinaculum tears and the articular surfaces of the patella and of the lateral femoral condyle may be damaged. The dislocation may spontaneously reduce, but sometimes the patella is 'locked', which might require reduction under anesthesia. Occasionally, a bipartite patella becomes symptomatic after a similar trauma. Following an acute dislocation, subsequent patella dislocations are not uncommon, especially in presence of patellofemoral dysplasia.

Hemarthrosis is a marked clinical sign of an acute patella dislocation. Although standard X-rays are diagnostic in the majority of the cases, MRI should be performed to exclude other associated injuries (e.g. osteochondral lesions).

Management

Arthroscopic evaluation and lavage is recommended in cases of osteochondral lesions for removal of small fragments and refixation of large osteochondral bodies (Dainer et al 1988). If arthroscopic intervention is required for the treatment of an osteochondral fracture, the suture of the medial retinaculum should be considered. Non-operative therapy consists of 3 weeks of immobilization in extension followed by bracing and rehabilitation.

Recurrent instability

Children with dysplasia of the patellofemoral joint may sustain patellar dislocations without obvious acute trauma. In this congenital disorder, dislocations occur medially or laterally in the same joint and are also reported bilaterally (Fig. 2.6).

Management

The management of children with congenital deficits of the patellofemoral joint includes bracing and physiotherapy for strengthening of the vastus medialis oblique muscle. Operative treatment should be delayed until the patients reach skeletal maturity. In cases of recurrent post-traumatic dislocation, surgical intervention with proximal and/or distal realignment should be performed to reduce the risk of early osteoarthritis.

Patellofemoral pain syndromes

Anterior knee pain is a relatively common sports-related knee disorder among adolescents. Several

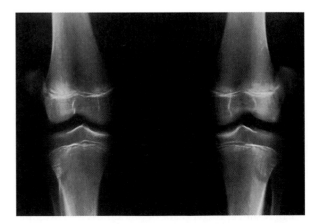

Figure 2.6 Bilateral patella dislocation.

syndromes of different etiology are associated with the anterior knee pain. Historically, disorders causing pain in the patellofemoral joint were all designated as chondromalacia patellae. Nowadays, this term is used for arthroscopic description of the softening or disruption of the articular cartilage.

Patella subluxation

Patella subluxation represents the largest subgroup of symptomatic patellofemoral dysplasia. This disorder often presents bilaterally and is usually diagnosed in female adolescents with no significant trauma. The affected individuals complain of painful locking or catching of the knee and experience episodes of giving way during sports activities. Axial radiographs of the patella reveal the typical configuration of lateral patellar translation and tilt that increase with quadriceps contraction. Physiotherapy approaching the restoration of muscle balance is essential. Temporarily, patella-restraining braces or tapes may be applied.

Lateral patellar compression syndrome

This represents the mildest form of patellofemoral dysplasia without instability symptoms. The pain is related to relatively tight lateral patellofemoral ligaments and is caused by continuous pressure of the lateral patellar facet against the lateral femoral condyle. Tight lateral retinaculum and chondromalacia of the lateral patellar articular surface are seen arthroscopically. After a failed physical therapy program, arthroscopic lateral release and shaving of the chondromalacic areas may be performed.

Plica syndrome

Plica syndrome is caused by superimposition of hypertrophic fibrotic synovial tissue between the medial patellar facet and femoral condyle. Synovial plicae originate from synovial septae which are exposed to repetitive microtrauma during running or jumping. Treatment of symptomatic plica is predominantly with local ice massage and anti-inflammatory medications combined with therapeutic exercise programs. In a small number of patients, arthroscopic plica resection is required. In those patients who require surgery, a tight lateral retinaculum may be released to improve the clinical results.

OSTEOCHONDRITIS DISSECANS OF THE KNEE

Osteochondritis dissecans (OCD) is a disorder of the subchondral bone and the overlying cartilage which can result in a partial or complete separation of chondral or osteochondral segments. This intra-articular lesion can affect many joints, but the most common locations are the knee and elbow. The juvenile OCD has a peak appearance at the age of 15 years, with a male predominance of 1:3 to 1:4. Incidence of bilateral involvement has been reported in about 20–30% of the cases.

Many factors, such as ischemia, abnormal epiphyseal ossification, trauma, cyclical strain or familiar predisposition, have been proposed to cause OCD, but there is still no agreement about the etiology of this joint disorder. The most plausible theories described by many authors are macro- and microtrauma. Both direct and indirect blows to the knee joint as well as continued cyclical strain were able to initiate OCD in experimental settings. For this reason, a differentiation is necessary between acute osteochondral fractures and osteochondritic lesions.

Clinical signs of OCD can include mechanical symptoms or be less specific with activity-related pain, swelling and tenderness. Because the classic OCD (70% of knee OCD) is localized at the lateral aspect of the medial femoral condyle, radiographic studies should include a tunnel view to obtain the best visualization of the lesions. MRI is recommended for evaluating the vitality of the fragment, for assessment of the articular cartilage and for staging of the disease (Fig. 2.7).

Management

The natural history of OCD in skeletally immature athletes is different from the clinical course in adults. While most adults with OCD develop a degenerative joint disease of the knee, there is a considerable amount of spontaneous healing in children. For this reason, conservative management, including non- or partial weight-bearing strategies, bracing and physiotherapy, may be sufficient for children with OCD. Usually, the progression of the disease is monitored by MRI, which helps to make the decision for an invasive procedure. Operative treatment is indicated in patients who have a loose fragment in the joint or in those for whom conservative treatment has failed (Cahill et al 1989). Arthroscopy has gained importance among various surgical options for the treatment of

OCD in children. Many operative procedures, such as retrograde drilling, fragment removal or fixation, and osteochondral transplantation, can today be performed arthroscopically by experienced arthroscopists (Glancy 1999) (Fig. 2.8).

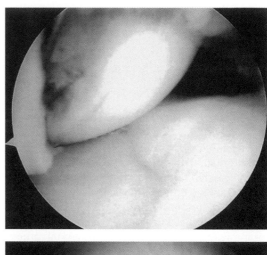

A

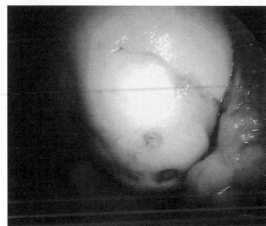

B

Figure 2.8 A: Arthroscopic photograph of a large OCD fragment from the lateral aspect of the medial femoral condyle. B: Arthroscopic photograph demonstrating the result after refixation of the OCD fragment with bioabsorbable 3.5 mm screws.

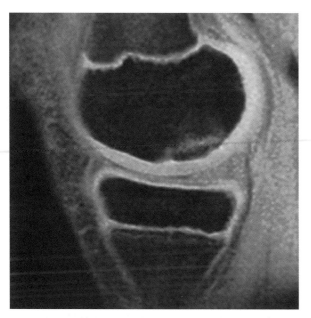

Figure 2.7 A T2-weighted MRI demonstrating osteochondritis dissecans of the medial femoral condyle.

CONCLUSIONS

1. The availability of new diagnostic tools (MRI) and arthroscopic techniques as well as increasing knowledge of joint biomechanics and the biology of soft tissue healing have influenced the management of knee disorders in children.

2. The incidence of ACL injuries is constantly increasing in immature athletes, due to the increased involvement of children in contact sports. Arthroscopic ACL reconstructions using soft tissue autografts, small transphyseal drill holes or the over-the-top position on the lateral femur are the treatments of choice.

3. Long-term results after meniscectomies in children are poor. Arthroscopic techniques should be used to repair and preserve the damaged meniscus as much as possible.

4. Physeal and epiphyseal injuries around the knee have a relatively high risk for growth disturbance. Anatomic reduction and minimally invasive fixation techniques are applied more frequently today than in the past.

5. Patellofemoral disorders represent a large number of pathologic conditions. When possible, anterior knee pain is managed conservatively or arthroscopically.

6. The etiology of osteochondritis dissecans is still not exactly known. This articular disorder, which mostly involves non-weight-bearing areas of the knee joint, can be treated conservatively in the majority of affected children. Arthroscopic techniques have gained importance as a treatment option after failed conservative management.

REFERENCES

Abdon P, Turner M S, Pettersson H, Lindstrand A, Stenstrom A, Swanson A J 1990 A long term follow-up study of total meniscectomy in children. Clinical Orthopaedics 257: 166–170

Arnoczky S P, Warren R F 1982 Microvasculature of the human meniscus. American Journal of Sports Medicine 10: 90–95

Binfield P M, Maffulli N, Good C I, King J B 2000 Anthroscopy in sporting and sedentary children. Bulletin of the Hospital for Joint Diseases 59: 125–130

Brief L P 1991 Anterior cruciate ligament reconstruction without drill holes. Arthroscopy 7: 350–357

Cahill B R, Phillips M R, Navarro R 1989 The results of conservative management of juvenile osteochondritis dissecans using joint scintigraphy. A prospective study. American Journal of Sports Medicine 17: 601–605

Dainer R D, Barrack R L, Buckley S L, Alexander A H 1988 Arthroscopic treatment of acute patellar dislocations. Arthroscopy 4: 267–271

DeHaven K E, Lintner D M 1986 Athletic injuries: comparison by age, sport, and gender. American Journal of Sports Medicine 14: 218–224

Glancy G L 1999 Juvenile osteochondritis dissecans. American Journal of Knee Surgery 12: 120–124

Grontvedt T, Engebretsen L, Benum P, Fasting O, Molster A, Strand T 1996 A prospective, randomized study of three operations for acute rupture of the anterior cruciate ligament. Five-year follow-up of one hundred and thirty-one patients. Journal of Bone and Joint Surgery (Am) 78: 159–168

Jaramillo D, Hoffer F A, Shapiro F, Rand F 1990 MR imaging of fractures of the growth plate. American Journal of Roentgenology 155: 1261–1265

Kellenberger R, von Laer L 1990 Nonosseous lesions of the anterior cruciate ligaments in childhood and adolescence. Progresses Pediatric Surgery 25: 123–131

Kujala U M, Kvist M, Heinonen O 1985 Osgood-Schlatter's disease in adolescent athletes. Retrospective study of incidence and duration. American Journal of Sports Medicine 13: 236–241

Maffuli N 1992 The growing child in sport. British Medical Bulletin 48: 561–568

Maffuli N, Chan K M, Miao M, Fu F H, Kurosaka M 1996 Athletic knee injuries. Similarities and differences between Asian and Western experiences. Clinical Orthopaedics 323: 98–105

McCarroll J R, Rettig A C, Shelbourne K D 1988 Anterior cruciate ligament injuries in the young athlete with open physes. American Journal of Sports Medicine 16: 44–47

McCarroll J R, Shelbourne K D, Porter D A, Rettig A C, Murray S 1994 Patellar tendon graft reconstruction for midsubstance anterior cruciate ligament rupture in junior high school athletes. An algorithm for management. American Journal of Sports Medicine 22: 478–484

Merchant A C 1988 Classification of patellofemoral disorders. Arthroscopy 4: 235–240

Meyers M H, McKeever F M 1959 Fracture of the intercondylar eminence of the tibia. Journal of Bone and Joint Surgery (Am) 41: 209–222

Nottage W M, Matsuura P A 1994 Management of complete traumatic anterior cruciate ligament tears in the skeletally immature patient: current concepts and review of the literature. Arthroscopy 10: 569–573

Raber D A, Friederich N F, Hefti F 1998 Discoid lateral meniscus in children. Long-term follow-up after total meniscectomy. Journal of Bone and Joint Surgery (Am) 80: 1579–1586

Ringer J L, Fay M J 1990 Acute posterior cruciate ligament insufficiency in children. American Journal of Knee Surgery 3: 192–203

Smith A D, Tao S S 1995 Knee injuries in young athletes. Clinical Sports Medicine 14: 629–650

Stanitski C L 1998 Correlation of arthroscopic and clinical examinations with magnetic resonance imaging findings of injured knees in children and adolescents. American Journal of Sports Medicine 26: 2–6

Steiner M E, Grana W A 1988 The young athlete's knee: recent advances. Clinical Sports Medicine 7: 527–546

Walker P S, Erkman M J 1975 The role of the menisci in force transmission across the knee. Clinical Orthopaedics 257: 184–192

Webber A 1988 Acute soft-tissue injuries in the young athlete. Clinical Sports Medicine 7: 611–624

3

Lower limb injuries in adolescence and childhood

John King

KEY POINTS

1. Ligaments and tendons are stronger than the growth plate.
2. Beware of the growth spurt.
3. Children will always give a history of injury despite spontaneous onset of pain.
4. Be prepared to radiograph the 'normal' side.
5. Injury patterns are different – children are not little adults.

INTRODUCTION

Children are for the main part subject to all the problems of the athletic adult but carry additional disadvantages. They are more active and less wise; their skeletons are changing shape and size, and they have the relatively weak physeal plate near the ends of the bones.

They have certain advantages over adults in that they are of a lower weight (usually) and have more elastic bones, so that the soft tissues are not subject to the same peaks of deformation as in adults, i.e. they have better shock absorbers.

Sports injuries in this group will occur during the sports active periods, which for the main part are the teenage years. Genuine sports-related injuries as opposed to accidents are rare below this age.

Injuries will be discussed by site with some division into bone, joint or soft tissue.

LESIONS OF AND AROUND THE HIP JOINT

There are various sites around the hip that are weak as a consequence of open physeal plates. Quite large

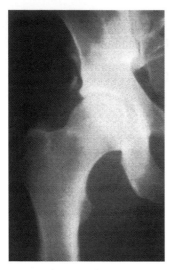

Figure 3.1 Avulsion of anterior inferior iliac spine.

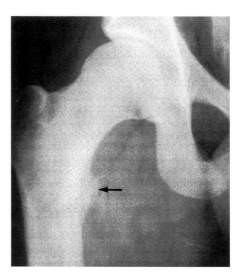

Figure 3.2 Lesser trochanter avulsion.

pieces can be pulled off, particularly with sudden unexpected loads. The *anterior-inferior iliac spine* tends to go in sports when the kicking foot is suddenly blocked, or as the consequence of a very powerful kick, such as shooting in soccer (Fig. 3.1). I have never seen it in a touch kick in rugby and I suspect that the hip has to be near extension to preload the insertion. This is not the position of kicking out of hand. The bone is pulled off by the reflected head of rectus femoris; there may be some separation and there is quite extensive bleeding. In very similar circumstances, the psoas muscle can pull off the lesser trochanter (Fig. 3.2).

The whole apophysis of the ischium can separate through the abnormal pull of the hamstrings; a good example is in cross country running when the ditch being jumped is wider than at first thought and the leading leg is suddenly overstretched. More rarely, the anterior superior iliac spine can be pulled off by sartorius in a bad gymnastic vault landing. The whole iliac crest apophysis can be pulled by the abdominal muscles, although displacement is most uncommon.

In all cases, there is a good history of injury associated with severe, immediate well-localized pain. Radiographs usually confirm the diagnosis if an awareness of the condition leads to a request for the appropriate views. Occasionally even good radiographs have failed to show the lesion and I have resorted to MRI scanning to show the bone bruise on the fat suppression sequence. Treatment is control of pain, rest and gradual resumption of activity as pain permits; this area is not amenable to the application of ice, as for the main part the avulsions are too deep.

There is no indication for immediate surgery and late surgery is exceptional, despite occasionally dramatic radiographic changes.

So-called *irritable hip* can occur at any age but is most common in children. It presents with a limp, and the localization of pain may be difficult. The child is usually brought along by worried parents, and only examination reveals painful restriction of motion of the hip joint. Full extension and/or abduction in flexion produce the pain. For the most part, a precise cause is never found and the pain settles during a period of bed rest and observation. For this reason the condition is often called *observation hip*. This is not an uncommon condition and there is no evidence that it and the sometimes associated Perthes' disease are related to sporting activity. It is advisable, however, to suggest avoidance of impact sport. Certainly running and jumping (impact sport) should be barred in a child with established Perthes' disease.

Between the ages of 10 and 16 years, slipping of the upper femoral epiphysis is the more common intra-articular problem (Fig. 3.3). It occurs mainly in boys and in two groups: the fat child with underdeveloped gonads (Frölich's syndrome) and the tall thin child in a growth spurt. West Indian females seem more common in the second group but are still a substantial minority.

The child is frequently brought to medical attention after an injury in which the lower thigh and knee have apparently become suddenly painful. Questioning often reveals some premonitionary discomfort, as in fact the 'acute' event is often an acute-on-chronic slip.

The pain is usually perceived at the knee because of the nerve supply of the hip (Hilton's law) and there are

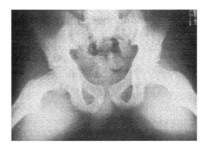

Figure 3.3 Slipped upper femoral epiphysis.

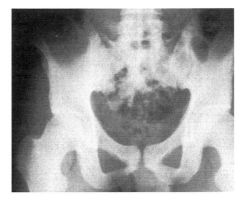

Figure 3.4 Erosion of the symphysis pubis.

very few cases in which there is not a radiograph of a normal knee in the envelope.

The physical signs are of loss of internal rotation or even fixed external rotation and shortening of the leg; the external rotation of the foot in stance is by far the most obvious, and with the child on the couch internal rotation will be restricted or even impossible. Such physical signs demand a radiograph of the hip in both anteroposterior and lateral projections. The deformity is much easier to see in the lateral, but there are well described criteria for its recognition in the antero-posterior radiograph. Treatment is surgical to prevent further displacement.

It has been suggested that minor degrees of slip, not noticed at the time, give rise to the loss of internal rotation often seen later in life with the so-called *pistol grip hips*. This can cause problems in later life where the foot pronates excessively. The consequence of pronation is internal rotation of the tibia. If that cannot be accommodated at the hip, lateral joint line pain at the knee may be the result. I have previously called this 'nebulous knee pain' and its treatment is with orthotics.

Another long term complication, brought about by the loss of hip rotation, can be erosion of the symphysis pubis as the twisting loads are transferred to this joint (Fig. 3.4).

Chondrolysis is another intra-articular lesion. It is, as the name suggests, a destructive lesion of the articular cartilage. It may be associated with a slipped epiphysis or, more commonly, the operation to fix it. It may be caused by dislocations of the hip or may come about spontaneously. In the apparent spontaneous chondrolysis that I have seen, there has been a history of injury in that region to the extent that I have wondered about a subluxation, but of course my practice is mainly sport injury. It is a rare injury; I have seen three cases in 20 years. Treatment has been traction, non-weight-bearing and mobilization of the very stiff hip in hydrotherapy. No patient of mine has returned to sport. This view is borne out by the literature.

The *snapping hip* usually presents with the parents saying that the hip keeps dislocating. There is a loud and frightening clunk. If it occurs with some adduction and in internal rotation, it will be the fascia lata slipping over the great trochanter. It can be blocked with firm pressure at this site or the movement can be felt under the finger. There is a deeper clunk, often in external rotation, with nothing to be felt under the finger on the trochanter. This is usually psoas flicking across the front of the femoral neck. My only indication for surgery is if there has been the formation of a painful bursa which does not respond to rest or injection. Usually it all gets better with explanation.

It must never be forgotten that activity-related pain can be caused by a stress fracture of the femoral neck (Fig. 3.5).

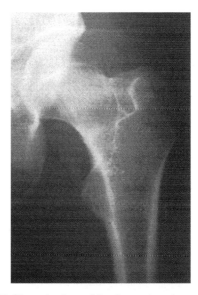

Figure 3.5 Stress fracture of the femoral neck.

Thigh injuries are non-specific to childhood except for the fact that the periosteum is more loosely attached and subperiosteal haematoma may occur more readily as a consequence of a direct blow.

The story of an injury followed by increasing pain, particularly with sleep disturbance, must alert the physician to a *bone tumour* or *infection*. A history of injury is very common. Children of this age are always banging themselves. They like order, so when they notice pain they mentally associate it with the injury, thus leading to the history given. Benign bone cysts (Fig. 3.6) on the verge of a fracture are the most likely cause, followed by osteosarcoma in this age group. Because of my working in a sports medicine practice, I have already seen more than four times the number of new osteosarcomas than I would be expected to see in a whole orthopaedic career. Early diagnosis may change the prognosis and sports physicians should be alert to the history, and radiograph early.

Hamstring and rectus femoris tears are generally held to be uncommon in this age group. The Football Association in England is screening all apprentices entering professional football and some clubs with centres and schools of excellence are doing similar surveys. From my own experience of these, it is clear that many young footballers do have significant periods of hamstring and rectus femoris discomfort (usually called strains) and that these are associated with growth spurts. Routine examination during a growth spurt will often reveal very tight hamstrings. Good club physiotherapy is the only, and essential, treatment.

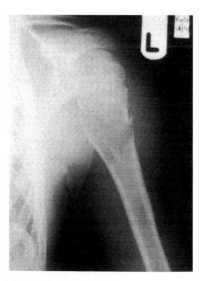

Figure 3.6 Unicameral bone cyst.

LESIONS OF AND AROUND THE KNEE JOINT

Ligaments

In the mature skeleton, valgus/varus stress tears the *collateral ligaments*; in the child, the physeal plate is weaker than the ligaments and more commonly gives way. The knee may appear unstable, and plain radiographs usually appear normal. A high index of suspicion is necessary and stress radiographs, under anaesthesia if the pain is great, must be done to show the growth plate opening. Treatment is immobilization for 4 weeks.

A similar disproportion of strength produces the classical *anterior cruciate lesion* of childhood. The ligament stays intact but a large piece of the proximal tibia is avulsed. The history of injury is a flexion twisting, or hyperextension injury with immediate pain and swelling. Radiographs are diagnostic and the fragment of bone can be fixed back. It is usual for full extension to be lost after this procedure, even with anatomical reduction. This may represent overgrowth from the fracture stimulus but I cannot find a study to confirm this. Fortunately there is some evidence that the slight lack of extension does not lead to the anterior knee pain that might be expected.

Tears of the ligament itself are less common; if symptomatic they must be treated as in an adult. The risk to the growth plate is, in fact, not high (Andrews et al 1994, Lo et al 1997).

Patella and extensor apparatus

The *patellofemoral joint* is often vulnerable especially if the patella is a bit high and thus does not fully engage the femoral groove. Twisting of the leg with the knee slightly flexed may cause sub- or dislocation of the patella. If it remains dislocated the diagnosis is easy, but spontaneous relocation can cause difficulties. The knee is swollen and the medial patellar margin is tender where the soft tissues have torn. Skyline radiographs are needed to exclude the marginal fractures of the femoral condyle which, if untreated, can lead to loose bodies (Nictosvaara et al 1994). The small medial separation from the edge of the patella is diagnostic of the injury, but as it is an avulsion, it does not cause loose bodies and can be left. A hypertrophic beak on the medial side of the patella is a sure sign of recurrent subluxations. As a basic rule in children, giving way on twisting is always patellar until proved otherwise. Osteochondral fractures of the back of the patella and margin of the lateral femoral condyle may occur. It is

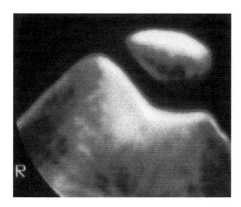

Figure 3.7 Osteochondral lesion of the patella.

advisable to CT scan these knees and, with early diagnosis, these lesions can be pinned back and consideration given to a concomitant soft tissue correction such as a lateral release and/or medial repair or plication. Delay means the osteochondral lesion (Fig. 3.7) cannot be reconstituted, with the obvious long-term problems that abnormal articular surfaces generate.

The *bipartite patella* may be a problem, but is not always associated with symptoms. It shows on radiographs as a separate piece of bone on the superolateral corner of the patella. The gap between it and the main part of the bone may be palpable. It is usually bilateral. It does not usually give rise to spontaneous pain, but if the patella has been damaged, usually by a blow on the front, the symptoms of that may not settle until the segment is removed.

The *extensor apparatus* above the patella is rarely injured in children. Distally, the so-called sleeve injury of the patella occurs in which the periosteal sleeve of the patella is stripped downwards in continuity with the patella tendon. The diagnosis is usually missed until the bone grows again in the empty pouch, producing the double patella appearance when it is too late to operate.

Traumatic cysts can occur in the patellar ligament in children, especially in board divers who kneel on the edge of the pool as they climb out. These cysts have proved resistant to the surgery of paratenon strip and excision of the central core lesion which is usually effective in older patients. Alteration of technique, local injection and meticulous stretching of the quadriceps, remembering that rectus femoris crosses the hip as well, seem to be the best treatment in this age group.

Perhaps the commonest lesion of the extensor apparatus is *Osgood–Schlatter's disease* in which the tip of the elongated proximal epiphysis is elevated by repetitive stress, resulting in a painful lump and radiological

fragmentation and elevation. Treatment is restriction of activity to acceptable pain levels and protection of the bone lump from daily trauma by a neoprene sleeve. Only very rarely does the fragmentation give rise to symptoms in later life. At the other end of the tendon at its patellar insertion (Sinding–Larsen–Johansson syndrome) there is pain and this can be associated with a small area of calcification which may respond to a carefully sited injection. Injection into normal tissue requires such high pressure as to be almost impossible, so low-pressure injection is pathognomonic of the needle in the lesion or the peritendinous tissues.

The knee joint

Within the knee, *osteochondral fractures* may affect the weight-bearing articular surface of the femur as a consequence of a twisting, weight-bearing injury. They present with a haemarthrosis which is by definition a rapid swelling of the knee. If in doubt, a fine-needle aspiration of the knee can be performed as an office procedure which will confirm the blood, and if fat globules are seen there is no doubt about the diagnosis (Stamitski et al 1993). Radiographs may be helpful but the diagnosis may only be clear on arthroscopy, although MRI is proving to be more and more helpful in my practice. It is important to emphasize that the best interpretation of the scan is by the clinician, simply because it can be married to the physical signs and history (unless you are lucky enough to have your radiologist attend the clinic and see the patient, which happens in my centre). The fragment must be fixed back as it can represent a major part of the weight-bearing articular surface.

Osteochondritis dissecans is a possibly atraumatic, definitely avascular lesion of the subchondral bone. Symptoms may become apparent during sport, because of the imposed loads, but there is no evidence that it is caused by sport. Symptoms are of giving way, usually induced by pain as in a painful arc when the damaged area is put under load. If the damaged segment of bone separates, then the symptoms are of a loose body. The consequences of removal are worse than at first thought, and an attempt to fix the fragment is advisable (Anderson & Pagrani 1997). An attempt to stabilize the lesion by drilling through it into the normal bone or by using biodegradable pinning should definitely be made in the active symptomatic child with the fragment still in situ. Fortunately, only a minority of osteochondritis dissecans extends significantly into the weight-bearing area of the femoral side of the knee joint, but if on the lateral side osteoarthritis may be accelerated (Tyman et al 1991). It can occur on the back of the patella where CT or MRI might be needed to confirm it.

Menisci

Meniscal lesions are not common but do occur. Some will be associated with a larger than normal or even completely discoid meniscus. Often the child will have had a history of painless clunking. This get worse and then is associated with pain and swelling, heralding the tear which will require surgery.

Some apparently normal-sized lateral menisci may produce a *cyst* on the periphery which gives symptoms through the pressure of the cyst on the surrounding structures, and indeed it may erode the margin of the bone. The cyst is almost always caused by some degree of intrameniscal degeneration associated with a 'fish-mouth' tear. I am very reluctant to remove much of the lateral meniscus in this age group, as a small and unpredictable proportion go on to get a severe lateral chondrolysis. In this age group, I do an MRI scan to be sure there is no damage to the articular surface, and then I will inject the cyst on up to two occasions. It seems to come and go, and may disappear for some years. This is a more pragmatic solution than immediate surgery, but there should be a review MRI at 6 months to check the articular cartilage status. If the articular cartilage is damaged at any point, then obviously meniscal surgery is essential.

THE LEG

The tibia (and more rarely the femur) may be the site of *stress fractures*. These come about as a consequence of repetitive load without adequate recovery time so that fatigue failure takes place. This is better described as a dys-coupling of the osteoclast and osteoblast axis, which is responsible for the normal bone turnover and response to activity. If viewed in this way, the input of diet and hormonal balance becomes more readily appreciated and must certainly be investigated in the female patient. The symptoms are of crescendo pain, i.e. pain coming on sooner and sooner after the commencement of activity. Initial radiographs are normal. If the fracture is seen on the original radiographs then the diagnosis has been delayed, a not uncommon situation where the child is desperate to compete and has not reported the pain until late. The fracture may become clear in later views. A technetium diphospho-

nate triple-phase bone scan is diagnostic with a well-localized transverse area of increased activity.

In the tibia, these changes must be distinguished from the *medial tibial stress reaction* where there is well-localized pain on the medial side of the junction of the middle and distal one-third of the tibia. This lesion appears to be inflammation of the tissues inserted at this site. The bone scan shows a vertical signal change just in that area of the medial tibia, and there is a significant association with a supinated foot which may be a bit stiff, or hyperpronation. Treatment of this condition may simply be with a well-fitting orthotic to protect the elevated medial arch, although I always add some degree of shock absorption. Treatment of a stress fracture is reduction of activity to a pain-free level with a very gradual increase in activity with adequate periods of rest for the bone to respond to the challenge of exercise.

Occasionally, both these conditions can be resistant to conservative management. Under those circumstances, I will perform a periosteal strip. The idea of this in a stress fracture is to promote a little subperiosteal new bone formation which increases the radius of the tibia by a small amount. This increases the stiffness quite significantly, although it is not a comfortable procedure. When doing a strip for medial tibial stress syndrome, I simply elevate the periosteum from the medial side of the tibia over the length of clinical tenderness.

Other causes of exercise-related calf injury again must be considered. If the pain is lateral and associated with numbness or paraesthesia in the outer foot then the diagnosis is irritation of the superficial peroneal nerve as it comes through the foramen in the fascia. This can be diagnosed by pressure over the fascial foramen reproducing the pain and the cure is a simple enlargement of the hole. There is no need to do a full, compartmental decompression.

Raised intracompartmental pressure is by no means unusual in this age group. It is certainly more common in athletes who are skeletally mature, but we have observed this condition on quite a number of occasions in professional soccer apprentices. It is essential to confirm the diagnosis before embarking on treatment. We do this with pressure studies and monitor the intracompartmental pressure during the activity which brings on the pain. It is essential to reproduce the activity, as otherwise the pressures may remain apparently normal. We have seen this problem in ballet dancers and underwater hockey players! It is now clear that orthotics do not help, and indeed make the symptoms worse on occasions. The treatment is decompression of the affected compartment and this may often be all four, i.e. both anterior and both posterior compartments. I use short incisions proximal and distal over each compartment and then split the fascia with a large pair of scissors. I put a finger in each incision to confirm that the split is complete. There are vessels around in the medial compartment which I routinely drain, and a small group of patients get some paraesthesiae over the dorsum of the foot, which is relatively short-lived. It is important to get the patient exercising as soon as possible to make sure that the muscle bulk keeps the edges of the fascia apart so that premature healing does not occur.

LESIONS OF AND AROUND THE ANKLE

The twisting injuries that cause the fractures in adults produce a different pattern of injury in the immature skeleton. Adduction force, instead of breaking the fibula, pulls off the distal fibular epiphysis. This almost always closes up, and the only way to make the diagnosis is to find the well-localized tenderness at the site of the physis. Treatment is immobilization for 2 or 3 weeks until the pain goes.

The other injuries fall more within the scope of orthopaedic surgery. They can be diagnosed from radiographs and are only mentioned here for reference. Inversion injury causing the talus to spin pulls off a piece of bone from the anterolateral corner of the epiphysis, the *Tillaux fracture*. Replacement of the bit of bone is necessary. Of more complexity is the *triplane fracture*, which looks initially like a Salter type 2 injury (Erl et al 1988). It is very difficult to reduce and may need to be opened.

Osteochondral fractures of the ankle can occur. They are much less frequent than in the knee. There is no obvious reason for this, as they are commonly seen in the young adult population. An MRI scan usually confirms them.

The adult problems of the Achilles tendon and the other tendons going around the pulley system of the malleoli do not seem to occur in the juvenile population that I see.

THE FOOT

Fractures can occur any time and are accidents rather than sports injuries. The foot is the site of stress lesions rather more commonly than is realized. There may be pain and radiological fragmentation of the calcaneal apophysis, which has been called *Sever's disease*. It presents with well-localized activity-related pain on the back of the heel. This has been described as stress fractures, but there is often a similar asymptomatic radiographic appearance of the other side. The pain responds to rest and a shock absorber under the heel but may be slow to settle, taking months in some cases. I do not use plaster immobilization, but in slow cases will use night splints to hold the ankle at 90° rather in the way I treat resistant plantar fasciitis in the adult, with the feeling that there is tightness in the continuum of the Achilles tendon, back of the heel and plantar fascia.

Although Sever's disease is not a stress fracture, the *navicular* is quite a common site of this lesion. The type of patient is a young fast bowler, sprinter or heptathlete, and the pain is well localized to the apex of the arch of the foot, which may be slightly supinated and stiff. Radiographs are almost always normal. A bone scan will show a hot navicular but the best test is a CT scan through the navicular which will show a linear fracture going up through the superior sclerotic quadrant. The transverse fracture of the inferior part of the navicular is traumatic. The treatment of the acute fracture is rest. Occasionally the stress fracture needs fixation and multiple drilling. We have used electrical stimulation in the form of capacitive coupling, but the data at this site are not yet significant, although anecdotally we have successes. The stress fractures of the *metatarsals* are common only in the 16+ age group; the history is diagnostic and the callus will show on the late radiographs. Treatment is as for stress fractures already described above.

There is an apparently similar lesion which occurs in the head of the second or third metatarsals. It is associated with local pain, there is swelling over the distal end of the metatarsal and radiographs show distortion and fragmentation of the bone at that site. Treatment is initially rest, in the hope that the lesion will harden up. Delayed surgery is often needed to reshape the distal end of the metatarsal, and indeed there may be loose bits in the joint. The condition is called Freiberg's disease and, if found in one foot, the other should be radiographed as there are likely to be changes there (Binck et al 1988). My philosophy is to await skeletal maturity before embarking on surgery unless there is a clear loose body giving symptoms (Sproul et al 1993).

Accessory bones may be a problem in both diagnosis and treatment. The os trigonum on the back of the talus is quite a frequent cause of symptoms. The symptoms often start after a soft tissue sprain. I suspect that there is a minimal increase in the allowed range of plantarflexion and this is enough to start the os trigonum impinging between the back of the tibia and the top of the calcaneum in full forced plantarflexion such as driving a football. Once this condition is established, conservative treatment does not appear to be effective. Excision of the accessory bone is necessary. I do that through a medial incision, and am intrigued by the frequency of inflammation in the tendon of flexor hallucis longus seen at the same time. The same clinical syndrome occurs with an enlarged posterior talar process and the prognosis and treatment are the same.

In the accessory navicular, problems are similar to those of the bipartite patella. There is a congenital separation of bone on the medial side of the navicular, lying usually within the tibialis posterior insertion.

This is symptom-free until injury irritates it. There has usually been a traction lesion from eversion injury and the pain may persist until excision of the extra bone. It can be shelled out from the tendon. If significant tendon damage has taken place, it is important to resecure the tibialis posterior tendon. There is no point in trying to screw back the accessory bone in the hope that it will fuse. It usually will not fuse and it leaves a bigger lump which rubs on the shoes. An almost identical situation exists at the base of the fifth metatarsal where there may be an os fibulare. Once symptoms are established, conservative treatment does not seem to be effective and indeed there may be quite aggressive erosive changes. Treatment is the same as for the accessory navicular.

CONCLUSIONS

1. Sports injury is difficult to separate from genuine accidents in this age group. What in adults is war, for children is play.
2. There is the pressure from the parents to be added to that of the coach and the peer group at a time when shape, size and hormonal balance are changing.
3. Muscles may tighten up during periods of rapid growth, bringing problems at apophyses, origins and insertions.
4. Physeal plates may give way before ligaments and tendons, causing difficulty in diagnosis but, fortunately, infrequent subsequent disorders of growth.

5. The consequences of apparently minor alterations of biomechanics, e.g. in the form of a supinated or pronated foot, may become apparent as the child increases the levels of activity, causing medial tibial stress syndrome or navicular stress fractures.
6. It is vital to remember that children/adolescents are not just small adults, but are entities with their own set of problems mainly reflected as a rapidly growing skeleton and a hormonal milieu, which make adjustment to change difficult.

REFERENCES

Anderson A F, Pagnani M J 1997 Osteochondritis dissecans of the femoral condyles. Long term results of excision of the fragment. American Journal of Sports Medicine 25(6): 830–834

Andrews M, Noyes F R, Barber-Westin S D 1994 Anterior cruciate ligament allograft reconstruction in the skeletally immature athlete. American Journal of Sports Medicine 22: 48–54

Binck R, Levisohn E, Bersani F et al 1988 Freiberg's disease complicating unrelated trauma. Orthopaedics 11: 753–757

Erl J P, Barrack R L, Alexander A H 1988 Triplane fracture of the distal tibial epiphysis. Long term follow up. Journal of Bone and Joint Surgery (Am) 70: 967–976

Lo I K Y, Krikley A, Fowler P J, Miniaci A 1997 The outcome of operativly treated anterior cruciate disruption in the skeletally immature child. Journal of Arthroscopic and Related Surgery 13(5): 627–634

Nictosvaara Y, Aalto K, Kallio P E 1994 Acute patellar dislocation in children; Incidence and associated osteochondral fractures. Journal of Pediatric Orthopedics 14: 513–515

Sproul J, Klaaren H, Mannarino F 1993 Surgical treatment of Freiberg's infarction in athletes. American Journal of Sports Medicine 21: 381–384

Stanitski C L, Harvell J C, Fu F 1993 Observations on acute knee haemarthrosis in children and adolescents. Journal of Pediatric Orthopedics 13: 506–510

Tyman R S, Desai K, Aicroth P M 1991 Osteochondritis dissecans of the knee; a long term study. Journal of Bone and Joint Surgery (Br) 53: 440–477

4

Spinal injuries in children's sports

Treg D. Brown Lyle J. Micheli

KEY POINTS

1. An increasing number of children and adolescents participating in organized sports are seeking medical attention for sports-related injuries – spine-related complaints account for approximately 10% of these.
2. The adolescent spine is uniquely different from that of the adult, and consequently the diagnosis and treatment of injuries to the spine differ between these two age groups.
3. Accurate diagnosis is crucial in spinal injuries in children, and, in the majority of cases, this can be achieved through history and physical examination.
4. It is important to distinguish between complaints of back pain in the athlete compared with the non-athlete, as failure to do so can result in misdiagnosis and treatment delay.
5. Trauma remains the primary cause of back pain in the adolescent athlete, but other etiologies (e.g. infection, neoplasms, and metabolic disorders) must be ruled out.

INTRODUCTION

The number of children and adolescents participating in organized sports has continued to rise over the years. As a result, an increasing number of these athletes are seeking medical attention for a variety of sports-related injuries (Maffulli 1992, Micheli 1994). The incidence of spinal injuries is no exception to this trend, with some studies suggesting that spine-related complaints comprise approximately 10% of the injuries seen in this patient population (Spencer & Jackson 1983). Sports such as gymnastics, dance, American football, rugby, rowing, racquet sports, and weight-lifting appear to be associated with a disproportionate number of spine-related complaints (Micheli & Mintzer 1998). As participation in these sports increases, it becomes incumbent upon physicians to recognize the unique risk factors associated with the adolescent spine and how this alters the diagnosis and treatment when compared with that of an adult. In addition to the injuries caused by direct contact and macrotrauma, there are also now overuse injuries of this population resulting from the repetitive flexion, rotation, and extension that repetitive sports training imposes on the immature axial skeleton.

The majority of spine-related complaints in adolescent athletes can be diagnosed with a thorough history and physical examination. Conservative management involving a brief alteration of activities and appropriate rehabilitation is often the only treatment required. While catastrophic neurologic sequelae resulting from an acute traumatic injury to the thoracolumbar spine is rare in sports, cervical spine injuries continue to be far too prevalent. All athletes having sustained an injury to the head, neck or thoracolumbar spine should be thoroughly evaluated, and proper stabilization and management protocols instituted if an unstable spinal injury is suspected. More commonly, though, the athlete will present to the clinic with a complaint of back pain that may or may not be associated with a specific injury. Micheli & Wood (1995) emphasize the need to distinguish between complaints of back pain in the athlete compared with the non-athlete. Failure to appreciate the differences in the etiology, pathoanatomy, and ultimate treatment plans for these two distinctly different populations can result in misdiagnosis, and delay in giving appropriate treatment.

Cervical spine injuries are usually the result of acute trauma, while thoracolumbar spine injuries are more often due to overuse. Acute traumatic injuries of the spine can be the product of both contact and noncontact injuries. Chronic overuse injuries are more commonly related to the repetitive microtrauma and musculoskeletal strain that result from excessive training. Distinguishing between these two etiologies is the first step in arriving at a correct diagnosis and subsequent treatment plan. However, one must be aware that on occasion an overuse injury may manifest itself after what may appear to be a trivial acute injury. Such injuries require initial management of the traumatic insult followed by a rehabilitation regimen tailored to address the overuse component.

While trauma, either acute or from overuse, remains the primary cause of back pain in the adolescent athlete, the physician must always rule out other etiologies such as infection, metabolic disorders, and neoplasms. Participation in athletics does not preclude a child developing back pain secondary to one of these more infrequent etiologies, even if the patient attributes the onset of the symptoms to a particular traumatic event.

Providing optimal care for the adolescent athlete requires the physician to observe the following six objectives:

- Be cognizant of the differences between adolescent and adult spine injuries.
- Perform a thorough history and physical exam.
- Use appropriate testing modalities to reach a timely and accurate diagnosis.
- Understand the natural history of the injury.
- Institute a specific treatment, rehabilitation, and prevention program.
- Determine when the athlete may safely return to play. Such decisions require careful analysis and a stepwise thought process. In addition, the physician must not allow the eagerness of the patient, or the urging of the coach or parents, to affect the treatment plan and return-to-play guidelines in any way.

ANATOMY AND BIOMECHANICS OF THE SPINE

Cervical spine anatomy and biomechanics in children, particularly those under 8 years of age, are significantly different from those of adults (Hill et al 1984, Hubbard 1974). The increased compliance and flexibility of its pedicles and the ongoing ossification process that occurs in children up to the age of 10–12 afford some protection from many of the injury patterns seen in adults. As a result, injuries in this region are rare and differ from those seen in the adolescent and adult population. In addition, certain anatomical variations can also cause confusion when interpreting radiographs of a child. For example, the cervical facet angles are only 30° in children under 8 compared with the 60° angles found in adults. This allows a greater degree of freedom in extension and flexion, thus contributing to the pseudo-subluxation appearance commonly seen in this age group at the C2–C3 and C3–C4 levels. Lateral flexion–extension views taken of children under 10 years of age may often reveal an atlantodens interval of up to 5 mm in comparison to the 3.5 mm limit established for adults. Also of note is the truncated odontoid and vertebral body wedging that is apparent until ossification is complete at age 10.

The upper cervical spine is the site of approximately 70% of the cervical spine fractures seen in children. This is in contrast to what is seen in adults. When interpreting radiographs of the child athlete, the physician must be cognizant of the differential in elasticity between the spinal column and the spinal cord. As was described by Pang & Wilberger (1982), such elasticity can result in a spinal cord injury without radiographic abnormality (SCIWORA) in children under the age of 8. These injuries can lead to serious necrologic sequelae and must always be ruled out in this age group.

The thoracolumbar spine of the child shares many of the same anatomical and biomechanical characteristics seen in the cervical region. The rigid support provided by the ribs T1–T10, as well as the orientation of the facet joints in this region, enables the thoracic spine to be relatively resistant to overuse injuries. Unfortunately, this rigid construction appears to transfer abnormal stresses to the cervical and lumbar spine segments, thus putting them at increased risk. These forces may be more pronounced if a hypo- or hyperkyphosis of the thoracic spine exists (the normal kyphus angle is 20–40°), as is seen in patients with atypical Scheuermann's and Scheuermann's disease, respectively (Micheli 1979).

The major components of lumbar motion occur near the L3–L4 through L5–S1 segments. As a result, stress concentrations occur predominantly across this region. Shear stresses in particular are selectively concentrated across the pars interarticularis of these vertebrae, leading to posterior element failure. Predisposing anatomical and biomechanical factors for such injuries include a pre-existing hyperlordosis of the lumbar spine, and repetitive hyperextension activities as seen in gymnastics, football, hockey, weight-lifting, and ballet. In addition, there is evidence showing a genetic predisposition to spondylolytic defects.

The biomechanical properties of the thoracolumbar spine in an 8- to 10-year-old are similar to those of an adult. However, the ring apophysis located at the vertebral end-plates remains open. This becomes relevant when axial loads across the intervertebral disc are coupled with forward flexion, particularly at the L3 through S1 segments, as mentioned above. Such force coupling, if of a significant nature, can fracture the end-plate and force the disc into the soft cancellous bone of the vertebral body as described by Techakapuch (1981) – an occurrence virtually unique to this age group. This is in contrast to frank disc herniation as seen in the adult, or less commonly in an adolescent.

Additional pathomechanical variables that may lead to spinal injuries in the athlete include poor technique, excessive training, and poor anatomy. The inability to alter the athlete's anatomy underscores the importance of optimizing extrinsic preventive measures such as adequate warm-up, close supervision, use of appropriate equipment, and a slow progression of conditioning exercises. In addition, an appropriate strengthening and flexibility program is a vital component in the training schedule of any rapidly growing adolescent athlete.

CERVICAL SPINE INJURIES

Trauma to the cervical spine can lead to fatal or catastrophic injury in the athlete. In fact, data from 1975 showed the incidence of catastrophic injuries in college level football players resulting from cervical spine trauma to approach 17 per 100 000 players (Albright et al 1985). Such injuries are not restricted to gridiron football. Sports such as rugby, gymnastics, ice hockey, diving, and wrestling also share a significant risk of acute cervical spine injury. Despite great strides in the acute evaluation, management, and rehabilitation phases of these injuries, the prognosis for athletes sustaining a catastrophic cervical spine injury remains poor. The potential for such significant impairment has prompted many health care providers to direct much of their attention to the prevention of these injuries. Micheli & Lynch (1994) have described five major types of preventive intervention:

- rules or policy changes
- equipment
- education
- exercise
- preparticipation evaluation.

Once again, though, it is incumbent upon the treating physician to be aware of the many differences that exist between the child's spine and that of an adolescent or adult. These variations often warrant an increased index of suspicion and a tailored acute care and definitive management regimen.

Recognition and acute management

The most important step in the treatment of a non-fatal catastrophic cervical injury is its timely recognition. Many of these injuries occur during practice sessions when a physician is not present, thus emphasizing the importance of educating both the coaching staff and the players to maintain a high index of suspicion for this type of injury in any patient sustaining a blow to the head or neck region. In addition, they should be aware of the potential dire consequences associated with movement of the athlete by persons other than trained personnel.

The physician and/or emergency medical technicians should be well versed in the acute on-field evaluation of the injured athlete. Prior preparation should ensure that all of the proper equipment is available, such as spine board, cervical collars or immobilization devices and a stretcher (Warren & Bailes 1998). An established hierarchy among the participating caregivers should exist, with a predetermined medical 'team captain' supervising the appropriate ABC management, immobilization techniques, log-rolling, and transport (Pizzutillo 1994). Of note is the athlete under 8–10 years of age who may be forced into hyperflexion of the spine if placed on an ordinary spine board. This is due to the increased size of the head in these children relative to their chest. Therefore, they should have a towel roll placed beneath the shoulders to create a more neutral position of the cervical spine (Herzenberg et al 1989). A predetermined protocol for the transportation of the injured athlete to a facility capable of managing catastrophic neurologic injury should exist far in advance of the traumatic event.

Concurrent management of a potential cervical injury in the emergency room should include the continuation of the appropriate ABCs and immobilization that were initiated in the field. The athlete should also be evaluated for a potential head injury; if suspected, a neurological consultation should be obtained. The diagnosis and management of the various potential cervical column injuries are beyond the scope of this review and are discussed in great detail in a number of texts on this topic (e.g. Rockwood et al 1996, Stanitski et al 1994).

Burners or stingers are a not too infrequent injury seen in American football players. These result from a brachial plexus stretch injury in the majority of the high school level players experiencing this phenomenon. The remainder manifest from a 'pinching' of a nerve root. The symptoms usually include pain, burning, or tingling down an arm, and it is occasionally accompanied by weakness. The C5–C6 nerve roots are most commonly affected. The symptoms usually resolve within minutes, but may on occasion persist for days or even weeks. Stingers are always unilateral, and therefore, if bilateral symptoms or concomitant lower extremity involvement are present, a burning hands syndrome must be ruled out. If the diagnosis of a stinger has been established, the athlete may return to play once pain-free with full range of motion of the neck, full motor strength, and normal sensation. Incomplete resolution of symptoms or recurrent episodes should warrant further evaluation with MRI and electromyography (Cantu et al 1998). Consideration should also be given to having the athlete wear elevated shoulder pads and a soft cervical roll to prevent excessive extension and lateral flexion of the cervical spine.

Transient quadriplegia suggests the presence of spinal cord compromise at some level. Much controversy currently exists regarding the role that spinal stenosis plays in this entity. In the past, radiographic bone measurements were advocated to determine the presence of spinal stenosis. At present, MR imaging or contrast computed tomography is advocated in order to better assess for disc protrusion, ligamentum flavum buckling or the presence of bony osteophytes (Cantu et al 1998). Currently we recommend the cessation of contact collision sports in athletes with documented spinal stenosis and a history of spinal cord symptoms.

Preventive intervention

Rules/policy changes

Developing protective rule changes for various sports first requires an understanding of the pathomechanics involved in cervical spine trauma. Axial loading applied to the vertex of the head has been described as the primary mechanism producing cervical spine injuries in athletes today. The normal cervical spine, when viewed from a lateral perspective, has a slightly extended posture due to its normal lordosis. However, with just 30° of neck flexion, the spine straightens and becomes a segmented column (Fig. 4.1). If an athlete assumes this position prior to making contact with another player or object, the spine will be compressed between the rapidly decelerating head and the continued force of the trunk. This force generation in a segmented column cannot be dissipated through motion of the spinal segments, and will therefore potentially result in a fracture and/or dislocation (Fig. 4.2). Unfortunately, axial loading in this position occurs frequently when athletes perform activities such as tackling in American football and rugby, diving, takedowns in wrestling, cross-checking or boarding in ice hockey, etc. A preventive solution to these injuries would obviously entail instituting rule changes

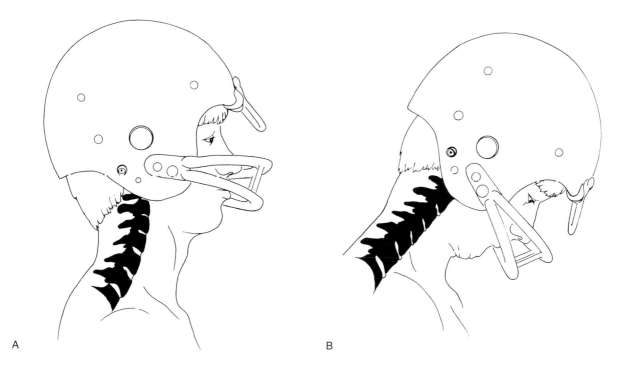

Figure 4.1 A: When the neck is in a normal, upright, anatomical position, the cervical spine is slightly extended due to natural cervical lordosis. B: When the neck is slightly flexed to approximately 30°, the cervical spine is straightened and converted into a segmented column. (From Torg et al 1990, with permission of the American Orthopedic Society for Sport Medicine.)

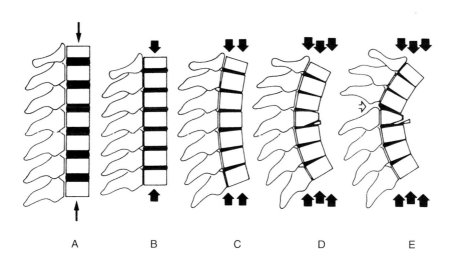

Figure 4.2 Biomechanically, a straight cervical spine responds to an axial load force like a segmented column. Axial loading of the cervical spine first results in compressive deformation of the invertebral discs (A, B). As the energy input continues and maximum compressive deformation is reached, angular deformation and buckling occur. The spine fails in a flexion mode (C) with resulting fracture, subluxation or dislocation (D, E). (From Torg et al 1990, with permission of J. S. Torg.)

prohibiting any type of contact involving an axial load to the vertex of the head. This was proven to be correct in 1976 when spearing rules were formulated that prohibited the intentional striking of an opponent with the crown of the helmet in American football. The number of catastrophic spinal cord injuries gradually dropped from the previously stated 17 per 100 000 college level athletes to 6.6 per 100 000 in 1984 (Albright et al 1985).

Recently, Torg et al (1993) described the 'spear tackler's spine', after discovering an association between spear-tackling and neurologic injury in four American football players. These athletes were found to share certain radiographic criteria:

- developmental narrowing of the cervical spinal canal
- straightening or reversal of the normal cervical lordotic curve
- pre-existing minor post-traumatic radiographic evidence of bony or ligamentous injury.

These findings suggest a possible cumulative effect and further emphasize the need for early intervention in the young athlete.

Rugby football also provides several examples of the potential benefits that preventive rules and regulations can offer. Scher (1987) published an excellent review of this topic, breaking down these injuries according to scrum injuries, injuries sustained while making a tackle, those sustained while being tackled, etc. The mechanism that appears to be most prevalent in rugby is hyperflexion of the cervical spine. This usually occurs to the hooker during a collapsing scrum. The unprotected hooker has little control of his or her neck position, and therefore if hyperflexion occurs while the scrum collapses and forward movement continues, a severe hyperflexion injury may result. Scher (1987) proposed rule changes and recommendations directed at reducing the incidence of these injuries, which included:

- staggering the scrum set-in to eliminate any posterior driving force to the initial front row at the time of set-in
- imposing a severe penalty for intentional collapsing of the scrum
- prohibiting the high tackle
- emphasis on safe tackling technique
- closer adherence to limiting loose ruck play.

The impact of these regulations remains to be seen but will be followed closely.

Equipment

The cervical spine is a difficult area to brace or protect in the athlete. Rigid immobilization would preclude most athletic participation. Numerous attempts have been made in American football to develop shoulder pads and neck rolls that would prevent dangerous extremes of motion of the cervical spine. Unfortunately, most cervical injuries result from axial loading, as previously mentioned, and therefore such equipment may decrease brachial stretch injuries or stingers but not cervical injuries *per se*. Nonetheless, Schneider et al (1985) have speculated on the potential benefits of well-fitting helmets that do not extend too far down the posterior aspect of the neck, and well-fitting shoulder pads that guard against excessive motion of the cervical spine.

Protective equipment is obviously not a panacea for the prevention of cervical trauma, and may inadvertently increase the risk of such injuries. Two such examples include the introduction of the face mask and helmet in ice hockey, and the face mask alone in football. Studies have suggested that these protective devices may have increased the number of cervical spine injuries in these sports. In ice hockey, explanations (Tator 1987) for the paradoxical rise in injuries include a diminished field of vision from the face mask, increased use of the head in play, and an alteration in the center of gravity. In football, the face mask can serve as an effective handle for a would-be tackler, or a dangerous lever arm for neck hyperextension if a player strikes the ground face first. The institution of rules addressing such abuses and their strict enforcement are requisite to obviate such risks.

Education

Educating coaches and athletes is essential for the pursuit of safe athletic competition. In addition, parents should also be included in the teaching process. Topics warranting mention range from the proper techniques necessary for safe participation to the potential catastrophic injuries associated with a particular sport.

Injury-reporting systems are a vital part of the education process. They can provide objective data to support the need for developing various precautionary measures and be an important tool for raising public awareness regarding problems that may be present in existing programs and/or sports. Reporting systems such as these were responsible for the successful implementation of the football spearing rules previously mentioned (Reid & Reid 1981, Torg &

Glasgow 1991). A similar example is Scher's recommendations for rule changes and altered playing technique in rugby. He emphasized the importance of coaches teaching correct tackling technique, in addition to pointing out the potential danger of charging into rucks. Also noted were the excessive hazards of high tackles, diving tackles and particularly late tackles which should be avoided at all costs. Similarly, all players must be educated about the tragic consequences of scrum collapse (Scher 1987).

The prevention of cervical spine injuries in water sports also relies heavily on patient education. Torg & Glasgow (1991) feel that the majority of these injuries can be prevented by strictly adhering to a set of eight guidelines developed to promote safe diving:

- Do not dive into water that is shallower than twice your height.
- Do not dive into unfamiliar water. Know the depth and be sure the water is free of submerged objects.
- Do not assume the water is deep enough. Familiar rivers, lakes, bays and swimming holes change levels. Remember at low tide there is 1.8–2.4 m (6–8 ft) less depth than at high tide.
- Do not dive near dredging or construction work. Water levels may change; dangerous objects may lie beneath the surface.
- Do not dive until the area is clear of other swimmers.
- Do not drink and dive. Alcohol distorts judgment.
- Do not permit or indulge in horseplay while swimming and diving.
- Do not dive into the ocean surf of front beaches.

Conditioning exercise

Strengthening the muscles of the neck and upper torso through directed resistive exercises is often recommended to prevent cervical spine injury. Surprisingly, there are presently no studies to support this recommendation. However, biomechanical observations derived from studies on other anatomical sites of the body, if extrapolated to the cervical spine, may support this recommendation. Studies performed by Lukoschek et al (1986) suggest that impact absorption around the knee and lower extremity is largely provided by the surrounding musculature and soft tissues. Reid & Reid (1981) also feel that improved conditioning plays a role in injury prevention through training and learned habitual responses to loads. They feel that, by repeatedly performing perfectly skilled

movements, successful repression of undesired contractions and delays in spinal readjustment is possible and may therefore result in decreased motor recruitment that might place the neck in danger.

Preparticipation evaluation

Structural variations exist in the cervical spine that appear to make some athletes more susceptible to injury than others. These anatomical and structural variations may be either congenital or acquired, and should be sought during the preparticipation physical examination. A review article by Torg & Glasgow (1991) discussed the various cervical abnormalities that appear to place the athlete at increased risk of injury. An emphasis was placed on performing a thorough preparticipation exam which should include any history of a previous cervical injury, pre-existing abnormality, or limitation in the cervical spine's range of motion.

THORACOLUMBAR SPINE INJURIES
Spondylolysis

Overuse injury to the pars interarticularis is quite common in the young athlete (Pizzutillo 1985). Micheli & Wood (1995) found a 47% incidence of spondylolysis in adolescents presenting to their sports medicine clinic. A spondylolysis is often the result of a stress fracture due to repetitive microtrauma across the pars interarticularis of the lumbar spine. This can result in a bony defect in the pars at one or both sides of a given vertebral level, with 85% located at the L5 vertebrae (Pizzutillo 1993). In addition to a genetic predilection in some individuals, there also appears to be some variation amongst races. It has been estimated in the general population that there is a 4.4% incidence of spondylolysis that increases to 6% with adulthood. However, amongst Blacks the figure drops to 2%, while in some Inuit communities the figure soars to nearly 50% (Pizzutillo 1985). The defect gives rise to instability and subsequent micromotion that may cause pain in the athlete, particularly with activities involving twisting and hyperextension as seen in American football linemen, gymnasts, ballet dancers, pole vaulters, and divers, to name a few (Goldstein et al 1991, Pizzutilllo 1993).

Spondylolysis has been classified into three types: dysplastic, isthmic (traumatic), and degenerative. It is generally believed that athletes sustain an isthmic lesion. This is supported by biomechanical studies demonstrating the presence of increased stresses at the pars interarticularis with extension of the spine, and accentuation of these stresses with lateral flexion, movements required for the execution of these sports.

These patients typically present with complaints of insidious-onset back pain, which may often coincide with an adolescent growth spurt. Initially the pain is exacerbated with strenuous activity, particularly with hyperextension maneuvers such as the back walkover in gymnastics or the arabesque in dance. Later, the pain becomes more progressive, is associated with activities of daily living and no longer responds to periods of rest. Occasionally, the pain may radiate to one or both buttocks. Rarely, radicular symptoms may be present.

On physical examination, these patients may have paraspinal spasm and associated tenderness of the affected paraspinal region. Phalen & Dickson (1961) found hamstring tightness and limited forward flexion in approximately 80% of the time. Forward flexion at the waist is relatively painless, while extension recreates the patient's symptoms. The patient is then asked to actively hyperextend while standing on one leg. This will specifically stress the ipsilateral pars and provoke pain if the lesion is present on this side. Standing on the contralateral leg is less painful or produces no pain at all, unless the lesion is bilateral. The thoracic spine should also be examined for any hyperkyphosis reflecting an underlying Scheuermann's disease (Ginsburg & Bassett 1997). The neurological examination is usually unremarkable.

As with most stress fractures, radiographs of this region will often be negative. Nonetheless, AP, lateral and, most importantly, oblique radiographs should be obtained. A narrow gap with irregular edges in the pars interarticularis is diagnostic of a spondylolytic lesion. If these are negative and the index of suspicion remains high, a SPECT (single-photon emission computed tomography) bone scan is indicated, which is highly sensitive for detecting early spondylolytic stress fractures. A positive scan does not always effectively rule out other possible etiologies such as osteoid osteoma, facet arthropathy, and infection. Therefore, if the diagnosis remains in question, a computed tomographic (CT) scan and/or appropriate blood work is indicated.

The management of a symptomatic, isthmic pars defect must first take into account the etiology behind this lesion. While some controversy surrounds the management of these lesions, we feel that, as a stress fracture, it should have the propensity to heal, particularly in the pre-adolescent and adolescent age groups.

A bracing regimen is therefore recommended using a rigid polypropylene lumbar orthosis. This brace has 0–15° of lumbar flexion acting to flatten the lumbar lordosis and reduce sheer stresses at the pars site. This brace is worn 23 out of 24 h/day for 6 months. The 1 h/day out of the brace is used for bathing, performing peripelvic strengthening, and antilordotic and lower extremity flexibility exercises. Patients are allowed to resume limited athletic activities with the brace only after resolution of their symptoms. Bone scans may be helpful in following the progress of the lesion. However, we currently recommend obtaining a focal CT scan of the involved level after 6 months of bracing in order to assess the lesion for bony healing more accurately. Patients with an initially cold scan may be allowed to discontinue wearing the brace upon resolution of their pain, usually after 3–4 weeks of brace wear. The remaining patients are warned to wean themselves slowly from the brace, taking as long as 4–6 months, as recurrence of symptoms is not uncommon with an abrupt cessation. Using this treatment protocol, Micheli & Steiner (1985) were able to achieve a 32% incidence of bony healing, and overall 88% of patients were able to return to their previous sport even if the lesion had not healed. Upon completion of the bracing program and resolution of all symptoms, it is incumbent on the athlete to continue the flexibility and strengthening exercises. This is especially important for the growing adolescent.

Patients who continue to have pain despite a carefully monitored bracing program may be candidates for surgery. If the pain is significant, a fusion of the posterolateral transverse process using bone graft is indicated, although direct osteosynthesis of the lesion has been described. Postoperatively, these patients are immobilized in a brace for 6 months, and heavy activities are not allowed for 12 months, or until a solid fusion mass is present radiographically.

Also of note are those patients with a clinical presentation suggestive of spondylolysis, but whose SPECT scans demonstrate diffuse posterior element uptake at several levels. This represents a stress reaction and not a true stress fracture. These patients begin the identical bracing and rehabilitation program as those with frank spondylolysis, but can usually be tapered from the brace after 3 months of treatment.

Spondylolisthesis

Spondylolisthesis refers to the anterior translation of one vertebral body on an adjacent vertebral body. These are often classified into one of four categories according to their etiology: type I, isthmic; type II, degenerative; type III, congenital; type IV, pathologic. They are graded according to the percentage of the vertebral body that has translated beyond the adjacent vertebrae's anterior margin, as measured in the sagittal plane. The five grades of spondylolisthesis are as follows: grade I, 0–25% translation; grade II, 25–50%, grade III, 50–75%; grade IV, 75–100%; grade V, >100% (also referred to as a spondyloptosis). As with spondylolysis, there appears to be a genetic predisposition, with studies showing an incidence of 27–69% in close relatives (Hensinger 1989). Overall, the development of a spondylolisthesis appears to be multifactorial, although women with the congenital form are noted to have a slightly higher risk of progression. This particular type is characterized by dysplastic or malformed facets of the involved vertebra(e), and has a higher incidence of slip progression (Seitsalo et al 1988). These patients are most often non-athletic females that present during their adolescent growth spurt. Overall, the incidence of high-grade (IV, V) spondylolisthesis is twice as high in females as it is in males. As with spondylolysis, the L5–S1 level is affected in 85–90% of cases.

These patients will often present in a similar manner to those patients with a spondylolysis. It is not uncommon for them to complain more of tight hamstrings than of pain. They will occasionally have a wide-based gait with a short stride length. Rarely a palpable step-off can be appreciated in patients with a severe slip (>100%); this is particularly true in the athletic population where such a slip would preclude participation in sports. The patient's pelvic tilt should also be observed, as it will often flex in an effort to compensate for the lumbosacral kyphosis.

The diagnostic work-up should include AP and lateral radiographs. As mentioned, slips most commonly occur at the L5–S1 juncture, and if seen at L4, a sacralization of L5 is usually present. The lateral view will enable the physician to grade and monitor the slip throughout the course of treatment.

The treatment of spondylolisthesis in the athlete remains somewhat controversial. Most studies have concluded that asymptomatic athletes with a grade I slip may return to contact sports providing they remain symptom-free. Management of grade II slips continues to be debated. Currently we treat mildly symptomatic patients with activity modification and a tailored rehabilitation program emphasizing peripelvic strengthening and hamstring stretching. Those patients who fail this treatment are then braced with a rigid, antilordotic, polypropylene lumbosacral ortho-

sis for 2–6 months until their symptoms resolve. They continue their physical therapy while in the brace and are allowed to return to athletic participation with the brace on once they are asymptomatic (Micheli & Steiner 1985). Children and adolescents should be monitored for progression of the slip once a year with a standing lateral radiograph until skeletal maturity.

Surgical indications for spondylolisthesis include patients with a documented progression, those who have failed a 6–12 month course of conservative management, slips in excess of 50% regardless of symptoms, and neurologic deficit. Grades I and II can be managed with an in situ posterolateral fusion between L5 and S1 (Bradford 1985). A resolution of symptoms usually heralds a solid fusion. Higher-grade slips should have their fusion extended from L4 to S1. Nerve root decompression is performed only in the presence of neurological compromise. Reduction and instrumentation remains highly controversial. The return to contact sports following a solid fusion is a decision that should be individualized for each athlete, and may be contraindicated.

Scheuermann's disease

During the adolescent growth spurt, the lumbodorsal fascia and hamstrings become tight as they are unable to keep up with the rapidly growing bony skeleton. This results in extension of the lumbar spine and pelvis relative to the lower extremities. The body will compensate for this by developing a round-back deformity. This is a self-limiting postural deformity that exhibits no structural abnormalities and is characterized by passive correction with extension. On the contrary, Scheuermann's disease is a structural entity that presents with a kyphotic deformity resistant to passive correction (Bradford 1987).

Classic Scheuermann's disease, or juvenile thoracic kyphosis, is a common cause for thoracic kyphosis in the adolescent population, but is rarely seen in the athletic population. The etiology remains unknown but has been attributed to juvenile osteoporosis, osteochondrosis, necrosis of the ring apophysis, and even tight hamstrings. The onset is most often spontaneous without any history of significant trauma, although repetitive flexion and a familial predilection have been mentioned as possible causes.

These patients rarely complain of pain, and instead present on the urging of parents or friends for cosmetic or postural complaints. Clinically, they have a round-back deformity that does not correct with passive extension. Typically there is a hyperlordosis of the lumbar spine and associated tight hip flexors, hamstrings and lumbar fascia. Radiographically, the presence of three or more adjacent vertebrae wedged more than 5° each is virtually pathognomonic for Scheuermann's disease (Sorenson 1964). The Scoliosis Research Society has stated that the accepted range of normal thoracic kyphosis for an adolescent is between 20° and 40° (Bradford 1987). Additional radiographic findings include irregular end-plates, Schmorl's nodes, and narrow disc spaces.

Treatment of Scheuermann's is warranted if the patient is symptomatic, finds the deformity cosmetically unacceptable, or if the deformity continues to progress. Initial efforts are directed at stretching the tight hamstring muscles, hip flexors, and lumbar fascia, in addition to strengthening the abdominal muscles. A progression of the thoracic kyphosis beyond 50° in a skeletally immature child warrants bracing with a Milwaukee brace or a modified Boston brace with thoracic uprights. The patients are allowed out of the brace to participate in sports; otherwise it is worn 16–18 h/day. Progression beyond 70° is an indication for anterior-posterior or posterior spine fusion with instrumentation. These patients are prohibited from doing all sports except swimming for approximately 1 year postoperatively or until a solid fusion is present. They are allowed to return to light-contact sports at this point, although gymnastics and contact sports are prohibited permanently (Micheli 1985).

Atypical Scheuermann's disease

Anterior vertebral wedging seen in the midthoracic to midlumbar region of the adolescent spine that is associated with pain may represent atypical or thoracolumbar Scheuermann's disease. The thoracolumbar junction is most often affected, although the entire lumbar spine may be involved. The pain that often accompanies this phenomenon is thought to result from multiple microfractures of the growth plates, or possible anterior disc herniation through the anterior ring apophysis, with secondary bony deformation of the vertebra. Athletes between the ages of 15 and 17 participating in sports requiring repetitive flexion–extension activities of the spine, such as rowing, gymnastics, and diving, are at most risk.

These young athletes may present clinically with complaints of transient non-descript pain that progressed to moderately severe pain over a period of 2–6 months. Commonly the symptoms are accentuated with forward flexion and relieved by rest. In contradistinction to Scheuermann's disease, atypical

Scheuermann's is characterized by thoracic hypokyphosis and lumbar hypolordosis (flat back) (D'Hemecourt & Micheli 1997). Tight lumbodorsal fascia and hamstrings are usually found, while radicular complaints are rare. Radiographs will often reveal vertebral end-plate irregularities with associated wedging and disc space narrowing.

Atypical lumbar Scheuermann's disease is thought to involve a disc rupture through the cancellous bone beneath the apophyseal ring. These repeated stress fractures can lead to the formation of Schmorl's node-type lesions of the vertebral body. The displaced apophyseal fragment at the anterior margin of the vertebral body seldom heals, thus leading to wedging and pain. Patients with these findings may benefit from a symptomatic bracing regimen. A semirigid thermoplastic brace with 15–30° of lumbar lordosis worn 18–23 h/day is recommended until sufficient vertebral body remodeling is present on radiographs (Micheli et al 1980). Peripelvic strengthening and flexibility exercises are instituted during brace wear once the pain has resolved. Athletes are allowed to return to sports while wearing the brace once they are asymptomatic.

DISCOGENIC BACK PAIN

Disc herniation in the pre-adolescent athlete is quite rare, accounting for 8–3.8% of all disc herniations that occur. However, the incidence rises dramatically as the child enters adolescence and adulthood (Hubbard 1974). An association between athletics and disc herniation has not been proven. In fact, many believe that physical fitness actually plays a role in the prevention of such injuries. The clinical presentation in children is variable and often differs from that seen in the adult population. Therefore the diagnosis is often difficult, warranting a high index of suspicion.

These children often have no radicular signs, and commonly complain of mild-to-moderate low back pain or pain that radiates to the buttock or posterior thigh region. Sciatica, with pain radiating below the knee and exacerbated by a Lesague test, may be present, but an epidural abscess or an intraspinal tumor may also cause sciatica pain and should be ruled out (Conrad et al 1992, Jacobsen & Sullivan 1994). The pain is exacerbated with any type of Valsalva maneuver and somewhat relieved by assuming the supine position. Parents and/or coaches may comment on the child's altered gait or running patterns in the absence of any complaints of pain. The child may also exhibit poor hamstring flexibility or trunk listing (sciatic scoliosis) which signals paravertebral spasm. A positive straight leg raise is present in 85% of these patients, and the presence of any motor or sensory changes, or decreased reflexes should be sought. A history of fever, weight loss, or malaise could signal a malignant condition, while a recent bacterial or viral infection may suggest a diagnosis of discitis. Although exceedingly rare in this population, cauda equina syndrome has been reported.

Upon completion of a thorough history and physical examination, lumbosacral films should be obtained to rule out a possible underlying osseous injury. Plain radiographs should be examined for avulsion fractures of the vertebral end-plate, which can also cause radicular symptoms. If these are negative, the physician should proceed to a MRI study. The L4–L5 and L5–S1 levels are those most commonly affected. At present, spinal MRI can demonstrate both disc degeneration and herniation. MRI findings should always be correlated with clinical findings. In patients with severe pain associated with constitutional symptoms, a complete blood count and erythrocyte sedimentation rate should be obtained. If these are elevated, a bone scan should follow to rule out a potential discitis or malignant process.

Conservative management is the standard of care for these patients. A non-steroidal anti-inflammatory regimen and an initial period of relative rest for 2–3 days are instituted. Patients should also be placed on a physical therapy program emphasizing flexibility, and spine and peripelvic strengthening. A gradual response should be noted within a few weeks. If these measures fail, or if the patient is markedly symptomatic, we recommend a bracing regimen using a semi-rigid thermoplastic brace with a 15° lumbar lordosis (Gerbino & Micheli 1995). The success rate of this bracing program is lower than that seen for spondylolytic processes, with only 50% of young athletes returning to sports without pain within the first year of treatment (Micheli et al 1980). Epidural injections may have a role in the treatment of more recalcitrant cases. Overall, successful management is often hindered by these young motivated athletes returning prematurely to sports.

Surgical indications for symptomatic herniated disc disease include failure of conservative management, posteriorly displaced disc with an attached apophysis, and the presence of a cauda equina syndrome. DeOrio & Bianco (1982) reported surgical success rates in the pre-adolescent and adolescent age groups ranging from 73 to 98%. During surgery, every effort should be made to preserve the facet joints and the interspinous ligaments in order to prevent segmental instability.

While there are no clear guidelines, most patients will be able to return to sports upon regaining full motor strength and pain-free range of motion. Gymnasts and those athletes involved in contact sports should be counseled that resumption of such activities may promote further degeneration at the involved level. Some athletes may find that they must alter their activities or even change to another sport altogether.

A condition that closely mimics that of a herniated lumbar disc is a slipped vertebral apophysis or end-plate fracture. These are usually associated with heavy lifting, with the patient's clinical examination suggesting a herniated disc as the etiology. Radiographs may demonstrate a displaced posterior inferior vertebral apophysis into the vertebral canal, with L4 being the most commonly affected. A CT study with metrizamide myelography is the procedure of choice, providing excellent bone visualization and documentation of anterior epidural compression (Ginsburg & Bassett 1997). MRI may also be useful and will reveal any extradural mass. The associated disc often remains attached to the apophysis by Sharpey's fibers. Treatment entails surgical excision of the disc and bony fragment.

SCOLIOSIS

Preparticipation physical examinations are an excellent opportunity for physicians to screen young athletes for scoliosis (Bradford 1987, Spencer & Jackson 1983). Idiopathic scoliosis does not cause pain or functional impairment in the athlete. Congenital scoliosis, differentiated by radiographs, should be evaluated for renal and cardiac abnormalities prior to allowing participation in sports. In addition, patients with congenital anomalies of the cervical spine or cervicothoracic junction should be evaluated carefully for participation in contact sports.

With the advent of school screening programs and a heightened awareness among coaches and parents, the early detection of scoliosis in skeletally immature children has improved. Most often, an asymmetry in the child's shoulders, an increased curvature of the spine, or a hump noted in the thoracic region upon forward bending prompts a referral to an orthopedic surgeon for further evaluation. Full-length spine radiographs should be obtained in order to document the type of curve present, and monitor the cobb angles for progression. Patients should be followed radiographically every 4–6 months, and a bracing regimen instituted if the curve progresses rapidly, or if it exceeds 25–30° in a skeletally immature child. The brace should be worn for a minimum of 18 h/day, and unrestricted participation in sports allowed with the brace on. Patients should be instructed in a flexibility and strengthening program to be performed while in the brace. Upon cessation of growth, they are weaned from their braces and allowed to return to full, unrestricted activities. Those patients progressing beyond 50° and remaining skeletally immature have a high incidence of further progression; therefore, an anterior and/or posterior fusion may be indicated. The fusion of multiple motion segments leads to increased bending moments at either end of the fusion mass; therefore, contact sports, gymnastics and diving are usually contraindicated following this treatment. Postoperatively, patients are prohibited from gym class for 1 year while the fusion mass is allowed to mature.

Young athletes presenting with painful scoliosis may actually have an underlying disc herniation. Additional etiologies to be ruled out include osteoid osteoma, osteoblastoma, spondylolisthesis, infection, intraspinal tumor, and discitis. The patient should be examined for hairy nevi or dermal sinuses, which are associated with congenital anomalies such as diastematomyelia. Appropriate laboratory work should be ordered if constitutional symptoms are present. An accurate diagnosis is essential when evaluating and treating a young athlete with painful scoliosis.

THORACOLUMBAR FRACTURES

Catastrophic injuries to the thoracolumbar spine with resultant neurologic sequelae are usually seen in association with motor vehicle accidents. As such, fractures, dislocations, and fracture-dislocations of the spine in young athletes are quite rare, with very few reports in the literature of neurologic sequelae resulting from a thoracolumbar injury in this population. Fortunately, musculotendinous strains and contusions are the predominate finding, while catastrophic neurologic injuries remain largely confined to the cervical spine. Most non-catastrophic fractures of the lumbosacral spine are transverse and spinous process fractures, and vertebral body compression fractures. These are relatively stable fractures and can be treated symptomatically with activity restrictions and oral analgesics until resolution of the pain. Occasionally, bracing is warranted to provide better immobilization and pain relief. Patients are allowed to perform conditioning activities while in the brace if they remain asymptomatic, with the brace being discontinued after 4–6 weeks.

The evaluation and management of acute thoracolumbar spine injuries in the adolescent athlete is beyond the scope of this chapter. Their treatment is outlined in numerous textbooks on pediatric fracture management (Rockwood et al 1996). Although the incidence of unstable thoracolumbar spine injuries is extremely rare, the physician should be well acquainted with on-field evaluation, immobilization, and transport protocols, as well as having pre-arranged access to a specialized acute-care facility (Leidholt 1973).

Most patients sustaining an unstable thoracolumbar spine injury will require an anterior and/or posterior spinal fusion. While each case must be evaluated individually, these patients are at an increased risk of re-injury should they return to sports. This is particularly true for those sustaining a concomitant neurologic injury. For this reason, Micheli (1985) recommends a discontinuation of contact sports for these patients.

MECHANICAL BACK PAIN

In the young athlete, mechanical back pain is generally a diagnosis of exclusion. The symptoms are frequently non-specific, exacerbated with activities and relieved with rest. It is commonly attributed to overuse or stretch injuries to the soft tissues, ligaments, joint capsules, and facets themselves (Spencer & Jackson 1983). It is often seen in the young athlete around the time of the adolescent growth spurt, prompting some to attribute the process to a transient overgrowth response (Micheli 1983).

These patients present with complaints of nondescript low back pain that is worse with activities. The patient usually describes a history of excessive athletic activity with poor conditioning, insufficient stretching, and improper technique. Physical examination reveals weak abdominal muscles, and tight lumbodorsal fascia, hip flexors and hamstrings. Paraspinous muscle spasm, increased lumbar lordosis, and occasionally a trigger point over a facet joint can be found. Radicular signs and neurologic findings are not present. Radiographs and skeletal imaging may be necessary to rule out any structural etiology.

Management includes an initial period of rest for 2–3 days; in addition, an icing and non-steroidal anti-inflammatory regimen may provide acute pain relief. Hydrotherapy, ultrasound, and electrical stimulation are useful adjuncts for addressing the paraspinal spasm. Upon resolution of the acute phase of pain, the patient is placed on an individualized rehabilitation and stretching program. This will include abdominal strengthening with pelvic tilts, antilordotic posturing, and stretching of the lumbodorsal fascia and hamstrings. Modifications of the athlete's training schedule and technique can help to prevent recurrence of the same injury (Gallagher et al 1995). Patients who are refractory to conservative measures are candidates for a bracing regimen using a semi rigid lumbar orthosis with a 0° or 15° lordosis (Micheli et al 1980). Mechanical back pain usually resolves within 3 weeks, and therefore continued pain despite these measures warrants further work-up. Additional etiologies to be entertained include ankylosing spondylitis, juvenile rheumatoid arthritis, infection, and neoplasms.

CONCLUSIONS

It is incumbent on the physician to recognize adolescent athletes as being uniquely different from adults. As such, the cervical and thoracolumbar injuries seen in this population often vary considerably from an etiologic, anatomic and biomechanical standpoint. An accurate diagnosis is crucial and begins with a thorough history and physical examination keeping in mind that rapid growth and open physis potentiate a host of injuries that often must be individually ruled out. Greater than 90% of the injuries can be accurately diagnosed by clinical examination and history; nonetheless, numerous diagnostic modalities are available to further aid the physician in arriving at a correct diagnosis. These studies should be used in a logical and stepwise fashion with the intent of confirming or monitoring the presumptive clinical diagnosis. Once the diagnosis has been established, an understanding of the injury's natural history is essential for instituting an effective treatment plan. This plan must not only address the acute management of these injuries, but also be directed to their prevention and rehabilitation with the goal of returning these athletes to their respective sports in a safe yet timely fashion.

REFERENCES

Albright J P, McCall E, Martin R K, Crowley E T, Foster D T 1985 Head and neck injuries in college football: an eight year analysis. American Journal of Sports Medicine 3(3): 147–152

Bradford D S 1985 Spondylolysis and spondylolisthesis in children and adolescents: current concepts in management. In: Bradford D S, Hensinger R M (eds) The pediatric spine. Thieme, New York, p 403–423

Bradford D S, Iza J 1985 Repair of the defect in spondylolysis or minimal degrees of spondylolisthesis by segmental fixation and bone grafting. Spine 10: 673–679

Bradford D S 1987 Juvenile kyphosis. In: Bradford D S, Lonstein J E, Moe J H, Ogilvie J W, Winter R B (eds) Moe's textbook of scoliosis and other spinal deformities, 2nd edn. W B Saunders, Philadelphia, p 347–368

Cantu R C, Bailes J E, Wilberger J E Jr 1998 Guidelines for return to contact or collision sport after a cervical spine injury. Clinics in Sports Medicine 17(1): 137–146

Conrad E U III, Olsewski A D, Berger M et al 1992 Pediatric spine tumors with spinal cord compromise. Journal of Pediatric Orthopaedics 12: 454–460

DeOrio J K, Bianco A J 1982 Lumbar disc excision in children and adolescents. Journal of Bone and Joint Surgery 64A(7): 991–995

D'Hemecourt P A, Micheli L J 1997 Acute and chronic adolescent thoracolumbar injuries. Sports Medicine and Arthroscopy Review 5: 164–171

Gallagher R M, Williams R A, Skelly J, Haugh L D 1995 Worker's compensation and return to work in low back pain. Pain 61: 299–307

Gerbino P G, Micheli L J 1995 Back injuries in the young athlete. Clinics in Sports Medicine 14: 571–590

Ginsburg G M, Bassett G S 1999 Back pain in children and adolescents: evaluation and differential diagnosis. Journal of the American Academy of Orthopaedic Surgeons 5(2): 67–78

Goldstein J D, Berger P E, Windler G E, Jackson D W 1991 Spine injuries in gymnasts and swimmers. An epidemiologic investigation. American Journal of Sports Medicine 19: 463–468

Hensinger R N 1989 Spondylolysis and spondylolisthesis in children and adolescents. Journal of Bone and Joint Surgery 71A: 1098–1107

Herzenberg J E, Hensinger R N, Dedrick D K et al 1989 Emergency transport and positioning of young children who have an injury of the cervical spine. Journal of Bone and Joint Surgery 71A: 15–22

Hill S A, Miller C A, Kosmik E J, Hunt W E 1984 Pediatric neck injuries. Journal of Neurosurgery 60: 700–706

Hubbard D D 1974 Injuries of the spine in children and adolescents. Clinical Orthopaedics 100: 56–65

Jacobsen F S, Sullivan B 1994 Spinal epidural abscesses in children. Orthopedics 17: 1131–1138

Leidholt J D 1973 Spinal injuries in athletes: be prepared. Orthopaedic Clinics of North America 4(3): 691–707

Lukoschek M, Boyd R D, Schaffler M B, Bur D B, Radin E L 1986 Comparison of joint degeneration models. Surgical instability and repetitive impulse loading. Acta Orthopaedica Scandinavica 57: 349–353

Maffulli N 1992 The growing child in sport. British Medical Bulletin 48: 561–568

Micheli L J 1979 Low back pain in the adolescent. American Journal of Sports Medicine 7: 362–364

Micheli L J 1983 Overuse injuries in children's sports: the growth factor. Clinical Orthopaedics 14(2): 337–360

Micheli L J 1985 Sports following spinal surgery in the young athlete. Clinical Orthopaedics 198: 152–157

Micheli L J 1994 The child and adolescent. In: Harries M, Williams C, Stanish W D, Micheli L J (eds) Oxford textbook of sports medicine. Oxford University Press, Oxford, ch 6, p 646–652

Micheli L J, Lynch M 1994 Spinal injuries. In: Renstrom P (ed) Clinical practice of sports injury prevention and care. Blackwell Scientific Publications, Oxford, ch 6, p 86–93

Micheli L J, Mintzer C M 1998 Overuse injuries of the spine. In: Harries M, Williams C, Stanish W, Micheli L (eds) Oxford textbook of sports medicine, 2nd edn. Oxford University Press, Oxford

Micheli L J, Steiner E M 1985 Treatment of symptomatic spondylolysis and spondylolisthesis with the modified Boston brace. Spine 10: 937–943

Micheli L J, Wood 1995 Back pain in young athletes. Archives of Pediatric and Adolescent Medicine 149: 15–18

Micheli L J, Hall J E, Miller M E 1980 Use of modified Boston back brace for back injuries in athletes. American Journal of Sports Medicine 8(5): 351–356

Pang D, Wilberger J E 1982 Spinal cord injury without radiographic abnormalities in children. Journal of Neurosurgery 57: 114–129

Phalen G S, Dickson J A 1961 Spondylolisthesis and tight hamstrings. Journal of Bone and Joint Surgery 43A(4): 505–512

Pizzutillo P D 1985 Spondylolisthesis: etiology and natural history. In: Bradford D S, Hensinger R M (eds) The pediatric spine. Thieme, New York, p 395–402

Pizzutillo P D 1993 Spinal considerations in the young athlete. Instructional Course Lectures 42: 463–472

Pizzutillo P D 1994 The cervical spine in pediatric and adolescent sports medicine. In: Stanitski C L, DeLee J C, Drez D (eds) Pediatric and adolescent sports medicine. W B Saunders, Philadelphia, ch 10, p 118–119

Reid S E, Reid S E Jr 1981 Advances in sports medicine. Prevention of head and neck injuries in football. Surgery Annals 13: 251–270

Rockwood C, Wilkins K, Beaty J (eds) Fractures in children, 4th edn. Lippincott-Raven, Philadelphia

Scher A T 1987 Rugby injuries of the spine and spinal cord. Clinical Sports Medicine 6(1): 87–99

Schneider R C, Peterson T R, Anderson R E 1985 Football. In: Schneider R C, Kennedy J C, Plant M C (eds) Sports injury mechanics, prevention, and treatment. Williams and Wilkins, Baltimore, p 1–61

Seitsalo S, Osterman K, Ponssa M, Laurent L E 1988 Spondylolisthesis in children under 12 years of age: long-term results of 56 patients treated conservatively or operatively. Journal of Pediatric Orthopaedics 8: 516–521

Sorenson K H (ed) 1964 Scheuermann's juvenile kyphosis: clinical appearances, radiography, aetiology and prognosis. Munksgaard, Copenhagen

Spencer G W, Jackson D W 1983 Back injuries in the athlete. Clinics in Sports Medicine 2: 191–216

Stanitski C, DeLee J, Drez D (eds) 1994 Pediatric and adolescent sports medicine. W B Saunders, Philadelphia

Tator C H 1987 Neck injuries in ice hockey: a recent, unsolved problem with many contributing factors. Clinical Sports Medicine 6(1): 101–114

Techakapuch S 1981 Rupture of the lumbar cartilage plate into the spinal canal in an adolescent. A case report. Journal of Bone and Joint Surgery 63A(3): 481–482

Torg J S, Glasgow S G 1991 Criteria for return to contact activities following cervical spine injury. Clinical Journal of Sport Medicine 4: 349–353

Torg J S, Vegso J, O'Neil M J, Senet B 1990 The epidemiologic, pathologic, biomechanical and cinematographic analysis of football-induced cervical spine trauma. American Journal of Sports Medicine 18(1): 50–57

Torg J S, Sennett B, Pavlov H, Leventhal M R, Glasgow S G 1993 Spear tackler's spine. American Journal of Sports Medicine 21: 640–649

Warren W L, Bailes J E 1998 On the field evaluation of athletic neck injuries. Clinics in Sports Medicine 17(1): 99–110

FURTHER READING

Jones E T, Hensinger R N 1996 Injuries of the cervical spine. In: Rockwood C, Wilkins K, Beaty J (eds) Fractures in children, vol 3, 4th edn. Lippincott-Raven, Philadelphia, ch 12, p 1024–1062

Loder R T, Hensinger R N 1996 Fractures of the thoracic and lumbar spine. In: Rockwood C, Wilkins K, Beaty J (eds) Fractures in children, vol 3, 4th edn. Lippincott-Raven, Philadelphia, ch 12, p 1062–1105

Pizzutillo P 1994 The cervical spine. In: Stanitski C, DeLee J, Drez D (eds) Pediatric and adolescent sports medicine. W B Saunders, Philadelphia, ch 10, pp 158–183

Whitecloud T S, Brinker M R, Butter J G et al 1997 The cervical spine. In: Frymoyer J W, Ducker T B, Hadler N M, Kostuik J P, Weinstein J N, Whitecloud T S (eds) The adult spine, principles and practices, vol 1, 2nd edn. Lippincott-Raven, Philadelphia, part III, p 1057–1320

5

Physical activity and cardiorespiratory fitness in young people

Neil Armstrong   Joanne R. Welsman

KEY POINTS

1. If rigorously determined, peak oxygen uptake (peak $\dot{V}O_2$) can be accepted as a maximum index of young people's cardiorespiratory fitness.
2. Peak $\dot{V}O_2$ increases with chronological age in both boys and girls, but boys' values are higher than those of girls from an early age.
3. The use of the ratio standard (mL/kg per min) to normalize for body size has clouded our understanding of growth and maturational changes in peak $\dot{V}O_2$.
4. The majority of children and adolescents seldom experience the intensity and duration of physical activity recommended for the promotion of health and well-being.
5. Boys are more active than girls and although both sexes reduce their physical activity as they move from childhood through adolescence and into adult life, the rate of decline is greater in girls.
6. There is little or no relationship between young people's habitual physical activity and their peak $\dot{V}O_2$.

INTRODUCTION

The Children's Health and Exercise Research Centre was established in 1987. During the subsequent decade, over 3000 young people had their cardiorespiratory fitness determined in the Centre, and over 1000 children and adolescents had their heart rate continuously monitored, over a period of at least 3 days, to estimate their habitual physical activity. This chapter will use these experiences to examine the assessment and interpretation of young people's cardiorespiratory fitness and physical activity patterns, and to explore any relationships between daily physical activity and cardiorespiratory fitness.*

CARDIORESPIRATORY FITNESS

Assessment of cardiorespiratory fitness

Maximal or peak oxygen uptake?

During exercise, oxygen uptake ($\dot{V}O_2$) increases with increasing exercise intensity up to a critical point beyond which no further increase in $\dot{V}O_2$ takes place, even though the person is still able to increase the exercise intensity. The point of levelling of $\dot{V}O_2$ (a $\dot{V}O_2$ plateau) is defined as the maximal $\dot{V}O_2$ ($\dot{V}O_{2\,max}$), and exercise beyond this point is supported by anaerobic energy sources resulting in lactate accumulation, acidosis and inevitable exhaustion. $\dot{V}O_{2\,max}$ is widely recognized as the best estimate of a person's cardiorespiratory fitness (US Department of Health and Human Sciences 1996). In contrast, only about 40% of children and adolescents demonstrate a $\dot{V}O_2$ plateau. The appropriate term to use is therefore peak $\dot{V}O_2$, the highest $\dot{V}O_2$ elicited during an exercise test to exhaustion, rather than $\dot{V}O_{2\,max}$ which conventionally implies the existence of a $\dot{V}O_2$ plateau (Armstrong & Welsman 1997).

It has been argued that many young people fail to demonstrate a $\dot{V}O_2$ plateau due to low levels of motivation or low anaerobic ability (Armstrong & Welsman 1994). However, although only a minority of children (Armstrong et al 1995) and adolescents (Armstrong et al 1991) exhibit a $\dot{V}O_2$ plateau, those who plateau do not have a higher peak $\dot{V}O_2$, heart rate or blood lactate than those who do not. Nevertheless, as exercise tests with young people are normally terminated when the subject, despite strong verbal encouragement, is unable or unwilling to continue, experimenters are left with the problem of deciding whether a maximal effort

was delivered. In our view, the ability of an experienced research team to interpret subjective criteria of intense effort (i.e. hyperpnoea, facial flushing, sweating, unsteady gait) is the vital ingredient in making this decision. Habituating the young subject to the laboratory environment and testing procedures is extremely important and, although no single subsidiary criterion can confirm a maximal effort, heart rate and respiratory exchange ratio (RER) at peak $\dot{V}O_2$ are valuable indicators when using a progressive, incremental test (Armstrong & Welsman 1994).

Some writers have recommended high post-exercise blood lactate levels (e.g. 6–7 mmol/L) as a criterion of maximal exercise (see Armstrong & Welsman 1994), but this is problematic given the extreme variability in young people's post-exercise blood lactates. Methodological factors such as the site of sampling, assay method and timing of post-exercise sampling will significantly influence the measured blood lactate (Welsman & Armstrong 1998, Williams et al 1992), but even where the same protocol, sampling and assay techniques have been used, blood lactates at peak $\dot{V}O_2$ ranging from less than 4.0 to over 13 mmol/L have been observed (Armstrong & Welsman 1995, Williams et al 1990).

Armstrong et al (1996b) provided further evidence of the validity of peak $\dot{V}O_2$ as a maximal index of young people's cardiorespiratory fitness. Twenty boys and 20 girls (mean age 9.9 ± 0.4 years) had their peak $\dot{V}O_2$ determined using a discontinuous, incremental test on a motorized treadmill. On two subsequent weeks, the children returned to the Centre and, following a warm-up, completed 2–3 min exercise bouts at the same treadmill speed but with the gradient raised to 2.5 and 5% greater than that which had elicited peak $\dot{V}O_2$ on the first test. Eighteen boys and 17 girls completed all three tests (Table 5.1). Tests 2 and 3 generated significantly higher peak lactate, RER and ventilation than test 1 in both boys and girls, but despite this increased anaerobic contribution, no significant increases in peak $\dot{V}O_2$ were detected.

Determination of peak $\dot{V}O_2$

The choice of laboratory ergometer for the determination of young people's peak $\dot{V}O_2$ lies between step bench, cycle ergometer and treadmill (see Armstrong & Welsman 2000a). Exercise intensity on a step bench depends upon step frequency, step height and the subject's body mass. It is difficult to teach children to step up and down with a consistent rhythm and problems may arise from differences in leg length.

* The excellent research and inspiration provided by friends and colleagues in the European Group of Pediatric Work Physiology and the North American Society of Pediatric Exercise Medicine are gratefully acknowledged but, at the request of the editors, this chapter will focus on data collected in the Children's Health and Exercise Research Centre. The suggested readings at the end of the chapter provide access to related research and comment by distinguished paediatric exercise scientists.

Table 5.1 Peak physiological data over three exercise tests. (Data are from Armstrong et al 1996b)

Test	One	Two	Three
Boys			
Oxygen uptake (L/min)	1.93 ± 0.23	1.95 ± 0.24	1.98 ± 0.17
Oxygen uptake (mL/kg per min)	62 ± 6	63 ± 8	64 ± 7
Minute ventilation (L/min)	63.6 ± 10.0	68.7 ± 11.1^{a}	69.9 ± 11.1^{a}
Respiratory exchange ratio	0.99 ± 0.05	1.15 ± 0.07^{a}	1.18 ± 0.09^{a}
Blood lactate (mmol/L)	5.7 ± 1.7	8.4 ± 2.2^{a}	9.3 ± 1.9^{a}
Girls			
Oxygen uptake (L/min)	1.85 ± 0.28	1.90 ± 0.26	1.91 ± 0.35
Oxygen uptake (mL/kg per min)	51 ± 6	52 ± 7	52 ± 7
Minute ventilation (L/min)	60.7 ± 7.1	66.2 ± 6.7^{a}	65.6 ± 11.2^{a}
Respiratory exchange ratio	1.00 ± 0.04	1.13 ± 0.06^{a}	1.13 ± 0.06^{a}
Blood lactate (mmol/L)	6.4 ± 1.3	8.3 ± 1.3^{a}	8.3 ± 2.1^{a}

Values are expressed as means ± standard deviation.
[a] Mean significantly different ($P < 0.05$) from test 1.

However, the major problem is the young subjects' lack of body mass. Stepping exercise is seldom terminated by cardiopulmonary insufficiency and, in our experience, peak $\dot{V}O_2$ on a step bench is 25–30% lower than that elicited during treadmill running.

Cycle ergometers often need to be modified for young children, who may find it difficult to maintain the required pedal cadence. They are, however, portable, relatively cheap, less noisy than a treadmill, and may induce less anxiety in young children. Nevertheless, treadmill running engages a larger muscle mass than cycling, and the peak $\dot{V}O_2$ obtained from the former is more likely to be limited by central rather than peripheral factors. In cycle ergometry, the effort required to pedal against a resistance may be high in relation to muscle strength, resulting in increased anaerobic metabolism as blood flow through the quadriceps is limited. Intramuscular lactate will accumulate and induce the subject to terminate the exercise before the limits of the cardiorespiratory system are reached. The treadmill is therefore the ergometer of choice in paediatric exercise physiology, and young people's peak $\dot{V}O_2$ is generally 8–10% higher than on a cycle ergometer, although correlations of about 0.9 have been reported between treadmill and cycle ergometer peak $\dot{V}O_2$ (Armstrong & Davies 1981).

In clinical settings, standardized exercise protocols (e.g. Balke, Bruce, James protocols) are common. In research laboratories, protocols tend to be developed according to the aims of the investigation. Although running protocols elicit higher peak $\dot{V}O_2$ than walking protocols, it appears to make little difference to the outcome whether a continuous or discontinuous protocol is adopted. We prefer discontinuous protocols, which accommodate the shorter attention span of many children and facilitate the collection of blood lactate between stages.

Peak $\dot{V}O_2$ and age

Peak $\dot{V}O_2$ in relation to chronological age has been well documented, at least from the age of 10 years, and Figure 5.1, drawn from published data representing 4000 peak $\dot{V}O_2$ determinations (Armstrong & Welsman 1994), illustrates a progressive, linear increase in peak $\dot{V}O_2$ with age in both boys and girls. Boys' peak $\dot{V}O_2$ is significantly higher than girls' peak $\dot{V}O_2$ throughout the teen years with the difference increasing to about 37% by the age of 16 years. Even in the prepubertal years, sex differences in absolute peak $\dot{V}O_2$ are apparent (Armstrong et al 1995). We measured peak $\dot{V}O_2$ in children aged 10 and 11 with Tanner (1962) stage one for both pubic hair and either breast or genital development. We reported boys' peak $\dot{V}O_2$ to be 18% higher than girls' peak $\dot{V}O_2$.

Cardiac output and arteriovenous oxygen difference are the determinants of peak $\dot{V}O_2$. Data describing maximal cardiac output are sparse due to the severe methodological limitations which surround its accurate determination, but age-related increases of 12.5–21.1 L/min in boys and 10.5–15.5 L/min in girls have been demonstrated over the age range 9–20 years (Miyamura & Honda 1973, Yamaji & Miyashita 1977). In contrast, heart rate at peak $\dot{V}O_2$ is independent of both age and sex (Armstrong & Welsman 2000b), suggesting that the increase in cardiac output at peak exercise is due solely to increases in stroke volume (Rowland 2000).

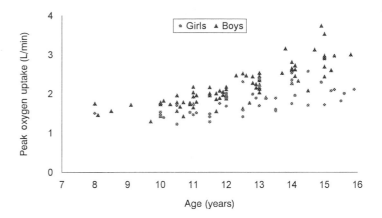

Figure 5.1 The relationship between peak $\dot{V}O_2$ and chronological age. (After Armstrong & Welsman 1994.)

Data describing changes in arteriovenous oxygen difference at peak $\dot{V}O_2$ are similarly sparse and, moreover, equivocal. Some authors have noted age-related increases in peak arteriovenous oxygen difference (Miyamura & Honda 1973, Rowland et al 1997), but others have not observed such a relationship (Yamaji & Miyashita 1977).

Peak $\dot{V}O_2$ and body size

Much of the increase in peak $\dot{V}O_2$ observed over the age range illustrated in Figure 5.1 may be accounted for by the general increase in body size which occurs over this period. Both stature and mass are highly correlated with peak $\dot{V}O_2$ in children and adolescents with coefficients typically in the range 0.6–0.8 (Armstrong et al 1991, 1995, 1998). As the correlation is normally stronger with mass than stature, and as physical activity most often requires the body mass to be moved, it is conventional to accommodate size differences by expressing peak $\dot{V}O_2$ in ratio with body mass, i.e. mL/kg per min. This, it is assumed, enables fair comparison between individuals and/or groups differing in body mass, e.g. children vs. adults, boys vs. girls etc.

When the data presented in Figure 5.1 are expressed relative to body mass, the pattern of change between the ages of 10 and 16 years in peak $\dot{V}O_2$ is markedly altered, and differences between the sexes are accentuated. In boys, mass-related peak $\dot{V}O_2$ remains virtually unchanged, with a mean value of approximately 50 mL/kg per min, whereas over the same period, girls' peak $\dot{V}O_2$ declines steadily from around 48 to 38 mL/kg per min (Armstrong & Welsman 1994). This decline in girls' mass-related peak $\dot{V}O_2$ is usually attributed to their increased levels of body fat during ado-

lescence which contrasts with the development in boys of relatively more muscle mass.

However, a series of studies from our laboratory has indicated that the expression of peak $\dot{V}O_2$ as a simple 'per-body-mass' ratio has clouded our understanding of the growth and maturation of peak $\dot{V}O_2$ relative to changes in body size. The aim of scaling is to produce a size-corrected variable which is truly independent of size, thus enabling valid comparisons between individuals of different size. This may be checked by correlating the derived variable (e.g. mL/kg per min) with the original size variable (i.e. mass), and the coefficient should be not significantly different from zero. In many cases, per-body-mass ratios for peak $\dot{V}O_2$ remain significantly negatively correlated with body mass, confirming that the mass-related variable is not, in fact, independent of mass (Welsman & Armstrong 2000a,b).

Allometric methods of normalizing for body size differences have been shown to be more appropriate for the interpretation of size-related changes in peak $\dot{V}O_2$ during the transition from childhood to adolescence (Welsman & Armstrong 2000a,b). Welsman et al (1996) examined age and sex differences in peak $\dot{V}O_2$ in prepubertal, circumpubertal and adult males and females using a log-linear (allometric) scaling model to remove the influence of body size. Briefly, this analysis involves the statistical comparison of the slopes and intercepts of the linear regression lines which describe the relationship between log-transformed body mass and peak $\dot{V}O_2$ data for the individual age and sex groups. Where the slopes of the log-linear regression lines are demonstrated to be parallel, differences in the intercept values reflect differences in magnitude between the groups under investigation. The results of this analysis demonstrated significant increases in peak $\dot{V}O_2$ throughout adolescence into adulthood in boys, and a significant increase in peak $\dot{V}O_2$ between prepuberty and circumpuberty in girls, with no evidence of subsequent decline in aerobic fitness into adulthood. In both sexes, these results differed notably from the conventional interpretation of age-related change in mass-related peak $\dot{V}O_2$ described above, although sex differences in peak $\dot{V}O_2$ remained in all age groups. Interestingly, when peak $\dot{V}O_2$ data from prepubertal children are scaled appropriately for body mass, boys retain a significantly higher peak $\dot{V}O_2$ than girls, with the discrepancy increasing from 13.3 to 16.2% (Armstrong et al 1995).

Until recently, the application of allometric modelling to longitudinal data has been problematic, but the emergence of multilevel modelling techniques (Goldstein 1995) has yielded some interesting insights into age- and sex-associated changes in size-related peak $\dot{V}O_2$. Multilevel modelling is best described as an extension of multiple regression which is suitable for nested or hierarchical data sets, i.e. where data can be seen to exist at different levels. Longitudinal data are one such example, as the repeated measurement occasions (the level 1 units) are nested within the individual, who represents the level 2 unit.

We applied multilevel modelling to the interpretation of 590 peak $\dot{V}O_2$ determinations in 11- to 13-year-old boys and girls obtained over three annual measurement occasions. A multiplicative, allometric model was applied as follows (Nevill et al 1998):

$$y = \text{mass}^{k_1} \times \text{stature}^{k_2} \times \exp(\alpha_j + b_j \times \text{age})\, \varepsilon_{ij}$$

The model was linearized by logarithmic transformation with multilevel regression analysis on $\log_e y$ used to solve for the unknown parameters:

$$\log_e y = k_1 \times \log_e \text{mass} + k_2 \times \log_e \text{stature} + \alpha_j + b_j \times \text{age} + \log_e(\varepsilon_{ij})$$

Multilevel modelling differs from traditional techniques in that, as well as describing underlying population trends (the fixed part of the analysis), random variation around the mean response is recognized and can be modelled at both levels of the analysis. Therefore, in the equation above, all parameters were fixed except for the intercept (α) and age terms, which were allowed to vary at level 2 (between individuals – denoted by the subscript j), and the error term (ε) which also varied at level 1 – denoted by the subscript i.

From this baseline model, additional effects were investigated, including sex and any age by sex inter-

action. The results of this model are presented in Table 5.2. Both mass and stature were significant, independent covariates yielding allometric exponents of 0.50 and 0.95, respectively. Peak $\dot{V}O_2$ was significantly higher in the boys than in the girls (the value of –0.14 would be deducted from the predicted $\dot{V}O_2$ for girls only), but increased significantly with age over and above any increases attributable to the growth in body size, although this age effect was greater for boys than for girls as shown by the negative age by sex interaction term. Thus, these results confirm the indications from the cross-sectional study described above (Welsman et al 1996) in contradicting conventional interpretation of the growth of peak $\dot{V}O_2$.

Table 5.2 Multilevel regression analysis for peak $\dot{V}O_2$ in 11- to 13-year-olds ($n = 590$) – model I. (After Armstrong et al 1999.)

	Estimate (SE)
Fixed parameters	
Constant	−1.3903 (0.0970)
$\log_e$ mass	0.5011 (0.0322)
$\log_e$ stature	0.9479 (0.1162)
Age	0.0585 (0.0111)
Sex	−0.1378 (0.0093)
Age × sex	−0.0134 (0.0068)
Random parameters	
Level 2	
Constant	0.0042 (0.0005)
Age	0.0007 (0.0003)
Covariance	Not significant
Level 1	
Constant	0.0030 (0.0004)

Age centred on group mean of 12.0 years.

Peak $\dot{V}O_2$ and maturity

The physiological responses of young people need to be interpreted in relation to maturation as well as age and body size. Few studies have examined the relationship between peak $\dot{V}O_2$ and maturation, but the available data indicate that, although the evidence is stronger in boys, the peak $\dot{V}O_2$ (in L/min) of both sexes increases with advancing maturity (Armstrong & Welsman 1997). However, when peak $\dot{V}O_2$ is expressed in ratio with body mass (i.e. in mL/kg per min), it remains unchanged with maturation in both sexes (Armstrong et al 1991). Until recently, no study had controlled for body mass using allometry and examined the relationship between peak $\dot{V}O_2$ and maturation.

Armstrong et al (1998) determined the peak $\dot{V}O_2$ of 93 boys and 83 girls, aged 12 years and classified according to Tanner's indices for pubic hair (Tanner 1962) to examine sex and maturational differences in peak $\dot{V}O_2$ expressed relative to body mass (i.e. mL/kg per min) and adjusted for mass using analysis of covariance (ANCOVA) on log-transformed data. Significant main effects for sex (P <0.01) but not for maturity (P >0.05) were demonstrated for peak $\dot{V}O_2$ in ratio with body mass. In contrast, the allometric analysis revealed significant main effects for both sex and maturity for peak $\dot{V}O_2$ adjusted appropriately for mass (P <0.01). A mass exponent of 0.65, common to both sexes, was identified, confirming the inability of the per-body-mass ratio to control for differences in body mass. Therefore, this study demonstrated that, although the conventional analysis, i.e. peak $\dot{V}O_2$ in ratio with body mass, indicated no main effect of maturity, a more appropriate method of controlling for body mass identified an increase in peak $\dot{V}O_2$ with maturation that was independent of increases attributable to any growth in body mass.

Armstrong et al (1999) added stage of maturity to the multilevel model previously presented (Table 5.2), and the results are presented in Table 5.3. Interaction terms 'maturity stage by sex' were also constructed to investigate any differential effects of maturity between the sexes. As demonstrated in Table 5.3, peak $\dot{V}O_2$ increased incrementally with advancing maturation – the positive parameter estimates ranging from 0.04 for stage 1 to 0.09 for stage 5 – with these effects over and above those already accounted for by changes in body size and chronological age. No maturity by sex interactions were significant, confirming that peak $\dot{V}O_2$ increases with maturation in both boys and girls similarly.

As previously mentioned, adolescence is characterized not only by changes in overall body size but also, more importantly, by changes in body composition. To ignore these changes in the interpretation of peak $\dot{V}O_2$ is likely to further confound the interpretation of differential patterns of growth in boys and girls. Armstrong et al (1999) added sum of triceps and subscapular skinfold thicknesses as an explanatory variable to the multilevel regression model previously described and the results are presented in Table 5.4. The incorporation of a measure of body fatness into the model had several interesting effects. Notably, the stature and age^2 terms became non-significant, and the value of the mass exponent almost doubled. The magnitude of the sex effect was reduced but the most striking effect was in explaining much of the previously observed maturity effects with estimates for stages 3 to 5 almost halved.

Table 5.3 Multilevel regression analysis for peak $\dot{V}O_2$ in 11- to 13-year-olds (n = 590) – model II. (After Armstrong et al 1999.)

	Estimate (SE)
Fixed parameters	
Constant	−1.2526 (0.0978)
$\log_e$ mass	0.4765 (0.0320)
$\log_e$ stature	0.8105 (0.1172)
Age	0.0428 (0.0116)
Age^2	−0.0073 (0.0035)
Sex	−0.1495 (0.0094)
Age × sex	−0.0177 (0.0068)
Maturity 2	0.0382 (0.0090)
Maturity 3	0.0548 (0.0106)
Maturity 4	0.0902 (0.0140)
Maturity 5	0.0892 (0.0221)
Random parameters	
Level 2	
Constant	0.0042 (0.0005)
Age	0.0008 (0.0003)
Covariance	0.0004 (0.0003)
Level 1	
Constant	0.0024 (0.0003)
Age	0.0004 (0.0005)
Covariance	−0.0006 (0.0002)

Age centred on group mean of 12.0 years.

Table 5.4 Multilevel regression analysis for peak $\dot{V}O_2$ in 11- to 13-year-olds (n = 590) – model III. (After Armstrong et al 1999.)

	Estimate (SE)
Fixed parameters	
Constant	−1.8735 (0.0945)
$\log_e$ mass	0.8629 (0.0317)
$\log_e$ stature	Not significant
$\log_e$ skinfolds	−0.1704 (0.0134)
Age	0.0450 (0.0108)
Sex	−0.1340 (0.0084)
Age × sex	−0.0177 (0.0065)
Maturity 2	0.0301 (0.0086)
Maturity 3	0.0372 (0.0105)
Maturity 4	0.0571 (0.0138)
Maturity 5	0.0435 (0.0212)
Random parameters	
Level 2	
Constant	0.0029 (0.0004)
Age	0.0006 (0.0003)
Covariance	0.0003 (0.0002)
Level 1	
Constant	0.0025 (0.0003)
Age	0.0004 (0.0005)
Covariance	−0.0007 (0.0002)

Age centred on group mean of 12.0 years.

Thus, the multilevel regression model of a large, representative longitudinal data set has indicated that changes in fat-free mass relative to total body mass account for much of the increase in peak $\dot{V}O_2$ between the ages of 11 and 13 years, but age and increasing maturity are independently associated with additional increases in aerobic fitness. These effects have been masked in previous studies by the reliance upon simple per-body-mass ratios to account for size difference and/or the failure to investigate the effects of covariates other than body mass.

Peak $\dot{V}O_2$ and sex

The previous research studies presented are consistent in revealing sex differences in peak $\dot{V}O_2$ which remain even when differences in body size and fatness are accounted for using appropriate statistical techniques. As previously mentioned, these differences are apparent even in the prepubertal years, broadening with increasing age and maturity. Secure explanations for the difference in cardiorespiratory fitness prior to puberty remain elusive, but factors such as haemoglobin concentration and body composition can be largely ruled out (Armstrong et al 1995) as sex differences do not emerge until later in puberty.

Similarly, the suggestion that girls' lower levels of physical activity are a causative factor in their lower peak $\dot{V}O_2$ has been refuted. Several studies have demonstrated that few children experience the intensity, frequency and duration of physical activity likely to be associated with increased levels of peak $\dot{V}O_2$ (Armstrong 1998, Armstrong & Welsman 1997).

When the components of $\dot{V}O_2$ are examined, no sex differences in heart rate or arteriovenous oxygen difference are evident in prepubertal children, but growing evidence indicates that boys have greater stroke volumes than girls. Obtaining measures of stroke volume at maximal exercise is notoriously difficult, but studies using carbon dioxide rebreathing (Miyamura & Honda 1973) and Doppler echocardiography (Rowland 2000) have observed higher values in boys than in girls within the age range 9–12 years. Data from submaximal exercise are more secure, and as stroke volume plateaus at around 60% of peak $\dot{V}O_2$, Rowland et al (1999) have suggested that maximal values can be predicted from submaximal data. Again, data from submaximal studies have tended to confirm that boys have greater stroke volume than girls at the same $\dot{V}O_2$ or exercise intensity (Godfrey et al 1971, Potter et al 1997). However, as stroke volume is a function of the complex interplay between ventricular preload, myocardial contractility and ventricular afterload, it would be premature to infer that girls simply have smaller hearts, and further research is required to confirm the mechanisms which contribute to girls' lower stroke volume and peak $\dot{V}O_2$.

In the pubertal years, changes in body composition are likely increasingly to contribute to sex differences in peak $\dot{V}O_2$ as boys' accelerated growth in muscle mass relative to total body mass contrasts with girls' accumulation of body fat. Indeed, the results presented in Tables 5.3 and 5.4 demonstrate this effect quite clearly, as the introduction of sum of skinfolds into the multilevel regression models explained a significant proportion of the sex and maturity effects observed prior to the inclusion of a measure of body fatness (compare Tables 5.3 and 5.4).

During adolescence, boys also experience a marked increase in haemoglobin levels which might be expected to augment peak $\dot{V}O_2$ and further accentuate the sex difference. Haemoglobin was entered into the multilevel model presented in Table 5.4 (Armstrong et al 1999), but a non-significant parameter estimate was obtained. However, as the largest sex differences in haemoglobin are not apparent until the mid- to late teens, it may be that the children in this study were just too young for a clear contribution from haemoglobin to be observed. It is therefore likely that, during the pubertal years, differences in stroke volume, fat-free mass and haemoglobin progressively contribute to the increasing sex difference in peak $\dot{V}O_2$ (Armstrong & Welsman 2000a,b).

The intriguing sex difference in cardiorespiratory fitness prior to puberty and the mechanisms behind the age and maturational influences on cardiorespiratory fitness recently confirmed invite further investigation and represent a fruitful avenue for future research.

PHYSICAL ACTIVITY
Assessment of physical activity

The accurate assessment of young people's habitual physical activity is extremely difficult. To obtain a true picture of physical activity patterns, the intensity, duration and frequency of activities should be monitored and, to take account of day-to-day variation, a minimum monitoring period of 3 days is required. Any equipment used must be acceptable to young people and it should not unduly influence their normal physical activity. Many methods of assessment have been proposed, but they can be grouped into four categories: self- or proxy report, observation, motion sensor monitoring and physiological analyses (including the use of doubly labelled water and heart rate monitoring).

Self-report is problematic because of the demands placed on young people's ability to recall specific events. Observation is acceptable for short periods, but it may cause subjects to alter their normal activity patterns (high subject reactivity) and it is not a feasible method of assessing habitual physical activity. Doubly labelled water provides an accurate measure of energy expenditure over several days, but it provides no information on physical activity patterns. Both heart rate and motion sensor monitoring have low levels of subject reactivity. Heart rate monitoring can provide an indication of the intensity, frequency and duration of physical activity, but it may be influenced by factors independent of exercise. Most motion sensors do not discriminate physical activity patterns, and their output in 'activity counts' is difficult to interpret. No single technique offers all the information necessary to provide a detailed picture of physical activity, and ideally a combination of methods should be used (Armstrong & Welsman 1997). However, the adoption of method(s) of assessing young people's physical activity is likely to continue to be dictated by the logistic and financial considerations of the research team.

Two recent reviews have analysed methods of assessing young people's physical activity (Armstrong & Welsman 1997, Armstrong & Van Mechelen 1998). Our own research has focused on the continuous monitoring of children's and adolescents' heart rate over several days (Armstrong 1998).

Heart rate monitoring offers an attractive, objective method of estimating physical activity in real-life situations, but the interpretation of heart rate in the context of physical activity is complex. Heart rate is not a direct measure of physical activity but a measure of the relative stress being placed on the cardiorespiratory system by the activity. Heart rate reflects not only the metabolism and posture of the subject, but also the transient emotional state, the prevailing climatic conditions, and the specific muscle groups which perform the activity. The relationship between heart rate and physical activity is therefore more secure at moderate to vigorous levels of physical activity than during low levels of physical activity. Nevertheless, a number of self-contained, computerized telemetry systems have been developed for the unobtrusive measurement of heart rate over several days. They are socially acceptable, permit freedom of movement, are not immediately noticeable, and therefore do not unduly influence children's normal physical activity patterns. The Polar Vantage NV is the instrument of choice and its use has been extensively tested and found to be reliable and valid in young people (Armstrong 1998, Armstrong & Welsman 1997).

Physical activity patterns assessed by heart rate monitoring

In a series of studies we have monitored the heart rates of over 1000 young people, aged 5–16 years, over three normal weekdays (Armstrong 1998). In this section, we will use these data to evaluate children's and adolescents' physical activity patterns in relation to established guidelines.

The NIH Consensus Development Panel on Physical Activity and Cardiovascular Health (1996, p. 243) recommended that:

all children and adults should set a long-term goal to accumulate at least 30 minutes or more of moderate-intensity physical activity on most, or preferably all, days of the week.

An earlier International Consensus Conference on Physical Activity Guidelines for Adolescents (Sallis & Patrick 1994) recommended that, in addition to participation in moderate physical activity for 30 min or more, on most days (p. 308):

adolescents should engage in three or more sessions per week of activities that last 20 minutes or more at a time and that require moderate to vigorous levels of exertion.

Moderate to vigorous activities were defined as those that require at least as much effort as brisk or fast walking (Sallis & Patrick 1994). To interpret our data in this context, we invited 10% of subjects to visit the centre to walk and run at various speeds on a horizontal treadmill. We noted that, regardless of age, brisk walking and jogging elicited steady-state heart rates of about 140 and 160 beats/min (bpm), respectively. We therefore defined moderate physical activity (equivalent to brisk walking) as generating a heart rate >139 bpm, and vigorous physical activity (equivalent to jogging) as generating a heart rate >159 bpm.

Twenty-minute periods of either moderate or vigorous physical activity were sparse in all age groups, illustrating that sustained periods of physical activity do not characterize young people's physical activity patterns: 84% of girls and 77% of boys did not experience a single sustained 20 min period of vigorous activity. Less than 3% of the boys and none of the girls

Table 5.5 Three-day heart rate monitoring studies of physical activity

Citation	Subject	Outcome
Armstrong et al (1990a)	163 girls, 103 boys, age 11–16 years	77% of boys and 88% of girls did not sustain a single 20 min period with HR >159 bpm 36% of boys and 52% of girls did not sustain a single 10 min period with HR >139 bpm 70% of boys and 53% of girls experienced the equivalent of a daily 5 min period with HR >139 bpm
Armstrong & Bray (1991)	65 girls, 67 boys, age 10.7 years	78% of boys and 78% of girls did not sustain a single 20 min period with HR >159 bpm 19% of boys and 25% of girls did not sustain a single 10 min period with HR >139 bpm 90% of boys and 85% of girls experienced the equivalent of daily 5 min period with HR >139 bpm
McManus & Armstrong (1995)	100 girls, 100 boys, age 11.1 years	75% of boys and 88% of girls did not sustain a single 20 min period with HR >159 bpm 22% of boys and 30% of girls did not sustain a single 10 min period with HR >139 bpm 89% of boys and 78% of girls experienced the equivalent of a daily 5 min period with HR >139 bpm
Welsman & Armstrong (1997)	31 girls, 26 boys, age 6–9 years	None of the children sustained a 20 min period with HR >159 bpm 23% of boys and 31% of girls did not sustain a single 10 min period with HR >139 bpm 89% of boys and 83% of girls experienced the equivalent of a daily 5 min period with HR >139 bpm

HR, heart rate.

experienced a daily 20 min period of vigorous activity. Ten-minute periods of moderate physical activity were more common, but over 50% of teenage girls and almost 40% of teenage boys did not experience a single 10 min period of moderate physical activity over 3 days of monitoring. Five-minute periods of moderate physical activity are more typical of the physical activity patterns of most children, but 5% of teenage boys and 14% of teenage girls did not exhibit a single 5 min period of moderate physical activity. Table 5.5 summarizes data from a selection of studies.

When the data were analysed in relation to the recommendation of the NIH Panel (1996), boys were noted to accumulate significantly more time per day with their heart rate >139 bpm than girls, at all ages studied. Figure 5.2 illustrates the percentage of young people who accumulated at least 30 min of moderate activity per day. Although the figure must be interpreted with caution (Armstrong 1998), it clearly illustrates the steady decline with age in the percentage of young people who achieve this target, with boys outscoring girls at all ages.

Data describing longitudinal changes in young people's physical activity using objective measures are sparse, but Armstrong et al (2000) collected 3-day heart rate data annually from a large, representative sample of 11- to 13-year-olds. The data were analysed using multilevel regression modelling, and the results for the percentage of time spent above moderate (>139 bpm) and vigorous (>159 bpm) activity thresholds are presented in Table 5.6. Broadly speaking, these longitudinal data supported the findings of cross-sectional studies in demonstrating for both activity thresholds a significant decline in physical activity with increasing age. Sex differences were also evident, with boys significantly and consistently more active than girls. The inclusion of Tanner stage of maturity into the model yielded some intriguing findings, with an additional significant decline in physical activity associated with later maturation. Interestingly, the rate of this decline was greater in the boys than in the girls, as indicated by the maturity 4 by sex interaction term. This would be added to the maturity 4 term for the girls only, thus reducing the magnitude of the maturity 4 effect for them from −2.530 to −1.317 and from −4.423 to −2.431 for % of time >159 bpm and 139 bpm respectively.

Whether young people are classified as active or inactive depends upon the criteria applied. Most children and a significant number of adolescents satisfy the recommendation of accumulating 30 min of daily moderate-intensity activity, but health benefits accruing from very short bursts of activity remain to be

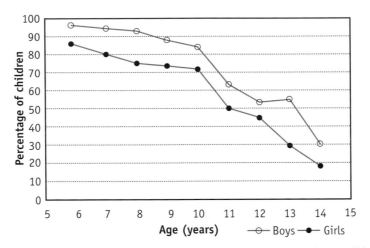

Figure 5.2 Percentage of children accumulating a daily 30 min with heart rate ≥140 bpm, by age. (After Armstrong 1998.)

Table 5.6 Multilevel regression analyses for percentage of time >139 bpm and >159 bpm in 11- to 13-year-olds (n = 505). (After Armstrong et al 2000.)

	Estimate (SE)
% time >139 bpm	
Fixed parameters	
Constant	10.069 (0.612)
Age	−1.370 (0.196)
Sex	−1.919 (0.394)
Maturity 4	−4.423 (1.501)
Maturity 4 by sex	1.992 (0.877)
Random parameters	
Level 2	
Constant	3.160 (0.877)
Level 1	
Constant	10.372 (0.913)
% time >159 bpm	
Fixed parameters	
Constant	5.119 (0.372)
Age	−0.729 (0.123)
Sex	−1.336 (0.240)
Maturity 4	−2.530 (0.937)
Maturity 4 by sex	1.213 (0.548)
Random parameters	
Level 2	
Constant	0.973 (0.328)
Level 1	
Constant	4.194 (0.367)

Age centred on group mean of 11.8 years.

elucidated. Few young people regularly experience 10 min or longer periods of moderate to vigorous physical activity. Boys are more active than girls from an early age and, although both sexes reduce their physi-

cal activity as they move from childhood through adolescence and into adult life, the rate of decline is greater in girls.

PHYSICAL ACTIVITY AND CARDIORESPIRATORY FITNESS

The effect of exercise training on young people's cardiorespiratory fitness has been investigated on numerous occasions, but few studies have reported the responses of children and adolescents to carefully controlled and well-defined programmes. Studies with girls are sparse. The optimum exercise prescription for young people is yet to be designed, and reliable dose–response data are not available. Nevertheless, exercise programmes of three to four sessions per week with an intensity of at least 80% of maximal heart rate and a duration of 8–12 weeks induce increases in young people's peak $\dot{V}O_2$. The size of the increase, however, is generally smaller than that which would be expected with adult subjects, although the existence of a critical period during growth and maturation for enhanced responses to exercise training remains to be proven (Armstrong & Welsman 1997).

Morrow & Freedson (1994) reviewed 17 studies which had investigated the relationship between habitual physical activity and cardiorespiratory fitness, and concluded that the majority of studies suggested no relationship, with a median correlation of $r = 0.17$. Only two substantial studies appear to have monitored physical activity for at least 3 days and related it to directly determined peak $\dot{V}O_2$ (Armstrong et al 1990b, 1996a). In an analysis of 154 boys and 171 girls, aged 11–16 years, no significant relationships between peak $\dot{V}O_2$ and heart rate estimates of physical activity were detected. In a similar study in 73 13-year-old children, Welsman & Armstrong (1992) reported no relationship between heart rate indicators of physical activity and submaximal measures of cardiorespiratory fitness. Armstrong et al (2000) entered peak $\dot{V}O_2$ as an explanatory variable into the multilevel regression model for their longitudinal activity data presented in Table 5.6 and discussed above. Again, a non-significant parameter estimate was obtained, confirming that the decline in physical activity observed in the 11- to 13-year-olds studied was unrelated to their cardiorespiratory fitness.

Intuitively, it may be expected that the most active youngsters should be the fittest or that high levels of cardiorespiratory fitness may encourage physical activity, but available data suggest that any relationship between habitual physical activity and peak $\dot{V}O_2$ is tenuous. The issue may be clouded by the methodological problems associated with the assessment of both physical activity and peak $\dot{V}O_2$. However, the simple explanation for the lack of relationship between habitual physical activity and peak $\dot{V}O_2$ is that few children and adolescents experience physical activity of the intensity, frequency and duration which has been shown to be necessary to increase peak $\dot{V}O_2$.

CONCLUSIONS

A $\dot{V}O_2$ plateau is not a requirement for defining a maximal assessment of young people's cardiorespiratory fitness, but if a $\dot{V}O_2$ plateau is not exhibited, the appropriate term to use is peak $\dot{V}O_2$ rather than the traditional $\dot{V}O_{2\,max}$. Peak $\dot{V}O_2$ increases with age in both boys and girls, both in absolute terms and with body size and composition accounted for, but boys' values are higher than those of girls even during the prepubertal years. Sex differences in peak $\dot{V}O_2$ increase as young people move through adolescence. The process of maturation exerts a significant influence on peak $\dot{V}O_2$ independent of body mass.

The assessment of children's and adolescents' habitual physical activity is complex, but data are consistent and indicate that sustained periods of moderate to vigorous physical activity are not typical of young people's physical activity patterns. Boys are more active than girls from an early age and, although both sexes reduce their physical activity as they get older, the rate of decline in physical activity during the teen years is more marked in girls.

Any significant relationship between young people's habitual physical activity and their peak $\dot{V}O_2$ remains to be proven, but the tenuous association may be explained by the fact that the majority of children and adolescents seldom experience physical activity of the intensity required to improve peak $\dot{V}O_2$.

REFERENCES

Armstrong N 1998 Young people's physical activity patterns as assessed by heart rate monitoring. Journal of Sports Science 16: S9–16

Armstrong N, Bray S 1991 Physical activity patterns defined by continuous heart rate monitoring. Archives of Disease in Childhood 66: 245–247

Armstrong N, Davies B 1981 An ergometric analysis of age group swimmers. British Journal of Sports Medicine 15: 20–26

Armstrong N, Van Mechelen W 1998 Are young people fit and active? In: Biddle S, Sallis J, Cavill N (eds) Young and active. Health Education Authority, London, p 69–97

Armstrong N, Welsman J 1994 Assessment and interpretation of aerobic fitness in children and adolescents. Exercise and Sport Sciences Reviews 22: 435–476

Armstrong N, Welsman J 1995 Laboratory testing of young athletes. In: Maffuli N (ed) A colour atlas of sports medicine in childhood and adolescence. Wolfe Medical, London p 112–125

Armstrong N, Welsman J R 1997 Young people and physical activity. Oxford University Press, Oxford

Armstrong N, Welsman J R 2000a Aerobic fitness. In: Armstrong N, Van Mechelen W (eds) Paediatric exercise science and medicine. Oxford University Press, Oxford, p 65–76

Armstrong N, Welsman J R 2000b Development of aerobic fitness during childhood and adolescence. Pediatric Exercise Science 12: 128–149

Armstrong N, Balding J, Gentle P, Kirby B 1990a Patterns of physical activity among 11 to 16 year old British children. British Medical Journal 301: 203–205

Armstrong N, Balding J, Gentle P, Williams J, Kirby B 1990b Peak oxygen uptake and physical activity in 11 to 16 year olds. Pediatric Exercise Science 2: 349–358

Armstrong N, Williams J, Balding J, Gentle P, Kirby B 1991 Peak oxygen uptake of British children with reference to chronological age, sex and sexual maturity. European Journal of Applied Physiology 62: 369–375

Armstrong N, Kirby B J, McManus A M, Welsman J R 1995 Aerobic fitness of pre-pubescent children. Annals of Human Biology 22: 427–441

Armstrong N, McManus A, Welsman J, Kirby B 1996a Physical activity patterns and aerobic fitness among pre-pubescents. European Physical Education Review 2: 7–18

Armstrong N, Welsman J, Winsley R 1996b Is peak $\dot{V}O_2$ a maximal index of children's aerobic fitness? International Journal of Sports Medicine 17: 356–359

Armstrong N, Welsman J R, Kirby B J 1998 Peak oxygen uptake and maturation in 12-year-olds. Medicine and Science in Sports and Exercise 30: 165–169

Armstrong N, Welsman J R, Nevill A M, Kirby B J 1999 Modeling growth and maturation changes in peak oxygen uptake in 11–13-year olds. Journal of Applied Physiology 87: 2230–2236

Armstrong N, Welsman J R, Kirby B J 2000 Longitudinal changes in 11–13-year-olds' physical activity. Acta Paediatrica, 89: 775–780

Godfrey S, Davies C T M, Wozniak E, Barnes C A 1971 Cardiorespiratory response to exercise in normal children. Clinical Science 40: 419–431

Goldstein H 1995 Multilevel statistical models. Arnold, London

McManus A, Armstrong N 1995 Patterns of physical activity among primary schoolchildren. In: Ring F J (ed) Children in sport. University Press, Bath, p 17–23

Miyamura M, Honda Y 1973 Maximum cardiac output related to sex and age. Japanese Journal of Physiology 23: 645–656

Morrow J R, Freedson P S 1994 Relationship between habitual physical activity and aerobic fitness in adolescents. Pediatric Exercise Science 6: 315–329

Nevil A M, Holder R L, Baxter-Jones A, Round J M, Jones D A 1998 Modeling developmental changes in strength and aerobic power in children. Journal of Applied Physiology 84: 963–970

NIH Consensus Development Panel on Physical Activity and Cardiovascular Health 1996 Physical activity and cardiovascular health. Journal of the American Medical Association 276: 241–246

Potter C R, Armstrong N, Kirby B J, Welsman J R 1997 An exploratory study of cardiac output responses to submaximal exercise. In: Armstrong N, Kirby B J, Welsman J R (eds) Children and exercise XIX: promoting health and well-being. E and FN Spon, London, p 440–445

Rowland T W 2000 Cardiovascular function. In: Armstrong N, Van Mechelen W (eds) Paediatric exercise science and medicine. Oxford University Press, Oxford, p 153–161

Rowland T W, Poposki B, Ferrone L 1997 Cardiac responses to maximal upright cycle exercise in healthy boys and men. Medicine and Science in Sports and Exercise 29: 1146–1151

Rowland T, Goff L, Martal L, Ferrone L 1999 Estimation of maximal stroke volume from submaximal values. Pediatric Exercise Science 11: 279

Sallis J F, Patrick K 1994 Physical activity guidelines for adolescents: a consensus statement. Pediatric Exercise Science 6: 302–314

Tanner J M 1962 Growth at adolescence, 2nd edn. Blackwell Scientific Publications, Oxford

US Department of Health and Human Services 1996 Physical activity and health: a report of the Surgeon General US Department of Health and Human Services. Centres for Disease Control and Prevention, National Centre for Chronic Disease Prevention and Health Promotion, Atlanta, GA

Welsman J, Armstrong N 1992 Daily physical activity and blood lactate indices of aerobic fitness. British Journal of Sports Medicine 26: 228–232

Welsman J R, Armstrong N 1997 Physical activity patterns of 5 to 11-year-old children. In: Armstrong N, Kirby B J, Welsman J R (eds) Children and exercise XIX: promoting health and well-being. E and FN Spon, London, p 139–144

Welsman J, Armstrong N 1998 Assessing post-exercise lactates in children and adolescents. In: Van Praagh E (ed) Pediatric anaerobic performance. Human Kinetics, Champaign, IL, p 137–154

Welsman J R, Armstrong N 2000a Interpreting exercise performance data in relation to body size. In: Armstrong N, Van Mechelen W (eds) Paediatric exercise science and medicine. Oxford University Press, Oxford, p 3–9

Welsman J R, Armstrong N 2000b Statistical techniques for interpreting body size-related exercise performance during growth. Pediatric Exercise Science 12: 112–127

Welsman J R, Armstrong N, Kirby B J, Nevill A M, Winter E 1996 Scaling peak oxygen uptake for differences in body size. Medicine and Science in Sports and Exercise 28: 259–265

Williams J, Armstrong N, Kirby B 1990 The 4 mmol.l^{-1} blood lactate level as an index of exercise performance in 11–13 year old children. Journal of Sports Sciences 8: 139–147

Williams J, Armstrong N, Kirby B 1992 The influence of site of sampling and assay medium upon the measurement and interpretation of blood lactate responses to exercise. Journal of Sports Science 10: 95–107

Yamaji K, Miyashita M 1997 Oxygen transport system during exhaustive exercise in Japanese boys. European Journal of Applied Physiology 36: 93–99

FURTHER READING

Armstrong N, Kirby B J, Welsman J R (eds) 1997 Children and exercise XIX: promoting health and well-being. E and FN Spon, London

Armstrong N, Van Mechelen W (eds) 2000 Paediatric exercise science and medicine. Oxford University Press, Oxford

Blimkie C J R, Bar-Or O (eds) 1995 New horizons in pediatric exercise science. Human Kinetics, Champaign, IL

Chan K-M, Micheli L J (eds) 1998 Sports and children. Williams and Wilkins, Hong Kong

Froberg K, Lammert O, Hansen H St, Blimkie C J R (eds) 1997 Exercise and fitness – children and exercise XVIII. University Press, Odense

Rowland T W 1996 Developmental exercise physiology. Human Kinetics, Champaign, IL

6

Strength training in young adults

David A. Jones   Jonathan P. Folland

KEY POINTS

1. Strength training is used extensively to enhance performance in athletic events that require strength and power.
2. There is little clear evidence that strength training leads to improvements in performance in complex athletic tasks.
3. The acquisition of skills, particularly for children, may be more important than strength training.
4. Strength gains as a result of training are due to a combination of changes in neural activation, muscle architecture and hypertrophy of individual fibres.
5. Little is known about what element of physical activity initiates and stimulates gains in muscular strength and size, but high forces and total duration of training are important factors.
6. The secretion of local muscle growth factors is increasingly recognized as an important stimulus for satellite cell division, which is required for muscle fibre growth.

INTRODUCTION

Strength training can result in considerable increases in the strength and power of human muscle and is used extensively to enhance athletic and sporting performance. Whilst the rationale for this form of training in events such as weight-lifting and sprinting is evident, it is difficult to find clear evidence in the literature that strength training leads to improvements in performance in the more complex physical skills involved in many sports. This should be borne in mind when considering the relative benefits of different types of training and this is especially true with respect to children, where the acquisition of skill is of prime importance, and the value of specific strength training may be questionable.

Despite the obvious popularity of strength training and body-building, remarkably little is known about what modulates strength in either the short or long term. There are major changes in muscle strength and size during childhood and adolescence that are largely independent of physical activity (Round et al 1999), but after the growth spurt and adolescence, the only way of increasing strength and size without resort to illegal substances is through exercise and training. The principle of progressive overload was first formalized by DeLorme (1946), and since then there has been much work examining different protocols of mechanical loading as well as nutritional and pharmacological influences on muscular strength. Nevertheless, the key question of what element of physical activity initiates and stimulates gains in muscular strength and size remains an enigma.

ADAPTATIONS TO STRENGTH TRAINING

The force produced by muscle contraction is proportional to the number of cross-bridges working in parallel (see, e.g., Jones & Round 1990). This implies that strength is determined by muscle cross-sectional area. In practice this can be demonstrated for simple muscles studied *in vitro*, but for complex human muscle groups the common finding is that cross-sectional area accounts for ~50% of the interindividual variance in strength (Chapman et al 1984, Hakkinen & Keskinen 1989). Other factors that may affect the strength of muscles working *in situ* include the mechanics of the joint over which the muscle acts (McCullogh et al 1984), fibre type composition (Grindrod et al 1987), the angle of insertion of the muscle fibres into the tendon (Alexander & Vernon 1975) and the activation of agonist (Herbert & Gandevia 1996) and antagonist muscles (Carolan & Cafarelli 1992).

Since muscle cross-sectional area is the largest single factor determining strength, any increase in strength might be expected to be reflected in muscle size. However, many studies have highlighted the greater increases in strength compared with size, particularly in the early stages of resistance training (up to ~8 weeks; Jones & Rutherford 1987, Young et al 1983).

Recent work employing magnetic resonance imaging (Hakkinen et al 1998) has reduced the disparity, but it is likely that morphological adaptations and neural factors still contribute to strength gains during training.

Neurogenic adaptations

Clearly, in complex motor tasks there is considerable potential for learning and coordination as a result of training, so that performance can improve without necessarily increasing the strength of individual muscles. It is often suggested that untrained individuals may not be able to fully activate their muscles during maximum voluntary contractions (Dudley et al 1990, Westing et al 1988), possibly because some fibres are not recruited at all, or are activated at an insufficient firing frequency to elicit maximum force. This may apply particularly to large, fast motor units that have both a high threshold of recruitment and a high maximum firing frequency. However, if this were the case, there should be a population of inactive fast fibres that would be expected to undergo atrophy. Whilst type II fibre atrophy is common in various pathological conditions, it is not a feature of normal muscle, where the fast fibres tend, if anything, to be larger than slow fibres. When tested with electrical stimulation, untrained healthy subjects have been found to achieve >95% full activation of major muscle groups (Allen et al 1995, Belanger & McComas 1981, Rutherford et al 1986). However, this may not be true for some small muscles or for unusual or unaccustomed movements (Belanger & McComas 1981, Herbert & Gandevia 1996). There have been no systematic studies of activation in children, and there is very little information on young adults less than 18 years.

Human motor units have discharge rates of 20–30 Hz during sustained maximum voluntary contractions (MVCs), yet with electrical stimulation maximum tetanic force requires frequencies of at least 50 Hz, suggesting that many fast fibres are submaximally activated during a voluntary contraction. The difference between the force–frequency relationships could be accounted for by the difference between synchronous (electrical) and asynchronous (voluntary) stimulation. With high force voluntary contractions there tend to be high initial discharge rates that decline rapidly (De Luca et al 1982). The initial high frequency may help rapid tension development and also potentiate force production for the next second or so. Strength athletes may be able to produce greater motor unit synchronization as a result of training, although it is not clear how an increase in synchronization can increase strength (Jones et al 1989).

The integrated EMG activity (iEMG) of muscle has been used as a measure of neural drive and in some cases has been reported to increase significantly with strength training, particularly during the first 3–4 weeks. Hakkinen & Komi (1983) found that the changes in force followed closely the changes in iEMG over 16 weeks of training and 8 weeks of detraining. In contrast a number of studies have found no change in iEMG after training (e.g. Narici et al 1996). This discrepancy may be partly due to the considerable technical problems of making repeated quantitative EMG measurement due to changes such as decreases in subcutaneous and/or intramuscular fat.

Myogenic adaptations

Hypertrophy

Muscle growth can be achieved by an increase in the size of muscle fibres (hypertrophy) or an increase in the number of fibres (hyperplasia). Although there continúes to be controversy as to whether hyperplasia occurs in human muscle (Antonio & Gonyea 1993, MacDougall 1992), it is unlikely to make a significant contribution to training-induced strength gains. Hypertrophy of individual muscle fibres is generally regarded as the primary myogenic adaptation to strength training as evidenced by numerous longitudinal studies (Hakkinen et al 1998, MacDougall et al 1980). Of the training studies that have included muscle biopsy, most have found significant muscle fibre hypertrophy, although there is considerable variation (reviewed by Jones et al 1989, McDonagh & Davies 1984).

Measurements of whole muscle size with training have generally shown significant hypertrophy even over relatively short training periods, even if this did not fully match the increase in strength. Magnetic resonance imaging (MRI) is probably the most reliable method of assessing skeletal muscle cross-sectional area and volume, and the reports of hypertrophy are typically greater when using this method. The extent of hypertrophy can vary between the constituent parts of a trained muscle group as well as along the length of each muscle (Housh et al 1992, Narici et al 1989). This is probably because the pattern of hypertrophy depends upon the extent of loading and the individual length–tension relationships of the component muscles.

The increase in muscle fibre size with strength training has been attributed to both more and larger myofibrils (MacDougall et al 1980). For muscle hypertrophy to take place, additional contractile proteins must be manufactured and functionally integrated into the existing fibres and myofibrils, and it has been shown that a bout of resistance exercise increases the net protein accretion for at least 24 h (Chesley et al 1992, Yarasheski et al 1992). An increase in the contractile material required to produce any substantial muscle hypertrophy appears to be largely dependent upon an increase in the DNA content of the muscle by the addition of nuclei. The only cells with mitotic potential, and hence the ability to furnish additional nuclei, are satellite cells. Their activation and division may be the key to skeletal muscle hypertrophy and increased strength.

Preferential hypertrophy

Greater hypertrophy of type II fibres has been frequently reported after strength training (Tesch et al 1987, Thorstensson et al 1977). There has been considerable debate about the force generating capacity of the different fibre types. Type II fibres may be able to generate higher specific tensions, and their preferential hypertrophy could account for the rise in the specific tension often observed for the whole muscle with training. Studies examining the relationship between strength per unit cross-sectional area contradict one another. Recently, work with skinned segments of human muscle fibres showed that the specific tension of the fast 2B fibres is approximately 50% greater than the slow type 1 fibres (Stienen et al 1996).

Fibre pennation

An increase in the angle of fibre pennation will allow more contractile material to attach to the tendon (Alexander & Vernon 1975), and although the force resolved along the tendon will be reduced, the net effect is that up to an angle of 45° there is an increase in force per unit anatomical cross-sectional area. A number of cross-sectional studies have demonstrated a relationship between muscle size and the angle of pennation in a variety of strength-trained and control groups (e.g. Abe et al 1998). This is strong evidence suggesting that hypertrophy involves an increase in the angle of fibre pennation and hence an increase in specific tension. It is surprising, therefore, that the only training study to evaluate the angle of pennation found no change after 12 weeks of training (Rutherford & Jones 1992).

OPTIMAL TRAINING AND THE STIMULUS FOR HYPERTROPHY

A number of possible stimuli for work-induced hypertrophy have been proposed. These include accumulation of metabolites, muscle damage and total neuromuscular activity. A high level of relative loading seems to be important, and an element of eccentric work may be advantageous, although mechanical stress *per se* does not seem to be critical. The role of paracrine hormones, especially insulin-like growth factor I (IGF-I) and fibroblast growth factor (FGF), has received considerable attention in the last decade, and their production may well be the link between the physical activity and a growth response.

The importance of high loads and duration of loading

DeLorme (1946) was the first to document the fact that exercise against high loads produced the greatest gains in strength. He devised the concept of the 10 repetition maximum (10 RM), i.e. a weight that can just be lifted 10 times. The 10 RM equates to ~70% of the maximum weight (1 RM) and, if the 1 RM is regularly measured, the training load can be increased proportionately. This is known as progressive overload and ensures that a high proportion of the muscle fibre population is recruited and exposed to a training stimulus (Schmidtbleicher 1992). In a review of 10 studies of isoinertial training, McDonagh & Davies (1984) concluded that loads of >66% of 1 RM were required to increase strength, suggesting that loading above a critical threshold is important. It is unclear whether high force is the stimulus *per se*, or simply that high force is a means of recruiting and subjecting the maximum number of fibres to a training stimulus. Atha (1981) also concluded that using a 6–8 RM was more effective at increasing muscle size and strength than 1–2 RM, while multiple sets at a submaximal load (70–80% of 1 RM) produced 50% greater gains in strength than a single set (Kraemer et al 1996). Therefore, the total duration of activity also appears important for strength gains and hypertrophy.

Mechanical stress and eccentric training

Mechanical stress, *per se*, has been suggested to be the critical stimulus for muscle hypertrophy (Goldberg et al 1975). Hence there has been considerable interest in eccentric, or stretching, movements that maximize mechanical stress. Several studies have found an eccentric component, used in addition to concentric contractions, to be beneficial to strength gains (Colliander & Tesch 1990, Hakkinen et al 1981) and hypertrophy (Hather et al 1991). This could simply be a result of performing more contractions, as the eccentric component in many of these studies was in addition to the concentric component. Hather et al (1991) found an additional eccentric component to be superior to simply doubling the number of the concentric contractions, but some studies have found no benefit (Carey Smith & Rutherford 1995, Jones & Rutherford 1987).

Metabolites

High force concentric and isometric contractions also involve considerable metabolic flux at a time when the blood supply is occluded by the high force contractions. Accumulation of metabolic by-products (H^+, La^-, Pi, Cr, K^+, together with smaller amounts of ADP, AMP, NH_3 and inosine) both inside and outside muscle fibres is associated with muscular fatigue and a reduction in force-generating capacity. It has been suggested that metabolite accumulation during high-resistance work may be the primary stimulus for gains in strength and muscle hypertrophy (Carey Smith & Rutherford 1995, Schott et al 1995). In contrast, two studies found high metabolite accumulation not to benefit strength gains. Robinson et al (1995) found that a rest interval of 3 min between sets, which minimized metabolic disturbance, produced significantly greater increases in squatting 1 RM than only 30 s of rest. In another study, Folland et al (1998) found a high metabolite accumulation protocol to be only marginally more effective than one with a low metabolite accumulation.

Creatine could also be the stimulus for muscle hypertrophy in response to training (Bessman & Savabi 1990). Creatine improves anaerobic work capacity and could facilitate more high force contractions and thus greater gains in strength and hypertrophy. Creatine may also stimulate the synthesis of myofibrillar proteins (Ingwall 1976). However, in healthy, sedentary individuals there is no evidence of a change in strength, at least over the short term (Bermon et al 1998, Greenhaff et al 1993).

HORMONAL INFLUENCES ON HYPERTROPHY AND STRENGTH GAINS

Endocrine hormones are undoubtedly important in skeletal muscle growth during childhood and maturation, especially in the period of rapid increase in strength and size around puberty. Growth hormone (GH) is clearly required for normal growth and testosterone is the principal reason that men are stronger and have larger muscles than women (Round et al 1999). However, it is not clear whether endocrine hormones are involved in work-induced increases in muscle strength and size. For example, hypophysectomized rats display normal work-induced hypertrophy despite the absence of all pituitary hormones (Goldberg et al 1975). The fact that the strength training response affects only those muscles used in the movement suggests that changes in circulating hormone levels, which would affect all muscles, are not the only, or major, stimulus for work-induced hypertrophy.

Testosterone

In healthy young men, supraphysiological doses of testosterone promote strength gains with or without training (Bhasin et al 1996). Testosterone is elevated following resistance training (Kraemer et al 1991), and it may therefore be involved in general hypertrophy and strength gains. Testosterone causes increased GH secretion and elevated IGF-I concentrations (Hobbs et al 1993), and these may mediate its anabolic properties. One factor that argues against testosterone being involved in work-induced hypertrophy is the fact that, where men and women have been compared, most studies have shown similar strength gains.

Growth hormone

Growth hormone is clearly important for normal growth, but it is not clear that giving GH to normal adults will result in useful strength gains. Acromegalics have larger but not stronger muscles and, in rats, the hypertrophy caused by excess GH appears to be very different from work-induced hypertrophy (Riss et al 1986). A recent review concluded that GH treatment of humans during training had not been shown to increase gains in strength or muscle mass (Zachwieja & Yarasheski 1999).

Insulin

Insulin stimulates the active transport system responsible for the uptake of amino acids into muscle cells, and in rats the anabolic response to resistance exercise appears to rely on sufficient insulin concentrations (Farrell et al 1998). In humans, there are complex interactions between the effects of exercise and insulin on protein synthesis and breakdown, the main effect of insulin after exercise being to reduce breakdown (Biolo et al 1999).

Recent work has shown post-exercise feeding to influence insulin levels, and Roy et al (1996) have shown that a post-exercise feed increases the rate of muscle protein accumulation after a bout of resistance exercise. This has led to considerable speculation in the popular strength training literature about the use of post-training feeds to manipulate insulin and maximize training-induced gains in muscle strength and size, but such long-term effects have yet to be demonstrated.

A considerable volume of work has demonstrated the importance of local growth factors in stimulating work-induced growth of healthy adult muscle, e.g. FGF (Clark & Feedback 1996) and IGF (DeVol et al 1990). The role of endocrine hormones may be to release or potentiate the release of local growth factors.

Insulin-like growth factors

In rats, Adams & Haddad (1996) found the increase in IGF-I during compensatory hypertrophy to precede increases in muscle protein and to correlate with the increase in DNA content. A later study from this group (Adams & McCue 1998) involved the infusion of IGF-I directly into the non-weight-bearing tibialis anterior of rats, leading to a 9% increase in muscle weight with a constant DNA:protein ratio. It was concluded that IGF-I may directly stimulate satellite cell proliferation. Injection of IGF-I increases muscle size and strength in young and old rats (Barton-Davis et al 1998). Recent work suggests that there may be a specific IGF isoform, named the *mechano growth factor*, that is the link between mechanical events and increases in protein synthesis (Goldspink 1999).

Oestrogen and the menstrual cycle

There are reports of fluctuations (~10%) in maximum voluntary force during the menstrual cycle (Phillips et al 1996, Sarwar et al 1996), although other investigators have found reproductive hormones to have no influence on muscle function (Greeves et al 1997). Reis et al (1995) examined the importance of timing training sessions with the phases of the menstrual cycle, and reported that training concentrated within the follicular phase produced more than twofold greater gains in strength than training at a fixed frequency.

HEALTH AND SAFETY ISSUES IN STRENGTH TRAINING

In any training programme, it is important both to assess the benefits of training and to take into account the potential risks. This is especially important when dealing with young people.

The spine

The spine is able to take loads that considerably exceed the mechanical strength of the intervertebral discs. This is because the load taken by intra-abdominal pressure can reduce the pressure on the discs by up to 40% (White & Panjabi 1990) and this is dependent on the strength of the muscles around the abdominal cavity. It is important, therefore, to include abdominal exercises in any strength training programme. Wearing a weight-lifting belt also helps to increase intra-abdominal pressure and protect the spine. High and potentially damaging loads on the spine can also be reduced by the use of good technique in all weight-lifting exercises. In general, this involves maintaining the natural curvature of the spine in all phases of the lift, so that loads on the intervertebral discs are kept even and not concentrated on one side of the disc.

The heart and circulatory system

As with other forms of physical training, high-resistance work has been suggested to cause potentially fatal cardiac hypertrophy. Strength training can lead to an improvement of left ventricular performance and a decrease in resting heart rate in previously sedentary individuals (Kanakis & Hickson 1980), although it may also cause an increase in the thickness of the left ventricular wall (Fagard 1997) that could be detrimental in subjects prone to hypertension or coronary vascular disease.

Strength training in children

Supervised strength training of children is a safe and beneficial physical activity resulting in increased strength, coordination and even flexibility, with no evidence that a sensible strength training programme is detrimental to bone or muscle growth (Lillegard et al 1997, Rians et al 1987). Whilst children can increase strength in response to training, their improvements seem to be particularly dependent on neurological adaptations (Ramsay et al 1990). The increase in muscle size appears to be significantly related to skeletal age, with larger gains in muscle size in older children (Fukunaga et al 1992).

CONCLUSIONS

A number of neurogenic and myogenic adaptations contribute to training-induced increases in strength, but muscle hypertrophy due to increase in fibre size appears to be the major adaptation, particularly in the longer term. High forces are required to increase strength and there is some evidence that an element of eccentric work optimizes the training stimulus. The transfer of training-induced gains in strength to complex motor tasks (e.g. javelin throwing and long jumping) clearly requires integration of the increased functional capacity of the muscle with the motor programme. In advocating strength training, it should be considered that, in many events, skill and coordination are of paramount importance. For the child and young adult, acquisition of skill and coordination is probably the most important aspect of training in many sports, and this should not be sacrificed for the more questionable benefits of weight training.

REFERENCES

Abe Y, Brechue W F, Fujita S, Brown J B 1998 Gender differences in FFM accumulation and architectural characteristics of muscle. Medicine and Science in Sports and Exercise 30(7): 1066–1070

Adams G R, McCue S A 1998 Localized infusion of IGF-I results in skeletal muscle hypertrophy in rats. Journal of Applied Physiology 84: 1716–1722

Alexander R McN, Vernon A 1975 The dimensions of the knee and ankle muscles and the forces they exert. Journal of Human Movement Studies 1: 115–123

Allen G M, Gandevia S C, McKenzie D K 1995 Reliability of measurements of muscle strength and voluntary activation using twitch interpolation. Muscle & Nerve 18: 593–600

Antonio J, Gonyea W J 1993 Skeletal muscle fibre hyperplasia. Medicine and Science in Sports and Exercise 25(12): 1333–1345

Atha J 1981 Strengthening muscle. Exercise and Sport Sciences Reviews 9: 1–73

Barton-Davis E R, Shoturma D I, Musaro A, Rosenthal N, Sweeney H L 1998 Viral mediated expression of insulin-like growth factor I blocks the ageing-related loss of skeletal muscle function. Proceedings of the National Academy of Science USA 95(26): 15 603–15 607

Belanger A Y, McComas A J 1981 Extent of motor unit activation during effort. Journal of Applied Physiology 51(5): 1131–1135

Bermon S, Venembre P, Sachet C, Valour S, Dolisi C 1998 Effects of creatine monohydrate ingestion in sedentary and weight-trained older adults. Acta Physiologica Scandinavica 164(2): 147–155

Bessman S P, Savabi F 1990 The role of the phosphocreatine energy shuttle in exercise and muscle hypertrophy. In: Taylor A W, Gollnick P D, Green H J, Ianuzzo C D, Noble E G, Metivier G, Sutton J R (eds) Biochemistry of exercise VII. Human Kinetics, Champaign, IL, p 167–178

Bhasin S, Storer T W, Berman N, Clavenger B, Bunnell T J, Tricker R, Casaburi R 1996 The effects of supraphysiological doses of testosterone on muscle size and strength in normal men. New England Journal of Medicine 335: 52–53

Biolo G, Williams B D, Fleming R Y, Wolfe R R 1999 Insulin action on muscle protein kinetics and amino acid transport during recovery after resistance exercise. Diabetes 48(5): 949–957

Carey Smith R, Rutherford O M 1995 The role of metabolites in strength training I. A comparison of eccentric and concentric contractions. European Journal of Applied Physiology 71: 332–336

Carolan B, Cafarelli E 1992 Adaptations in coactivation after resistance training. Journal of Applied Physiology 73: 911–917

Chapman S J, Grindod S R, Jones D A 1984 Cross-sectional area and force production of the quadriceps muscle. Journal of Physiology 353: 53P

Chesley A, MacDougall J D, Tarnopolsky M A, Atkinson S A, Smith K 1992 Changes in muscle protein synthesis after resistance exercise. Journal of Applied Physiology 73(4): 1383–1388

Clark M S, Feedback D L 1996 Mechanical load induces sarcoplasmic wounding and FGF release in differentiated human skeletal muscle cultures. FASEB Journal 10: 502–509

Colliander E B, Tesch P A 1990 Effects of eccentric and concentric muscle actions in resistance training. Acta Physiologica Scandinavica 140: 31–39

De Luca C J, LeFever R S, McCue M P, Xenakis A P 1982 Behaviour of human motor units in different muscles during linearly varying contractions. Journal of Physiology 329: 113–128

DeLorme T L 1946 Heavy resistance exercises. Archives of Physical Medicine 27: 607–630

DeVol D L, Rotwein P, Sadow J W, Bechtel P J 1990 Activation of insulin-like growth factor gene expression during work-induced skeletal muscle growth. American Journal of Physiology 259: E89–95

Dudley G A, Harris R T, Duvoisin M R, Hather B M, Buchanan P 1990 Effect of voluntary vs. artificial activation on the relationship of muscle torque to speed. Journal of Applied Physiology 69: 2215–2221

Fagard R H 1997 Impact of different sports and training on cardiac structure and function. Cardiology Clinics 15(3): 397–412

Farrell P A, Fedele M J, Vary T C, Kimball S R, Jefferson L S 1998 Effects of intensity of acute-resistance exercise on rates of protein synthesis in moderately trained diabetic rats. Journal of Applied Physiology 85(6): 2291–2297

Folland J P, Irish C, Roberts J C, Tarr J E, Jones D A 1998 Fatigue is not essential in strength training. Journal of Physiology 506: 102–103P

Fukunaga T, Funato K, Ikegawa S 1992 The effects of resistance training on muscle area and strength in prepubescent age. Annals of Physiological Anthropology 11(3): 357–364

Goldberg A L, Etlinger J D, Goldspink D F, Jablecki C 1975 Mechanisms of work-induced hypertrophy of skeletal muscle. Medicine and Science in Sports and Exercise 7: 248–261

Goldspink G 1999 Changes in muscle mass and phenotype and the expression of autocrine and systemic growth factors by muscle in response to stretch and overload. Journal of Anatomy 194: 323–334

Greenhaff P L, Casey A, Short A H, Harris R, Soderlund K, Hultman E 1993 Influence of oral creatine supplementation of muscle torque during bouts of maximal voluntary exercise in man. Clinical Science 84: 565–571

Greeves J P, Cable N T, Luckas M J, Reilly T, Biljan M M 1997 Effects of acute changes in oestrogen on muscle function of the first dorsal interosseus muscle in humans. Journal of Physiology 500: 265–270

Grindod S, Round J M, Rutherford O M 1987 Type 2 fibre composition and force per unit cross-sectional area in the human quadriceps. Journal of Physiology 390: 154P

Hakkinen K, Keskinen K L 1989 Muscle cross-sectional area and voluntary force production characteristics in elite strength-trained and endurance-trained athletes and sprinters. European Journal of Applied Physiology 59(3): 215–220

Hakkinen K, Komi P V 1983 Electromyographic changes during strength training and detraining. Medicine and Science in Sports and Exercise 15(6): 455–460

Hakkinen K, Komi P V, Tesch P A 1981 Effect of combined concentric and eccentric strength training and detraining on force-time, muscle fibre, and metabolic characteristics of leg extensor muscles. Scandinavian Journal of Sports Science 3: 50–58

Hakkinen K, Newton R U, Gordon S E et al 1998 Changes in muscle morphology, electromyographic activity, and force production characteristics during progressive strength training in young and old men. Journal of Gerontology 53A: B415–423

Hather B M, Tesch P A, Buchanan P, Dudley G A 1991 Influence of eccentric actions on skeletal muscle adaptations to resistance training. Acta Physiologica Scandinavica 143: 177–185

Herbert R D, Gandevia S C 1996 Muscle activation in unilateral and bilateral efforts assessed by motor nerve and cortical stimulation. Journal of Applied Physiology 84(4): 1351–1356

Hobbs C J, Plymate S R, Rosen C J, Adler R A 1993 Testosterone administration increases insulin-like growth factor-I levels in normal men. Journal Endocrinology and Metabolism 77: 776–779

Housh D J, Housh T J, Johnson G O, Wei-Kom C 1992 Hypertrophic response to unilateral concentric resistance training. Journal of Applied Physiology 73(1): 65–70

Ingwall J S 1976 Creatine and the control of muscle specific protein synthesis in cardiac and skeletal muscle. Circulation Research 38(5): I115–123

Jones D A, Round J M 1990 Skeletal muscle in health and disease. Manchester University Press, Manchester

Jones D A, Rutherford O M 1987 Human muscle strength training: the effects of three different training regimes and the nature of the resultant changes. Journal of Physiology 391: 1–11

Jones D A, Rutherford O M, Parker D F 1989 Physiological changes in skeletal muscle as a result of strength training. Quarterly Journal of Experimental Physiology 74: 233–256

Kanakis C, Hickson R C 1980 Left ventricular responses to a program of lower-limb strength training. Chest 78(4): 618–621

Kraemer W J, Fleck S J, Evans W J 1996 Strength and power training: physiological mechanisms of adaptation. Exercise and Sport Sciences Reviews 24: 363–397

Kraemer W J, Gorden S E, Fleck S J, Mello R, Freidl K 1991 Endogenous anabolic hormonal and growth factor responses to heavy resistance exercises in males and females. International Journal of Sports Medicine 12: 228–235

Lillegard W A, Brown E W, Wilson D J, Henderson R, Lewis E 1997 Efficacy of strength training in prepubescent to early postpubescent males and females: effects of gender and maturity. Pediatric Rehabilitation 1(3): 147–157

McCullogh P, Maughan R J, Watson J S, Weir J 1984 Biomechanical analysis of the knee in relation to measured quadriceps strength and cross sectional area in man. Journal of Physiology 346: 60P

McDonagh M J N, Davies C T M 1984 Adaptive response of mammalian skeletal muscle to exercise with high loads. European Journal of Applied Physiology 52: 139–155

McDougall J D 1992 Hypertrophy or hyperplasia. In: Komi P V (ed) Strength and power in sport. Blackwell Science, London

MacDougall J D, Elder G C B, Sale D G, Moroz J R, Sutton J R 1980. The effects of strength training and immobilisation on human muscle fibres. European Journal of Applied Physiology 43: 25–34

Narici M V, Roi G S, Landoni L, Minetti A E, Cerretelli P 1989 Changes in force, cross sectional area and neural activation during strength training and detraining of the human quadriceps. European Journal of Applied Physiology 59: 310–319

Narici M, Binzoni T, Hiltbrand E, Fasel J, Terrier F, Cerretelli P 1996 In vivo human gastrocnemius architecture with changing joint angle at rest and during graded isometric contraction. Journal of Physiology 496(1): 287–297

Phillips S K, Sanderson A G, Birch K, Bruce S A, Woledge R C 1996 Changes in maximal voluntary force of human adductor pollicis muscle during the menstrual cycle. Journal of Physiology 496: 551–557

Ramsay J A, Blimkie C J, Smith K, Garner S, MacDougall J D, Sale D G 1990 Strength training effects in prepubescent boys. Medicine and Science in Sports and Exercise 22(5): 605–614

Reis E, Frick U, Schmidtbleicher D 1995 Frequency variations of strength training sessions triggered by phases of the menstrual cycle. International Journal of Sports Medicine 16(8): 545–550

Rians C B, Weltman A, Cahill B R, Janney C A, Tippett S R, Katch F I 1987 Strength training for prepubescent males: is it safe? American Journal of Sports Medicine 15(5): 483–489

Riss T, Novakofski J, Bechtel P 1986 Skeletal muscle hypertrophy in rats having growth hormone secreting tumor. Journal of Applied Physiology 61: 1732–1735

Robinson J M, Stone M H, Johnson R L, Penland C M, Warren B J, Lewis R D 1995 Effects of different weight training exercise/rest intervals on strength, power, and high intensity exercise endurance. Journal of Strength Cond Research 9(4): 216–221

Round J M, Jones D A, Honour J W, Nevill A M 1999 Hormonal factors in the development of differences in strength between boys and girls during adolescence: a longitudinal study. Annals of Human Biology 26: 49–62

Roy B D, Tarnopolsky M A, MacDougall J D, Fowles J, Yarasheski K E 1996 The effect of oral glucose supplements on muscle protein synthesis following resistance exercise training. Medicine and Science in Sports and Exercise 28: S129

Rutherford O M, Jones D A 1992 Measurement of fibre pennation using ultrasound in human quadriceps in vivo. European Journal of Applied Physiology 65: 433–437

Rutherford O M, Jones D A, Newham D J 1986 Clinical and experimental application of the percutaneous twitch superimposition technique for the study of human muscle activation. Journal of Neurology, Neurosurgery and Psychiatry 49: 1288–1291

Sarwar R, Niclos B B, Rutherford O M 1996 Changes in muscle strength, relaxation rate and fatiguability during the human menstrual cycle. Journal of Physiology 493: 267–272

Schmidtbleicher D 1992 Training for power events. In: Komi P V (ed) Strength and power in sport. Blackwell Science, Oxford

Schott J, McCully K, Rutherford O M 1995 The role of metabolites in strength training II. Short versus long isometric contractions. European Journal of Applied Physiology 71: 337–341

Stienen G J M, Kiers J L, Bottinelli R, Reggiani C 1996 Myofibrillar ATPase activity in skinned human skeletal muscle fibres: fibre type and temperature dependence. Journal of Physiology 493: 299–307

Tesch P, Komi P V, Hakkinen K 1987 Enzymatic adaptations consequent to long-term strength training. International Journal of Sports Medicine 8(S1): 66–69

Thorstensson A, Larsson L, Tesch P, Karlsson J 1977 Muscle strength and fiber composition in athletes and sedentary men. Medicine and Science in Sports and Exercise 9(1): 26–30

Westing S H, Seger J Y, Karlson E, Ekblom B 1988 Eccentric and concentric torque velocity characteristics of the quadriceps femoris in man. European Journal of Applied Physiology 58: 100–104

White A A, Panjabi M M 1990 Clinical biomechanics of the spine. Lippincott, Philadelphia

Yarasheski K E, Campbell J A, Smith K, Rennie M J, Holloszy J O, Bier D M 1992 Effect of growth hormone and resistance exercise in young men. American Journal of Physiology 26: E261–267

Young A, Stokes M, Round J M, Edwards R H T 1983 The effect of high resistance training on the strength and cross sectional area of the human quadriceps. European Journal of Clinical Investigation 13: 411–417

Zachwieja J J, Yarasheski K E 1999 Does growth hormone therapy in conjunction with resistance exercise increase muscle force production and muscle mass in men and women aged 60 years and older? Physical Therapy 79(1): 76–82

7

The physiology of exercise in children

Colin Boreham

KEY POINTS

1. Children are being exposed to competitive sport at ever younger ages – an appreciation of paediatric exercise physiology is a necessity for those in positions of responsibility over young athletes.
2. Adolescence is a key phase in the physical development of children. The processes of maturation and growth which take place during adolescence have profound influences on performance. Both boys and girls improve in most aspects of fitness, but boys do so at a faster rate, leading to a widening of the gender gap in performance.
3. The early maturing male remains at a physical advantage compared with his average or late maturing peers throughout childhood. The situation is reversed for the female, particularly in activities involving weight control, such as gymnastics or ballet, in which the leaner, more linear late maturer is at an advantage.
4. Aerobic endurance performance, as measured by a maximal, progressive running test, improves for boys and remains stable for girls over adolescence. The improvements for boys seem to be due more to changes in anaerobic metabolism and running economy than to maximal oxygen uptake. Any such changes in girls may be negated by their relative increase in body fat.

5. Anaerobic performance over adolescence follows roughly the same pattern as aerobic performance. Improvements are largely, but not wholly, due to the increased muscle bulk observed over adolescence, particularly in boys. Hormonal and neural changes also seem to contribute to improvements in anaerobic performance over this period.
6. The ability of children to thermoregulate metabolic heat generated during exercise may be compromised by a reduced sweating efficiency and a greater skin surface area to body mass ratio. It is thus important for children to follow appropriate guidelines relating to drinking, clothing and acclimatization practices.

INTRODUCTION

Children are being exposed to competitive sport and associated training practices at younger and younger ages, and it is important that those responsible for these young athletes understand how children respond physiologically to exercise and training, and how these responses differ from those of the adult athlete (Maffulli & Helms 1988). Secondly, the experiences and responses of the childhood athlete are invariably dominated by the profound physical and behavioural changes that occur during adolescence, and some knowledge of the processes and features of maturation and its interaction with performance is required. Finally, it could be argued that childhood is the seedbed of virtually all sporting prowess, and that, without the necessary scientific background, coaches and others involved with young sportspersons run the risk of, at best, squandering potential champions, and at worst, doing harm through inappropriate practices and attitudes.

Postnatal growth can be divided into four phases: infancy (from birth to 1 year), early childhood (pre-school years), middle childhood (to adolescence) and adolescence (8–18 years for females and 10–22 years for males). As most exercise taken by children prior to adolescence may be classified as play, this chapter will con-centrate on the adolescent years, when regular exercise and training may begin to feature prominently.

PHYSICAL PERFORMANCE DURING ADOLESCENCE

Adolescence is characterized primarily by a rapid rate of growth and the accompanying processes of sexual maturation known as 'puberty'. Growth is ultimately under neuroendocrine and genetic control, with 60% of final stature estimated to be under genetic influence (Malina & Bouchard 1991). Many hormones interact in a complex way to stimulate and control growth during adolescence, including growth hormone (GH), somatomedin C, insulin, thyroid hormone and the pre-eminent oestrogens and androgens (e.g. testosterone). Before adolescence, levels of testosterone and oestrogen are relatively low, and there is no sex difference (Fig. 7.1). However, in parallel with increasing sexual maturity, levels of both hormones rise dramatically, promoting the development of secondary sex characteristics and, through their primary effects on protein metabolism and other growth hormones, a general increase in growth. In boys, the effect of testosterone is particularly manifested in the increase of muscle mass, while in girls higher concentrations of oestrogen promote an accumulation of body fat, from approximately 20% of body mass to 25%. Boys, on the other

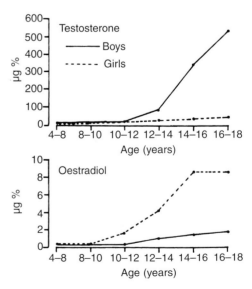

Figure 7.1 Changes in serum concentrations of testosterone and oestrogen (oestradiol) in boys and girls with chronological age. (From Malina & Bouchard 1991, with permission of Human Kinetics.)

hand, generally become leaner during adolescence, with body fat decreasing from 18 to 16% of body mass.

Indeed, adolescence is characterized by a widening of sex differences which, in turn, affect physical performance. Girls, on average, start their adolescent growth spurt 2 years before boys (12 and 14 years, respectively), so for a period of 1 or 2 years, it is not uncommon for girls to be bigger, heavier and even stronger than boys of the same age. Boys eventually surpass girls in most dimensions during their growth spurt, to attain, on average, a larger stature by young adulthood. At the age of 18, the average male is about 12 cm taller and 10 kg heavier than his female counterpart (Riddoch et al 1991).

During the early phase of the growth spurt, rapid growth of the lower extremities is evident, followed by an increased trunk length, and a greater muscle mass later still. It may be appropriate to mention the phenomenon of 'adolescent awkwardness' – a perceived temporary disruption of balance and coordination which occurs during the growth spurt. There is some evidence (Beunen & Malina 1988) that such clumsiness may become apparent especially in boys, lasting for approximately 6 months. This can affect up to one-third of boys, and is probably a result of the disproportionate growth of trunk over legs. There are dramatic changes in lean tissue between the ages of 12 and 16 years, with boys nearly doubling their muscle mass, and girls showing a 50% increase. Boys display only a slightly greater increase in calf muscle mass than girls, but nearly double the muscle mass of the arm during adolescence (Malina & Bouchard 1991). Differential growth of the skeleton also takes place, with girls generally displaying a broader pelvis and hips, with a slightly greater trunk:leg ratio. Boys develop relatively broader shoulders and narrower hips (the shoulder:hip ratio is 1.40 in prepubertal children, but 1.45 in postpubertal boys and 1.35 in postpubertal girls). Taken together, these differences between the sexes – the boys being relatively leaner, more muscular, broader shouldered and narrower hipped – have obvious implications for physical performance, reflected in results from simple fitness tests over the adolescent period (Fig. 7.2). Other factors, such as changes in attitude and motivation and the well documented decline in physical activity (Boreham et al 1993) over adolescence, may also affect the performance in such tests.

INDIVIDUAL DIFFERENCES IN MATURATION

Although the previous section may give the impression that the processes of maturation and their conse-quences for performance occur in a fixed pattern for all children, this is far from true. In fact, there is considerable interindividual variation, and an early maturer may start puberty even 5 years before a late maturing peer. Not surprisingly, given the influence of maturation and growth on performance, such individual variation in the timing and rate of biological maturation can have profound repercussions for the adolescent athlete. This is illustrated in Figure 7.3, which shows that, for most measures of performance, the early maturing male is at a distinct advantage over the late maturer during childhood.

The practical implications of such differences in levels of maturity were elegantly illustrated by Brewer et al (1995) who investigated selection policies for national junior soccer squads. They reported a significant bias in the distribution of players' birthdays towards the beginning of a given selection year, presumably reflecting the physical advantages the 6–10 months of growth and development would confer on these individuals. For females, the situation is reversed, with the leaner, lighter and more linear late maturers – who also tend to be better coordinated – being at a distinct advantage, particularly in sports and activities which emphasize weight control, such as diving, gymnastics, running and ballet (Claessens et al 1992).

AEROBIC ENDURANCE

Between the ages of 5 and 10 years, there is little difference between the aerobic endurance of boys and girls. However, from early adolescence, it is apparent that boys' performance, as measured on a progressive shuttle running test, improves steadily into their late teens, while that of girls remains static throughout this period (Fig. 7.2A). How can these changes and differences be accounted for physiologically?

Aerobic endurance performance is largely determined by three factors (Sjodin & Svedenhag 1985):

- aerobic power, defined as maximal oxygen uptake, or $\dot{V}O_{2\,max}$
- aerobic capacity, or maximum *sustainable* aerobic power, which is governed primarily by an individual's 'anaerobic threshold'
- exercise economy, defined as the oxygen cost of exercising at a given submaximal workload.

$\dot{V}O_{2\,max}$

$\dot{V}O_{2\,max}$ has traditionally been expressed relative to body weight, i.e. millilitres of oxygen consumed per

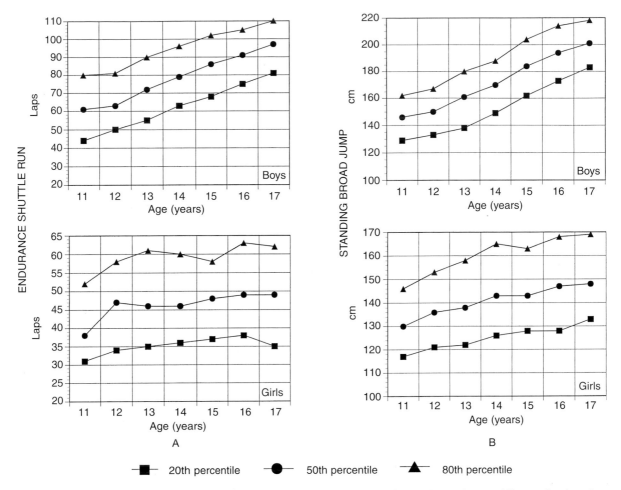

Figure 7.2 Changes in physical performance throughout the adolescent period for running endurance (A), standing broad jump (B), grip strength (C) and speed/agility (D). Results are taken from the Northern Ireland Health and Fitness Survey (Riddoch 1990) and are presented as 20th, 50th and 80th percentiles for approximately 200 children per age and sex group.

minute *per kilogram* of body weight. The use of this so-called ratio scaling method in children has been criticized due to the confounding effects of body size on $\dot{V}O_{2\,max}$ (Welsman 1997). However, as Nevill (1997) has pointed out, the traditional ratio standards still provide the best prediction of weight-bearing running performance in children. It can be seen, however (Fig. 7.4), that $\dot{V}O_{2\,max}$ relative to body weight does not follow the same trends as running performance (Fig. 7.2A) over the adolescence period. For boys, $\dot{V}O_{2\,max}$ stays relatively stable, while for girls it declines steadily. It seems, therefore, that changes in $\dot{V}O_{2\,max}$ cannot account for the observed development of aerobic running performance over childhood.

Aerobic capacity

Skeletal muscle of children appears to be metabolically geared to aerobic rather than anaerobic energy production. This is clear from the pioneering work done by Professor P.-O. Åstrand in Sweden (Fig. 7.5). He demonstrated that maximal blood lactate concentrations are considerably lower in prepubertal than in post-pubertal children. Subsequent studies have indicated that lower levels of the rate-limiting glycolytic enzyme phosphofructokinase in male adolescents compared with adults might explain this phenomenon (Fournier et al 1982). The increasing ability to produce energy from glycolysis over adolescence (Fig. 7.5), coupled with a higher

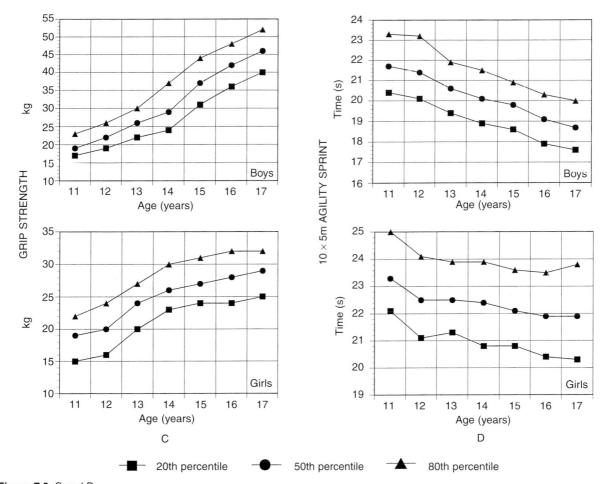

Figure 7.2 C and D.

maximal lactate steady state (the highest level of blood lactate that can be sustained during exercise without progressive accumulation), may combine to enhance maximal running performance.

Exercise economy in children

Running economy may be defined as the metabolic cost, measured as oxygen uptake per kilogram per minute, of exercising at a given treadmill speed and slope. A reduced oxygen uptake at a given running speed may be interpreted, therefore, as an improved running economy. On this basis, children clearly become more efficient as they grow and mature.

This was first shown in the 1950s by P.-O. Åstrand, and is illustrated in Figure 7.6 for running exercise in children aged 5–18 years indicating an approximate 15% improvement in running economy between these

ages. Interestingly, such improvements are not apparent for cycling, suggesting that biochemical factors may be less important than biomechanical factors in explaining these changes. It is likely that the single greatest contribution to the improvement in children's running economy is made simply by the reduction in stride frequency with increasing leg length as the child grows (Unnithan & Eston 1990).

Thus, it seems that the observed changes in aerobic running performance over adolescence are due more to changes in aerobic capacity and running economy than to changes in maximal oxygen uptake.

ANAEROBIC POWER

Exercise patterns in children are characterized by short bursts of physical activity, relying, by definition, on anaerobic sources of energy rather than aerobic

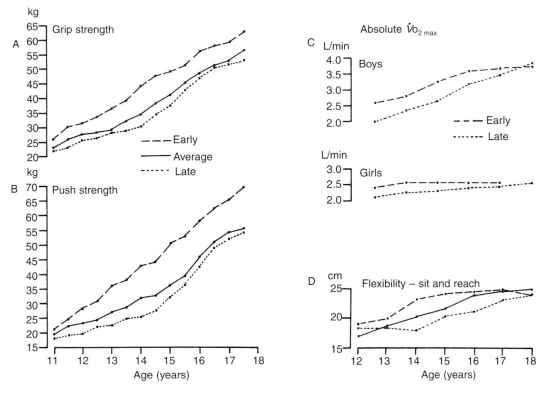

Figure 7.3 The effects of early, average and late maturing on physical performance throughout adolescence for grip strength (A), push strength (B), maximal oxygen uptake ($\dot{V}o_{2\,max}$) (C) and flexibility (D). (From Malina & Bouchard 1991, with permission of Human Kinetics.)

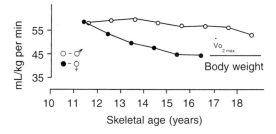

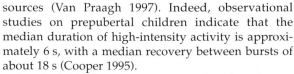

Figure 7.4 Mean relative maximal oxygen uptake ($\dot{V}o_{2\,max}$) of boys and girls. (From Kemper 1985, with permission of Karger.)

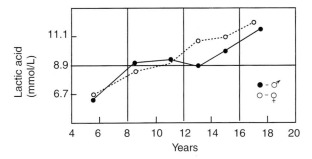

Figure 7.5 Maximal exercise blood lactate concentration in relation to age. (From Åstrand 1952, with permission of Munksgaard.)

sources (Van Praagh 1997). Indeed, observational studies on prepubertal children indicate that the median duration of high-intensity activity is approximately 6 s, with a median recovery between bursts of about 18 s (Cooper 1995).

Simple field tests, such as the standing broad jump and the 10×5 m shuttle sprint test give good approximations of instantaneous and anaerobic (glycolytic)

power, respectively. A glance at Figures 7.2B and D reveals the essential characteristics of power development from 11 to 17 years. There is steady improvement throughout adolescence, and, at all ages, boys outperform girls, with an accelerated rate of improvement in boys after the onset of puberty.

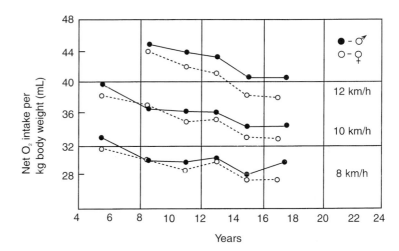

Figure 7.6 Changes in running efficiency with age at three different speeds. (From Åstrand 1952, with permission of Munksgaard.)

Such features can be largely explained by changes in muscle mass over adolescence, but not wholly so. For example, Ferretti et al (1994) observed that, while peak power values were 65% lower in children than in young adults, the cross-sectional areas of lower limb muscles were only 45% lower in the children. Similarly, Inbar (1996) has reported that, while the absolute upper arm power of young females may be 50% of that of their male counterparts, a deficit of 25% remains when power is normalized for body mass differences between the sexes. Thus it seems that age and sex-related differences in anaerobic power are partly due to qualitative factors such as hormonal variation and neural factors such as differences in motor coordination or motor unit recruitment. Possible biochemical mechanisms, including a reduced capacity for anaerobic glycolysis in muscle from prepubertal children, have been described previously (see Fig. 7.6). However, it is fair to comment that much of the discussion on underlying mechanisms explaining age- and sex-related differences in anaerobic power production in children remains speculative (Inbar 1996, Van Praagh 1997).

HEAT BALANCE

Although children produce more metabolic heat per kilogram during exercise than adults, their ability to thermoregulate may be compromised by two characteristics. Firstly, the rate at which children sweat (evaporation of sweat is the main thermoregulatory mechanism in adults) is lower by about one-third in comparison with adults, due primarily to a reduced sweating rate per sweat gland rather than a reduced density of sweat glands (Bar-Or 1989). Secondly, children have a larger skin surface area to body mass ratio.

For example, a young adult 1.77 m tall and weighing 64 kg will have a surface area of 1.80 m^2, while an 8-year-old child 1.28 m tall and weighing 25 kg will have a surface area of 0.95 m^2 – an increase in skin surface area of 36% per kilogram of weight compared with the adult (Sharp 1986). Because the skin's surface is the interface for heat transfer between the environment and the body, the child will tend to absorb relatively more heat from the environment in hot conditions. These problems may be compounded by the relative delay in acclimatization to heat displayed by children (Wagner et al 1972), and children exercising in such conditions should take precautionary measures, particularly in relation to appropriate clothing and drinking practices (Box 7.1). Conversely, in cold conditions, children will lose heat more rapidly.

Box 7.1 Guidelines for young people exercising or training in the heat. (From Armstrong & Welsman 1997, with permission of Oxford University Press)

- Ensure acclimatization
- Ensure full hydration before exercise (e.g. 300–400 mL fluid 20–30 min prior to activity for a 12-year-old)
- Drink periodically throughout prolonged activities (e.g. 100 mL every 15 min)
- Fluids should be chilled, flavoured and not too concentrated (e.g. 0.3 g/L NaCl and 25 g/L glucose)
- Discourage 'making weight' by dehydration
- Make sure activities suit the prevailing climate: take account of children's special problems
- Make sure clothing is appropriate
- Children need to be educated about maintenance of body fluid balance and should learn to drink beyond their subjective needs

The latter situation may become more apparent for young swimmers, as the heat conductance of water is 25 times that of air. While most indoor pools are heated at 25°C or above, much outdoor swimming occurs at temperatures below 20°C. Caution is required in such circumstances, as young children may begin to show distress within 18–20 min of swimming at such low temperatures (Sharp 1986).

CONCLUSIONS

As children become involved with competitive sports at ever younger ages, an appreciation of the physiology of exercise in children becomes essential for successful outcomes. Adolescence, in particular, is a key phase in the physical and sporting development of children. It is during this period that the gender gap widens in favour of boys' performance, and the effects of early and late maturation are manifested. For boys, the early maturers often remain at a physical advantage throughout childhood, while the opposite is invariably the case for females, with the leaner, more linear late maturers holding the physical advantage. During adolescence, aerobic endurance performance improves steadily in boys, but remains stable in girls, the latter largely reflecting the increases in female adiposity throughout adolescence. Anaerobic performance follows a similar developmental pattern, with improvements reflecting increases in muscle bulk over this period, especially in boys. Finally, thermoregulation during exercise may be compromised in children, who should therefore be encouraged to follow appropriate preventive measures.

REFERENCES

Armstrong N, Welsman J 1997 Young people and physical activity. Oxford University Press, Oxford

Åstrand P-O 1952 Experimental studies of physical working capacity in relation to sex and age. Munksgaard, Copenhagen

Bar-Or O 1989 Temperature regulation during exercise in children and adolescents. In: Gisolfi C V, Lamb D R (eds) Perspectives in exercise science and sports medicine, vol 2. Youth, exercise and sport. Benchmark Press, IN, p 335–367

Beunen G, Malina R M 1988 Growth and physical performance relative to the timing of the adolescent growth spurt. Exercise and sports sciences reviews, vol 24. American College of Sports Medicine Series. Williams and Wilkins, Baltimore, ch 15

Boreham C, Savage J M, Primrose D et al 1993 Coronary risk factors in schoolchildren. Archives of Disease in Childhood 68: 182–186

Brewer J, Balsom P, Davies J 1995 Seasonal birth distribution amongst European soccer players. Sports Exercise and Injury 1: 154–157

Claessens A L, Malina R M, Lefevre J, Beunen G, Stijnen V, Maes H, Veer F M 1992 Growth and menarcheal status of elite female gymnasts. Medicine and Science in Sports and Exercise 24: 755–763

Cooper D M 1995 New horizons in pediatric exercise research, In: Blimkie C J R, Bar-Or O (eds) New horizons in pediatric exercise science. Human Kinetics. Champaign, IL, p 1–24

Ferretti G, Narici M V, Binzoni T, Gariod L, Le Bas J F, Reutenauer H, Ceretelli P 1994 Determinants of peak muscle power: effects of age and physical conditioning. European Journal of Applied Physiology 68: 111–115

Fournier M, Ricci J, Taylor A W, Ferguson R J, Monpetit R R, Chaitman B R 1982 Skeletal muscle adaptation in adolescent boys: sprint and endurance training and detraining. Medicine and Science in Sport and Exercise 14: 453–456

Inbar O 1996 Development of anaerobic power and local muscular endurance. In: Bar-Or O (ed) The child and adolescent athlete. Encyclopaedia of Sports Medicine, vol VI. Blackwell Science, Oxford, ch 3

Kemper HCG (1985) Medicine and Sports Science, vol 20. Growth, health and fitness of teenagers. Karger, Basel

Maffulli N 1992 The growing child in sport. British Medical Bulletin 48: 561–568

Maffulli N, Helms P 1988 Controversies about intensive training in young athletes. Archives of Disease in Childhood 63: 1405–1407

Malina R M, Bouchard C 1991 Growth, maturation and physical activity. Human Kinetics, Champaign, IL

Nevill A M 1997 The appropriate use of scaling techniques in exercise physiology. Pediatric Exercise Science 9: 295–298

Riddoch C 1990 Northern Ireland Health and Fitness Survey 1989. Division of Physical and Health Education, The Queen's University of Belfast, Belfast

Riddoch C, Savage J M, Murphy N, Cran G W, Boreham C 1991 Long-term health implications of fitness and physical activity patterns. Archives of Disease in Childhood 66: 1426–1433

Sharp N C C 1986 Some aspects of the exercise physiology of children. In: Gleeson G (ed) The growing child in competitive sport. Hodder and Stoughton, London, ch 9

Sjodin B, Svedenhag J 1985 Applied physiology of marathon running. Sports Medicine 2: 83–99

Unnithan V G, Eston R G 1990 Stride frequency and submaximal treadmill running economy in adults and children. Pediatric Exercise Science 2: 149–155

Van Praagh E 1997 Development aspects of anaerobic function. In: Armstrong N, Kirby B, Welsman J R (eds) Children and exercise XIX. E and FN Spon, London, p 267–290

Wagner J A, Robinson S, Tzankoff S P, Marino R P 1972 Heat tolerance and acclimatization to work in the heat in relation to age. Journal of Applied Physiology 33: 616–622

Welsman J R 1997 Interpreting young people's exercise performance: sizing up the problem. In: Armstrong N, Kirby B J, Welsman J R (eds) Children and exercise XIX. E and FN Spon, London, p 191–203

8

Endurance training in young athletes

Adam D. G. Baxter-Jones
Nicola Maffulli

KEY POINTS

1. Although children and youth are physiologically adaptive to endurance training, the volume and depth of scientific literature in this field are very limited.
2. Despite a significant genetic component, maximum oxygen uptake, physical work capacity and performance levels can be modified through training programmes.
3. Most information related to the outcomes of endurance training is based on changes in maximal aerobic power. Typically, an increase of 10–14% is observed in children.
4. The few studies available in girls show that they are able to undergo the same adaptations as boys.
5. The adaptive responses to endurance training may be less pronounced in prepubertal compared with more mature children.

INTRODUCTION

As children grow, the many factors determining endurance fitness develop in a progressive, predictable fashion. The pattern of development follows not only physical growth but functional maturation as well. Performance abilities in endurance sports (running, swimming, cycling, rowing etc.) steadily improve throughout childhood. Although studies suggest that children are capable of improving endurance with training, given an adequate training intensity, there is also growing evidence that genetic determination plays a prominent role in both a child's endurance exercise capabilities and response to training. In fact, some experts have questioned the effects that endurance training have on youngsters at certain developmental ages, suggesting that these effects are minimal.

The technical complexity and physical and psychological preparation of certain sports require training to start at an early age. However, our understanding of the endurance 'trainability' of youngsters is limited. This is due in part to ethical considerations, methodological constraints and study designs. Protocols, apparatus and physiological end-points to determine endurance characteristics in adults are not always suitable for use with children. The type of analysis used to scale for differences in body size may also have contributed to our lack of understanding of training effects. With regard to study design, most studies have been cross-sectional, and the interpretation of training effects is therefore clouded by the effects that growth, development and maturation have on the physiological variables under investigation.

PHYSIOLOGY OF ENDURANCE EXERCISE

Although the effect of training on various physiological systems of adults and adolescents are well documented, comparisons of physiological variables between adults and children need to be assessed with caution.

Most sports can be classified into one of two broad categories:

- endurance – those involving prolonged periods of submaximal exercise
- multisprint – those which involve brief periods of high-intensity exercise interspersed with intervals of submaximal exercise.

In simple terms, endurance sports are supported by utilization of oxygen as the main energy fuel (aerobic metabolism), whereas multisprint sports rely on intramuscular stores of phosphagens and the anaerobic metabolism of muscle glycogen.

The highest rate at which the body consumes oxygen during a given time period involving a significant portion of muscle mass (maximal oxygen consumption, $\dot{V}O_{2\,max}$) has for long been considered as the key determinant of endurance exercise. However, only a minority of children and adolescents fulfil the adult criteria for true $\dot{V}O_{2\,max}$ measurements, a plateau in $\dot{V}O_2$. The appropriate index for maximal aerobic power

measurements in children is peak oxygen uptake (peak $\dot{V}O_2$), where peak $\dot{V}O_2$ represents the highest oxygen consumption elicited during an exercise test to exhaustion.

The ability to sustain a high rate of aerobic energy expenditure for prolonged periods is a function of peak $\dot{V}O_2$, and another important physiological variable for endurance performance. The anaerobic threshold is the rate of aerobic expenditure at which the fatiguing by-product of anaerobic metabolism, lactic acid, begins to accumulate in the blood. In adults, a fixed blood lactate reference level of 4.0 mM is used for this purpose. The ability to sustain a high rate of aerobic energy expenditure can be enhanced by increasing either or both peak $\dot{V}O_2$ and the anaerobic threshold. Exercise at the same relative intensity elicits a lower blood lactate response in children than in adults. There is growing evidence to suggest that a 2.5 mM reference level is more appropriate in children, but the cut-off age of when this is applicable is uncertain, as anaerobic capacity improves during childhood.

Thus, training would enhance endurance performance by increasing peak $\dot{V}O_2$ and the anaerobic threshold. In practice, these physiological variables operate in combination to determine endurance exercise performance. Of these variables, by far the most information is available for development of aerobic power.

DEVELOPMENT OF AEROBIC POWER

Aerobic uptake and age

Current research suggests that the improvements in peak aerobic power which occur as a child ages are an expression of both increased body size and improved function. A number of comprehensive reviews (Armstrong & Welsman 1994, Krahenbuhl et al 1985) have concluded that, in normal healthy children, absolute peak $\dot{V}O_2$ (L/min) increases roughly proportionally to body size. In general, prior to puberty, absolute values for aerobic power are approximately the same for boys and girls. When expressed as mL/kg per min, sex differences have been observed. In males, peak $\dot{V}O_2$ (mL/kg per min) remains relatively stable throughout childhood and adolescence, but in females it decreases. Unfortunately, scaling peak $\dot{V}O_2$ to account for body size differences using a 'per-body-mass' ratio standard is theoretically limited and it is more appropriate to express peak $\dot{V}O_2$ relative to mass$^{0.67}$. Such loglinear scaling methods have shown that, in boys, peak

$\dot{V}O_2$ actually continues to increase throughout adolescence, and in girls increases into puberty before levelling as they approach adulthood (Armstrong & Welsman 1997).

Aerobic power development in children and adolescents must always be assessed together with growth and maturation, as it is important to determine whether changes are a result of training or growth, or both, since an increase in body size may result in changes similar to the training effect. However, as most studies of aerobic development in children have been cross-sectional, until recently it has not been possible to separate the effects of training from growth and maturation (Baxter-Jones et al 1993).

Heritability of aerobic power

High levels of aerobic power are most likely the result of intensive endurance training and genetic predisposition. The response of a given athlete to a particular training regimen is due in part to an inherited genotype, as only approximately 30% of the $\dot{V}O_{2\,max}$ can be accounted for by training (Åstrand & Rodahl 1986). Studies of adult twins have shown that genetic variance of peak $\dot{V}O_2$ intake is very significant (Fagard et al 1991). Other twin studies have shown that genetic factors account for 93% of the variability of aerobic power (Mirwald & Bailey 1986). However, critics of such studies have pointed to potential errors associated with experimental procedures and study designs. Weber et al (1976) concluded from their study of twins that 42% of the variance in $\dot{V}O_{2\,max}$ was attributed to training, 51% to heredity and 7% to environment/heredity interaction. More recent reports suggest that the sensitivity to aerobic training is largely genotype-dependent (Bouchard et al 1990), and individuals who possess high aerobic capacities are likely to select themselves for participation in endurance sports (Andersen et al 1984, Baxter-Jones & Helms 1996).

Effects of training on aerobic power

Although resting oxygen uptake is very similar in trained and untrained individuals, there is at least a twofold higher maximal oxygen uptake in the trained versus the untrained individual (Åstrand & Rodahl 1986), in both sexes (Krahenbuhl et al 1985). The rate and magnitude of increased maximal oxygen uptake in adults are related to baseline levels of $\dot{V}O_{2\,max}$ prior to training, and the frequency, duration and intensity of the exercise programme undertaken (Raven & Hagan 1994). Young adults typically demonstrate a 5–30% rise

with training. The effect that training has on the development of peak $\dot{V}O_2$ during childhood and adolescence is still contentious (Armstrong & Welsman 1997, Pate & Ward 1996, Rowland 1990). Although there are some conflicting results as to whether aerobic training in prepubescent children can cause an improvement in $\dot{V}O_{2\,max}$ (Bar-Or 1983), most studies conclude that such an effect does exist (Armstrong & Welsman 1997, Pate & Ward 1996, Rowland 1990). One explanation for this child/adult difference is the greater habitual activity levels found in children, which maintain them closer to their maximal oxygen intake potential. However, they seldom undertake the amount of physical activity believed necessary to benefit the cardiopulmonary system (Armstrong & Welsman 1997).

The general consensus is that children and adolescents are physiologically more apt to endurance exercise training, if the training stimulus is adequate (Armstrong & Welsman 1997, Pate & Ward 1996, Rowland 1990). However, there are three main areas of contention, namely: is endurance training limited by a ceiling effect in maximal arteriovenous oxygen difference?; do genetic programmes promote a high level of functionality?; and does trainability vary with developmental status? Studies of elite prepubertal athletes have shown that, on average, they have superior cardiovascular function and higher $\dot{V}O_{2\,max}$ values when compared with their untrained peers (Baxter-Jones et al 1993, Baxter-Jones & Helms 1996). However, it is not known whether these observations are a result of training or of genetic predisposition (Rowland 1990). The reason why there is still much debate relates in part to the fact that few studies are carefully controlled and/or have well-defined exercise training programmes (Armstrong & Welsman 1997).

Pate & Ward (1996) recently reviewed 11 studies which met the following stringent inclusion criteria:

- use of a control group (random or pair-matched)
- provision of a clear description of the training protocol
- applications of physiological measures as indicators of training outcomes
- publication in a peer-reviewed research journal
- use of a training protocol administered outside of the physical education class
- use of subjects with no known health problems
- use of endurance training without any supplementary modes of training such as weight training.

They found an average net increase in peak $\dot{V}O_2$ of 10% in the training group(s) over the control group (range 1–16%). They tentatively concluded that adolescent girls (15–16 years of age) appeared to be at least as adaptive to endurance training as boys, although due to limited studies, this is still to be proven. More work is still needed with regard to younger age groups, particularly during the prepubertal and pubertal years. Recently, Armstrong et al (1999), working with untrained 11- to 13-year-olds found that, when body size and maturational differences were accounted for, gender difference was apparent at 11 years of age, a difference that increased with increasing age. Our own study of young athletes undergoing systematic training (gymnasts, swimmers, soccer and tennis players) suggested that age and gender differences are present within sports, but that, when comparisons are made between sports, these differences disappear. However, our study included no non-training control subjects (Baxter-Jones et al 1993, Baxter-Jones & Helms 1996).

Effects of training during puberty

Although maximum oxygen uptake ($\dot{V}O_{2\,max}$) in relation to chronological age has been studied extensively, very few studies have considered the relationship between $\dot{V}O_{2\,max}$ and sexual maturity (Armstrong & Welsman 1994, Baxter-Jones et al 1993, Mirwald & Bailey 1986). Although previous workers have suggested that aerobic training does not influence levels of $\dot{V}O_{2\,max}$ prior to puberty (Yoshida et al 1980), our own studies suggest otherwise (Baxter-Jones et al 1993).

Boys show a spurt in aerobic power development at puberty that is closely aligned with the adolescent growth spurt (Mirwald & Bailey 1986), whereas development in girls is slower after puberty. Two popular hypotheses have been presented to explain the relationship of maturation to a child's aerobic capacity. Gilliam & Freedson (1980) hypothesized that a maturational threshold exists whereby prepubescent children are unable to elicit physiological changes in response to training, although this view is disputed (Rowland 1990). The second hypothesis states that adolescence is a critical period during which the child is particularly susceptible to aerobic training. Training initiated 1 year prior to the period of rapid growth induces remarkable increases in $\dot{V}O_{2\,max}$, and a number of genetic, environmental and endocrinological reasons could explain this effect (Mirwald & Bailey 1986). This theory has been questioned by, amongst others, Weber et al (1976) who studied the effects of aerobic training on 12 pairs of identical twins (aged 10–16 years). They found that 10- and 16-year-old twins improved their $\dot{V}O_{2\,max}$ with training, but 13-year-olds did not, thus making the rapid growth theory untenable. In a review of the aerobic capacity of children, Zwiren (1989) concluded that there was limited evidence to suggest that training during prepubescence increased peak $\dot{V}O_2$ beyond that attributed to growth, a view that conflicts with others who have concluded that peak $\dot{V}O_2$ did respond to endurance training in prepubescent children (Armstrong & Welsman 1997). These reviews clearly indicate the continuing uncertainty regarding the separate effects that training and maturation have on the development of aerobic power in children and adolescents. Although evidence does exist that young athletes beginning serious training already have marked functional advantages, this may relate to findings that young athletes regularly training in endurance sports in general have early sexual maturation (Malina 1994).

Pulmonary function

Pulmonary function is a key component of oxygen uptake. Numerous studies have shown that athletes have larger pulmonary function values than their height-, age- and sex-matched peers (Armstrong & Welsman 1997). In particular, they have larger lung volumes.

During growth, the thorax and lungs expand considerably, and as a result so does vital capacity. Forced vital capacity (FVC) increases almost linearly with age, with the most rapid increase during the pubertal years. This rapid period of growth is associated with a rapid increase in stature, although lung growth lags behind increases in standing height. Similar to stature, FVC has distinct growth phases, with puberty again having a dramatic effect on lung function.

In general, children involved in high levels of physical activity have larger lung volumes than untrained children at comparable ages and body size (Eriksson et al 1980). Young swimmers undergoing intensive training have larger lung volumes than other similarly aged land-based athletes (Baxter-Jones & Helms 1996) and non-athletes (Bradley et al 1985). To what extent these differences are the consequence of training and to what extent they are due to natural endowment is not known. Whilst some investigators have found evidence linking the degree and duration of training to increases in FVC, others have not. There is also some evidence of a relationship between the physical process of lung stretching and lung growth. Andersen et al (1984) related the growth of lung volumes to physical performance capacity, and reported that physical performance capacity did not affect the development of lung volume. These results were in agreement with earlier work by Eriksson et al (1980) who found that champion swimmers at 12–16 years of age were physiologically superior to normal swimmers and that, even after cessation of training, their lung volumes remained at their previously high level. These findings have recently been confirmed by Bloomfield et al (1990), but it is still not clear whether the observed larger lung volumes in athletes are a result of physical training.

DEVELOPMENT OF ANAEROBIC THRESHOLD

A child's performance at anaerobic-type activities at supramaximal levels is significantly lower than that of an adult. Studies on anaerobic threshold during child-hood are limited. In general, blood lactate levels are lower in children and adolescents than in adults at any given exercise intensity. Theoretical issues related to standardization of lactate criteria have hindered the understanding of anaerobic threshold determination. The adult-derived 4.0 mM reference criteria is likely to be too high, and a lower value of 2.5 mM has been proposed. Although this may be due to hormonal difference, muscle metabolic difference, faster oxygen transients or levels of increased habitual physical activity, there are insufficient data to confirm these explanations (Armstrong & Welsman 1997). When ventilatory measures have been used to measure anaerobic threshold, much larger increases were observed in the training group compared with the control group (Pate & Ward 1996). Thus, it is likely that top-performing endurance child athletes, at given absolute exercise intensities, have lower lactate levels which are cleared faster than in less fit individuals.

CONCLUSIONS

Exercise training is designed to enhance exercise tolerance and ultimately to improve sports performance. The two major physiological variables thought to determine exercise performance in an individual are maximal oxygen uptake and anaerobic threshold. Of these two variables, by far the most information is available for peak oxygen uptake (peak $\dot{V}o_2$). Peak $\dot{V}o_2$ has been widely studied in young athletic and non-athletic populations, and has remained remarkably consistent over the last 50 years, an indication of its close association with growth. Although limited in number, those studies which have investigated the effects of exercise programmes have shown increases in peak $\dot{V}o_2$. However, the size of change is smaller in magnitude than that observed in adults (Pate & Ward 1996) and the effects of exercise training on prepubescent children is still debatable (Rowland 1990).

Although those with the highest peak oxygen uptake will, in general, be able to perform best, additional factors will also determine who crosses the finish line first. For example, effects of training may be largely genotype-dependent. This would be in accord with the hypothesis that children with natural ability self-select for specific sports.

Interpretation of peak $\dot{V}o_{2\,max}$ in children is further confounded by the changes brought about by growth and development. The methods previously used to interpret these effects have been questioned, especially the use of ratio standards normalizing absolute peak $\dot{V}o_2$ to body mass. Alternative scaling methods are now suggested (Armstrong & Welsman 1997).

More research is needed to fully understand the endurance trainability of children. Future studies must avoid the methodological pitfalls of previous work. They need to include (i) adequate numbers of subjects; (ii) subjects who are not overly fit; and (iii) subjects who are randomly assigned to an exercise programme. The exercise needs to be of adequate frequency, intensity and duration to induce increases in peak aerobic power and other beneficial adaptations. Ideally, the design of the study should be longitudinal and span the prepubescence, pubescence and postpubescence periods, so that training effects can be distinguished from those of growth and maturation.

REFERENCES

Andersen K L, Ilmarinen I, Rutenfranz J, Ottmann W, Kylian H, Ruppel M 1984 Leisure time sport activities and maximal aerobic power during late adolescence. European Journal of Applied Physiology and Occupational Physiology 52: 431–436

Armstrong N, Welsman J 1997 Young people and physical activity. Oxford University Press, Oxford

Armstrong N, Welsman J R 1994 Assessment and interpretation of aerobic fitness in children and adolescents. Exercise and Sport Sciences Reviews 22: 435–476

Armstrong N, Welsman J, Nevill A M, Kirby B 1999 Modeling growth and maturation changes in peak oxygen uptake in 11–13 yr olds. Journal of Applied Physiology 87: 2230–2236

Åstrand P-O, Rodahl K 1986 Textbook of work physiology. McGraw-Hill, Kogakusha

Bar-Or O 1983 Pediatric sports medicine for the practitioner. Springer-Verlag, New York

Baxter-Jones A, Goldstein H, Helms P 1993 The development of aerobic power in young athletes. Journal of Applied Physiology 75: 1160–1167

Baxter-Jones A D G, Helms P J 1996 Effects of training at a young age: a review of the Training of Young Athletes (TOYA) Study. Pediatric Exercise Science 8: 310–327

Bloomfield J, Blanksby B A, Ackland T R 1990 Morphological and physiological growth of competitive swimmers and non-competitors through adolescence. The Australian Journal of Science and Medicine in Sport 22: 4–12

Bouchard C, Boulay M R, Dionne F T, Perusse L, Thibault M C, Simoneau J-A 1990 Genotype, aerobic performance to training. In: Beunen G, Ghesquiere J, Reybrouck T, Claessens A L (eds) Children and exercise. Enke, Stuggart, p 124–135

Bradley P W, Troup J, van Handel P J 1985 Pulmonary function measurements in US elite swimmers. Journal of Swimming Research 1: 23–26

Eriksson B O, Freychuss U, Lundin A, Thoren C A R 1980 Effect of physical training in former female top athletes in swimming. In: Berg K, Eriksson B O (eds) Children and exercise IX. University Park Press, Baltimore, p 116–127

Fagard R, Bielen E, Amery A 1991 Heritability of aerobic power and anaerobic energy generation during exercise. Journal of Applied Physiology 70: 357–362

Gilliam T B, Freedson P S 1980 Effects of a 12 week school physical fitness program on peak VO_2, body composition and blood lipids in 7 to 9 year old children. International Journal of Sports Medicine 1: 73–78

Krahenbuhl G S, Skinner J S, Kohrt W M 1985 Developmental aspects of maximal aerobic power in children. Exercise and Sport Sciences Reviews 13: 503–538

Malina R M 1994 Physical growth and biological maturation of young athletes. Exercise and Sport Sciences Reviews 22: 389–434

Mirwald R L, Bailey D A 1986 Maximal aerobic power. Sports Dynamics, London, Ontario, p 1–80

Pate R R, Ward D S 1996 Endurance trainability of children and youths. In: Bar-Or O (ed) The child and adolescent athlete. Blackwell Science, Oxford, p 130–137

Raven P B, Hagan R D 1994 Cardiovascular responses to exercise and training. In: Harries M, Williams C, Stanish W D, Micheli L J (eds) Oxford textbook of sports medicine. Oxford University Press, Oxford, p 161–172

Rowland T W 1990 Exercise and children's health. Human Kinetics Books, Champaign, IL

Weber G, Kartodihardjo W, Klissouras V 1976 Growth and physical training with reference to heredity. Journal of Applied Physiology 40: 211–215

Yoshida T, Ishiko I, Muraoka I 1980 Effect of endurance training on cardiorespiratory functions of 5-year-old children. International Journal of Sports Medicine 1: 91–94

Zwiren L D 1989 Anaerobic and aerobic capacities of children. Pediatric Exercise Science 1: 31–44

9

Nutrition in children's sports

Gabe Mirkin

KEY POINTS

1. Healthy children should be encouraged to eat as much food as they want because it takes tremendous amounts of food to supply energy for training, growth and tissue repair. Food supplements offer no advantage over food.
2. Except for common table salt, athletes rarely suffer from deficiencies of minerals unless they lack iron because of bleeding, or calcium from excessive protein intake.
3. Children who want to lose weight should do so by increasing training, rather than restricting total food intake.
4. Children with diabetes or lipid abnormalities should follow the recommendations of their physicians, but restriction of calories will result in a deterioration of training and prevent them from reaching their maximum efficiency on the playing field.
5. Maximum endurance comes from starting an event with liver and muscles loaded with glycogen, and this cannot be accomplished without eating 3 h or less before an event. Endurance can be maintained by drinking fluids of choice and eating heavily salted foods during the event.
6. Recovery is hastened by eating as soon as the athlete finishes competition.

INTRODUCTION

The nutritional needs of child and adolescent athletes are the same as those for their adult counterparts. This chapter will review the physiologic principles that can be employed as a foundation for advising young athletes on how to use sound nutritional principles to maintain their health and maximize their performance in sports.

NUTRIENTS

Humans require approximately 46 nutrients to be healthy (Box 9.1). Lack of even one nutrient can impair performance, but taking massive doses of any single nutrient will not improve performance.

How food is utilized by the body

Carbohydrates, proteins and fats are the only nutritional sources of energy. Before they can pass into the bloodstream, they must first be separated from other components of food and be catabolized into their basic building blocks: carbohydrates into single sugars, proteins into single and small chains of amino acids, and fats to monoglycerides, glycerol and fatty acids.

Only four sugars can pass into the bloodstream: glucose, fructose, galactose and mannose. Three are immediately taken up by the liver and converted to the fourth, glucose. All cells can use glucose for energy. Glucose that is not used immediately can be stored only as glycogen in muscle and liver cells. When these tissues are saturated with glycogen, all excess glucose is converted to triglycerides. Liver glycogen can be released into the bloodstream, while muscle glycogen can be utilized only by that specific muscle.

Most of the ingested protein is used to form structural components. It can also be used to supply as much as 15% of energy during exercise, with more than half coming from one amino acid, leucine. Most

leucine does not come from ingested protein. The nitrogen comes from other branched-chain amino acids (isoleucine and valine) and most of the carbon comes from glucose and other amino acids. Before amino acids can be used for energy, deamination and transamination must occur to remove the nitrogen.

Epithelial cells lining the intestines combine glycerol and fatty acids to form triglycerides which can be used immediately for energy or be stored for future use in fat, muscle and other cells.

MAXIMIZING ENDURANCE

Endurance is the ability to continue exercising muscles for an extended period of time. The major sources of energy are triglycerides and glycogen in muscles, and triglycerides and glucose in blood. Most blood triglyceride comes from fat stores. Most blood glucose is synthesized by the liver.

There is a virtually unlimited amount of fat stored in the body. Fat cells of athletes contain enough fat to support exercise for 119 h. However, muscles contain only enough glycogen to last 1.5 h, and the liver contains only enough glycogen to last 6 min. As exercise intensity increases, the percentage of energy from muscle glycogen also increases. When muscles become depleted of glycogen, they hurt and become more difficult to coordinate.

Until recently, scientists thought that running out of glycogen caused 'hitting the wall', the severe muscle stiffness and pain that occurs in many runners between the 18th and 25th miles of a marathon, causing them to work much harder to maintain pace. No chemical explanation for this effect is evident (Green 1991). The explanation that lack of glycogen causes fatigue by blocking the regeneration of adenosine triphosphate (ATP) is not supported by experimental data. Low muscle glycogen levels cause only a minimal decrease in ATP levels, and cyclists do not 'hit the wall' after they use up muscle glycogen from pedaling many hours, because pedaling is done with a smooth rotary motion that does not tear muscle fibers. Dr Tim Noakes of the University of Cape Town in South Africa has shown that running causes damage to muscle fibers. The leg muscles are stretched violently when they contract at the moment the feet hit the ground, causing great damage to fibrous connective tissue that surrounds muscles (Grisdale 1990). This makes leg muscles feel stiff and heavy. Runners can protect their muscles against 'hitting the wall' by doing eccentric training once a week, repeat bursts of running downhill very fast.

Box 9.1 Essential nutrients

- Water
- Linoleic acid
- Alpha-linolenic acid
- Nine amino acids
- 13 vitamins
- Approximately 21 minerals
- Glucose (for energy)

Athletes can increase endurance by maximizing muscle glycogen prior to competition, and by conserving glycogen by burning more fat (and less glycogen), eating food and drinking energy-rich fluids during competition. Ninety-eight per cent of the energy for the brain comes from circulating blood glucose. However, there is only enough glucose in blood to last 3 min at rest, so the liver must provide constant replacement. The liver contains enough glycogen to supply glucose for only 6 min, so it must constantly synthesize glucose from protein.

Most conditioned athletes can tolerate low blood sugar levels during exercise without experiencing untoward effects (Felig et al 1982). However, when blood levels of glucose fall below 30 mg/dL, some can feel tired or dizzy and even suffer a syncopal episode. This is called 'bonking'. Bicyclists who do not eat during endurance races may experience this after 2 h or more of racing.

Athletes can increase endurance prior to competition by using special training methods and manipulating their diet, and during competition by taking in additional foods and supplements and using certain techniques such as starting out slowly, maintaining a relatively constant intensity, and choosing mid-temperature and low-humidity weather.

Training to increase endurance

To improve the ability of muscles to increase stores of glycogen and conserve available stores, athletes in endurance events utilize a training technique called 'depletion' (Mirkin 1983). Once a week, they exercise for an extended period after their muscles ache and feel heavy. This increases production of muscle glycogen synthetase (Karlsson et al 1974). When depletion training is done more often than once a week, recovery is delayed, restricting the amount of intense training that can be done during the rest of the week.

Eating to increase endurance

When athletes ingest food, the carbohydrates are stored as glycogen in the liver and muscle. When these stores are filled, the liver converts all extra calories to fat, which is stored in the body. Extra fat means extra weight, which can slow the athlete during competition. Any dietary manipulation that advocates increased energy intake or decreased energy expenditure for more than 3 days will usually increase fat stores.

Eating during the week before competition

In 1939, Swedish researchers showed that a high carbohydrate diet will increase muscle glycogen stores (Christensen & Hansen 1939). In the mid-1960s, Per Olaf Åstrand (1968) recommended the following dietary maneuver. Seven days prior to competition, athletes should perform a long depletion workout. For the next 3 days, they should keep the glycogen content of their muscles low by eating a very low-carbohydrate diet, and for the following 3 days, they should eat their regular diet plus extra carbohydrate-rich foods.

Most top athletes have abandoned this regimen because more recent research shows that athletes can load their muscles maximally with glycogen just by markedly reducing their workouts for the 3 days prior to competition. A further limitation of the regimen is that athletes cannot train effectively during the depletion phase. Furthermore, the ingestion of very large amounts of carbohydrates has been reported to cause chest pain (Mirkin 1973), myoglobinuria and nephritis (Banks 1977). For 6 days prior to major competitions, most athletes restrict intense workouts, and for 3 days prior to competition they eat their regular meals plus a little extra carbohydrate (Sherman et al 1981) (Box 9.2).

Eating the night before competition

For the 'last supper', athletes usually eat a high-carbohydrate meal (Box 9.3). This helps to maximize muscle glycogen stores. The pre-game meal cannot serve this function since it takes at least 10 h to replenish muscle glycogen (Piehl 1974). The meal can contain either simple sugars or complex carbohydrates, or any combination of each. It can be either high or low in fat, and should contain fiber to facilitate evacuation. Pre-competition constipation is common in athletes who eat low-fiber suppers, such as pasta and lots of bakery products, on the night before competition. To prevent

---

Box 9.2 High-carbohydrate foods

- Pasta
- Fruits
- Vegetables
- Beans and seeds
- Grains and cereals
- Most bakery goods
- Candies
- Many desserts

Box 9.3 High-carbohydrate foods for the 'last supper'

High-fat meal
● Pasta with tomato sauce and meatballs or pizza
● Milk, juice
● Garlic bread
● Apple pie
● High-fiber foods: vegetable salad, seeds, nuts, beans or whole grains

or

Low-fat meal
● Large vegetable salad
● Bean and eggplant casserole
● Bread, rolls
● Juice
● High-fiber source: fruit, seeds, nuts, beans, whole grains

---

this from happening, they should include nuts, seeds, vegetables, fruit and whole grains.

The pre-competition meal

Athletes can eat anything they want before a competition, provided that it will pass through the stomach by the time competition starts. A high-fat meal has not been shown to increase endurance by causing muscles to utilize increased amounts of fat with resultant sparing of muscle glycogen. A high-sugar meal has not been shown to decrease endurance by increasing muscle utilization of glycogen. Fructose can harm athletic performance by causing diarrhea. Glycerol solutions, ingested either before or during exercise, have not been shown to increase endurance or hydration or to improve tolerance to exercise in the heat (Murray et al 1991).

The pre-competition meal should be eaten not more than 5 h prior to competition. Liver glycogen is necessary to maintain blood glucose levels. There is only enough glycogen in hepatocytes to last 12 h when the athlete is at rest (Hultman & Nilson 1971). If more than a few hours elapse between the pre-competition meal and the time of competition, considerable amounts of liver glycogen will be catabolized. Eating replenishes liver glycogen stores. Athletes can eat right up to the time of competition if that meal can pass from the stomach by the time they start to compete.

Fasting before competing

Athletes who advocate fasting before competition have misinterpreted basic research. Fasting causes muscles to burn more fat and thus spare glycogen, but this is irrelevant if the athlete does not have enough glycogen stored when starting to exercise. Instead, the athlete will run out of stored muscle sugar faster and tire earlier.

Eating during competition

Most athletes do not need to eat during events lasting less than 90 min. However, in events lasting longer than that, athletes can benefit from ingesting additional food or drinking fluids that contain carbohydrates (Tsintzas & Williams 1998). The more fit athletes are, the better able they are to utilize ingested carbohydrates during exercise (Krzentowski et al 1984). One of the leading researchers on energy requirements during exercise is Dr David Costill of Ball State University in Muncie, Indiana. He feels that to enhance endurance, the very least amount of carbohydrate required is 40 g/h. The optimum amount is closer to twice that level. That would explain why cyclists eat solid foods during competition. Otherwise, they would have to drink at least 800 mL of a 10% carbohydrate drink per hour. This would pose a problem because only 600 mL can pass through the stomach in 1 h.

Athletes should eat small amounts of carbohydrate-rich foods frequently, rather than large amounts occasionally (Table 9.1). This will result in less variation in blood sugar levels and give enhanced sprint performance at the end of competition (Fielding et al 1985). While optimum frequency has not been determined, it may be prudent to eat 10 g of carbohydrate every 15 min, or 20 g every 30 min.

Drinking to increase endurance

Drinking during training

During training, particularly in hot weather, some athletes become increasingly dehydrated and suffer

Table 9.1 Examples of easily digested foods to be eaten during competition

Item	Carbohydrate (g)
1 slice bread	13
1 water bagel	30
4 graham crackers	21
1 fig bar	11
1 orange	16
1 cup grapes	20
1 banana	26

progressive weakness and deterioration in performance. Thirst is not a dependable signal of dehydration. Furthermore, training for hot weather competition by repeatedly dehydrating yourself will not improve endurance in hot weather any more than being hit repeatedly with a stick will make you resistant to being hit. To prevent dehydration during early season workouts in hot weather, the athlete should be weighed before and after practice. For every pound (0.5 kg) an athlete loses, he or she needs to ingest 2 cups (500 mL) of fluids immediately after practice.

Drinking before competition

Although most athletes do not benefit from eating in events that last less than 1 h, virtually all benefit from maintaining hydration. Competitive athletes can lose up to 2 L/h of fluid during intense exercise in warm weather. The maximum rate of stomach emptying is 600 mL/h (10 mL/min). Therefore, no matter how much fluid athletes ingest during competition, they will not be able to replenish their fluid losses completely during intense exercise.

An athlete can increase hydration during the week prior to competition and immediately before competition. Doubling the athlete's daily intake of fluid for 1 week, from 1 to 2 L, can increase blood volume by 10%. The extra fluid is not lost completely as urine (Kristal-Boneh et al 1988).

After fluid leaves the stomach, it is absorbed almost immediately. The only way to increase the rate that water is absorbed is to make it leave the stomach faster. Nancy Rehrer of the University of Limberg in the Netherlands has shown that filling the stomach with water markedly accelerates stomach emptying (Rehrer et al 1990).

If athletes drink large amounts of water 30 min before competition, they will start the race with full bladders. However, if they drink 600 mL of water just before the race starts, their stomachs will be full and their bladders empty. Almost 400 mL will pass into the intestines in 20 min (Rehrer et al 1990). They should then try to ingest 3 oz (~90 mL) of water every 10 min.

Drinking during competition

Athletes should drink before they feel thirsty. They will not feel thirsty until they have lost 1–2 L of fluid. By that time, performance will be compromised and it will not be possible to replace the fluid completely.

Athletes lose water during exercise primarily through sweating. Sweat contains a far lower concentration of salt than blood. Therefore, athletes lose far more water than salt, causing the concentration of salt in the blood to rise. A person will not feel thirsty until the concentration of salt in the blood rises high enough to trip off thirst osmoreceptors in the brain, and by that time the person will have already lost 2–4 pints (0.95–1.9 L) of fluid.

What to drink

Many athletes do not need to drink for competitions lasting less than 30 min. Water is the drink of choice for competitions lasting less than 1 h (Costill et al 1981, Hargreaves et al 1981). However, athletes who exercise longer than that need energy sources and minerals as well. The rules for energy-containing fluids have changed dramatically in the last few years. In 1968, studies showed that 2.5% was the highest concentration of sugar that could be contained in an exercise drink and still be absorbed (Costill & Saltin 1974). This posed a problem because drinks taste best when they contain a 10% concentration of sugar, as do, for example, soft drinks and fruit juices. Soon after these studies, many exercise drinks containing 2.5% sugar appeared on the market. They did not taste good because the concentration of sugar was too low, so some of the manufacturers added saccharin to sweeten the taste.

Twenty years later, new studies refuted the 1968 report. The 1968 data were collected on resting subjects, whereas in fact exercise increases gastric emptying of both solid meals and liquids (Moore et al 1990). When the same studies were repeated using people who were exercising at an intense level, 10% sugar drinks were absorbed rapidly. Based on the most recent evidence, special exercise drinks are not necessary, although many athletes may prefer them. All 10% drinks are equally effective in supplying energy (10% drinks are made by dissolving 8 tblsp of sugar in 1 L of water; 1 tblsp contains 12 g sucrose). These recent data seem to conflict with previous data showing the need for special drinks that contain polymers of five glucose molecules bound together. Polymers are supposed to provide a lot of sugar at a low osmotic pressure, thereby not delaying absorption. However, they are not superior to free glucose for maintaining hydration and blood glucose levels, and they have not been shown to increase endurance (Massicotte et al 1989).

Electrolytes

Additional minerals are not needed in exercise that takes less than 1 h. Sweat is so dilute, when compared with blood, that blood levels of sodium and potassium rise during exercise, calcium stays the same, and only magnesium levels drop. However, this drop in the blood level of magnesium is caused by that ion leaving the bloodstream to enter red blood cells (Casoni et al 1990), and taking magnesium oxide pills does not raise blood or muscle concentrations of magnesium and it does not help athletes to recover faster from exercise (Weller et al 1998). Dilute mineral drinks may improve performance in events lasting longer than 1 h. As long as they are hypotonic in comparison to blood, they are absorbed almost as rapidly as pure water (Schneider et al 1991). Sodium also increases sugar absorption. Hypertonic drinks markedly delay stomach emptying (Rehrer et al 1990). However, athletes need extra calories during events lasting longer than 2 h, and in these events most athletes replace minerals by eating solid food.

Salt is essential in hot weather

Exercising in hot weather requires lots of water and salt. Dr James Gamble, a professor at Harvard Medical School, spent most of World War II studying people lying on rafts under a very hot sun. He wanted to find out the best way to protect American pilots from the ravages of fighting in very hot weather. His landmark studies showed that exercisers have to take in large amounts of salt to survive in very hot weather, so salt tablets were prescribed for everyone who had to exercise or work at such temperatures. But salt tablets caused occasional nausea or vomiting, side-effects which do not occur when salt is taken with foods such as peanuts and potato chips during exercise. To better understand how important salt is for endurance, all physicians, athletes and coaches should read Dr Gamble's outstanding first text, written in 1942 (Gamble 1958).

As a result, many athletes and recreational exercisers are not taking in adequate amounts of salt in hot weather. They become dehydrated and exhausted, can't finish their workouts or competitions, and may pass out or even die. When you exercise in hot weather, eat salty food and drink plenty of water. During hot weather exercise, it really does not make much difference what you drink, as long as you take in enough fluid and sodium. Obviously, avoid sea water! Sodium makes you thirsty so you drink enough to replace the fluid that you lose during exercise. As mentioned earlier, thirst is caused by high salt levels in the blood flowing to your brain. If you drink and do not take in adequate amounts of salt, you will dilute salt levels in your brain, not feel thirsty and falsely think that you have replaced your lost fluid. If you eat salty food along with your drink during exercise, you will not need salt in the drink and will get by drinking just plain water.

What's the best exercise drink?

The best drinks for recreational exercisers and competitive athletes are those that they like best (Greenleaf et al 1998). If you feel thirsty while you're exercising, you have already lost more than 2 pints (0.95 L) of fluid. It doesn't make much difference what you drink as long as you get plenty of fluid, along with calories and salt in your food or drink (Box 9.4).

Carbonated beverages are okay

During exercise lasting more than 1 h, you have to drink lots of fluid, and the more fluid you drink, the less likely you are to become exhausted. The most important factor that determines how much you drink is how much you like the taste of the drink. More than half of the cyclists in the 1997 US Professional Championship drank cola soft drinks. Researchers at Washington University in St Louis showed that bubbles in soft drinks do not affect blood acidity and therefore do not limit endurance.

Another concern was that the caffeine in many soft drinks, being a diuretic, would increase fluid loss, but research at the University of Guelph has shown that it is not a diuretic during exercise. It appears that the caffeine in soft drinks helps muscles to burn more fat and less carbohydrate, so that muscles preserve their stored sugar and can be exercised longer. The only theoretical concern is that a person with a weak heart might develop irregular heartbeats from the increased stimulation of caffeine. In the 1960s, data showed that cold drinks (4°C) are absorbed faster than warm ones. The theory was that cold water causes the stomach to contract and push fluids rapidly into the intestines.

Box 9.4 Drinks for competition

- Most carbonated soft drinks
- Most fruit juices
- 5–10% sugared water or tea
- Drink water and eat any salted foods

However, more recent studies have shown that temperature does not make much difference (McArthur & Feldman 1989, Maughan & Lambert 1991).

What not to drink

Alcohol harms athletic performance by reducing the force of the heart's contractions so that less blood is pumped to the body. This may increase oxygen needs and tire the athlete sooner, increase sweating and dehydrate the athlete earlier, and may cause muscles to burn up more carbohydrate, thus fatiguing the athlete sooner (Mangum 1986).

Eating and drinking after competition

Much of post-competition tiredness is caused by depletion of body water and muscle glycogen. It makes no difference whether the carbohydrate replenishment is with simple sugars found in fruits or more complex sugars found in grains and beans. The average athlete takes in 250 g of carbohydrate each day. Recovery can be maximized by taking in three times that amount for a day or two (Costill et al 1981) (Table 9.2).

The timing and amount of carbohydrate intake also significantly affect glycogen replenishment. Two hours after competition, athletes who ate immediately were shown to have three times as much muscle glycogen as those who did not eat (Ivy et al 1988a). Furthermore, the maximal amount of glycogen replenishment comes from eating 225 g of carbohydrate. Eating more carbohydrate than that does not increase the rate of glycogen replenishment further (Ivy et al 1988b).

Replacing fluid in hot weather

In 1967, the try-outs for the United States Pan American games marathon team were held in Holyoke, Massachusetts, at high noon with the temperature above 100°F. Eighty-seven out of the 125 entrants dropped out. Most mediocre runners could have made

Table 9.2 225-g carbohydrate post-exercise meal

	Carbohydrate (g)
2 rolls, each with 3 tablespoons of jelly	120
2 bananas	60
2 cups orange juice	52
Total	**232**

the United States national team on that day if they knew how to drink during competition. When you exercise intensely in temperatures above 80°F, you lose more than 2 pints (0.95 L) of fluid each hour. You can replace fluid by drinking, but your stomach will only allow a little more than 1 pint (0.47 L) of fluid, or half your losses, to pass through it each hour. So, no matter how much or how often you drink during intense exercise, you will always lose more fluid than you can take in. As you lose fluid, your body temperature rises and you become weaker and more tired.

As mentioned earlier, you can markedly increase water absorption by making it leave the stomach faster. Immediately after water leaves your stomach, it is absorbed through your intestines. If you drink a large amount of water a half-hour before a competition, you will start a race with a full bladder and be the worse off. However, if you drink 20 oz (0.6 L) or a little more than a pint of water just before the race starts, your stomach will be full and your bladder empty. Almost a pint (0.47 L) will pass into the intestines in 20 min. You should then take in about 3 oz (90 mL) of water every 10 min if possible.

THE ATHLETE'S DIET

To maintain muscle glycogen, athletes in endurance sports need to take in at least 600 g of carbohydrates each day, so young athletes should eat all the food they want (Box 9.5). To protect their health, they should avoid eating excessive amounts of the harmful saturated or partially hydrogenated fats that increase their risk of developing coronary artery disease and certain cancers as adults. They should eat unrestricted amounts of polyunsaturated vegetable fats, including the essential fatty acids – omega-3, alpha-linoleic acid, and omega-6, linoleic acid – that are found in whole grains, cereals made from whole grains, beans, other seeds and nuts. Lack of the essential fatty acids raises blood levels of LDL cholesterol and increases a person's chances of suffering a heart attack (Jenkins et al 1999). No data show that eating large amounts of omega-3-rich foods, such as almonds, soybeans, flax seeds, hemp seeds or deep-water fish, is more effective in preventing heart attacks than adding a small amount of these foods to regular meals. Nobody has shown that once you meet your needs for essential fatty acids, more is better. Some lay publications advocate a high-fat diet to increase endurance and improve athletic performance. There are no data to support this view and there are data to refute it (Kosich et al 1986).

Box 9.5 Sample 4000 kcal carbohydrate-rich menu (60% carbohydrate, 15% protein and 25% fat)

Breakfast
1 orange
4 cups of cereal
1 cup of skim milk
2 pieces of toast

Snack
Banana

Lunch
Pitta bread
Lettuce and tomato salad topped with crushed peanuts or flaxseeds
4 oz tuna fish
Apple
Skim milk

Snack
2 slices of bread with peanut butter and jelly

Dinner
2 cups mashed potatoes
2 4-oz breasts of chicken
Large vegetable salad topped with seeds and nuts
Apple pie
4 slices of bread

Snack
2 slices of bread
Jelly

Trans fatty acids

In 1952, Ancel Keys' ground-breaking studies showed that a lack of polyunsaturated fats in vegetable oils causes heart attacks. Scientists recommended substituting vegetable oils for the saturated fats that are found in meat, chicken and dairy products. However, over the next 35 years, the rate of breast cancer doubled. Polyunsaturated fats in vegetable oils are healthful when left in vegetables, but removed from their natural sources and exposed to light, heat and oxygen, they turn rancid rapidly. To prevent this from happening, manufacturers convert healthful polyunsaturated fats to partially harmful hydrogenated fats. About 7.5% of the fat in our diets comes from partially hydrogenated fats (Allison et al 1999). The amount of partially hydrogenated fat stored in a woman's buttocks predicts her susceptibility to breast cancer (Simonsen et al 1998a,b). Partially hydrogenated fats increase risk for heart attacks by lowering blood levels of HDL cholesterol, raising levels of the bad LDL cholesterol and very bad Lp(a) and blocking arachidonic acid to cause clotting (Koletzko & Decsi 1997).

The United States government requires food manufacturers to list partially hydrogenated fat content on labels. Current recommendations are to eat unrestricted amounts of vegetables for their polyunsaturated oils, and reduce intake of foods containing partially hydrogenated oils, e.g. many bakery products, breakfast cereals and prepared meals, and foods that are fried in partially hydrogenated oils such as french fries and hamburgers.

Phytochemicals

Of the countless plants that have been on earth during the past 3.5 billion years, the vast majority have become extinct. Surviving plants contain insecticides, antibiotics, fungicides and chemicals that protect them from animals, including humans. They also contain other phytochemicals that help them to heal when they are damaged and may protect them from cancers and degenerative diseases. When you eat plants, you consume these phytochemicals and they are used by your body to help keep you healthy and protect you from disease (Box 9.6).

Minerals

With the exception of sodium, calcium and iron, mineral deficiencies rarely occur in athletes. Sodium needs can be met by salting foods liberally. Iron levels can be checked by measuring serum ferritin. Low iron reserves, even in the absence of anemia, can interfere

---

Box 9.6 Phytochemicals

Help prevent cancer
- Peppers contain *capsaicin*
- Citrus fruits and tomatoes contain *coumarins*
- Berries, peppers, carrots, tomatoes contain *flavinoids*
- Tomatoes and many fruits contain *lycopenes*
- Broccoli contains *sulforophane*
- Garlic, onions and chives contain *S-allycysteine*
- Licorice contains *triterpenoids*
- Cabbage family contains *indoles* and *isothiocyanates*
- Soybeans, beans, peas and lentils contain *genistein*

Help prevent heart attacks
- Barley, wheat and flaxseed contain *lignins*
- Beans, peas and lentils contain *genistein*
- Onions and garlic contain *allicin*

> **Box 9.7** Foods that contain 250 mg of calcium
>
> - 1 glass milk (240 cc)
> - 1 cup yogurt (120 cc)
> - $1\frac{1}{2}$ cups cottage cheese
> - $1\frac{1}{2}$ cups ice cream
> - $1\frac{1}{2}$ slices hard cheese
> - 2 ounces sardines with bones
> - 4 ounces canned salmon with bones
> - 1 250-mg calcium carbonate pill

with lactic acid clearance during exercise (Finch et al 1979). If low, daily iron supplements or a high meat–fish–chicken diet may be prescribed. Iron tablets should not be prescribed to athletes who are not deficient in that mineral. Excessive iron intake can cause zinc deficiency (Solomons 1986) and damage to internal organs. Amenorrheic female athletes may need to take in 1500 mg of calcium each day, instead of the usual 1000 mg. They can do this by taking in extra high-calcium foods such as dairy products, seeds, nuts, and vegetables (Box 9.7), or by taking calcium supplements.

Vitamins

Young athletes can get the vitamins that they need from the foods that they eat. Most vitamins are parts of enzymes that start chemical reactions in the body, and certain enzymes, particularly from the B vitamins, are needed to convert foods to energy. Athletes have markedly increased needs for the energy-producing vitamins, such as thiamine, niacin, riboflavin, biotin and pantothenic acid, but they rarely suffer from vitamin deficiencies. Athletes should be aware that the B vitamins are found in the germ in whole grains and that grinding whole grains produces a flour that turns rancid rapidly. To prolong shelf-life, the miller removes the germ from whole grains before grinding. Most countries have laws requiring commercial flour to have thiamine, niacin and riboflavin added back in, but not biotin and pantothenic acid. So athletes should eat a diet containing the germ of plants such as whole grains and their cereals, nuts, other seeds and beans. Even though a varied diet should supply adequate amounts of all the vitamins necessary for health, scattered data show some advantage to taking in doses of vitamins that are substan-

tially greater than necessary for health (Bucci 1993). However, megavitamin nutrition is highly controversial. It appears safe for athletes to take a supplement containing the Recommended Dietary Allowances (RDAs) for vitamins.

Protein supplements are no better than food

Protein supplements are made from foods such as milk powder, tuna fish and soybeans. No process has been devised that can make a protein extract from food more effective in building muscles than the food itself. It is illegal in many countries for a manufacturer to claim that protein supplements will make you stronger, give you larger muscles or make you a better athlete. To support this position, the Food and Drug Administration of the United States commissioned a study by the Federation of American Societies for Experimental Biology (FASEB). They found no scientific reason for healthy people to take protein supplements.

Several other studies have shown that protein supplements do not help athletes become stronger or develop larger muscles. Protein supplement manufacturers promoted 'free form' amino acids, but adding acid to protein to separate the amino acids offers no benefit, since your stomach and intestines do that efficiently. Some manufacturers claim that the specific amino acids, arginine, ornithine and lysine, raise growth hormone levels, which makes muscles larger and stronger. Recent studies have shown that these amino acid supplements do not affect insulin, testosterone, cortisone or growth hormone levels, they do not make athletes stronger and they do not build larger or stronger muscles.

A simple guide for healthful eating is to have unlimited amounts of fruits, vegetables, whole grains, cereals, beans, seeds and nuts, and reasonable amounts of other foods, except for those that are high in saturated or partially hydrogenated fats.

WEIGHT LOSS AND WEIGHT GAIN
Losing weight

The most effective way for most athletes and regular exercisers to lose weight is to increase the intensity and duration of their workouts without altering their diets. However, some athletes cannot lose weight unless they also manipulate their diets.

Calorie restriction does not work

Calorie restriction is rarely an effective means for athletes to lose weight and keep it off. First, athletes do not like to follow a program that markedly restricts the duration and intensity of their training, and second, they do not like to feel hungry when they leave the table after each meal and go to bed each night.

Fat restriction works sometimes

Some athletes can follow a fat-restricted diet without a deterioration in their training and feeling of well-being. Restricting fat without also restricting caloric intake will not cause weight loss (Miller et al 1990). Although North Americans have reduced their intake of fat from an average 43 to 32% in the last 20 years, they are 11 pounds (5 kg) fatter. Scientists at the University of North Carolina at Chapel Hill reviewed 28 well-controlled studies on how dietary fat affects weight and found that a 10% reduction in fat intake is associated with a weight loss of a little more than 1 lb (0.45 kg) per month (Bray & Popkin 1998). You expect this because fats are the densest source of calories, containing twice as many calories as carbohydrates and proteins. However, this result came from scientific studies. In the real world, losing weight depends on what you substitute for fat. If you reduce your intake of foods made from butter, margarine, fatty meats, chicken and whole milk dairy products, and eat lots of foods made from flour, such as bakery products and pastas, you will gain weight because flour-based foods are not very filling. On the other hand, substituting fiber-rich foods such as whole grains and their cereals, beans, vegetables and fruits is more effective in suppressing appetite.

Restricting refined carbohydrates works most often

Obese teenagers eat far more when meals raise their blood sugar to high levels than when they raise blood sugar only a little (Ludwig et al 1999). A high rise in blood sugar causes the pancreas to release large amounts of insulin, inducing hunger. The glycemic index measures how high a person's blood sugar level rises after eating a certain food compared with eating sugar. Foods that raise blood sugar to high levels include sugar, bread, spaghetti, macaroni, bagels, crackers, cookies, white rice, rolls and root vegetables such as potatoes. Meals that raise blood sugar levels only a little are loaded with vegetables, whole grains, seeds and beans. A weight-reduction diet should include whole grains instead of bakery products and pastas, and vegetables, beans and fruits instead of dense sources of calories, such as meat and chicken. A healthful diet should include small amounts of fatty nuts and seeds, which can be added to salads.

Bulimia

Some athletes try to restrict caloric intake by sticking their fingers down their throats to induce vomiting. Girls are far more likely than boys to do this. Bulimic athletes are often brought for medical attention with a chief complaint of a deterioration in athletic performance, weakness and tiredness. They usually deny that they are vomiting. They often appear emaciated and can have severe dental problems. Laboratory tests reveal reduced blood potassium levels and increased 24-h urine potassium levels. Vomiting causes a loss of large amounts of hydrogen, resulting in a metabolic alkalosis, which prompts the kidneys to try to conserve hydrogen by increasing their output of potassium.

Gaining weight

Some athletes can gain weight just by forcing themselves to eat when they are not hungry. However, much of their weight gain is fat, and force-feeding tends to elevate blood fat levels, which can increase susceptibility to coronary artery disease in later life.

Although most sedentary people store extra fat when they eat more food than they need, many competitive athletes do not. First, vigorous exercise that is required for competitive sports suppresses appetite far more than less intense exercise of shorter duration (Oscai 1973). Second, a vigorous exercise program can increase thermogenesis markedly (Stern & Lowney 1986). Furthermore, there is no evidence that eating when not hungry will cause an athlete to grow large muscles.

The only effective way to gain lean body mass is to exercise muscles against progressively greater resistance. To grow large muscles, athletes also need to ingest 1.5 g of protein per kg each day (Paul 1989). This can be accomplished by most athletes without paying particular attention to protein needs (Table 9.3). Physicians and coaches should avoid recommending a high-protein diet. Eating large amounts of protein could limit carbohydrate intake and decrease endurance during workouts and recovery from them.

Table 9.3 A 50 kg adolescent needs 75 g of protein

	Protein (g)
1 chicken breast (4 oz)	25
4 cups of milk	36
6 oz can of tuna	48
1 cup dried beans	14
1 cup peanuts	37
3 oz salmon	17
3 oz hamburger	25

CHRONIC FATIGUE IN ATHLETES

Competitive athletes often reach a point in their training when they feel tired and can't get through their workouts. Outdated texts claim that tiredness is caused by low mineral levels and recommend that athletes eat lots of fruit for potassium, nuts for magnesium, and salt tablets for sodium. However, healthy athletes can suffer from lack of salt, but they rarely suffer from deficiencies of potassium, magnesium or calcium. Viruses and other infectious agents will certainly cause athletes to feel fatigued, but most of the time, chronic fatigue in athletes is caused by muscle damage.

Athletes train by taking a very hard workout on one day, which causes minute tears in muscle fibers and makes them feel sore on the next day. They are then supposed to take easy workouts until the soreness disappears. However, many athletes are so obsessed with training that they attempt hard workouts before their muscles have recovered. This prevents muscle fibers from adequately storing muscle sugar for fuel, so they contract with less force and tire earlier. If athletes continue to train intensely, either their muscles stay sore and fatigued for several days and weeks or these tear the muscles completely. Exhaustion then forces rest. Exhausted competitive athletes should check with their doctors, and if no cause is found, they should stop training for a few weeks.

CONCLUSIONS

Child athletes should follow the same rules of eating as recommended for adults. Healthy children should be encouraged to eat as much food as they want because it takes tremendous amounts of food to supply energy for training and tissue repair. Eating extra carbohydrates after hard exercise has been shown to hasten recovery. No extract of food is more healthful than that food, so it is nonsensical to think that protein supplements taken from food offer any advantage over milk, soy, tuna or any other protein source. There is no evidence that vitamins extracted from food, or chemical copies of natural vitamins, offer any advantage over taking vitamins in food. Several disturbing studies have shown that large doses of vitamins E or beta-carotene pills increase the risk of heart attacks and cancer. Except for common table salt, athletes rarely suffer from deficiencies of minerals unless they lack iron from bleeding, or calcium from excessive protein intake.

Since almost all foods are loaded with potassium, lack of that mineral is not a concern for athletes.

Some children may want to lose weight. They should do this by increasing training, rather than restricting total food intake. Children with diabetes or lipid abnormalities should follow the recommendations of their physicians, but restriction of calories will result in a deterioration of training and prevent them from reaching their maximum efficiency on the playing field. Maximum endurance comes from starting an event with liver and muscles loaded with glycogen and this cannot be accomplished without eating 3 h or less before an event. Fasting before competing causes early fatigue. Child athletes can maintain endurance by drinking fluids of choice and eating heavily salted foods during their event. Recovery is hastened by eating as soon as the athlete finishes competition.

REFERENCES

Allison D B, Egan S K, Barraj L M, Caughman C, Infante M, Heimbach T 1999 Estimated intakes of trans fatty and other fatty acids in the US population. Journal of the American Dietetic Association 99(2): 166–174

Åstrand P O 1968 Something old and something new – very new. Nutrition Today 3(2): 9

Banks W J 1977 Myoglobinuria in marathon runners: possible relationship to carbohydrate and lipid metabolism. Annals of the New York Academy of Sciences 301: 942

Bray G A, Popkin B M 1998 Dietary fat intake does affect obesity. American Journal of Clinical Nutrition 68(6): 1157–1173

Bucci L 1993 Nutrients as ergogenic aids for sports and exercise. CRC Press, Ann Arbor, MI

Casoni I, Guglielmini C, Graziano L, Reali M G, Mazzotta D, Abbasciano V 1990 Changes of magnesium concentrations in endurance athletes. International Journal of Sports Medicine 11: 234–237

Christensen E H, Hansen O 1939 Hypoglykamie, Arbeitsfahigkeit und Ermudung. Scandinavian Archives of Physiology 81: 172

Costill D, Sherman W M, Fink W J, Maresh C, Witten M, Miller J M 1981 The role of dietary carbohydrates in muscle glycogen resynthesis after strenuous running. American Journal of Clinical Nutrition 34: 1831–1836

Costill D L, Saltin B 1974 Factors limiting gastric emptying during rest and exercise. Journal of Applied Physiology 37: 679

Costill D L, Cote R, Fink W J et al 1981 Muscle water and electrolyte distribution during prolonged exercise. International Journal of Sports Medicine 3: 130

Felig P, Cherif A, Minagawa A et al 1982 Hypoglycemia during prolonged exercise in normal men. New England Journal of Medicine 306: 895

Fielding R A, Costill D A, Fink D S, King M, Hargreaves M, Kovaleski J E 1985 Effect of carbohydrate feeding frequencies and dosage on muscle glycogen use during exercise. Medicine and Science in Sports Exercise 17(4): 472–476

Finch C A, Gollnick P D, Hlastala M P et al 1979 Lactic acidosis as a result of iron deficiency. Journal of Clinical Investigations 64: 129–137

Gamble J L 1958 Chemical anatomy physiology and pathology of extracellular fluid: a lecture syllabus. Harvard University Press, Cambridge, MA

Green H J 1991 How important is endogenous muscle glycogen to fatigue in prolonged exercise? Canadian Journal of Physiology and Pharmacology 69: 290–297

Greenleaf J E, Looft-Wilson R, Wisherd J L et al 1998 Hypervolemia in men from fluid ingestion at rest and during exercise. Aviation Space and Environmental Medicine 69(4): 374–386

Grisdale J 1990 Relative effects of glycogen depletion and previous exercise on muscle force and endurance capacity. Applied Physiology 69(4): 1276–1282

Hargreaves M, Costill D L, Cogan A et al 1981 Effects of carbohydrate feeding on muscle glycogen utilization and exercise performance. Medicine and Science in Sports Exercise 16: 219

Hultman E, Nilson L H 1971 Liver glycogen in man: effect of different diets on muscular exercise. In Saltin B, Pernow B (eds) Muscle metabolism during exercise. Plenum, New York, p 143–163

Ivy J L, Katz A L, Cutler C L, Sherman W M, Coyle E F 1988a Muscle glycogen synthesis after exercise: effect of time on carbohydrate ingestion. Journal of Applied Physiology 64: 1480–1485

Ivy J L, Lee M C, Brozinick J T and Reed M J 1988b Muscle glycogen storage after different amounts of carbohydrate ingestion. Journal of Applied Physiology 65: 2018–2023

Jenkins D J A, Kendall C W C, Vidgen E et al 1999 Health aspects of partially defatted flaxseed, including effects on serum lipids, oxidative measures, and ex vivo androgen and progestin activity: a controlled crossover trial. American Journal of Clinical Nutrition 69(3): 395–402

Karlsson J, Nordesjo L O, Saltin B 1974 Muscle glycogen utilization during exercise after physical training. Acta Physiologica Scandinavica 90: 210

Koletzko B, Decsi T 1997 Metabolic aspects of trans fatty acids. Clinical Nutrition 16(5): 229–237

Kosich D, Conlee R, Fischer A G et al 1986 The effects of exercise and a low-fat diet or a moderate-fat diet on selected coronary risk factors. In: Dotson C, Humphrey J (eds) Exercise physiology: current selected research, vol 2. AMS Press, New York, p 173

Kristal-Boneh E, Glusman J G, Chaemovitz C, Canuto Y 1988 Improved thermoregulation caused by forced water intake in human desert dwellers. European Journal of Applied Physiology 57: 220–224

Krzentowski G, Prinary F, Luyckx A S et al 1984 Effect of physical training on utilization of a glucose load given orally during exercise. American Journal of Physiology 246: E412

Ludwig D S, Majzoub J A, Al-Zahrania A, Dallal G E, Blanco I, Roberts S B 1999 High glycemic index foods, overeating and obesity. Pediatrics 103(3): e26–39

Massicotte D, Peronnet F, Brisson G, Bakkouch K, Hillaire-Marcel C 1989 Oxidation of a glucose polymer during exercise: comparison with glucose and fructose. Journal of Applied Physiology 66(1): 179–183

Maughan R J, Lambert C P 1991 Effects of beverage temperature on the appearance of a deuterium tracer in the blood. Medicine and Science in Sports Exercise 23(4): S84

McArthur K E, Feldman M 1989 Gastric acid secretion, gastric release and gastric emptying in humans as affected by liquid meal temperature. American Journal of Clinical Nutrition 89: 51–54

Mangum J, Gatch W, Cocke T B, Brooks E 1986 The effect of beer consumption on the physiological responses to submaximal exercise. Journal of Sports Medicine and Physical Fitness 26(3): 301–305

Miller W C, Linderman A K, Wallace J, Niederman M 1990 Diet composition, energy intake, and exercise in relation to body fat in men and women. American Journal of Clinical Nutrition 52: 426–430

Mirkin G B 1973 Carbohydrate loading: a dangerous practice. Journal of the American Medical Association 223: 1511

Mirkin G B 1983 Food and nutrition for exercise. In: Bove A A, Lowenthal D T (eds) Exercise medicine: physiological principles and clinical applications. Academic Press, New York

Moore J G, Datz F L, Christian B S 1990 Exercise increases solid meal gastric emptying in men. Digestive Diseases and Sciences 35(4): 428–432

Murray R, Eddy D E, Paul G L, Seifert J G, Halaby G A 1991 Physiological responses to glycerol ingestion during exercise. Journal of Applied Physiology 71(1): 144–149

Oscai L B 1973 The role of exercise in weight control. In: Wilmore J H (ed) Exercise and Sport Sciences Reviews, vol 1. Academic Press, New York, p 103

Passe D H, Horn M, Murray R 1997 The effects of beverage carbonation on sensory responses and voluntary fluid intake following exercise. International Journal of Sport Nutrition 7(4): 286–297

Paul G L 1989 Dietary protein requirements in physically active individuals. Sports Medicine 8: 154–176

Piehl K 1974 Time course for refilling of glycogen stores in human muscle fibers following exercise-induced glycogen depletion. Acta Physiologica Scandinavica 90: 297–302

Rehrer N J, Brouns F, Beckers E J, ten Hoor F, Saris W H M 1990 Gastric emptying with repeated drinking during running and bicycling. International Journal of Sports Medicine 11: 238–243

Schneider H, Brouns F, Saris W H M 1991 A rationale for electrolyte replacement during endurance exercise. Medicine and Science in Sports Exercise 23(4): 768–773

Sherman W M, Costill D L, Fink W et al 1981 The role of dietary carbohydrates in muscle glycogen resynthesis after strenuous running. American Journal of Clinical Nutrition 34: 1831–1836

Simonsen N, Fernandez Crehuet Navajas J, Martin-Moreno J M et al 1998a Tissue Stores of individual mono-unsaturated fatty acids and breast cancer: the EURAMIC Study. American Journal of Clinical Nutrition 68: 134–141

Simonsen N, van't veer P, Strain J J et al 1998b Adipose tissue omega-3 and omega-6 fatty acid content and breast cancer in the EURAMIC study. American Journal of Epidemiology 147(4): 342–352

Solomons N W 1986 Competitive interaction of iron and zinc in the diet: consequences for human nutrition. Journal of Nutrition 116: 926–935

Stern J S, Lowney P 1986 Obesity: the role of physical activity. In: Brownell K D, Foreyt J P (eds) Handbook of eating disorders: physiology, psychology, and the treatment of obesity, anorexia, and bulimia. Basic Books, New York, p 145

Tsintzas K, Williams C 1998 Human muscle glycogen metabolism during exercise: effect of carbohydrate supplementation. Sports Medicine 25(1): 7–23

Weller E, Bachert P, Meinck H M et al 1998 Lack of effect of oral Mg-Supplementation on Mg in serum, blood cells, and calf muscle. Medicine and Science in Sports Exercise 30(11): 1584–1594

10

Growth and maturation issues in elite young athletes: normal variation and training

Adam D. G. Baxter-Jones
Robert M. Malina

KEY POINTS

1. There is very wide variation amongst children in size, physique and body composition, in rate of growth, and in the timing and tempo of biological maturation at any given age.
2. There is similar variation in the growth and maturity characteristics observed among young athletes.
3. Successful young athletes are a highly selected group in terms of skill, size and physique, and socioeconomic status.
4. Comparison of young athletes with reference data for the general population indicate that, in general, young athletes grow and mature in a similar manner to non-athletes, allowing for variation among sports.
5. Observed short stature and decreased body mass in some elite young athletes (primarily gymnasts of both sexes, with less data for figure skaters) are likely to reflect the selection practices of specific sports that focus on presumably desirable physical and maturational characteristics.
6. It is difficult to attribute the observed variation in the growth and maturation of young athletes to the effects of training. The presently available data do not meet the criteria for causality, and many factors which are known to influence growth and maturation are ordinarily not considered in studies of young athletes.

INTRODUCTION

Parents, coaches, sport administrators, and sports medicine practitioners often show considerable interest in the growth and maturation of children and adolescents involved in sport. This interest has its basis in several perspectives. The primary concern is that of the child's health and well-being, and therefore measures of growth and maturation are routinely accepted as indicators of health and nutritional status. Secondly, there is an interest in physical characteristics associated with success in some sports and in identifying these characteristics at an early age in youngsters who may have the potential for success. Thirdly, there is an interest in the influence of regular training for sport on growth and maturation. Claims of both positive and negative influences of intensive training for sport on the growing and maturing individual have been expressed.

As young people grow, they also mature and develop. They experience three interacting processes: growth, maturation and development. Often, these terms are treated as the same. Yet, they are three distinctive tasks in the daily lives of children and youth for approximately the first two decades of life (Malina & Bouchard 1991).

Growth refers to the increase in the size of the body as a whole and of its parts. Thus, as children grow, they become taller and heavier, they increase in lean and fat tissues, their organs increase in size, and so on. Heart volume and mass, for example, follow a growth pattern similar to that for body weight, while the lungs and lung functions in normal healthy children grow proportionally to height. Different parts of the body grow at different rates and at different times. This results in changes in body proportions. The legs, for example, grow faster than the trunk during childhood. Hence, the child becomes relatively longer-legged.

Maturation refers to progress towards the biologically mature state. It is an operational concept because the mature state varies with body systems. Maturation differs from growth in that, although biological systems mature at different rates, all individuals reach the same end-point and become fully mature. In contrast, there may be wide variations in growth endpoints, i.e. adult stature, physique, and so on. Studies of growing children commonly focus on sexual and skeletal maturation. Maturation, i.e. the process of maturing, has two components: timing and tempo. The former refers to when specific maturational events occur, e.g. age at the beginning of breast development in girls, age at the appearance of pubic hair in boys and girls, or age at maximum growth during the adolescent growth spurt. Tempo refers to the rate at which maturation progresses, e.g. how quickly or slowly the youngster passes from the initial stages of sexual maturation to the mature state. Timing and tempo vary considerably among individuals.

Development refers to the acquisition of behavioral competence, i.e. the learning of appropriate behavior expected by society, and is culture-specific. As children experience life at home, school, church, sports, recreation, and other community activities, they develop cognitively, socially, emotionally, morally, and so on. They are learning to behave in a culturally appropriate manner.

It is important to recognize that the three processes – growth, maturation and development – occur simultaneously and interact. They proceed in concert, but may operate on different timescales. These processes interact to influence the child's self-concept, self-esteem, body image, and perceived competence. The demands of specific sports are superimposed upon those associated with normal growth, maturation and development. A mismatch between the demands of a sport and those of normal growth, maturation and development may be a source of stress among elite young athletes.

The focus of this chapter is normal variation in growth and maturation and the potential influence of training for sport on these processes. Growth and maturation are characterized by individual variation both between and within sexes. Although under genetic and neuroendocrine control, growth and maturation may also be influenced by environmental factors (Bouchard et al 1997, Malina & Bouchard 1991, Tanner 1962).

Physical activity, especially as in intensive training for sport, is often indicated as one such environmental factor. Although widely discussed and to a lesser extent systematically investigated, its exact role is still to be confirmed. Nevertheless, concern is periodically expressed about potential negative influences of intensive training on the growth and maturation of elite young athletes in some sports, especially females (Baxter-Jones & Helms 1996, Malina 1998a).

GROWTH AND MATURATION
Growth

Normal growth is in general a very regular process and refers to increase in size, either of the body as a whole or of its parts. Stature and weight (mass) are the two body dimensions most commonly used to monitor the growth of children and adolescents. With age, children are expected to become taller and heavier. The growth status (size attained at a given age) and progress (rate of growth) of a child are usually monitored by making comparisons with reference percentiles (Freeman et al 1995, Malina & Bouchard 1991, Tanner 1989). These are based on cross-sectional data derived from large, representative samples of children from infancy to young adulthood. Such charts are useful for comparison or for the assessment of growth status of a child or a sample of children at a given age or across several ages. However, growth rates are not linear during childhood and adolescence, so that interpretation may at times be difficult.

Size at birth is determined largely by the intrauterine environment. Linear growth velocity rapidly decelerates from birth to 2 years (approximately 9 cm/year) and from 2 to 5 years (approximately 7 cm/year). Linear growth then continues on average at approximately 5–8 cm/year until the onset of puberty (the terms 'puberty' and 'adolescence' are used interchangeably). The typical girl is slightly shorter than the typical boy at all ages until adolescence. By about 9–10 years in girls and 11–12 years in boys, the rate of growth in height begins to increase. This marks the beginning of the adolescent growth spurt, a period of rapid growth highly variable among individuals. The rate of growth increases until it reaches a peak (age at maximum growth increment or peak height velocity [PHV]); then it gradually decreases and growth in height eventually stops. Girls, on average, start their growth spurts, reach PHV, and stop growing about 2 years earlier than boys. Nevertheless, when the growth spurt starts, when PHV is reached, and when growth stops are quite variable among individuals.

Statural gain from birth to adulthood can be viewed as a form of motion where the increase in height between these two time periods is the distance travelled and height gain per year represents the speed of the journey. The rate of growth, therefore, reflects the child's state at any particular time better than does the distance achieved or size attained.

The growth spurt in body mass begins slightly later than that of stature. Body mass is a composite measure of many body tissues. It is most often partitioned in terms of its lean (fat-free) and fat components. Thus, body mass is the sum of fat-free mass (FFM) and fat mass (FM). FFM has a growth pattern like that for body mass and there is a clear adolescent spurt. FM increases more gradually during childhood and adolescence.

Box 10.1 Guidelines for expected changes in height, weight and body composition during childhood and adolescence. (Based on materials reported in Malina & Bouchard 1991)

Pre-adolescence (about 6–10 years of age)
Children are expected to grow, i.e. increase in weight and height. Although there is much variation among individuals, children gain, on average, about 5–8 cm/year and about 2–3 kg/year between 6 and 10 years of age. As adolescence and puberty begin, growth rates increase, first in height and then in weight.

Adolescence
Adolescence is characterized by the growth spurt and sexual maturation. It is a time of considerable variation in terms of when events occur (timing) and the rate at which children pass through them (tempo). The following highlights general trends that characterize the growth spurt:
- Girls
  — begins around 9–10 years
  — reaches maximum around 12 years
  — growth rate then slows, but growth continues to about 16–18 years.
- Boys
  — begins around 11–12 years
  — reaches maximum around 14 years
  — growth rate then slows, but growth continues to about 18–20 years.
- Growth in height continues into the early 20s in some girls and in many boys.
- There is considerable variation among individuals in
  — timing: when the adolescent spurt occurs
  — tempo: rate of progress through the spurt.
- Body weight, fat-free mass, and muscle mass also show adolescent spurts; they occur, on average, several months after the maximum rate of growth (peak height velocity) in height.
- During the interval of maximum growth in height (about 11–13 years in girls and 13–15 years in boys), girls gain about 7 kg in fat-free mass while boys gain double this value, 14 kg; girls gain a bit more fat than boys during the interval of the growth spurt, 3 vs. 1.5 kg.

Guidelines for expected changes in stature, mass and body composition are shown in Box 10.1. Other body dimensions follow growth patterns that are generally similar to those for stature and mass.

Maturation

Biological maturation differs fundamentally from the measurement of growth in that every child completes it by becoming fully mature. Maturation refers to the timing and tempo (rate) of progress to the mature state. It is most often viewed in the context of skeletal

(skeletal age), sexual (secondary sex characteristics) and somatic (age at PHV) maturation (Beunen & Malina 1996, Malina & Beunen 1996, Malina & Bouchard 1991). The processes of growth and maturation are intimately linked as differential growth creates form.

Maturation of the skeleton focuses on the bones of the hand and wrist, which generally reflect the remainder of the skeleton. A plain radiograph of the hand and wrist is needed to assess skeletal maturation. As such, the method may have limited utility outside of a clinical setting. Several different methods are available to assess the skeletal maturity of the hand and wrist, and they do not all provide equivalent estimates (Malina & Bouchard 1991). Skeletal maturation, nevertheless, is a valuable tool that is useful throughout childhood and adolescence. It is also used along with height at a given age to predict adult height.

Somatic (body) maturation is based on the timing of the growth spurt in height, i.e. the inflection in the growth curve leading to maximum growth in height during adolescence (PHV). It is available only in longitudinal studies in which the height of the individual is measured on a regular basis from about 9 through 16–17 years of age. Although this indicator of maturation is valuable, it has limited utility unless good longitudinal data are available. This is important because many studies of young athletes are short-term and rarely span the entire period of the adolescent spurt. Hence, estimates of the age at PHV may be of limited utility.

The most obvious feature of biological maturation during adolescence is puberty or sexual maturation. The first overt sign of sexual maturation in girls is usually the initial development of the breasts, followed by the appearance of pubic hair. The first overt sign of sexual maturation in boys, on average, is the initial enlargement of the testes, followed by the appearance of pubic hair. Each of these secondary sex characteristics goes through a series of changes as the individual passes through puberty to maturity (Malina & Bouchard 1991, Tanner 1962). They are usually assessed at clinical examination, although self-administered scales are being increasingly used in the sport and exercise literature (Malina & Beunen 1996). The assessment of secondary sex characteristics requires invasion of the adolescent's privacy at a time of life when the youngster is learning to cope with the physiological changes that are occurring. Hence, monitoring of these characteristics requires utmost care and sensitivity toward the youngster involved.

Age at menarche, the first menstrual period, is limited to girls. Male puberty has no corresponding, overt physiological event. Menarcheal status (i.e. whether or not menarche has occurred) and age at menarche in individual girls can be obtained with a careful and sensitive interview. At times it may be appropriate to interview the girl's mother to obtain this information. In addition, familial effects can be investigated by obtaining information with regard to the mother's own age of onset (Baxter-Jones et al 1994, Malina et al 1994). The normal range of variation for the occurrence of menarche is 9 through 17 years of age. Estimated median ages at menarche for European girls from the mid-1960s through the 1980s range between 12.5 and 13.5 years (with two exceptions). There is a geographic gradient in the distribution of menarcheal ages within Europe; median ages decline from the north to the south. The estimate for girls in the United States is 12.8 years (Eveleth & Tanner 1990).

Guidelines for ranges of normal variation in sexual maturation are summarized in Box 10.2. It is important that physicians and sports medicine personnel be aware of such variation as well as the significance of sexual maturation for physical growth and behavioral development. Sexual maturation in boys is accompanied by marked gains in muscle mass and strength, and broadening of the shoulders relative to the hips. In girls, it is accompanied by smaller gains in muscle mass and strength, by a widening of the hips relative to the shoulders, and by gains in fatness. The net result is sex differences in strength, physique and body composition in late adolescence and young adulthood. Sexual maturation also influences behavioral development, e.g. increased self-consciousness about overt manifestation of sexual maturation, concern with weight gain in girls, relationships with the opposite sex, and so on.

PHYSICAL PERFORMANCE

Sports demand a variety of physical performances, and young athletes are characterized by highly skilful performances that are specific to their respective sports. As such, it is difficult to compare athletes in different sports, or athletes and non-athletes. Nevertheless, the outcomes of the performance of tasks done under specified conditions are commonly used in growth studies to document changes associated with growth and maturation. Examples of such tasks include the distance or height jumped (power), the distance a ball is thrown (power and coordination), the time elapsed in completing a 30 m dash (speed) or a shuttle run (speed and agility), the number of sit-ups performed in 20 s (abdominal strength), the force expressed against a fixed resistance (strength), power

Box 10.2 Guidelines for normal variation in sexual maturation. (Based on materials in Malina & Bouchard, 1991)

Girls
- The first overt sign of sexual maturation of girls is the initial enlargement of the breasts, which occurs, on average, at about 10 years of age, but may occur before 9 years in about 10% of girls, and not until after 12 years in another 10%.
- Pubic hair tends to appear at the same time or shortly after initial enlargement of the breasts, but in some girls it may appear before breast development begins.
- Mature breast and pubic hair development occurs, on average, between 14 and 15 years of age. However, maturity may occur as early as 12 years in some girls and not until 16 or 17 years in others.
- Progress from initial to mature breast or pubic hair development is highly variable among girls. Some girls may pass through the process in 2 years, while others may take 5 or more years.
- Menarche, the first menstrual period, is a rather late maturational event of puberty. It ordinarily occurs after maximum growth in height (peak height velocity).

Boys
- Initial enlargement of the genitals (testes and penis) marks the first overt sign of sexual maturation in boys. It occurs, on average, at about 11 years of age, but may occur around 9 years in about 10% of boys, and not until after 13 years in another 10%.
- Pubic hair tends to appear at the same time or shortly after initial enlargement of the genitals, but in some boys it may appear before genital development begins.
- Mature genital and pubic hair development occurs, on average, at about 15 years of age. However, maturity may occur as early as 13 years and after 18 years of age.
- Progress from initial to mature genital and pubic hair development is highly variable among boys. Some boys may pass through the process in 2 years, while others may take about 5 or more years.

off or improve slightly or more gradually. The overall pattern of age- and sex-associated changes in a variety of performance tasks during childhood and adolescence is summarized in Box 10.3. The trends are based on group averages. Girls can improve their performances through adolescence, and instruction and practice are important contributing factors. Further, the sex difference in the performances of elite young athletes within the same sport (e.g. diving) is not as great as that between non-athlete boys and girls (Eisenmann et al 1999, Geithner et al 1999a, Klika & Malina 1999).

Box 10.3 Guidelines for changes in physical performance during childhood and adolescence. (Based on materials reported in Malina & Bouchard 1991)

- Performances in tasks requiring strength, power, speed, endurance, agility, and coordination tend to increase with age. Sex differences are relatively small on most tasks during middle childhood.
- With the onset of the adolescent growth spurt, most performance items show an accelerated rate of development, more so in boys than in girls. In many tasks, performances of girls increase, but not to the same magnitude as those in boys. As a result, sex differences in performance are magnified.
- In contrast to performance items, flexibility tends to decline from childhood until the early stages of the adolescent spurt, and then increases in later adolescence. Girls are more flexible than boys at all ages. Flexibility tends to be joint-specific, and flexibility exercises (stretching) may have the potential to offset the decline noted with age.
- Performance tasks also show well-defined adolescent spurts in boys. Static strength (arm pull), power (vertical jump) and functional strength (flexed arm hang) show peak gains after peak height velocity, while flexibility (sit and reach), speed and agility (shuttle run) and speed of arm movement (plate tapping) show peak gains before peak height velocity.
- Arm strength shows peak gain after maximum growth in height in girls, but the peak gain in strength is only about one-half of that in boys. Data on growth spurts in other performances of girls show peak velocities of growth in the standing long jump and medicine ball throw (power) after peak height velocity, and in the dash (speed) and shuttle run (speed and agility) before peak height velocity.
- Power output at a heart rate of 170 beats per minute (PWC$_{170}$) and maximal aerobic power ($\dot{V}O_{2\,max}$) show an adolescent spurt in boys and girls. The spurts occur at about the same time as the adolescent growth spurt in height in boys. The spurt in $\dot{V}O_{2\,max}$ occurs at peak height velocity in girls, but that in PWC$_{170}$ occurs later.

output at a heart rate of 170 beats/min (PWC$_{170}$), and maximal aerobic power ($\dot{V}O_{2\,max}$).

Data are available for a number of tasks which provide a good indicator of how performances change with age from childhood through adolescence. Performances improve with age during childhood, and boys perform, on average, better than girls. There is considerable overlap between the sexes during childhood. With the onset of adolescence, the performances of boys show an acceleration, while those of girls improve up to about 14–15 years of age, and then level

Performances during adolescence are influenced by individual differences in the timing of the adolescent growth spurt. In boys, performances in a variety of tasks show well-defined adolescent spurts relative to PHV. Measures of static strength (grip, arm pull), power (vertical jump), and functional strength (flexed arm hang) show their peak gains, on average, after PHV (Beunen et al 1988). At PHV, boys become stronger in the quadriceps and biceps in proportion to body size (Nevill et al 1998). On the other hand, measures of speed and agility (shuttle run), speed of arm movement (as in the number of times two plates, 20 cm in diameter and separated by 60 cm, are tapped in 20 s), and lower back flexibility (sit and reach) show their peak gains before PHV (Beunen et al 1988). The trends for measures of strength and power are similar in timing to those for body mass and muscle mass, both of which experience their maximum growth after PHV. The earlier adolescent spurts for running speed and lower back flexibility may be related to growth of the lower extremities. Height comprises the legs, trunk, neck and head, and the legs experience maximum growth first. Thus, boys have relatively longer legs for their height early in the adolescent spurt, and this may influence running speed and lower trunk flexibility.

With regard to aerobic power development in boys undergoing systematic training in sport, age, height and weight contribute to changes in $\dot{V}O_{2\,max}$ over time, but there is also a significant positive independent effect of puberty (Baxter-Jones et al 1993). It has been inferred that this pubertal effect may be due to higher haemoglobin concentrations and greater muscle mass as boys mature.

Data relating performances of girls to the adolescent spurt are limited largely to strength. Girls show an adolescent spurt in static strength of the arm after PHV, but this trend is not consistent across studies. The magnitude of the adolescent spurt in strength in girls, however, is only about one-half of the maximum adolescent gain in boys (Beunen & Malina 1988). Trends for Spanish girls based on a mixed-longitudinal design show peak velocities of growth in the standing long jump and medicine ball throw (power) after PHV, and in the dash (speed) and shuttle run (speed and agility) before PHV (Heras Yague & de la Fuente 1998). These trends are consistent with observations for boys. In contrast to boys, however, sexual maturation does not seem to independently influence the development of $\dot{V}O_{2\,max}$ in girls (Baxter-Jones et al 1993). When performances of girls are related to the time before and after menarche, there are no consistent trends. Menarche is a late maturational event which occurs after PHV. Major gains in growth and performance have already occurred.

GROWTH AND MATURITY STATUS OF YOUNG ATHLETES

In considering the maturity status of athletes, it should be kept in mind that the analyses are beset with a number of difficulties. The definition of what constitutes a young athlete is often vague and includes a wide variety in age groups, skill and competitive levels. Young athletes are also a highly select group with regard to skill and performance levels. Size and physique are likely to have important interactions with skill and performance, as are many other factors in the child's environment. Many studies of young athletes, however, include youth who can be classified as select, elite, or junior national caliber (Malina 1994, 1998a).

Body size

Trends in the mean heights and weights of athletes in a variety of sports are summarized in Table 10.1. Young athletes of both sexes in a variety of sports have, on average, statures that equal or exceed reference medians from childhood through adolescence. Gymnastics is the only sport that consistently presents a profile of short stature in both sexes. More recent samples of elite female gymnasts are, on average, shorter than those of 20 years ago (Malina 1997). Figure skaters of both sexes also present shorter statures, on average, although data are not extensive. Female ballet dancers tend to have shorter statures during childhood and early adolescence, but catch up to non-dancers in late adolescence.

Body mass presents a similar pattern with several exceptions. Young athletes in a variety of sports tend to have body masses that, on average, equal or exceed the reference medians. Gymnasts, figure skaters and ballet dancers of both sexes consistently show lighter body mass. Gymnasts and figure skaters have appropriate mass-for-height, while ballet dancers have low mass-for-height. A similar trend is indicated in female distance runners.

Physique

Physique is a often a selective factor in sport. Physique, or body build, refers to the configuration of the entire body as opposed to emphasis on specific

Table 10.1 Heights and weights of young athletes relative to percentiles (P) of United States reference values. (Adapted from Malina 1998a)

Sport	Males		Females	
	Stature	Weight	Stature	Weight
Basketball	P 50 to >P 90	P 50 to >P 90	P 75 to >P 90	P 50–P 75
Volleyball			P 75	P 50–P 75
Soccer	P 50±	P 50±	P 50	P 50
Ice hockey	P 50±	P 50		
Distance runs	P 50±	≤P 50	≥P 50	<P 50
Sprints	≥P 50	≥P 50	≥P 50	≤P 50
Swimming	P 50–P 90	>P 50–P 75	P 50–P 90	P 50–P 75
Diving	<P 50	≤P 50	≤P 50	P 50
Gymnastics	≤P 10–P 25	≤P 10–P 25	≤P 10 to <P 50	P 10 to <P 50[a]
Tennis	P 50±	≥P 50	>P 50	P 50±
Figure skating	P 10–P 25	P 10–P 25	P 10 to <P 50	P 10 to <P 50
Ballet	<P 50	P 10–P 50	≤P 50	P 10–<P 50

[a] More recent samples of gymnasts are closer to P 10.

features. Assessment of physique focuses on external dimensions and characteristics of the body. It is most often quantified as somatotype, which is defined by the contributions of endomorphy (roundness of contours, fatness), mesomorphy (dominance of muscular and skeletal development), and ectomorphy (linearity). The three components together describe the individual's physique. Treating a component of somatotype independent of the other two, or without statistically controlling for the other two, is not correct.

Athletes in a given sport tend to have reasonably similar somatotypes and also to show a more limited range of variability compared with the general population (Carter & Heath 1990). With the exception of throwing events in track and field, and the higher weight categories in weight-lifting and related activities, endomorphy is rather low in most athletes and mesomorphy is well developed, while ectomorphy is more variable. Data for early adolescent and adolescent athletes (about 12–18 years of age) suggest that those who are successful tend to have, on average, somatotypes that are similar to adult athletes in the respective sports (Carter 1988, Geithner & Malina 1993). As in adult athletes, somatotypic variation is smaller among younger athletes compared with the general population of youth. Young athletes tend to be less endomorphic, particularly females, less mesomorphic and more ectomorphic than adult athletes. The latter, of course, reflects the role of growth in the transition from late adolescence into young adulthood.

Physique is also a significant contributor to success in many sports, and may be of particular importance in aesthetic sports. Performance scores in subjectively evaluated sports, such as gymnastics, figure skating and diving, may be influenced by the athlete's physique as perceived by the judges. For example, in a sample of elite gymnasts participating in the 1987 World Championships Artistic Gymnastics (Rotterdam), about 41% of the variance in the total competition score could be explained by endomorphy (negative coefficient) and chronological age (positive coefficient) (Claessens et al 1999). The positive influence of chronological age suggests an important role for experience in international competition. On the other hand, the negative effect of endomorphy is more difficult to explain. It may reflect a real influence of endomorphy on performance, or perhaps a negative perception of endomorphy by gymnastics judges, or some combination of the two factors. Mean endomorphy in this international sample of elite gymnasts is uniformly low and homogeneous in the age range 13–20 years, ranging from 1.4 to 1.9 (Claessens et al 1992), which markedly contrasts the trend toward increasing endomorphy with age across adolescence in non-athlete females. Among a national sample of Flemish girls, mean endomorphy increases from 2.9 at 10 years of age to 4.1 at 18 years of age (A L Claessens, personal communication). Thus, it may be difficult to detect a negative influence of such low endomorphy on competition scores. The issue of the perception of fatness or endomorphy by gymnastics judges, or the aesthetic demands of the sport which place an emphasis on petiteness and leanness, should perhaps be systematically addressed. This, of course, has relevance for the health of young gymnasts, many of whom are in negative energy balance in an attempt to limit weight gain and fat accumulation when the normal course of growth, and especially sexual maturation, is to gain in both.

A similar trend is suggested for elite young divers. In a sample of 121 male and 151 female Junior Olympic divers aged 11–18 years, observed in 1991 and 1992, 12 males and 17 females were identified as eventually successful in national and international competitions. In their youth, the successful female divers were more muscular (greater estimated arm and calf muscle circumferences) and had less relative fatness and lower endomorphy than those who were not successful. Females divers as a group are higher in endomorphy than gymnasts, mean values ranging from 2.5 to 3.5 among divers aged 11–18 years (Geithner & Malina 1993). In contrast, the successful male divers were shorter and lighter, lower in ectomorphy and higher in mesomorphy, and had relatively broad shoulders compared with those who were not successful (Geithner et al 1999b).

The results of these two analyses suggest a need for further study of the influence of the selective criteria of specific sports and perhaps the judging criteria on the physique and body composition of young competitors. Undue emphasis on leanness can potentially have a negative influence on the health of the young athletes, in particular females. The same applies to other sports in which coaches and/or the sport system place undue emphasis on fatness in female athletes, e.g. distance running, ballet, swimming, and so on.

Maturation

Information on the maturity status and progress of young athletes is not as extensive as that for stature and mass. Maturity differences are most apparent during the transition into adolescence and the adolescent spurt, and reflect extreme individuality in timing and tempo of maturation.

Male athletes in a variety of sports, with few exceptions, tend to be average (on time for chronological age, i.e. skeletal age is within ±1 year of chronological age) or advanced in biological maturation (skeletal age is in advance of chronological age by more than 1 year). Other than gymnasts, who show later skeletal maturation, there is a striking lack of late maturing boys (skeletal age lags behind chronological age by more than 1 year) who are successful in sport during early adolescence. However, late maturing boys are often successful in some sports in later adolescence (16–18 years), e.g. track and basketball, which emphasizes the catch-up in skeletal maturation and reduced significance of maturity-associated variation in body size in the performances of boys in late adolescence (Malina 1994, 1998a).

Information on the maturity status and progress of young female athletes is not extensive, except for the age at menarche (see below). Like boys, maturity differences among young female athletes are most apparent during the transition into adolescence and the adolescent spurt, and reflect the individuality in timing and tempo of maturation. Data on skeletal age are most available for female gymnasts and swimmers, with less data for ballet dancers and track athletes. The data for track and field are to some extent confounded by event.

During childhood, gymnasts have skeletal ages that can be classified as average or on time for chronological age. As gymnasts span the age range of puberty, most gymnasts are classified as average and late, and few early maturing girls are in the samples. In later adolescence, most gymnasts are late maturing (Malina 1994). The data suggest that early and average maturing girls are systematically less represented among gymnasts as girls pass from childhood through adolescence. This trend probably reflects the selection criteria of the sport, and perhaps the performance advantage of later maturing girls in gymnastics activities. Corresponding data for secondary sex characteristics are less extensive, but are consistent with the trends in skeletal age. Although data are not as extensive as for gymnasts, female ballet dancers and distance runners show a similar maturity gradient in adolescence. In contrast, young female swimmers tend to have skeletal ages that are average or advanced in childhood and adolescence (Malina 1994, 1998a). The data for later adolescence are difficult to evaluate, because maturity status at this time is influenced by the early attainment of maturity by youth advanced in maturation and the catch-up of average and later maturing youth, i.e. all youth eventually reach skeletal and sexual maturity.

Discussions of biological maturation of female athletes focus on menarche, which is a late pubertal event. There is confusion about later ages at menarche in athletes, which is related in part to the methods of estimating age at which this indicator of maturity occurs (Malina & Beunen 1996). Age at menarche can be estimated in three ways. In longitudinal studies, girls are ordinarily examined at 3 month intervals so that interviewing the girl or her mother on each occasion can usually provide a reasonably accurate estimate of when menarche occurs. This is the prospective method. Sample sizes in prospective studies are generally small. Longitudinal studies of athletes followed from prepuberty through puberty are ordinarily short-term and limited to small, select samples; a potentially confounding issue is selective drop-out.

The status quo method provides a sample or population estimate for the age at menarche. It is a statistical method (based on probits) which requires a sample that spans approximately 9–17 years of age. Two pieces of information are needed: the exact age of each girl, and whether or not she has attained menarche. Status quo data for young athletes actively involved in systematic training provide estimates for the sample, but these samples often include athletes of different skill levels and training histories. Only prospective and status quo data deal with maturing athletes.

The vast majority of data on the age at menarche of athletes are retrospective and are based on samples of post-menarcheal late adolescent and adult athletes. Retrospective data, of course, include potential error associated with accuracy of recall.

Prospective and status quo data for adolescent athletes are summarized in Table 10.2. Retrospective data for athletes in a variety of sports are summarized elsewhere (Beunen & Malina 1996, Malina 1983, 1996, 1998b, Skierska 1998). Prospective and status quo data for gymnasts and ballet dancers, and status quo data for Junior Olympic divers and soccer players are generally consistent with the retrospective data. The limited prospective and status quo data for tennis players, rowers, and track athletes, and the more available data for age group swimmers indicate earlier mean ages at menarche than retrospective estimates for each sport, i.e. late adolescent and young adult athletes (retrospective data) in these sports tend to attain menarche later than those involved in the respective sports during the pubertal years (prospective and/or status quo data). The differences probably represent the interaction of several factors, including the longer growth period associated with later maturation, selective success and persistence of late maturing girls in some sports, selective drop-out of early maturing girls, and increased opportunity in sport at the collegiate level or older ages.

DOES REGULAR TRAINING FOR SPORT INFLUENCE GROWTH AND MATURATION?

Over the last 100 years or so, many investigators have attempted to study the effect of systematic exercise on growth. Early discussions focus on a stimulatory or accelerating influence on growth, while more recent commentaries focus on a potentially negative influence on growth and maturation. Although early studies suggested that exercise increases the rate of growth, and in particular height, in males, the results are limited. The apparent acceleration in height observed in some studies is likely to be related to early biological maturation of the young male athletes

Table 10.2 Prospective and status quo ages at menarche in samples of adolescent athletes.[a] (Adapted from Malina 1998a)

Athletes – prospective	Age (years)	Athletes – status quo	Age (years)
Gymnasts, Polish	15.1 ± 0.9	Gymnasts, world[c]	15.6 ± 2.1
Gymnasts, Swiss	14.5 ± 1.2	Gymnasts, Hungarian	15.0 ± 0.6
Gymnasts, Swedish	14.5 ± 1.4	Swimmers, age group, US	13.1 ± 1.1
Gymnasts, British[b]	14.3 ± 1.4	Swimmers, age group, US	12.7 ± 1.1
Swimmers, British	13.3 ± 1.1	Divers, Junior Olympic, US	13.6 ± 1.1
Tennis players, British	13.2 ± 1.4	Ballet dancers, Yugoslavia	13.6
Track, Polish	12.3 ± 1.1	Ballet dancers, Yugoslavia	14.1
Rowers, Polish	12.7 ± 0.9	Track, Hungarian	12.6
Elite ballet dancers, US	15.4 ± 1.9	Soccer players, age group, US	12.9 ± 1.1
		Team sports, Hungarian	12.7

[a] Prospective data report means, while status quo data report medians based on probit analysis.
[b] Among the British athletes, 13% had not yet attained menarche, so that the estimated mean ages will be somewhat older. Small numbers of Swiss and Swedish gymnasts and ballet dancers also had not reached menarche at the time of the studies.
[c] This sample is from the 1987 world championships in Rotterdam. It did not include girls under 13 years of age so that the estimate may be biased towards an older age.

studied and sampling variation rather than to the intensity of training program. More recently, the literature dealing with the potential effects of training for sport on maturation has concentrated on female athletes and, in particular, the age at which menarche is attained (Baxter-Jones et al 1994, Malina 1994, 1998b).

Physical activity is not the same as regular training. Training refers to systematic, specialized practice for a specific sport or sport discipline for most of the year, or to specific short-term experimental programs. Training programs are ordinarily specific (e.g. endurance running, strength training, sport skill training, etc.), and vary in intensity and duration.

Body size

Sport participation and training for sport have no apparent effect on growth in height and the rate of growth in height in healthy, adequately nourished children and adolescents. With few exceptions, athletes of both sexes in a variety of sports have, on average, heights that equal or exceed data for non-athletes (Table 10.1). Exceptions among athletes are gymnasts and figure skaters, participants in sports in which successful participants present shorter heights than average. This trend probably reflects the selection criteria of the sports. The smaller size of elite gymnasts is evident long before any systematic training started (Peltenburg et al 1984) and is part familial, i.e. gymnasts have parents who are shorter than average (Malina 1999). There is also a size difference between those who persist in the sport and those who drop out (Malina, 1999, Tönz et al 1990, Ziemilska 1981). Corresponding data are not available for female figure skaters, but given the emphasis on early entry into this sport, one might expect similar trends.

Short-term longitudinal studies of athletes in several sports in which the same youngsters are followed on a regular basis over time (volleyball, diving, distance running, basketball) indicate rates of growth in height that, on average, closely approximate rates observed in non-athlete children and adolescents (Malina 1994). The growth rates are well within the range of normally expected variation among youth.

In contrast to height, body mass can be influenced by regular training for sport, resulting in changes in body composition. Training is associated with a decrease in fatness in both sexes and occasionally with an increase in fat-free mass, especially in boys. Young athletes also have thinner skinfold thicknesses compared with reference samples. It should be noted that individual skinfolds change differentially during growth. This is especially evident in boys, as skinfolds on the extremities (but not those on the trunk) generally decline during adolescence. The trunk–extremity contrast is not as apparent in girls, although some extremity skinfolds may show a reduced rate of adipose tissue accumulation during adolescence. Changes in fatness depend on continued, regular activity or training (or caloric restriction, which often occurs in sports like gymnastics, ballet, figure skating and diving in girls and wrestling in boys) for their maintenance. When training is significantly reduced, fatness tends to accumulate.

It is difficult to separate specific effects of training on fat-free mass from expected changes that occur with normal growth and sexual maturation during adolescence. This is especially so in boys because they almost double their estimated fat-free mass during the adolescent growth spurt and sexual maturation (Box 10.1). Bone and skeletal muscle are major components of the fat-free mass. Short-term, high-resistance training studies of small samples indicate muscular hypertrophy in adolescent boys. Hypertrophy may not occur, or may occur to a much lesser extent, in pre-adolescent boys and girls, and in other forms of training. On the other hand, regular training during childhood and adolescence is associated with increased bone mineral content and mass. The beneficial effects are more apparent in weight-bearing (e.g. running, soccer, gymnastics) than in non-weight-bearing (e.g. swimming) activities. Of particular importance to physical activity and the integrity of skeletal tissue is the observation that bone mineral levels established during childhood and adolescence may be an important determinant of bone mineral status in adulthood (Bailey et al 1996).

Physique

Information on the effects on physique of regular training for sport during childhood and adolescence is limited. In small samples of boys (total $n = 39$) participating in different training programs from 11 to 18 years of age (6, 4 and 2.5 h/week), distributions of somatotypes did not differ among the three activity groups (Parizkova & Carter 1976). Somatotypes changed over adolescence in a random manner and were not associated with training. Thus, there does not appear to be a significant effect of regular training on somatotype during growth and puberty. In a follow-up analysis of a small sample of the original series at 24 years of age ($n = 14$), mesomorphy increased from 18 to 24 years even though the boys had ceased regular training (Carter & Parizkova 1978).

In the preceding longitudinal study, specific intensities of the training programs were not indicated. Some forms of training may, however, result in muscular hypertrophy of the body parts specifically exercised, e.g. thoracic and arm measurements in male gymnasts, shoulder musculature in young swimmers, or arm musculature responses to weight-training programs. Such changes may, at times, be rather extreme, and give the impression of altered physique. However, the changes are rather localized and do not markedly alter an individual's somatotype (Meleski & Malina 1985, Tanner 1952). For example, changes in somatotype components during a specific weight-training program among young adult males (18–25 years) and during a competitive swim season, which included high-repetition, low-resistance weight training, among elite university level swimmers (18–23 years) were minor. Among the males, on average, mesomorphy increased slightly in response to weight training, while endomorphy and ectomorphy were unchanged. Changes with weight training occurred primarily in the upper arm and shoulder girdle, but were not sufficient to alter estimates of somatotype. All changes in somatotype components varied within +0.5 and –0.5 units, and the majority were unchanged with training (Tanner 1952). Among the female swimmers, on average, small changes occurred in endomorphy (decrease) and ectomorphy (increase), while mesomorphy was virtually unchanged. Changes in somatotype components ranged between +1.5 and –1.0 units, but most of the changes occurred in endomorphy and ectomorphy. Mesomorphy was unchanged in the majority of swimmers (Meleski & Malina 1985). The preceding thus suggests limited, if any, changes in somatotype with training in young adults.

Biological maturation

Does regular training for and participation in sport influence the timing and tempo of biological maturation? As noted earlier, there is a wide range of normal variation among youth in the timing and tempo of biological maturation. It is a highly individual characteristic that often shows a tendency to run in families, i.e. mothers and their daughters may both be early or late maturers. The following summarizes the general trends in the literature for young athletes.

Skeletal maturation

Short-term longitudinal studies of boys and girls in several sports indicate similar gains in skeletal maturation in both athletes and non-athletes; on average, skeletal age proceeds in concert with the child's chronological age (Malina 1994, 1998a). It should be noted that in later adolescence, differences in maturity status among participants at younger ages are reduced and are eventually eliminated as skeletal maturity is attained by all individuals.

Somatic maturation

Available data indicate no effect of training for sport on the age at PHV and on growth rate in height during the adolescent spurt in boys and girls (Malina 1998a). It has been suggested that intensive training may delay the timing of the growth spurt and stunt the growth spurt in female gymnasts. Unfortunately, the data are not sufficiently longitudinal to warrant such a conclusion. Many confounding factors are not considered, especially the rigorous selection criteria for gymnastics, marginal diets, short parents, and so on. Female gymnasts as a group show the growth and maturation characteristics of short, normal, slow maturing children with short parents (Malina 1999). Interestingly, male gymnasts also present consistently short statures and late maturation, but these trends are not attributed to intensive training (Malina 1994, 1998a).

Sexual maturation

Longitudinal data on the sexual maturation of either girls or boys who are regularly active or training for sport are not extensive. The available data are largely cross-sectional so that it is difficult to make clear statements on the potential effects of training for sport. The limited longitudinal data for boys and girls active in sport indicate no effect of training on the timing and progress of breast and pubic hair development in girls, and genital and pubic hair development in boys compared with non-athletes. Mean intervals for progression from one stage to the next or across two stages of secondary sex characteristics are similar to those for non-active youth, and are well within the range of normal variation in longitudinal studies of non-athletes (Malina et al 1997b). The interval between ages at PHV and menarche for girls active in sport and non-active girls also does not differ, and is similar to those for several samples of non-athletic girls, with mean intervals of 1.2–1.5 years (Geithner et al 1998).

Most discussions of the potential influence of training on sexual maturation focus on the later mean ages at menarche which are often observed in female athletes (Table 10.2). Training for sport is indicated as the factor which is responsible for the later mean ages at menarche, with the inference that training 'delays' the onset of this maturational event. Unfortunately, studies of athletes ordinarily do not consider other factors which are known to influence menarche. For example, there is a familial tendency for later maturation in athletes (Malina et al 1994). Mothers of athletes in several other sports attain menarche later than mothers of non-athletes, and sisters of elite swimmers and university athletes attain menarche later than average. In addition, age at menarche in athletes varies with number of children in the family (Malina et al 1997a). Athletes from larger families attain menarche later than those from smaller families.

Allowing for the many factors that are known to influence menarche, it is exceedingly difficult to implicate training *per se* as the causative factor (Malina 1998b). The conclusions of two comprehensive discussions of exercise and reproductive health of women summarize the situation as follows:

although menarche occurs later in athletes than in nonathletes, it has yet to be shown that exercise delays menarche in anyone.

(Loucks et al 1992, p. 5288)

the general consensus is that while menarche occurs later in athletes than in nonathletes, the relationship is not causal and is confounded by other factors.

(Clapp & Little 1995, pp 2–3)

TRAINING AND POTENTIAL GROWTH DISORDERS

In the few young athletes who present problems related to growth and maturation, there is a need for more systematic and comprehensive evaluation. Factors other than training for sport must be more closely scrutinized. In many cases of short stature, the shortness is largely familial, i.e. short children tend to have short parents. Shortness may also be related to constitutionally late maturation, which may also be familial. In some sports, the growth of young athletes may be compromised by chronic marginal or poor nutritional status, to which coaches, parents and the specific sport system may be significant contributors. Some young athletes also present clinical eating disorders. It is possible that intensive training for sport may interact with or may be confounded by these factors and others in the sport and home environments of the young athlete. Hence, the effect of physical training on growth and maturation may be difficult to extract.

SPORT SELECTION, GROWTH AND MATURATION

As has been continually emphasized in the chapter, sport is extremely selective and exclusive at elite levels. Most community-based programs emphasize mass participation, but some programs have as their objective the identification and subsequent training of young athletes with potential for success in regional, national and/or international competition. The selection/exclusion process begins early and appears to be a closed one, excluding many children from entering sport at a later age.

Much time and effort have been spent trying to identify the particular physical and psychological characteristics which contribute to the selection and development of talent (Malina 1998b). The debate often focuses the relative contributions of genetic, environmental and social factors. As can be seen from the research presented in this chapter, it would seem that training does not affect growth and maturation. It is more likely that young athletes select themselves, or are selected by coaches and sport systems, into their specific sports. This implies that, in general, sporting success in the young athlete has a large genetic component and that the differences observed in growth and maturation between athletes and non-athletes are mainly the result of nature rather than nurture. Genetic considerations in growth, maturation and performance are discussed in more depth elsewhere (Bouchard et al 1997).

Young potentially talented athletes have to be introduced to their sport. A major limiting factor to organized sport participation is the availability of local resources, in particular human resources in the form of adults to coach, supervise and administer programs. Parental support in terms of both time and finance is very important. In a study of young British athletes, parents played the main role in introducing children into sport; further, most of these parents had participated in sport themselves when younger (Rowley 1992). Similarly, among university athletes in the United States, parents were most often indicated as the primary persons responsible for getting them involved in sport, and the majority of athletes had one or both parents who were involved in sport at the high school level or above (R M Malina, unpublished data).

Economic considerations are an additional factor. Young athletes often have to travel considerable distances to get to a training facility and are dependent on their parents for transport. Further, the cost of intensive training can be considerable and, for the most part, is met almost exclusively by parents (Rowley &

Baxter-Jones 1995). Systematic training in sports such as gymnastics, swimming, diving, tennis and figure skating is often limited to private clubs and requires a substantial economic investment by parents and possibly sponsors. Economic considerations are therefore likely to limit access to sports for children and adolescents in many countries.

CONCLUSIONS

Given the presently available data, there is limited evidence to suggest that intensive training for sport has a negative effect on the growth and maturation of young athletes. In those few young athletes who present problems related to growth and maturation, factors other than physical training must be more closely scrutinized. Observed differences between elite young athletes and non-athletes of similar chronological age are likely to reflect the self-selective nature of elite youth sport. Although growth and maturation do not seem to be influenced by regular intensive training, regular training for sport has the potential to influence body composition favorably, by increasing bone mineral and skeletal muscle and by decreasing fatness.

REFERENCES

Bailey D A, Faulkner R A, McKay H A 1996 Growth, physical activity, and bone mineral acquisition. Exercise and Sport Sciences Reviews 24: 233–266

Baxter-Jones A D G, Helms P J 1996 Effects of training at a young age: a review of the Training of Young Athletes (TOYA) Study. Pediatric Exercise Science 8: 310–327

Baxter-Jones A, Goldstein H, Helms P 1993 The development of aerobic power in young athletes. Journal of Applied Physiology 75: 1160–1167

Baxter-Jones A D G, Helms P J, Baines Preece J, Preece M 1994 Menarche in intensively trained gymnasts, swimmers and tennis players. Annals of Human Biology 21: 407–415

Beunen G, Malina R M 1988 Growth and physical performance relative to the timing of the adolescent spurt. Exercise and Sport Sciences Reviews 16: 503–540

Beunen G, Malina R M 1996 Growth and biological maturation: relevance to athletic performance. In: Bar-Or O (ed) The child and adolescent athlete. Blackwell Science, Oxford, p 3

Beunen G, Malina R M, Van't Hof M A et al 1988 Adolescent growth and motor performance: a longitudinal study of Belgian boys. Human Kinetics, Champaign, IL

Bouchard C, Malina R M, Perusse L 1997 Genetics of fitness and physical performance. Human Kinetics, Champaign, IL

Carter J E L 1988 Somatotypes of children in sports. In: Malina R M (ed) Young athletes: biological, psychological, and educational perspectives. Human Kinetics, Champaign, IL, p 153

Carter J E L, Heath B H 1990 Somatotyping – development and applications. Cambridge University Press, Cambridge

Carter J E L, Parizkova J 1978 Changes in somatotypes of European males between 17 and 24 years. American Journal of Physical Anthropology 48: 251–254

Claessens A L, Lefevre J, Beunen G, Malina R M 1999 The contribution of anthropometric characteristics to performance scores in elite female gymnasts. Journal of Sports Medicine and Physical Fitness 39: 355–360

Claessens A L, Malina R M, Lefevre J et al 1992 Growth and menarcheal status of elite female gymnasts. Medicine and Science in Sports and Exercise 24: 755–763

Clapp J F, Little K D 1995 The interaction between regular exercise and selected aspects of women's health. Am Journal of Obstetrics and Gynecology 173: 2–9

Eisenmann J C, Seefeldt V D, Haubenstricker J L, Malina R M 1999 Sex differences in selected motor performances of elite young distance runners. In: Malina R M (ed) Organized sport in the lives of children and adolescents: abstracts. Institute for the Study of Youth Sports, Michigan State University, East Lansing, MI, p 57

Eveleth P B, Tanner J M 1990 Worldwide variation in human growth, 2nd edn. Cambridge University Press, Cambridge

Freeman J V, Cole T J, Chinn S, Jones P R M, White E M, Preece M A 1995 Cross sectional stature and weight reference curves for the UK, 1990. Archives of Disease in Childhood 73: 17–24

Geithner C A, Malina R M 1993 Somatotypes of junior Olympic divers. In: Malina R M, Gabriel J L (eds) Proceedings of the U.S. Diving Sport Science Seminar 1993. United States Diving, Indianapolis, p 36

Geithner C A, Woynarowska B, Malina R M 1998 The adolescent spurt and sexual maturation in girls active and not active in sport. Annals of Human Biology 25: 415–423

Geithner C A, O'Brien R O, Gabriel J L, Malina R M 1999a Sex differences in the motor performances of elite young divers. Medicine and Science in Sports and Exercise 31: 5170

Geithner C A, O'Brien R O, Gabriel J L, Malina R M 1999b Characteristics of successful junior Olympic divers. In: Malina R M (ed) Organized sport in the lives of children and adolescents: abstracts. Institute for the Study of Youth Sports, Michigan State University, East Lansing, MI, p 56–57

Heras Yague P, de la Fuente J M 1998 Changes in height and motor performance relative to peak height velocity: a mixed-longitudinal study of Spanish boys and girls. American Journal of Human Biology 10: 647–660

Klika R J, Malina R M 1999 Sex differences in motor performance in elite young alpine skiers. Medicine and Science in Sports and Exercise 31: 5319

Loucks A B, Vaitukaitis J, Cameron J L et al 1992 The reproductive system and exercise in women. Medicine and Science in Sports and Exercise 24: S288–293

Malina R M 1983 Menarche in athletes: a synthesis and hypothesis. Annals of Human Biology 10: 1–24

Malina R M 1994 Physical growth and biological maturation of young athletes. Exercise and Sport Sciences Reviews 22: 389–433

Malina R M 1996 The young athlete: biological growth and maturation in a biocultural context. In: Smoll F L, Smith R E (eds) Children and youth in sport: a biopsychosocial perspective. Brown and Benchmark, Dubuque, IA, p 161

Malina R M 1997 Growth and maturation of female gymnasts. Spotlight on Youth Sports (Institute for the Study of Youth Sports, Michigan State University) 19(3): 1–3

Malina R M 1998a Growth and maturation of young athletes: is training for sport a factor? In: Chan K-M, Micheli L J (eds) Sports and children. Williams and Wilkins, Hong Kong, p 133

Malina R M 1998b Physical activity, sport, social status and Darwinian fitness. In: Strickland S S, Shetty P S (eds) Human biology and social inequality. Cambridge University Press, Cambridge, p 165

Malina R M 1999 Growth and maturation of elite female gymnasts: is training a factor? In: Johnston F E, Zemel B, Eveleth P B (eds) Human growth in context. Smith-Gordon, London, p 291

Malina R M, Beunen G 1996 Monitoring growth and maturation. In Bar-Or O (ed) The child and adolescent athlete. Blackwell Science, Oxford, p 647

Malina R M, Bouchard C 1991 Growth, maturation, and physical activity. Human Kinetics, Champaign, IL

Malina R M, Ryan R C, Bonci C M 1994 Age at menarche in athletes and their mothers and sisters. Annals of Human Biology 21: 417–422

Malina R M, Katzmarzyk P T, Bonci C M et al 1997a Family size and age at menarche in athletes. Medicine and Science in Sports and Exercise 29: 99–106

Malina R M, Woynarowska B, Bielicki T et al 1997b Prospective and retrospective longitudinal studies of the growth, maturation, and fitness of Polish youth active in sport. International Journal of Sports Medicine 18 (suppl 3): S179–185

Meleski B W, Malina R M 1985 Changes in body composition and physique of elite university-level swimmers during a competitive season. Journal of Sports Science 3: 33–40

Nevill A M, Holder R L, Baxter-Jones A, Round J M, Jones D A 1998 Modelling developmental changes in strength and aerobic power in children. Journal of Applied Physiology 84(3): 963–970

Parizkova J, Carter J E L 1976 Influence of physical activity on stability of somatotypes in boys. American Journal of Physical Anthropology 44: 327–340

Peltenburg A L, Erich W B M, Zonderland M L et al 1984 A retrospective growth study of female gymnasts and girl swimmers. International Journal of Sports Medicine 5: 262–267

Rowland T W 1996 Developmental exercise physiology. Human Kinetics, Champaign, IL

Rowley S 1992 Training of Young Athletes (TOYA) Study: Identification of talent. The Sports Council, London

Rowley S, Baxter-Jones A D G 1995 Training of Young Athletes (TOYA) Study: Identification of talent II. The Sports Council, London

Skierska E 1998 Age at menarche and prevalence of oligo/amenorrhea in top Polish athletes. American Journal of Human Biology 10: 511–517

Tanner J M 1952 The effect of weight-training on physique. American Journal of Physical Anthropology 10: 427–461

Tanner J M 1962 Growth at adolescence, 2nd edn. Blackwell Scientific Publications, Oxford

Tanner J M 1989 Foetus into man. Physical growth from conception to maturity. Castlemead Publications, London

Theintz G E, Howald H, Weiss U, Sizonenko P C 1993 Evidence for a reduction of growth potential in adolescent female gymnasts. Journal of Pediatrics 122: 306–313

Tofler I R, Stryer B K, Micheli L J, Herman L R 1996 Physical and emotional problems of elite female gymnasts. New England Journal of Medicine 335: 281–283

Tönz O, Stronski S M, Gmeiner C Y K 1990 Wachstum und Pubertät bei 7-bis 16 Jährigen Kunstturneirinnen: eine prospektive Studie. Schweizerische Medizinische Wochenschrift 120: 10–20

Ziemilska A 1981 Wplyw intensywnego treningy gimnastycznego na rozwoj somatyczny i dojrzewanie dzieci. Akademia Wychowania Fizycznego, Warsaw

11

Competitive stress and coping in young sport performers

Nickolas C. Smith   Bryan Jones
Neil K. Roach

KEY POINTS

1. Appraisal-based models of stress that highlight the transactional nature of the coping process represent the most satisfactory way of examining the effects of competitive stress on sport performers.
2. Pre-competitive anxiety states have been the focus of extensive research in sport. Well validated measures of multidimensional competitive state anxiety exist that can be used with a range of athletic groups and ages.
3. The antecedents of cognitive anxiety differ among sports, gender of the participants, the perceived ability of performers, and the manner in which success is evaluated. The antecedents of somatic anxiety are less influenced by such variables.
4. Differences in competitive stress experienced by performers are strongly influenced by the coping strategies employed in such settings. Little is known, however, about how such coping strategies develop in young athletes.
5. Differences between performers in goal orientation (i.e. task versus goal) exert a strong influence on the level of stress experienced during competition. This influence of goal orientation is mediated by changes in the level of competence and personal control perceived by performers.

6. The majority of research in the area covered by this chapter has focused on either competitive anxiety in sub-elite performers or older athletic groups. Consequently, the study of competitive stress in elite young performers can be considered a research priority.

INTRODUCTION

One of the attractions of high-level competitive sport is its power to provide a test of the psychological skills of those involved as much as it does their physical preparation and technical skills. The settings in which athletic events are played out usually involve a contest conducted in the presence of socially significant others, normally in the form of an audience, often for high rewards in the face of an uncertain outcome. As a consequence, they have the potential to be experienced by performers as either highly challenging or highly threatening. Not surprisingly, such settings have provided sport psychologists with ideal opportunities to study the cognitions, emotions and behaviours of performers when faced by such potentially stressful situations and to gain an understanding of their impact on athletic performance.

Whilst much research has been conducted into the effect of competitive stress on sporting performance in older athletes, far less is known about its impact on younger performers. This is the case despite the fact that in many sports the age of performers at elite level has reduced significantly during the last two decades.

This chapter provides an overview of the literature that has examined competitive stress in sport, the coping strategies used by performers, and their emotional consequences. Where data exist, it also focuses on the young performer involved at the elite end of the performance spectrum and compares these findings with those obtained in older athletic groups.

STUDYING COMPETITIVE STRESS IN SPORT PERFORMERS

Sport psychologists have tended to approach the study of competitive stress in performers in one of three ways. One approach has been to examine the frequency of life stress and daily hassles experienced by performers, often with the aim of examining the

potential link between such life stressors and athletic injury (Andersen & Williams 1988, Petrie 1992). A second approach has been to study the emotional reactions of athletes to sport competition and the performance consequences that result. A final, but by no means as extensively researched, area can also be identified in the study of coping behaviours of athletes and their emotional impact. This chapter will focus on the latter two of these approaches.

The emotional, physiological and behavioural responses of performers to competition can best be viewed as the consequence of a process of cognitive appraisal. Appraisal is the process whereby individuals assess the significance of a situation and evaluate their own capabilities to cope with the demands faced (Folkman et al 1986). Appraisal involves a comparison between the demands that performers believe they face in competition, a process termed primary appraisal, and the resources they feel they have to meet them, termed secondary appraisal. Primary and secondary appraisal processes are then evaluated via a process of reappraisal based on the emotional reactions and performance consequences that arise (Fig. 11.1). The perceived intensity of the stressful event in conjunction with the coping resources available and the control the performer perceives he or she has over the situation determine the emotional consequences of appraisal for the performer. Although these emotional and behavioural consequences can be viewed as outcomes of cognitive appraisal, via the process of reappraisal they can in turn also act as antecedents of future coping efforts.

THE ASSESSMENT OF PRE-COMPETITIVE ANXIETY IN SPORT

An extensive body of research has emerged that has examined the effect of competition as a potential source of stress on the pre-competitive emotional state of performers. The majority of this research has focused on the study of pre-competitive anxiety (Jones 1995).

The main objective of this research has been to better understand the factors that produce anxiety in performers prior to competition and, to a lesser extent, the subsequent performance impact. These lines of inquiry have been accompanied within mainstream psychology by considerable progress in understanding the nature of anxiety and its impact on cognitive function (Eysenck 1997). Concurrent with these developments have come refinements in the way in which anxiety is assessed in sporting contexts.

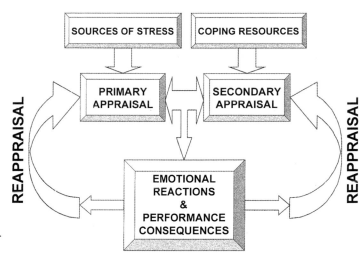

Figure 11.1 The nature of appraisal and its relationship to sources of stress, coping resources, and the emotional and performance consequences. The role of reappraisal is also highlighted.

A clearer understanding of the emotional impact of competitive stress on athletes has been gained as a result of the development of sport-specific anxiety measurement scales. Typical of such scales are questionnaires that attempt to identify those features within competitive settings that signal threat and prompt worry and nervousness in performers. Essentially these questionnaires are used to measure the intensity of symptoms experienced by performers that are assumed to reflect the underlying anxiety state. By focusing on situation-specific features of competitive sport, these questionnaires generally achieve greater sensitivity and specificity of measurement compared with more general anxiety questionnaires.

The item content of these scales normally focuses on the performer's thoughts and feelings as competition approaches, probing areas such as self-doubts over personal performance, personal concerns about how others will view the performance, as well as the physical sensations experienced. Typical of this type of measure is the Competitive State Anxiety Inventory-2 (CSAI-2; Martens et al 1990), the most widely used measure of multidimensional competitive anxiety in sport. As such measurement scales are easy to administer and are easily understood, they are ideal for use with young performers from age 12 upwards.

The measurement of pre-competitive anxiety states is not without its problems. A most significant problem associated with the measurement of anxiety reactions in performers is often their reluctance or inability to accurately report the more negative cognitions and feelings experienced. Most sport-specific anxiety measurement scales attempt to reduce this problem by the use of anti-social desirability instructions that

acknowledge the potency of such settings to prompt concerns within performers whilst emphasizing the importance of athletes responding openly and honestly to each item. Despite attempts to reduce the tendency of performers to provide socially desirable responses, it is likely that athletes may still misreport, deny or repress their feelings and cognitions. As a consequence, the valid and reliable measurement of competitive anxiety states may be more difficult to achieve than is generally assumed. Future developments in the area of measurement of the emotions experienced prior to competition are likely to see a combination of scales that measure sport-specific anxiety together with the tendency towards a defensive coping style or a strong motive to protect self-esteem. Once developed, such scales would provide one method of distinguishing genuinely anxious performers from their repressive counterparts.

Anxiety states have both cognitive and somatic components, and the symptoms that characterize these components can be experienced by performers relatively independently of each other (Morris et al 1981). Cognitive anxiety is normally experienced as self-doubt and worry over poor performance and the likely consequences, and is sometimes associated with both negative images and self-talk linked to failure. Somatic anxiety refers to the athlete's awareness of physical symptoms such as nervousness, trembling hands or a racing heart.

As mentioned, the most widely employed questionnaire measure of competitive state anxiety used in sport is the CSAI-2. The CSAI-2 measures the intensity of both cognitive and somatic symptoms of anxiety as well as the self-confidence experienced by performers.

Recently, researchers in the UK have argued that, in addition to the intensity of the anxiety symptoms experienced, the athletes' interpretation of the likely influence of such symptoms on their performance should also be determined (Jones & Swain 1992). To obtain this information, a modified version of the CSAI-2 has been developed. Data are collected in the normal way, but each of the 27 items on the CSAI-2 is modified by adding an additional seven-point scale (−3 to +3) that asks performers whether the symptoms experienced are perceived as likely to be debilitative or facilitative to performance. When using this modified scale, it is possible for two performers to report similar symptom intensities but to interpret the symptoms very differently in terms of their impact on performance. Preliminary findings using this facilitative/debilitative measurement approach suggest that the tendency to view anxiety symptom intensity as facilitative or debilitative may be an important determinant of athletic success (Jones et al 1994). How such symptom interpretation develops in athletes is poorly understood, as are the links between such interpretation and other psychological attributes of performers.

Although there are some encouraging aspects of a measurement approach that differentiates potentially facilitative from potentially debilitative anxiety symptoms, there are also inherent concerns. These concerns are threefold. Firstly, information regarding the validity and reliability of the modified CSAI-2 scale has yet to be published and, as a consequence, its psychometric properties remain unclear. Secondly, concerns have also been expressed by some authors (Burton & Naylor 1997) that a measurement strategy that presupposes a potential for anxiety symptoms to be interpreted as facilitative risks confounding anxiety with other more positive emotions. Finally, by advocating a measurement approach that gathers information on both intensity and direction of symptoms simultaneously, important processes involved in situational appraisal and coping efforts that occur across time are obscured. In the light of these concerns, it could be argued that, rather than focusing on the potential for anxiety symptoms to be experienced as either debilitative or facilitative to performance, the function of different coping behaviours exhibited by performers provides a more appropriate focus of study.

COPING STRATEGIES AND THEIR USE BY SPORT PERFORMERS

Recent years have seen a growing interest in the study of coping strategies used by performers and their emotional and performance consequences (Ntoumanis & Biddle 1998). This interest has stemmed from the recognition of the importance that such strategies play in moderating the impact of stressful events on performers. Early work by Pearlin & Schooler (1978) attempted to identify the nature of coping in adults when faced by stressful events, and concluded that three general styles of coping strategies could be identified, as follows:

- strategies aimed at changing the situation
- strategies aimed at modifying the meaning or appraisal of the source of stress
- strategies aimed at controlling the negative emotional reactions to the situation.

This exploratory work led other researchers to attempt to classify the coping strategies reported within a taxonomy based on the assumed function of each coping strategy. The most widely accepted taxonomy of coping strategies was developed by Folkman & Lazarus (1985), who classified coping behaviours in one of two ways: emotion-focused or problem-focused. Emotion-focused coping describes those strategies designed to reduce the emotional distress experienced, often in situations where the source of stress remains unaffected. Problem-focused coping refers to cognitive or behavioural attempts to manage or eliminate a source of stress. Endler & Parker (1990) subsequently proposed a third form of coping, termed avoidance, that referred to strategies aimed at withdrawal from, or evasion of, stressful events. Coping strategies that fall into each of these three categories can be reliably identified in elite performers in sport prior to and during competition. Such research also suggests that in sport competition performers more often use problem-focused strategies than either emotion-focused or avoidance strategies (Gould et al 1993). This tendency to use problem-focused coping strategies also predicts positive affect in sport performers, whilst emotion-focused coping has been linked to negative affective reactions (Ntoumanis & Biddle 1998).

Whilst instructive at the descriptive level, the system of classification developed by Folkman & Lazarus (1985) can be criticized as being rather atheoretical. Implicit within this system of classification is the assumption of a mutually exclusive role for any coping strategy. An example of the problem produced by this assumption is provided in the following. Seeking social support is widely recognized as a coping strategy used by many performers. However, the role served by this strategy is less clear when the possible functions served by social support are considered. Social support may provide a source of information that assists the problem-solving efforts made by the performer. In this context, seeking social support would be seen to provide a good example of a problem-focused coping strategy. However, such support can also serve to reduce the experience of negative emotions as a consequence of the empathy and understanding provided by significant others. In this context, these coping efforts would most commonly be identified as an example of emotion-focused coping. Equally plausibly, social support can be seen to serve an avoidance function, as it may provide an opportunity to withdraw from the source of stress. Consequently, the classification system proposed by Folkman & Lazarus (1985) based on the assumed function of each behaviour can often lead to interpretive problems. The example provided above highlights the importance of studying coping strategies from an idiographic perspective in an attempt to understand the unique function served by a particular strategy for the individual at any one time within a given context.

In addition to the concerns over the reliable classification of coping strategies, a further concern exists in sport research regarding attempts to explore the causal links between specific coping strategies and their sometimes conflicting emotional and performance consequences. To examine such links, variables relating to both the emotional impact (i.e. the assumed intervening process) and performance outcome (i.e. the assumed behavioural consequence) should be both measured and differentiated. For example, the use of stimulant drugs as a coping strategy for withstanding high training demands may serve to improve performance in the short term and, as a consequence, could be considered an effective coping strategy if performance-related measures provide dependent variables. However, if dependent variables linked to the psychosocial health and well-being of the performer are considered, it seems unlikely that such a strategy would be considered effective in the longer term.

As is the case in a number of areas of research covered by this chapter, our understanding of the role served by different coping strategies in elite sport performers is limited. More limited still is our understanding of how such strategies are acquired and refined in developing athletes. One related area in which progress has been made, however, is in the identification of the links between potential sources of stress in sport and their emotional impact. These sources of stress provide the focus for the next section.

SOURCES OF STRESS IN SPORT AND THEIR LINKS TO COMPETITIVE ANXIETY

Considerable importance has been attached to identifying what it is about the competitive situation that gives rise to the worry and nervousness experienced by athletes. To address this question is to attempt to address the subjective meaning of sport competition to the performer. Some *a priori* assumptions can be made about what may concern performers in such situations, based on the nature of competitive sport at a high level. In general terms, sport competition presents an opportunity for individuals or groups to demonstrate public achievement and competency in a context where social comparison plays an important role. This opportunity for social comparison takes place in a context where success or failure is often judged on the outcome of the competition in circumstances where outcome uncertainty is often high. Finally, the contest is normally enacted in the presence of significant others who possess a strong evaluation potential.

To address the question posed above regarding the focus of performers' worries, research has attempted to identify those factors within the competitive environment most strongly associated with cognitive and somatic symptoms. Although a consensus has yet to be reached, some agreement over the antecedents of competitive anxiety in sport is apparent. The antecedents that most strongly predict cognitive anxiety are those that influence the performer's expectations of success. In competitive sport, these are normally beliefs about the quality of the performer's preparation, perceptions of competence and personal control given the challenge faced, and the performer's appraisal of the opponent's ability. The antecedents of somatic anxiety differ from those for cognitive anxiety and appear more closely linked to physical characteristics of the performance environment (i.e. the sights, sounds and smells encountered). Thus they appear less evaluative in nature than the antecedents of cognitive anxiety and are more akin to conditioned responses to the actual or imagined performance settings. Whilst little evidence is available regarding the antecedents of anxiety experienced by elite young athletes, that available on younger athletes suggests some consistency with those reported by older performers (Hall & Kerr 1997).

The antecedents of cognitive and somatic anxiety in competition have been found to differ between sports depending on how successful performance is judged. In sports where the success of a performance is assessed using objective criteria (e.g. goals scored, distance thrown), the cognitive anxiety levels reported by performers are generally lower than in sports where outcome is judged on more subjective grounds (e.g. gymnastic and artistic criteria). One plausible explanation for this difference between objectively and subjectively scored sports is the additional worry generated in performers over the control of the impression their performance makes on judges. Consequently, in addition to focusing on the technical aspects of their performance, athletes devote additional resources and effort to worries relating to how officials will interpret their performance efforts. In more objectively determined sports, these potential sources of stress are less conspicuous or often absent.

The cognitive anxiety experienced by athletes during competition is strongly influenced by the perceived ability of the performers involved. Elite performers demonstrate high levels of technical competence in their chosen sport. Faced by situations of high demand, it may be predicted that highly competent performers would perceive such situations as challenging rather than stressful. However, this is not always the case, and even highly competent performers face crises of confidence linked to perceptions of their ability which are often disproportionate to more objectively derived judgements. This serves to illustrate the importance of the process of appraisal and reappraisal in determining subjective estimates of competence. Factors within competition that are likely to influence performers' perceptions of competence will be closely linked to their underlying motivations for involvement in sport and the outcomes they most value. Principally within competitive settings in sport, uncertainty surrounding the control of outcome and changes in the perceived importance of performing well provide powerful influences on performers' perceived competence, processes that, in turn, provide powerful stimuli for worry.

Gender differences are also apparent in the antecedents of cognitive anxiety, and these have been linked to differences in goal orientation between males and females. In male performers, the antecedents of cognitive anxiety seem more closely linked to concerns over ego-centred social comparisons and winning, whilst in females personal performance standards seem more often to provide the focus of worry. Whilst it is premature to conclude from these findings that the antecedents of cognitive and somatic anxiety differ in elite performers as a function of gender, they do highlight the need for further research into the motivational climate of male and female sport and the cognitive and emotional consequences that arise.

In addition to the potential sources of stress reported by older athletes, young performers also have to contend with developmental stressors of both a physical and a psychological nature. One such stressor faced by young performers is parental pressure. Retrospective accounts from young performers of the influence of parents on sport training and competition (Hellstedt 1990, 1995, Scanlan 1995) highlight both positive and negative aspects of parental involvement. On the one hand, parents were often cited as being the main source of encouragement, positive role models and providers of support. Parents, however well meaning, also provided a source of stress as a result of criticism of performance, financial 'blackmailing' based on the financial 'investment' made by them, and unrealistic expectations. Presently, our understanding of the point at which parental involvement becomes a source of added stress rather than a means of social support rests on findings from a limited number of cross-sectional studies. Continued research in this area remains a priority.

COMPETITIVE STRESS AND GOAL ORIENTATION IN SPORT

A clearer descriptive understanding of what performers worry about prior to and during competitive sport has been gained from examining the antecedents of pre-competition anxiety, but progress at the explanatory level has been limited. This can be attributed to the descriptive and often atheoretical nature of much of the work conducted in the area. A potentially more fruitful approach has been provided by research conducted in sport from a social cognitive perspective (Duda 1993). A social cognitive perspective emphasizes the importance of understanding the complex relationship between the social context of competitive sport, the athletes' achievement goal orientation, subjective construal of success and failure, and the emotions experienced prior to and during competition. This perspective appears to hold considerable promise for researchers in their quest to unravel the complex relationships between athletes' motivation for involvement in competitive sport and their emotional reaction to such involvement. Equally important is the influence of the motivational climate created during training on a performer's psychological development. In such settings, the principal influences consistently to emerge are coaches, peers and parents.

Gaining an understanding of performers' motives for involvement in training and competition is important in the process of creating the optimal motivational climate. Coaches, peers and parents all have a major role to play in ensuring that these motives are satisfied. It has been shown that the primary sporting influence on performers shifts from parents to coaches and peers at approximately 13 years of age (Hellstedt 1995). This is typically a strained transition and often leads to coach–parent and performer–parent conflict. These sources of conflict provide another potential source of stress faced by young performers. Hellstedt (1990) examined perceptions of parental pressure in ski racers and its emotional impact on performers across two different age groups (i.e. 13- and 15-year-old groupings). The main findings to emerge from this study were that 13-year-old skiers reported higher perceptions of parental pressure than the 15-year-old group. When perceptions of parental pressure were examined across both age groups, a significant correlation was found between perceptions of pressure and the dissatisfaction experienced with sport involvement.

To achieve a clearer understanding of the motives of performers for engaging in sport competition, research has examined the influence of differences in goal orientation on such involvement. This research has also examined how emotional reactions to competition vary between groups who differ in goal orientation. Goals are viewed as powerful motivators and directors of behaviour, with goal-setting programmes widely acknowledged in the sport psychology literature as powerful motivational devices that can influence athletes' behaviour.

Goal orientation describes a tendency within performers to interpret their involvement in an activity (e.g. competition) in a particular way. Two such goal orientations within performers have been identified and these have been termed ego and task. Ego-orientated performers are assumed to engage in competition as a way of demonstrating ability, often with reference to that shown by others. It is further assumed that performers who are ego-involved when competing place high value on winning as a way of demonstrating ability. Task-involved performers, on the other hand, show a preoccupation with demonstrating self-referenced improvement and eventual mastery of the task rather than defining success with reference to others.

Why these differences in goal orientation have attracted the research attention of sport psychologists interested in competitive stress in sport can be attributed to Roberts' (1986) proposal regarding the relationship between goal orientation and competitive anxiety. Essentially, Roberts (1986) argued that, in competitive situations, ego-orientated performers are likely to worry to a greater extent than task-orientated performers over the threat posed to their chances of demonstrating superior ability. Task-orientated performers are less likely to worry in such settings, as they view the demonstration of ability as less important. Task-orientated performers are also less likely to experience cognitive anxiety during competition as their self-worth is less threatened in such settings.

The influence of goal orientation on the somatic anxiety experienced by performers is less clear. Evidence suggests that attributional biases performers make about the causes of such somatic symptoms combined with other dispositional factors exert stronger influences than goal orientation on whether they are experienced as unpleasant or, alternatively, as an indication of the body's readiness for competitive engagement.

Crucially, the prediction that ego-orientated performers are more likely to experience heightened cognitive anxiety during competition rests on the assumption that competition exerts a powerful influence on the performer's perceived ability to achieve valued outcomes. As one of the defining characteristics of competition in sport is uncertainty of outcome, ego-involved performers in such settings are more likely to experience a stronger sense of threat to their demonstration of superior ability than task-involved performers. This sense of threat is predicted to heighten as the uncertainty over the control of the outcome of the contest increases. The conundrum here is that ego-orientated performers appear likely to seek out competitive settings as they provide ideal opportunities to demonstrate superior ability over opponents.

It must be stressed that much of the evidence regarding the influence of goal orientation on competitive anxiety has been gained from young performers involved in youth sport at the sub-elite level, and any extrapolation to higher-level performers must be only tentative at this point. However, a similar pattern of findings may emerge in elite groups who differ in goal orientation. If such is the case, then important implications for practitioners arise regarding how different motivational climates and coaching practices may serve to foster the disposition towards ego or task orientation in young performers. Whilst some may argue that young performers should be encouraged to adopt an ego orientation in both training and competition if they are to become elite, the reverse seems to be the case when the goal orientations of elite athletes are compared with less proficient performers (Duda 1997). Again it is the case, however, that longitudinal data that would permit stronger conclusions to be drawn regarding the influence of different motivational climates on goal orientation are lacking.

CONCLUSIONS

This chapter has highlighted how an approach based on the athlete's cognitive appraisal of the demands faced in competition represents the most satisfactory framework for studying stress in sport. This approach emphasizes the importance of understanding individual differences in coping behaviour and the function served by such behaviours in a particular context at any one time. The difficulty of classifying coping strategies in a valid manner using existing taxonomies was also highlighted (e.g. that proposed by Folkman & Lazarus 1985). Furthermore, we considered the strengths and limitations of using existing psychometric measures to examine the relationship between competitive anxiety and performance, and again reinforced the importance of appraisal in the stress process. The antecedents of multidimensional competitive anxiety were described, and differences highlighted between sports, gender and other contextual factors.

Whilst the nature of coping efforts was recognized as an important mediator of the affective reaction to a stressful event, little is known about how such strategies are developed in young athletes. Longitudinal and hypothesis-driven research in this area remains a priority.

One fruitful avenue of under-explored research is the role played by goal orientation in mediating differences in the affective reaction of performers to competition. By placing emphasis on understanding performers' goals and motives for engaging in competition, a clearer appreciation can be gained of how goals may serve to heighten or reduce the stress experienced. The effects of different motivational climates in training and competition, combined with the influence of significant others on young athletes, appear to be particularly important areas for research attention.

There is a paucity of research in young elite athletes, despite the fact that in many sports the age of elite performers continues to decline. Future priorities have been identified to serve as a stimulus for research that will help us better understand competitive stress in sport, the acquisition of coping strategies and the emotional and behavioural consequences for the developing athlete.

REFERENCES

Andersen M B, Williams J M 1988 A model of stress and athletic injury: Prediction and prevention. Journal of Sport and Exercise Psychology 10: 294–306

Burton D, Naylor S 1997 Is anxiety really facilitative? Reactions to the myth that cognitive anxiety always impairs sport performance. Journal of Applied Sport Psychology 9: 295–302

Duda J 1993 Goals: a social cognitive approach to the study of motivation in sport. In: Singer R N, Murphey M, Tennant L K (eds) Handbook of research in sport psychology. Macmillan, New York, p 421–436

Duda J 1997 Perpetuating myths: a response to Hardy's 1996 Coleman Griffith Address. Journal of Applied Sport Psychology 9: 303–309

Endler S E, Parker J D A 1990 Multidimensional assessment of coping: a critical evaluation. Journal of Personality and Social Psychology 58: 844–854

Eysenck M W 1997 Anxiety and cognition: a unified theory. Psychology Press, Hove

Folkman S, Lazarus R S 1985 If it changes it must be a process: a study of emotion and coping during three stages of a college examination. Journal of Personality and Social Psychology 48: 150–170

Folkman S, Lazarus R S, Dunkel-Schetter C, DeLongis A, Gruen R J 1986 Dynamics of a stressful encounter: cognitive appraisal, coping and encounter outcomes. Journal of Personality and Social Psychology 50: 992–1003

Gould D, Eklund R C, Jackson S A 1993 Coping strategies used by U.S. Olympic wrestlers. Research Quarterly for Exercise and Sport 64: 83–93

Hall H K, Kerr A W 1997 Motivational antecedents of precompetitive anxiety in youth sport. The Sport Psychologist 11: 24–42

Hellstedt J C 1990 Early adolescent perceptions of parental pressure in the sport environment. Journal of Sport Behavior 13: 135–144

Hellstedt J C 1995 Invisible players: a family systems model. In: Murphy S (ed) Sport psychology interventions. Human Kinetics, Champaign, IL, ch 5, p 117–146

Jones J G 1995 More than just a game: Research developments and issues in competitive anxiety in sport. British Journal of Psychology 86: 449–478

Jones J G, Swain A B J 1992 Intensity and direction as dimensions of competitive state anxiety and relationships with competitiveness. Perceptual and Motor Skills 74: 467–472

Jones J G, Hanton S, Swain A B J 1994 Intensity and interpretation of anxiety symptoms in elite and non-elite sports performers. Personality and Individual Differences 17: 657–663

Martens R, Vealey R S, Burton D 1990 Competitive anxiety in sport. Human Kinetics, Champaign, IL

Morris L W, Davis M A, Hutchings C H 1981 Cognitive and emotional components of anxiety: literature review and a revised worry-emotionality scale. Journal of Educational Psychology 73: 541–555

Ntoumanis N, Biddle S J H 1998 The relationship of coping and its perceived effectiveness to positive and negative affect in sport. Personality and Individual Differences 24: 773–788

Pearlin L I, Schooler C 1978 The structure of coping. Journal of Health and Social Behavior 19: 2–21

Petrie T A 1992 Psychosocial antecedents of athletic injury: the effects of life stress and social support on women collegiate gymnasts. Behavioral Medicine 18: 127–138

Roberts G C 1986 The perception of success. A potential source and its development. In: Weiss M R, Gould D R (eds) Sport for children and youths. Human Kinetics, Champaign, IL, p 251–281

Scanlan T K 1995 Social evaluation and the competition process: a developmental perspective. In: Smoll F L, Smith R E (eds) Children and youth in sport: a biopsychosocial perspective. Brown & Benchmark, Dubuque, p 298–308

12

Overuse injuries in gymnastics

Julie Sparrow

KEY POINTS

1. Gymnastics is a complex sport placing a high physical demand on the gymnast.
2. Prolonged and often intensive training load on the developing skeleton predisposes the gymnast to overuse injury.
3. In the gymnast, all major body systems are vulnerable to injury.
4. An understanding of the core skills of gymnastics is important in developing effective assessment and treatment protocols.
5. Effective treatment should be based on a model of prevention.
6. Communication between therapist, gymnast and coach is an important component of a successful prevention strategy.

INTRODUCTION

The sport of artistic gymnastics is complex, combining elements of balance, coordination, power, strength and flexibility. It incorporates six disciplines for the men and four for the women (Box 12.1).

Whilst there are many common factors involved in both male and female gymnastics, they are, in fact, very different in the demands they place on the athlete. Male gymnastics is primarily a strength and power sport, whilst female gymnasts are more dependent on balance and flexibility.

Performed at its best, gymnastics makes compelling viewing. However, the road to success is long.

Box 12.1 Disciplines of male and female artistic gymnastics

Men
- Vault
- Floor
- High bar
- Parallel bars
- Rings
- Pommel horse

Women
- Vault
- Floor
- Uneven bars
- Balance beam

Figure 12.1 Distribution of overuse injuries. A: Male gymnasts. B: Female gymnasts.

Children with dreams of becoming champion gymnasts often begin their training as young as 6 years old but do not achieve their full potential until 10–15 years later. Training and competing with immature skeletons over prolonged periods can result in the potential for overuse injury. This early start and prolonged development course therefore pose a significant challenge to all who are involved with the gymnasts' well-being.

Traditionally gymnastics has been associated with a high injury rate. This association is in part due to the media coverage of the relatively rare catastrophic head and spinal injuries. However, the number, distribution and nature of injuries within the sport has not been well defined due to poor injury definition reporting. Meeusen & Borms (1992) attempted to develop a comprehensive review of injuries in gymnastics by pooling data from numerous gymnastic studies. They demonstrated a wide variation in rate, incidence, distribution and nature of the injuries. Dixon & Fricker (1993), in a survey of the incidence and nature of injuries at the Australian Institute of Sport, found that the majority of injuries were as a result of overuse. Their findings did, however, show a slightly different pattern in men compared with women (Fig. 12.1).

Overuse disorders can be considered injuries to normal tissue as a result of cumulative, repetitive submaximal microtrauma due to inadequate time for recovery between stress episodes (Krivickas 1997). They are characterized by slow insidious onset, suggesting antecedent sub-threshold spectrum of structural damage (Leadbetter 1992).

The aetiology of overuse injury is multifactorial, involving both intrinsic and extrinsic factors. Intrinsic factors are related to the athletes themselves, including anatomical alignment, growth/age, muscle tendon imbalance, genetic endowment, general health, nutri-

tional status and prior injury. Extrinsic factors include training error, equipment inadequacy and environmental factors (Brukner & Khan 1997). The impact of each of these factors on the clinical presentation needs to be evaluated in order to gain an accurate diagnosis around which the treatment can be planned.

Gymnastics, more than any other sport, demands the total integration of trunk and limb movements. All spinal and peripheral musculoskeletal structures are therefore vulnerable to injury. The high repetition of activity necessary to develop and perfect gymnastic skill produces the potential for chronic overuse injury. The epiphyses and apophyses of the growing skeleton are specifically at risk. Poor technique, coupled with the anomalies of growth, produce skill errors which, if not appreciated and accommodated by the coach, may result in an increased stress on the musculoskeletal tissues. The tissue produces pain in response to microtrauma or overload. In order to minimize the pain response, the body adopts compensatory mechanisms. These compensatory mechanisms ultimately add to the skill errors, and the vicious circle of overload is established (Fig. 12.2). If this cycle is not recognized and broken, it will continue until the gymnast is forced to stop and seek treatment.

The poor recognition, localization and reporting of pain by young gymnasts can often delay access to appropriate and timely intervention to prevent injury chronicity. The first requirement for effective management of gymnastic injury is therefore prevention, based on an understanding of the factors involved in overuse injuries generally, and gymnastic injuries specifically.

Factors in gymnastic injuries

- Age and sex of gymnast
- Anatomy and genetics
- Gymnast experience and skill
- Exposure to training and competitive level
- Flexibility/strength/power
- Coach technique and experience
- Equipment.

Factors contributing to overuse injuries

- Excessive training load
- Poor technique

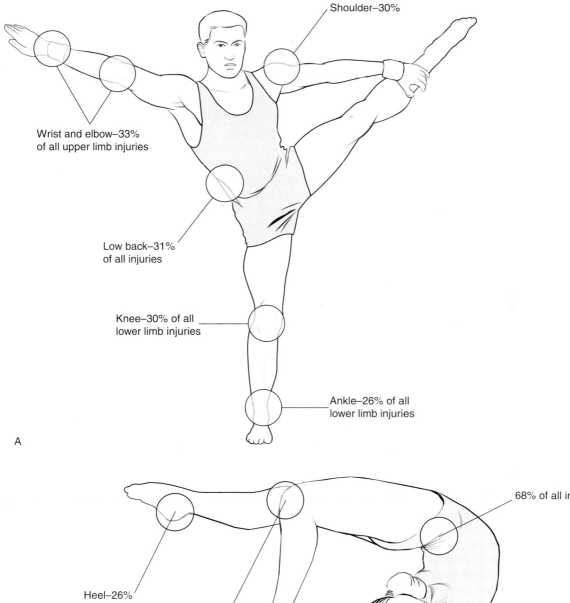

Shoulder–30%

Wrist and elbow–33%
of all upper limb injuries

Low back–31%
of all injuries

Knee–30% of all
lower limb injuries

Ankle–26% of all
lower limb injuries

A

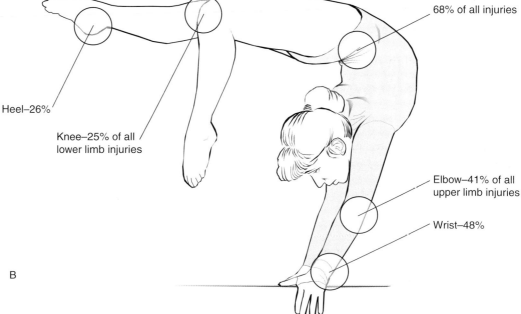

68% of all injuries

Heel–26%

Knee–25% of all
lower limb injuries

Elbow–41% of all
upper limb injuries

Wrist–48%

B

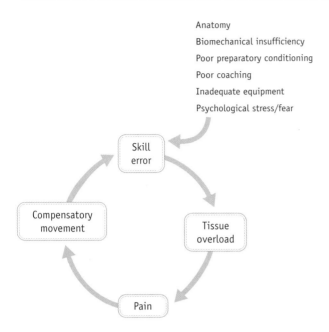

Anatomy
Biomechanical insufficiency
Poor preparatory conditioning
Poor coaching
Inadequate equipment
Psychological stress/fear

Skill error

Tissue overload

Pain

Compensatory movement

Figure 12.2 Skill error and overload cycle.

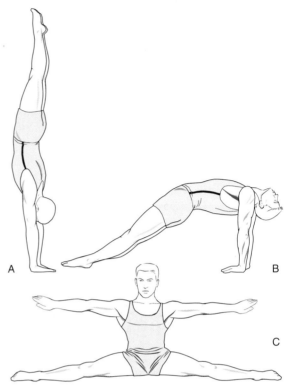

Figure 12.3 A: Handstand. B: Bridge. C: Side split.

- Inadequate conditioning
- Inadequate warm-up
- Anatomical abnormalities
- Incomplete rehabilitation
- Poor equipment and facilities.

This chapter aims to introduce some of the components of gymnastic skill and to consider their potential for overuse injury and the implications for effective physiotherapy management of the injured gymnast.

COMPONENTS OF GYMNASTIC SKILL

There are three common core gymnastic elements that form the basis of most technical high-performance skills (Fig. 12.3):

- handstand
- bridge
- side split.

The young gymnasts need to have a sound mastery of these skills if they are to successfully develop in the sport. Gymnastic skill relies on the ability of the individual to balance articular flexibility with control and stability. As a consequence, while the naturally flexible child may be successful in the early stages of gymnastics, any hypermobility soon becomes a disadvantage. It is important that all who are involved in the management of the gymnast remain sensitive to the problems of hypermobility, as range without control can result in significant tissue damage. Changes in flexibility associated with growth should also be borne in mind. Attempts to force a range of motion that is reduced as a natural consequence of growth can be detrimental to the individual.

Optimum mobility must therefore be the goal of all gymnastic skill preparation and the final goal of all rehabilitation for the injured gymnast (Fig. 12.4).

Along with the common core elements, there are three other major components of gymnastic skill that must be considered:

- Support – in which the body's weight is taken by either the hands or the feet
- Swing – in which the body travels about a fixed point (in the ring discipline, the gymnast must swing against a mobile base as the rings hang free from an overhead gantry)

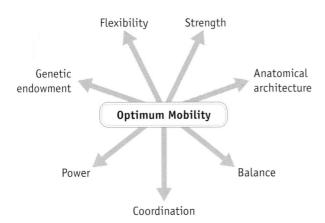

Figure 12.4 A model of the components of optimum mobility.

- Flight – in which the unsupported body travels through space.

Each of these skills places specific stresses on the musculoskeletal system of the gymnast. Performance of a gymnastic routine demands that the gymnast be able to combine and perform these component skills in variable sequence, often at great speed.

THE TRUNK

Swing and flight are often coupled in gymnastic skill, with the swing acting as a preparation for the flight. The most spectacular examples of this are high bar release and catch activities.

Three basic body positions are essential components of all swing and flight activities: the open, closed and straight body positions (Fig. 12.5). Control of these three shapes, and rapid transition between them, are essential to successful and safe performance. In gymnastic performance, both the arms and legs are involved in the generation and transmission of force. The trunk is therefore significantly involved in the control, translation and coordination of force between the upper and lower extremities. Consequently, trunk integrity and control are paramount to the safe execution of gymnastic skill. Any factor that reduces the range of motion or impairs the muscle control of the trunk inhibits the efficient transference of force, leading to compensation and potential injury. Careful monitoring and evaluation of the components of the spinal stabilizing triad are therefore essential in the overall screening and management of the gymnast (Fig. 12.6).

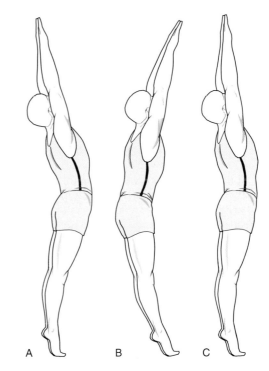

Figure 12.5 Basic body positions of swing and flight activities. A: Open shape. B: closed shape. C: Straight shape.

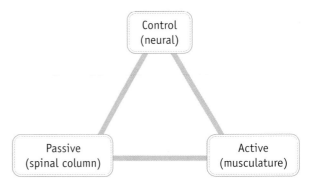

Figure 12.6 Spinal stabilizing triad (Panjabi 1992).

Accurate figures for the incidence and nature of low back pain and injury in gymnastics are difficult to establish due to the limited prospective sport-specific research. The consensus of opinion among authors, however, would be to agree that back pain is common amongst gymnasts although direct causation is yet to be fully proven.

Several pathologies have been associated with the developing gymnast:

- soft tissue injury
- facet syndrome
- spondylolysis
- vertebral end-plate fracture.

It must, however, be remembered that tumour and infection should always be excluded in any complaint of back pain in the child and adolescent.

The extremes of flexion and extension found in gymnastic skills, especially in the handspring and backflick derived actions, demonstrate that hyperextension and hyperflexion are major components of the sport. The effect of these extremes of movement is significantly amplified when impact forces through the hands or feet, high-velocity swinging actions and twisting movements are superimposed. Failure of the trunk control mechanisms can therefore lead to a significant potential for injury.

Compression load on the normal lumbar spine is taken predominantly on the anterior vertebral endplates and the annulus fibrosis. In a healthy disc, axial compression does not result in annular disruption as pressure in the disc can be evenly distributed from the nucleus to the annulus. Excessive compressive loading can, however, result in end-plate fracture. If the frac-

ture does not heal spontaneously then the normal compression-absorbing capacity of the disc will be disturbed, leading to annular disruption, and potential herniation can occur (Bogduk & Twomey 1991; Fig. 12.7).

Torsional stress is poorly tolerated by the vertebral structures. Farfan et al (1970) found that relative resistance of torsion is 65% from ipsilateral facet joint impaction and 30% from the annulus on the disc. The orientation of the facet articulations in the lumbar spine allows only 2–3° of pure rotation. When rotation of more than 3° is imparted, the resulting ipsilateral facet joint impaction can lead to facet joint injury and pars interarticularis stress reaction, including fracture (spondylolysis; Jackson et al 1976) (Fig. 12.8).

Spondylolysis is the most commonly reported cause of pain in the low back in the gymnast. Adolescence itself predisposes to the development of spondylolysis, as there is a plastic quality of the bone and an immaturity of the pars. The strong disc in the adolescent increases the shear potential through the pars.

The therapist must naturally consider not only the multifactorial causes of back pain, but also the multifaceted components of the sport in working up a treatment plan. The age, level of ability and training load, as well as the history, must all be considered in arriving at a diagnosis.

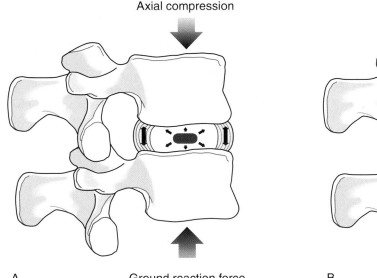

Figure 12.7 A: Normal distribution of compression forces across the intervertebral disc. B: Disturbance of normal disc compression distribution with loss of annular rigidity.

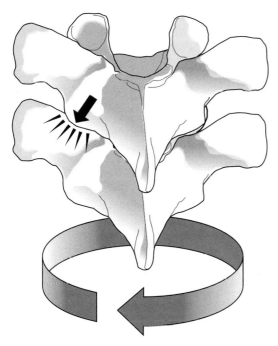

Figure 12.8 Extension with rotation: leads to impaction at the facet articulation; tissue irritation may develop.

THE UPPER LIMB

Gymnastics is unique among sports in the repetitive use of the upper limb for load-bearing. These loads are both compressive and distractive. The swing and support components of the skills are particularly stressful, combining strength, flexibility and speed, and impart high-impact load, rotational stress and compression loads to the tissues, respectively. This can lead to a high potential risk for injury at the wrist, elbow and shoulder. Respect for the stage of skeletal maturity, the stage of skill development and the level of physical preparation is crucial in minimizing the risk of injury in the upper limb.

The shoulder complex

The integrated functions of the rotator cuff muscles and the scapular stabilizers, coupled with the large multiplanar movements inherent in gymnastic skills, make the shoulder complex vulnerable to injury.

Shoulder pathology seen in the gymnast can be described along a continuum, ranging from minor overuse microtrauma tendinosis at one end to macro-traumatic full-thickness tears at the other. Shoulder pathology in the gymnast can therefore be considered under the following headings:

- impingement
- instability
- tensile overload leading to macroscopic tendon failure.

Impingement

Impingement involves a spectrum of lesions of the tissues in the suprahumeral space. The space beneath the acromion allows only a small margin for the normal passage of the suprahumeral tissues under the acromion process. Any factor that reduces the subacromial space or enlarges the suprahumeral tissues will significantly impair this mechanism. The structures most often involved in impingement are the supraspinatus tendon and the long head of biceps tendon.

Peak forces against the acromion have been measured between 85° and 136° of elevation (Wuelker et al 1994). Swinging through handstand, when the shoulder is carried into elevation through flexion, with associated rotation, can potentiate subacromial impingement, as in this position the suprahumeral tissues are effectively driven under the anterior one-third of the acromion.

Instability

Impingement can occur as a consequence of an instability of the glenohumeral joint and/or loss of scapular stabilization, resulting in increased anterior head translation.

Attenuation of the static stabilizers of the glenohumeral joint, such as the capsular ligaments and labrum, from the excessive demands of swinging actions can lead to anterior instability. A progressive loss of glenohumeral stability is created when the dynamic stabilizing functions of the rotator cuff are diminished from fatigue, tendon injury or growth-related muscle imbalance.

The dynamic control of the scapula and humerus is achieved through a series of force couples. The scapular force couple is formed by the upper fibres of trapezius, the levator scapulae muscle, and the upper fibres of serratus anterior. The lower component of the force couple is formed by the lower fibres of trapezius and the lower fibres of serratus anterior (Kapandji 1989). The simultaneous contraction of these muscles produces a smooth motion of scapula protraction around the thoracic wall as the arm is carried into elevation. The scapula thereby functions as a stable base, allowing the humeral head to maintain its normal position within the glenoid. Disturbance of this force couple mechanism produces an unstable base of support for the humerus with a resultant overload stress on the rotator cuff mechanism.

The coordinated action of the scapular muscles is therefore essential for the efficient and safe performance of all upper limb support and swing activities of the gymnast. As growth can have a marked effect on posture and muscle length, it is important that the gymnast be regularly monitored. Specific parascapular function should therefore be incorporated into the conditioning and preparation profile of the gymnast. The lateral scapular slide test described by Kibler (1991) can be used as a basic evaluation tool. Kibler found that an increase of 1 cm or more in two of the three test positions correlated with shoulder impingement. It may be necessary in the evaluation of the gymnast to develop the test positions to make the screening more sport-specific. This is an area awaiting future research.

Tensile overload

Heavy repetitive eccentric forces incurred by the rotator cuff musculature during high-speed swinging actions can lead to overload failure of the tendon. The presence of either acquired or congenital capsular laxity along with labral insufficiency can greatly increase the tensile stresses to the rotator cuff muscle–tendon units.

Cofield (1985) suggested that normal tendons do not tear and that 30% or more of the tendon must be damaged to produce a significant reduction in strength. The consequence of cumulative microtrauma and degenerative changes in the matrix of the tendon over time may therefore increase the vulnerability to total tendon failure.

Treatment considerations

Successful rehabilitation programmes for injury to the shoulder complex must be tailored to the individual, based on accurate diagnosis of the tissue damage and pathomechanics, clinical signs, stage of growth and specific sports skill demands.

As many gymnasts experience pain only during specific skill execution, normal physical testing of the shoulder is often not sufficient to reproduce the gymnast's pain. The therapist must therefore use functional testing in order to identify the pain-provoking position with an estimation of the force, direction and magnitude of muscle activity. It should be remembered that the underlying dysfunction influencing the shoulder mechanics may not be evident in the shoulder girdle but may result from a weakness in another link of the kinetic chain producing excessive load on the shoulder.

As the shoulder in the gymnast functions in both open and closed chain activity the selection of rehabilitation exercises should include both to be effective.

The elbow

Overuse injuries at the elbow in the gymnast are strongly related to the use of the upper limb for load-bearing. The swing phase of gymnastic skill can be likened to the acceleration phase of throwing. The valgus forces that occur during the acceleration phase are maximized at the elbow, as the trunk and shoulder rotate faster than the arm and forearm on the downward phase of the swing.

Elbow injury has the potential for significant functional disability and should therefore be avoided at all costs. Sound technique and meticulous preparation are key elements in injury prevention at the elbow.

The average female gymnast has been shown to have an extension range of between 3° and 12° of recurvarum and an accentuated valgus inclination (Weiker 1995). The female gymnast takes advantage of the hyperextension to lock the elbow into a mechanically stable position to accept the weight-bearing load. The male gymnast appears to use the strength of the triceps to achieve and then control extension.

The repeated load-bearing coupled with forceful extension and valgus stress indicative of many gymnastic skills place a significant demand on the anterior, posterior and medial musculotendinous structures. Such repeated overload, left unchecked, is likely to result in microtrauma and subsequent injury.

The anterior band of the medial (ulnar) collateral ligament has been shown to be the primary structure resisting valgus stress at the elbow. Microtrauma as a result of repetitive valgus stress can lead to compromise of the integrity of the medial collateral ligament which may lead to instability and further injury.

The valgus stress to the joint produces tension forces medially and compression forces laterally. The lateral compartment is therefore subjected to significant compressive stress in gymnastics when load-bearing is added to the valgus stress. The lateral compressive forces involve the radial head and the capitellum. This repetitive compressive stress across the radiocapitellar joint can lead to damage of the articular cartilage of the radial head or capitellum, or both. The development of osteochondral defects in the capitellum or radial head can lead to long-term disability (Maffulli et al 1992).

The wrist

The wrist is a complex functional unit. In gymnastics, it is required to provide multi-axial motion while bearing weight across its many articulations. It also provides a narrow passage for the nerves, vessels and tendons of the hand. As the wrist is without intrinsic musculature, it is dependent for both its dynamic and static stability on the intercapsular and interosseous ligaments and the inherent stability of the joint configurations. As a consequence, any injury that disturbs these stability mechanisms can lead to significant functional instability and impairment.

The potential for both direct and indirect trauma to the growth plates at the wrist is also a major concern in the overall management of the skeletally immature athlete. While acute injuries can, and do, occur, the greatest presentation is for non-specific wrist pain often associated with chronic stress-related reaction implicating the growth plates. The support and swing activities of gymnastics demand that the growth plates withstand combinations of tension, compression, shear and torsion. As the growth plate is least resistant to torsion, swing and support, with rotation, put the growth plate at further risk.

Stress-related injury to the distal radial and ulnar growth plates has been described in gymnasts as a consequence of hyperextension and rotation in support. This is a common mechanism associated with vaulting incorporating a twisting component, the wrist on the side of the twist being forced into a position of hyperextension and ulnar deviation. The ulnar stabilizing structures of the lunotriqueteral and mid-carpal joints will also be placed under stress by this mechanism. Injury to the triangular fibrocartilage complex can also occur as a consequence of weight-bearing rotation with hyperextension.

The compression of the radial epiphysis from repeated load-bearing may be sufficient to cause a permanent growth disturbance, resulting in deformity of the distal radius (Caine 1992). As a consequence, the length of the ulna in relation to the radius is increased (positive ulnar variance). In upper limb support, the radius normally accepts 80% of the load and the ulna 20% (Zuluaga 1995). Positive ulnar variance alters this ratio, increasing the load on the triangular fibrocartilage.

As in all gymnastic injury, evaluation, accurate history and functional evaluation are essential to the successful management of the gymnast. Grip strength testing can be used as a useful screening and evaluation tool in managing chronic wrist pain, as a positive correlation has been demonstrated between a decrease in grip strength and the presence of a confirmed injury.

THE LOWER LIMB

All gymnastic routines require landing, often with a rotational component, either to dismount from apparatus or to complete a tumble or vault. The distraction and shear forces, which must be absorbed by the lower limb kinetic chain, are considerable, as the gymnast is required to execute these manoeuvres without taking a step. The peak ground reaction force generated during take-off and landing from a double back somersault, a standard element of all elite level floor routines, can be as much as 14 times body weight. As a consequence, the potential for overload and overuse injury in the lower limb is considerable.

The knee

The knee is a common site of injury in the gymnast. The demand on the knee mechanism from repeated take-off and landing activities is naturally high, and therefore any disturbance of optimal function can potentiate injury.

Aside from traumatic injury, the most common presentation is that of vague non-specific anterior knee pain with a minimum of objective signs at the knee. Common sites of overuse injury are:

- patellofemoral pain syndrome
- fat pad inflammation
- Osgood–Schlatter's apophysitis
- Sinding–Larsen Johansson apophysitis
- patellar tendinopathy.

It is not uncommon for a combination of patellar tendinopathy and patellofemoral pain syndrome to coexist. The high demand on the apophyses of the tibial tubercle and the apex of the patella can leave them vulnerable to injury, especially during periods of rapid growth.

The anterior fat pad of the knee can also become chronically inflamed by irritation of the inferior pole of the patella during maximum extension activities. This is accentuated in gymnasts with a genu recurvatum or posterior tilting of the patella.

Effective management is dependent on accurate diagnosis, based on a careful history establishing the precise provoking mechanisms and their impact on the underlying tissues.

Factors to consider are:

- anatomical alignment
- developmental postural stress
- girdle stability
- technique error.

Anatomical alignment

The arc of normal patellar tracking in functional range is important if injury is to be avoided. Patellar tracking can be influenced by several factors: patella shape, patella position, muscle balance, resultant line of pull, and the quality and arrangement of the non-contractile tissue.

There are several other alignment factors that need to be considered when evaluating patellar tracking. They include femoral rotation, femoral neck anteversion, genu valgum, genu recurvatum, tibial torsion, excessive pronation and leg length discrepancy.

Evaluation of patellar alignment and arc of patellar tracking through functional range should therefore be included in the screening of the gymnast and in the assessment of knee pathology (Reid 1992).

Developmental postural stress

In the pre-adolescent child, the normal standing posture tends to demonstrate an increase in internal rotation at the hip, resulting in an increase in 'in-toeing'. There is also an increase in valgus at the knee and an increase in pronation. Repeated take-off and landing during this period can result in patellofemoral pain as a consequence of patellar maltracking.

Girdle stability

Stability of the pelvic girdle is essential in controlling the direction of weight transference through the lower limb. The integrity of the glutei as lateral stabilizers plays an important part in controlling the positioning of the knee over the foot for effective take-off and landing. Muscle control of the low back and pelvic girdle will be altered throughout the growth period and therefore regular evaluation and conditioning of the girdle stabilizers is essential.

Technique error

High repetition of poor technique will naturally exacerbate any biomechanical fault, as will landing onto hard surfaces. Evaluation of all knee pain must, as far as is reasonably practicable, incorporate an evaluation of the individual technique and training pattern.

Foot and ankle

The complex structure and function of the foot and ankle are essential for effective take-off and controlled impact during landing. Like the wrist, the ankle has little local muscle support, relying for its function on mechanical efficiency of its capsular and ligamentous structures. As much of gymnastics is performed either barefooted or with only thin gymnastic slippers, the integrity of the foot is essential, as shoe support and orthotic devices cannot be used to modify poor foot biomechanics.

Heel pain (Sever's disease)

Young gymnasts are susceptible to apophysitis because of the repetitive jumping and landing from a height. The posterior portion of the calcaneus develops as an independent centre of ossification separated from the main bone by a cartilaginous apophyseal plate. This centre appears at approximately 10 years of age and fuses with the main bone at 15 years of age. The vertical alignment of the apophyseal plate causes it to be subjected to large shearing stresses by the gastrocnemius. During the period of the prepubertal growth spurt, the epiphyseal–diaphyseal junction may be weaker and vulnerable to circulatory compromise, resulting in a traumatic avascular necrosis. This may explain the typical X-ray appearances of fragmentation and altered density of the calcaneal apophysis. The take-off and landing demand during this period of growth should be carefully monitored to minimize the potential for injury.

Plantar fasciitis

The plantar fascia has a major role to play in take-off and landing activities. On landing, it assists with the lowering and flattening of the medial longitudinal arch, while on take-off the windlass effect allows the medial arch to be reformed and provide a rigid lever for effective push-off. This dual function leaves the plantar fascia vulnerable to the potential for overuse injury. Early identification and management of this condition are important in order to prevent the gymnast developing compensatory increased weight-bearing on the lateral aspect of the foot. Such compensation can lead to subsequent overload on structures along the lower limb kinetic chain.

Talar anterior impingement syndrome

The talar anterior impingement syndrome is related to the presence of osteophytes on the neck of the talus.

Repeated plantarflexion may cause a chronic overload stress reaction at the tibia and talar attachments of the anterior capsule, resulting in osteophyte formation at either or both attachments.

Repeated landings into forced end-range dorsiflexion, especially in 'short landing' (in which backward tumbles are under-rotated) produce repeated impingement stress of the bony surfaces resulting in osteophyte formation. Continued end-range dorsiflexion causes impingement of the bony spurs along with pinching of hypertrophied and chronically swollen synovium.

REHABILITATION OF THE GYMNAST

Rehabilitation in gymnastics must be based on a model of prevention:

- primary prevention
- secondary prevention
- tertiary prevention.

Primary prevention

Primary prevention is the first step in effective management. Appropriate and regular screening is an essential component of primary prevention. It ensures a sound foundation on which all training and skill acquisition components can be built without damage to the musculoskeletal system. To be successful, screening needs to be sport skill-specific and related to age and sex-related norms. Individual flexibility, muscle balance and growth factors need to be evaluated against known risk factors. The information gathered should then be fed back to the coach so that skill-specific conditioning can be implemented and deficits corrected.

Gymnastics demands a high-intensity training response from the immature skeleton and supporting structures. Any screening or evaluation process must therefore take both training effect and developmental process into account.

The establishing of a definitive model for screening is, however, complicated by a lack of agreement over risk factors facing the developing athlete. Further research is needed in this area.

Secondary prevention

Secondary prevention requires that the injured gymnast be rehabilitated sufficiently to ensure that full recovery is achieved and that recurrence is prevented.

Treatment must first of all be targeted at removing the provoking factors to allow recovery of the implicated tissue. This is done by evaluating the evidence gathered from the subjective assessment of the extrinsic factors. Rest is the key feature of effective treatment, but absolute rest is rarely indicated and poorly tolerated by the athlete. Active rest, avoiding the provoking activity, needs to be explained to the athlete and, where necessary, the coach, to gain compliance at an early stage with what may be a lengthy rehabilitation programme.

Once the programme of active rest is established, treatment is aimed at facilitating the repair of the implicated tissue. Clinical signs and the history will indicate the presence of active inflammation or determine whether the condition is a chronic alteration in the tissue matrix with focal degeneration. When inflammation is present, local treatment modalities can be delivered in the form of ice, electrotherapy and topical NSAIDs. Supportive strapping may also be employed to 'unload' the affected tissue. When chronic alteration in the cell matrix is present, local treatment is unlikely to be successful. In this instance, treatment should move straight on to preventive measures. The overall musculature in the affected kinetic chain must be carefully assessed for functional muscle balance and, where necessary, rehabilitated appropriately (Grace 1985, Kibler 1987).

Tertiary prevention

Specific rehabilitation programming is essential to prevent recurrence of the problem. The planning and staging of the rehabilitation programme are based on the findings of the objective evaluation coupled with an understanding of the demands of the skills of the sport the gymnast is engaged in, and the level of participation.

The correction of identified contributing alignment faults must be addressed. In the lower limb, orthotics worn during periods outside the gym may be effective in reducing the load on the implicated soft tissues. Careful prescription is important and a progressive introduction essential if resolution of one injury is not to lead to another.

Where loss of tissue extensibility is found to be a contributor, stretching protocols need to be implemented (Sapega et al 1981). These may take the form of soft tissue mobilization, manipulation, massage, proprioceptive neuromuscular facilitation (PNF) and active stretching regimes. Local heat may be employed to enhance tissue extensibility.

Alteration in muscle balance and disturbed movement patterning must be dealt with sequentially so that normal movement is restored and appropriate strength and extensibility are achieved (Richardson et al 1999).

Throughout the rehabilitation process, the athlete and, where appropriate, the coach and/or parent must fully understand the rationale behind the treatment and the extended time-frame needed for recovery, if compliance is to be maintained and the outcome is to be successful.

CONCLUSIONS

1. The complex sport of gymnastics poses many challenges for the therapist.
2. A sound understanding of the impact of overload on the kinetic chain is important in designing prevention strategies.
3. Effective management of the injured gymnast is dependent on sound communication with all involved in the gymnast's preparation.
4. Regular screening of the gymnast should be undertaken to prevent long-term problems developing.

REFERENCES

Bogduk N, Twomey L T 1991 Clinical anatomy of the lumbar spine, 2nd edn. Churchill Livingstone, New York
Brukner P, Khan K 1997 Clinical sports medicine. McGraw-Hill, Sydney
Caine D, Roy S, Singer K M, Brrekhoff J 1992 Stress changes of the distal radial growth plate: a radiographic survey and review of the literature. American Journal of Sports Medicine 20: 290
Cofield R 1985 Current concepts review of rotator cuff disease of the shoulder. Journal of Bone and Joint Surgery 67A: 974
Dixon M, Fricker P 1993 Injuries to elite gymnasts over 10 years. Medicine and Science in Sport 25(12): 1322–1329
Farfan H F, Cossette J W, Robertson G H, Wens R V, Krans H 1970 The effects of torsion on the lumbar intervertebral joints: the role of torsion in the production of disc degeneration. Journal of Bone and Joint Surgery 52A: 468

Grace T G 1985 Muscle imbalance and extremity injury: a perplexing relationship. Sports Medicine 2: 77
Jackson D W, Wiltse L L, Ciricone R J 1976 Spondylolysis in the female gymnast. Clinical Orthopedics and Related Research 117: 68
Kapandji I A 1989 The physiology of the joints, vol 1. The upper limb. Churchill Livingstone, Edinburgh
Kibler W B 1987 Strength and flexibility findings in anterior knee pain. American Journal of Sports Medicine 15: 410
Kibler W B 1991 Role of the scapula in the overhead throwing motion. Contemporary Orthopaedics 22: 525
Krivickas L S 1997 Anatomical factors associated with overuse sports injuries. Sports Medicine 24(2): 132–146
Leadbetter W B 1992 Cell matrix response in tendon injury. Clinical Sports Medicine 11: 533–578
Maffulli N, Chan D, Aldridge M J 1992 Derangement of the articular surfaces of the elbow in young gymnasts. Journal of Pediatric Orthopaedics 12: 344–350
Meeusen R, Borms J 1992 Gymnastic injuries. Sports Medicine 13(5): 337
Panjabi M M 1992 The stabilising system of the spine. Part 1. Function, dysfunction, adaptation and enhancement. Journal of Spinal Disorders 5: 383–389
Reid D C 1992 Sports injury assessment and rehabilitation. Churchill Livingstone, Edinburgh
Richardson C, Jull G, Hodges P, Hides J 1999 General considerations in motor control and joint stabilisation: the basis of assessment and exercise techniques. In: Therapeutic exercise for spinal segmental stabilisation in low back pain. Churchill Livingstone, Edinburgh
Sapega A A, Quedenfeld T C, Moyer R A 1981 Biophysical factors in range of motion exercises. Physician and Sports Medicine 9: 57
Weiker G G 1995 Upper extremity gymnastic injuries. In: Nicholas J A, Hershman E B (eds) The upper extremity in sports medicine, 2nd edn. Mosby, St Louis, MO
Wuelker N, Plitz W, Roetman B 1994 Biomechanical data concerning shoulder impingement syndrome. Clinical Orthopedics 303: 242
Zuluaga M 1995 Sports physiotherapy. Applied science and practice. Churchill Livingstone, Edinburgh

FURTHER READING

Donatelli R A (ed) 1997 Clinics in physical therapy. Physical therapy of the shoulder, 3rd edn. Churchill Livingstone, Edinburgh
Mandelbaum B R, Bartolozzi A R, Davis C A, Tentlings L, Bragonier B 1989 Wrist pain syndrome in the gymnast: pathogenic, diagnostic and therapeutic considerations. American Journal of Sports Medicine 17: 305
Richardson C, Jull G, Hodges P, Hides J 1999 Therapeutic exercise for spinal segment stabilisation in low back pain. Churchill Livingstone, Edinburgh

Women athletes

13

Endocrinological changes in exercising women

Bruno Arena   Nicola Maffulli

KEY POINTS

1. The physical activity required to participate in sports at an elite competitive level can produce significant, albeit temporary, hormonal disturbances.
2. Hormonal problems are becoming an important issue in female athletes, particularly among younger age groups.
3. Hormones regulating the reproductive system may become involved and cause, for example, delay in menarche, irregularity of the menstrual cycle and infertility.
4. An unbalanced diet can worsen the effects of intensive training on the endocrine system – at its most extreme, an abnormally low body fat content may interfere with pituitary function.
5. Younger female athletes, particularly in the peripubertal age group, require close and expert supervision.

INTRODUCTION

Sport is practised with the expectation of maintaining good health and physical fitness. The effects that it produces, such as muscular hypertrophy or decrease in body fat and body weight in particular, are seen as positive physiological changes, and are often actively sought. While leisure sport rarely produces dramatic body changes, demanding physical activity, as may occur when participating in sports at a high competitive level, can produce alterations in some physiological parameters at very pathological levels. The endocrine system can often be affected, as the delicate balance between hormonal production and catabolism may be altered with significant changes in circulating hormonal levels. The number of women practising sport has increased, and hormonal problems are becoming an important and frequent issue, particularly among younger athletes. Most hormones can be affected, albeit temporarily: when those regulating the reproductive system are involved, there can be delay in the age of menarche, irregularity of menstrual cycles with oligomenorrhoea or amenorrhoea, and infertility. The mechanisms involved are psychological as well as physical: the stress of the competition may be quite significant, particularly in younger athletes who are often overconcerned with their diet. Unbalanced diets, sometimes self-prescribed by adolescent athletes to achieve a rapid weight loss, can determine caloric and nutritional deficits that worsen the effects of intensive training on the endocrine system. In more extreme cases, prolonged fasting can enhance the overproduction of cortisol and prolactin induced by exercise and, as fat tissue is the site of conversion of androgen precursors to oestrone, and gonadotrophin release is affected by circulating sex steroid levels, an abnormally low body fat content may interfere with normal pituitary function.

In this following chapter, we examine the effects of physical training on the hormones in female athletes.

EXERCISE AND SEX STEROID HORMONES

Exercise can alter plasma levels of oestrogens and progesterone (Montagnani et al 1992): anovulation and a short luteal phase with a monophasic basal body temperature are frequent in women involved in intensive physical training. A significant increase in core temperature may inhibit the binding of sex steroid hormones to plasma proteins, producing an increase in the metabolically active free hormonal fraction (Lata et al 1980). Anovulation, associated with low oestrogens and progesterone levels (Ellison & Lager 1986), is a cause of infertility. This condition, which may not represent a problem in a young adolescent athlete, may certainly become so in an adult athlete who plans to start a family while still actively engaged in sport. The decreased plasma levels of oestrogens and progesterone linked to anovulation, which often coexist with higher relative levels of oestrone due to increased peripheral conversion of androgens, may, in more severe cases, determine amenorrhoea which, if protracted, may be responsible for the skeletal changes usually found in the post-

menopause, particularly bone decalcification and remodelling (Arena et al 1998, Prior et al 1990). Bone formation markers (osteocalcin, carboxyterminal propetide of type 1 collagen and bone alkaline phosphatase), as well as bone resorption markers (pyridinoline and deoxypyridinoline), are lower in amenorrhoeic runners compared with eumenorrhoeic or sedentary controls, but in the first group bone resorption occurs at a higher rate than bone formation (Zanker & Swaine 1998). Low blood levels of oestrogens appear to be more critical than low progesterone levels for the onset of bone decalcification (De Souza et al 1997).

In postmenopausal women, moderate physical exercise produces a reduction in sex hormone binding globulin (SHBG) levels, with a protective effect against bone decalcification (Caballero et al 1996). Maximal aerobic capacity increases significantly, and plasminogen activator inhibitor type 1 and tissue plasminogen activator decrease with exercise. Fasting plasma insulin and glucose are also lower, and lipid and lipoprotein profiles improve (Stevenson et al 1995). The hormonal response to exercise may differ according to the individual level of training: trained healthy women show an increase in plasma oestradiol during an acute bicycle ergometer bout and a decrease in its metabolic clearance rate which is higher than untrained controls. This may depend on decreased splanchnic blood flow as a consequence of exercise and a decrease in hepatic clearance rate. The menstrual cycle phase when moderate exercise is performed can also affect the hormonal response, as oestradiol tends to remain stable following moderate exercise in the follicular phase, and to increase if the same exercise is performed in the mid-luteal phase (Jurkowski et al 1978, Loucks & Horvath 1984). Intensive exercise is also associated with increased blood levels of adrenocortical hormones, dehydroepiandrosterone sulphate (DHEA-S), androstenedione (A) and testosterone (T), but only the first one remains elevated for more than 2 h. This may depend on prolonged adrenocorticotrophin stimulation or reduced hepatic clearance (Hale et al 1983, Keizer et al 1987a). Increased levels of androgens may enhance the muscular hypertrophy produced by exercise, and DHEA-S is positively associated with high-density lipoprotein cholesterol (HDL-C), which has a protective effect on cardiovascular disease (Thompson et al 1997).

THYROID AND PARATHYROID HORMONES

Fasting blood levels of T_3, FT_3, FT_4 and RT_3 are lower in amenorrhoeic adolescent athletes than in eumenorrhoeic controls. The latter show lower levels of T_4 (Baer 1993, Loucks et al 1992). Low levels of thyroid hormones are often associated with high prolactin levels, which may interfere with ovulation. Parathormone (PTH) secretion is stimulated by exercise but basal levels are low in subjects with a high level of physical fitness (Brahm et al 1997).

BETA-ENDORPHINS

Beta-endorphins are higher in exercising women compared with sedentary controls. The pattern of beta-endorphin production appears to be independent of the phase of menstrual cycle when the exercise is performed (Harber et al 1997). A higher secretion of endorphins during exercise can interfere with the gonadotrophin-releasing hormone (GnRH) production, and therefore reduce significantly the luteinizing hormone (LH) pulsatility (Prior 1982, Veldhuis et al 1985): this effect is counteracted by naloxone in eumenorrhoeic, but not in amenorrhoeic, athletes (Samuels et al 1991). Conversely, opioid peptides may increase blood levels of growth hormone and prolactin (Howlett et al 1984).

GROWTH HORMONE

Exercise stimulates growth hormone (GH) production and enhances statural growth. Hypertrophic muscle growth produced by exercise is mainly a consequence of mechanical strain, but GH appears to have an important role in reparative muscle growth (Borer 1995). In addition, low-volume resistive exercise produces a luteal phase-induced increase in GH and androstenedione (Kraemer et al 1995).

MELATONIN

Melatonin, an indole derivative of serotonin, is produced in the pineal gland, located in the roof of the third ventricle. It is normally produced with a circadian rhythm, decreasing during light and increasing during darkness. Precocious puberty has been found in children affected by tumoral or infective destruction of the pineal gland. Melatonin increases during exercise (Highnet 1989) and is unresponsive to either dopaminergic or opioidergic blockade.

PROLACTIN

Increased opioid production during exercise can stimulate prolactin release (Howlett et al 1984), which can

stimulate adrenal release of androgens (Schiebinger et al 1986) and interfere with the ovarian aromatization of androgen precursors to oestrogens (Keizer et al 1989). Prolactin increase during exercise is higher in eumenorrhoeic than in amenorrhoeic runners (De Souza et al 1991).

CORTISOL

— Cortisol and adrenalin increase may alter the balance between facilitating and inhibiting neurotransmitters on pulsatile LH release.
— ACTH and cortisol response to exercise is blunted in lactating women.

Cortisol levels increase during exercise, particularly in amenorrhoeic athletes (Ding et al 1988). This increase, together with adrenaline, during daily intensive physical exercise can inhibit the pulsatile release of luteinizing hormone by disrupting the balance between facilitating and inhibiting brain neurotransmitters (Bergen & Leung 1986). In a recent study (Rupprecht et al 1997), subjects with atopic eczema, who show a poor adrenocorticotrophic hormone (ACTH) and cortisol response to the administration of human corticotrophin-releasing hormone, showed a significant ACTH and cortisol increase induced by the same incremental graded bicycle exercise performed by normal controls. This difference has been attributed to the possible effects of neuropeptides released during exercise on the hypothalamic– pituitary–adrenal axis. ACTH and cortisol responses appear to be impaired in lactating women following 20 min of graded treadmill exercise compared with non-lactating controls (Altemus et al 1995).

GONADOTROPHINS

The pulsatile release of luteinizing hormone (LH) may disappear in women with regular periods as a consequence of prolonged intensive physical training (Keizer et al 1987b), while follicle-stimulating hormone (FSH), which has a longer half-life, may increase following endurance exercise. Blood levels of LH, SHBG and oestradiol are generally lower following exercise compared with eumenorrhoeic controls and the increase in prolactin is less significant (Loucks & Horvath 1984).

Gonadotrophin release following administration of GnRH after a training programme consisting of running increasing mileage can be impaired in eumenorrhoeic runners, while it can be quite marked in amenorrhoeic runners (Boyden et al 1984, Veldhuis et al 1985). The rise of LH in the 2 h following an acute exercise and the decrease in its pulsatile pattern can be further enhanced by the stress of the competition, and luteal phase dysfunction is the direct consequence of impaired LH release (Fries et al 1974).

MENSTRUAL DISTURBANCES IN EXERCISING WOMEN

The first menstrual cycle (menarche) represents the most significant event of puberty, when a clear definition of secondary sexual characteristics is achieved, and reproductive capacity is established with the onset of ovulation. The neuroendocrine mechanism determining the onset of puberty is an increase in amplitude and frequency of GnRH release which stimulates production of the gonadotrophins, FSH and LH from the pituitary gland. Gonadotrophins stimulate the ovaries and enhance maturation of follicles, with a consequent increase in blood levels of oestrogens and progesterone. In the presence of oestradiol, GnRH production is stimulated by dopamine, adrenaline and noradrenaline, and inhibited by beta-endorphin and serotonin. In the absence of oestradiol, these hormones may have the opposite effect on GnRH production (Sizonenko & Aubert 1986). Intensive physical exercise during the prepubertal years may produce a delayed onset of menarche (Frisch et al 1981), which is associated with lower serum oestradiol and higher SHBG levels, and a later establishment of ovulatory cycles (Apter 1996). The delay in the closure of epiphyses can determine excessive growth in long bones, and has been associated in some ballet dancers with an eunuchoid-like condition (Warren et al 1986).

There are conflicting reports on the influence of menstrual status on the level of physical performance (De Souza et al 1990, Galliven et al 1997, Maffulli & Arena 1993), and often amenorrhoea is more common in female athletes with a history of menstrual disturbances preceding commencement of training activity (Schwartz et al 1980), in those younger than 30, in those who run more than 40 miles per week, and in parous athletes (Dale et al 1979). Functional hypothalamic amenorrhoea is more common in women with a low fat body mass and a high lean body mass and who follow a low-fat, high-fibre and high-carbohydrate diet compared with regular cycling controls. They also show an abnormal pattern of GH production, with blunted pulse amplitude, accelerated pulse frequency and elevated interpulse concentrations. GH-binding protein levels are also low (Laughlin et al 1998).

Some sports (such as running) tend to be associated with menstrual disturbances more often than others (such as swimming), and athletes with a lower than normal body weight are more prone to develop amenorrhoea (Sanborn et al 1982). A reduction in the intensity of training can often allow menstrual cycles to return, as has been reported in ballet dancers (Pearson 1985). When this is not possible, cyclic administration of progesterone can be useful both to resume menstrual cycles and to protect the bone (Prior et al 1992).

CONCLUSIONS

Leisure physical exercise is not associated with significant hormonal changes, and is definitely to be recommended for its positive effects on general health and fitness in all age groups. The intensity of training required to participate in sports at a competitive level is generally much higher and in some athletes, often with predisposing conditions, can produce significant, albeit temporary, hormonal disturbances. Younger female athletes, particularly in the peripubertal age group, are more at risk and therefore require close and expert supervision.

REFERENCES

Altemus M, Deuster P A, Galliven E, Carter C S, Gold P W 1995 Suppression of hypothalamic-pituitary-adrenal axis responses to stress in lactating women. Journal of Clinical Endocrinology and Metabolism 80(10): 2954–2959

Apter D 1996 Hormonal events during female puberty in relation to breast cancer risk. European Journal of Cancer Prevention 5(6): 476–482

Arena B, Santori L, Lauri A, Morleo M A 1998 Urinary excretion of pyridinolines as an index of bone remodelling: influence of hormone replacement therapy. Tutorial System International 5(1): 10–13

Baer J T 1993 Endocrine parameters in amenorrhoeic and eumenorrhoeic adolescent female runners. International Journal of Sports Medicine 14(4): 191–195

Bergen H, Leung P C K 1986 Norepinephrine inhibition of pulsatile LH release: receptor specificity. American Journal of Physiology 250 (Endocrinology and Metabolism 13): 205–211

Borer K T 1995 The effects of exercise on growth. Sports Medicine 20(6): 375–397

Boyden T W, Pamenter Stanforth P 1984 Impaired gonadotropin responses to gonadotropin releasing hormone stimulation in endurance-trained women. Fertility and Sterility 41: 359–363

Brahm H, Piehl-Aulin K, Ljunghall S 1997 Bone metabolism during exercise and recovery: the influence of plasma volume and physical fitness. Calcified Tissue International 61(3): 192–198

Caballero M J, Mahedero G, Hernandez R, Alvarez J L, Rodriguez J, Rodriguez I, Maynar M 1996 Effects of physical exercise on some parameters of bone metabolism in postmenopausal women. Endocrinology Research 22(2): 131–138

Dale F, Gerlach D M, Wilwhite A L 1979 Menstrual dysfunction in distance runners. Obstetrics and Gynecology 54: 47–53

DeSouza M J, Maguire M S, Rubin K R, Maresh C M 1990 Effects of menstrual cycle and amenorrhoea on exercise performance in runners. Medicine and Science in Sports and Exercise 22: 575–580

DeSouza M J, Maguire M S, Maresh C M 1991 Adrenal activation and the prolactin response to exercise in eumenorrhoeic and amenorrhoeic runners. Journal of Applied Physiology 70(6): 2378–2387

De Souza M J, Miller B E, Sequenzia L C et al 1997 Bone health is not affected by luteal phase abnormalities and decreased ovarian progesterone production in female runners. Journal of Clinical Endocrinology and Metabolism 82(9): 2867–2876

Ding K H, Scheckter C B, Drinkwater B L 1988 Higher serum cortisol levels in exercise associated amenorrhoea. Annals of Internal Medicine 108: 530–534

Ellison P T, Lager C 1986 Moderate recreational running is associated with lowered salivary progesterone profiles in women. American Journal of Obstetrics and Gynecology 154: 1000–1003

Fries H, Nillius S J, Petterson F 1974 Epidemiology of secondary amenorrhoea. American Journal of Obstetrics and Gynecology 118: 473–479

Frisch R E, Gotz-Welbergen A V, McArthur J W 1981 Delayed menarche and amenorrhoea of college athletes in relation to age of onset of training. Journal of the American Medical Association 246: 1559–1563

Galliven E A, Singh A, Michelson D, Bina S, Gold P W, Deuster P A 1997 Hormonal and metabolic responses to exercise across time of day and menstrual cycle phase. Journal of Applied Physiology 83(6): 1822–1831

Hale R W, Kosasa T, Krieger J 1983 A marathon: the immediate affect on female runners' luteinizing hormone, follicle stimulating hormone, prolactin, testosterone and cortisol levels. American Journal of Obstetrics and Gynecology 146: 550–556

Harber V J, Sutton J R, MacDougall J D, Woolever C A, Bhavnani B R 1997 Plasma concentrations of beta-endorphin in trained eumenorrhoeic and amenorrhoeic women. Fertility and Sterility 67(4): 648–653

Highnet R 1989 Athletic amenorrhoea: un update on aetiology, complications and management. Sports Medicine 7: 82–108

Howlett T A, Tomlin S, Ngahfoong L 1984 Release of beta-endorphin and met-enkephalin during exercise in normal women: response to training. British Medical Journal 288: 1950–1952

Jurkowski J E, Jones N L, Walker W C 1978 Ovarian hormonal response to exercise. Journal of Applied Physiology 44: 109–114

Keizer H A, Beckers E, Des Haan J 1987a Exercise induced changes in the percentage of free testosterone and estradiol in trained and untrained women. International Journal of Sports Medicine 8: 151–155

Keizer H A, Menheere P, Kuipers H 1987b Changes in pulsatile LH secretion after exhaustive exercise and training. Medicine and Science in Sports and Exercise 19(suppl): 216

Kraemer R R, Heleniak R J, Tryniecki J L, Kraemer G R, Okazaki N J, Castracane V D 1995 Follicular and luteal phase hormonal responses to low-volume resistive exercise. Medicine and Science in Sports and Exercise 27(6): 809–817

Lata G F, Hu H K, Bagshaw G 1980 Equilibrium and kinetic characteristics of steroid interactions with human plasma sex binding protein. Archives of Biochemistry and Biophysics 199: 220–227

Laughlin G A, Dominguez C E, Yen S S 1998 Nutritional and endocrine-metabolic aberrations in women with functional hypothalamic amenorrhoea. Journal of Clinical Endocrinology and Metabolism 83(1): 25–32

Loucks A B, Horvath S M 1984 Exercise-induced stress responses of amenorrheic and eumenorrheic runners. Journal of Clinical Endocrinology and Metabolism 59: 1109–1120

Loucks A B, Laughlin G A, Mortola J F, Girton L, Nelson J C, Yen S S 1992 Hypothalamic-pituitary-thyroidal function in eumenorrhoeic and amenorrhoeic athletes. Journal of Clinical Endocrinology and Metabolism 75(2): 514–518

Maffulli N, Arena B 1993 Menstrual cycle and performance in female athletes. Obstetrics and Gynaecology Today 4(1): 6–9

Montagnani C F, Arena B, Maffulli N 1992 Estradiol and progesterone during exercise in healthy untrained women. Medicine and Science in Sports and Exercise 24(7): 764–768

Pearson R M 1985 Bionic ballerinas. Lancet 1: 481–482

Prior J C 1982 Endocrine 'conditioning' with endurance training, a preliminary review. Canadian Journal of Applied Sport Science 7: 148–157

Prior J C, Vigna Y M, Schechter M T 1990 Spinal bone loss and ovulation disturbances. New England Journal of Medicine 323: 1221–1227

Prior J C, Vigna Y M, McKay D W 1992 Reproduction for the athletic woman: new understandings of physiology and management. Sports Medicine 14(3): 190–199

Rupprecht M, Salzer B, Raum B et al 1997 Physical stress-induced secretion of adrenal and pituitary hormones in patients with atopic eczema compared with normal controls. Experiments in Clinical Endocrinology and Diabetes 105(1): 39–45

Samuels M H, Sanborn C F, Hofeldt F 1991 The role of endogenous opiates in athletic amenorrhoea. Fertility and Sterility 55(3): 507–512

Sanborn C F, Martin B J, Wagner W W 1982 Is athletic amenorrhoea specific to runners? American Journal of Obstetrics and Gynecology 143: 859–861

Schiebinger R J, Chrousos G P, Cutter G B 1986 The effect of serum prolactin on plasma adrenal androgens and the production and metabolic clearance rate of dehydroepiandrosterone sulphate in normal and hyperprolactinemic subjects. Journal of Clinical Endocrinology and Metabolism 62: 202–209

Schwartz B, Rebar R W, Yen S S C 1980 Amenorrhoea and long distance runners. Fertility and Sterility 34(3): 306

Sizonenko P C, Aubert M L 1986 Neuroendocrine changes characteristics of sexual maturation. Journal of Neural Transmission (Supplement) 21: 159–181

Stevenson E T, Davy K P, Seals D R 1995 Hemostatic, metabolic and androgenic risk factors for coronary heart disease in physically active and less active postmenopausal women. Arteriosclerosis Thrombosis and Vascular Biology 15(5): 669–677

Thompson D L, Snead D B, Seip R L, Weltman J Y, Rogol A D, Weltman A 1997 Serum lipid levels and steroidal hormones in women runners with irregular menses. Canadian Journal of Applied Physiology 22(1): 66–77

Veldhuis J D, Evans W S, Demers L M 1985 Altered neuroendocrine regulation of gonadotropin secretion in women distance runners. Journal of Clinical Endocrinology and Metabolism 61: 557–563

Warren M P, Brooks-Gunn J, Hamilton L H 1986 Scoliosis and fractures in young ballet dancers. New England Journal of Medicine 314: 1348–1353

Zanker C L, Swaine I L 1998 Bone turnover in amenorrhoeic and eumenorrhoeic women distance runners. Scandinavian Journal of Medicine and Science in Sports 8(1): 20–26

14

Special gynecological problems of the young female athlete

Marisa Z. Rose   C. Terence Lee
Nicola Maffulli   Pasquale Patrizio

KEY POINTS

1. The association between exercise and menstrual cycle regulation is multifactorial and complex.
2. Competitive athletes have several contributing factors to their hypothalamic–ovarian dysfunction: intensity of physical exercise, decreased body fat, inappropriate dieting and stress.
3. The consequences of amenorrhea include osteoporosis, increased risk of fracture, deleterious lipid changes and infertility.
4. Special considerations should be made when a female athlete chooses contraception.
5. Prevention of breast injury and irritation is a concern for many athletes.
6. The literature to date on athletic amenorrhea is limited by poor study design and paucity of subjects.

INTRODUCTION

In the last quarter of the 20th century, female participation in sports increased over 600% to an estimated total of 2 million female athletes at the high school collegiate level in the USA (West 1998). Increased physical fitness has excellent health benefits. However, the female athlete faces a unique set of challenges, including an increased risk of menstrual dysfunction and its consequences, performance considerations when choosing contraception, and sport-related breast injury and irritation. This chapter will review the special problems faced by young female athletes. A basic review of normal menstrual cycle physiology will provide the foundation for understanding the pathophysiology associated with exercise.

MENSTRUAL CYCLE PHYSIOLOGY

Regular menstrual cycling requires normally functioning anatomy and an intact central nervous system. The anatomic structures are the vagina, uterus and ovaries, which are located in the pelvis. The central control involves the hypothalamus and pituitary, both located in the brain. The hypothalamus secretes gonadotrophin-releasing hormone (GnRH) in a pulsatile pattern from ventromedial neurons. Pulsatile release of GnRH (every 60–90 min) stimulates the pituitary to secrete follicle-stimulating hormone (FSH) and luteinizing hormone (LH). FSH and LH promote ovulation and production of estrogen and progesterone. Estrogen stimulates development of the endometrial lining of the uterus. Withdrawal of estrogen and progesterone initiates menses, the cyclical shedding of the endometrium.

MENSTRUAL DISORDERS

In general, the majority of women of reproductive age have regular menses at intervals of every 25 to 35 days. In women who undertake chronic strenuous exercise (marathon running, competitive biking, ballet dancing), a wide range of menstrual disturbances is seen, ranging from complete amenorrhea (no menses) to oligomenorrhea (fewer than nine menstrual cycles per year) to irregular, erratic menstruation. In certain groups of athletes, particularly those with very low body fat, such as ballet dancers, endurance athletes and gymnasts, abnormal menstruation may be the rule rather than the exception. These menstrual irregularities often originate in the hypothalamic–pituitary unit rather than from the ovaries or the uterus. Amenorrheic and oligomenorrheic women have a low body mass index and a low percentage of body fat, which in turn, through abnormal pulsatility of GnRH, decreases FSH concentrations and LH pulse frequency. The decrease of FSH and LH is associated with an increase in growth hormone (GH), cortisol and free fatty acids and with a decrease in insulin, insulin-like growth factor I (IGF-I) and glucose. The potential health risks of abnormal menstruation include infertility, increased risk of oxidative damage, and problems usually seen in menopause such as hypoestrogenism, osteoporosis and predisposition to fractures.

Women contemplating a vigorous training schedule should be counseled that, even if they have normal menstrual cycles before training, the adoption of an intense exercise regimen could cause them to experience irregular menses. Those who already have irregular menses before training risk complete cessation of menses. Although likely, these trends are by no means absolute. Many women continue to have regular cycles despite increasing their exercise intensity. Furthermore, some women with irregular cycles may normalize their cycles by increasing their level of exercise.

The least severe form of menstrual dysfunction is the condition known as luteal phase defect. Follicular development occurs and proceeds through ovulation. However, the follicular development is suboptimal and, as a result, progesterone secretion after ovulation is low. The main problem associated with this disorder is decreased fertility during the cycles in which it occurs.

With more severe menstrual dysfunction, women still develop follicles, but their development ceases prior to ovulation. In this state of normoestrogenic anovulation, there is no progesterone produced and an environment of unopposed estrogen is created. The health hazard created by this situation is one of increased risk to endometrial cancer. These patients usually have irregular menses or oligomenorrhea. The most severe manifestation of menstrual dysfunction occurs when there is no follicular development and a low estrogen/low progesterone state is created. Without estrogen, the endometrial lining does not proliferate, leading to amenorrhea or cessation of menstrual cycling. This situation can lead to some of the manifestations of menopause, such as vaginal dryness and decreased bone density. This condition, known as hypothalamic amenorrhea, differs from menopause, although both are classically hypoestrogenic states. In menopause, the brain sends the appropriate stimulation to the ovaries, but the ovaries are devoid of follicles, and therefore do not secrete estrogen. Women in menopause typically have high levels of GnRH, LH and FSH and low levels of estrogen. In hypothalamic amenorrhea, the ovaries are normal and have the full capacity to secrete estrogen in response to normal stimulation. However, the hypothalamic–pituitary hormone secretion is decreased and there is insufficient stimulation of the ovaries for estrogen production. Women with hypothalamic amenorrhea typically have low levels of GnRH, LH, FSH and estrogen.

Treatment differs for the mild, moderate and severe types of menstrual irregularities. With luteal phase dysfunction, no treatment is necessary unless the patient is actively trying but unable to get pregnant. As long as the patient is ovulating and menstruating regularly, no intervention is necessary. Patients with oligomenorrhea experience periodic anovulation. It is important to supplement these women with progesterone on a regular basis. Otherwise, the prolonged unopposed action of estrogen could lead to the development of endometrial hyperplasia and endometrial cancer. Since the duration of the anovulation is unpredictable, patients who are sexually active require contraception in case they have an ovulatory cycle. The oral contraceptives pill (OCP) provides both contraception and prevention of unopposed estrogen action. The progesterone component of the OCP protects the endometrium, while the overall actions protect against unplanned pregnancy. For anovulatory patients who are not sexually active, supplementation with progesterone alone, instead of the combination OCP, is sufficient. Progesterone withdrawal induces menses, and can be achieved by prescribing medroxyprogesterone acetate (Provera) 10 mg daily for the first 10 days of every other month.

In the most severe form of menstrual dysfunction, the patient ceases menstruating and becomes hypoestrogenic. Treatment in these cases is aimed at restoring estrogen levels. Estrogen and progesterone supplementation with the combination OCP restores regular menses and protects the bones as well as the endometrium. However, it does not restore ovulation. In order to become pregnant, these patients require ovulation induction, not with oral agents such as clomiphene citrate, but with injectable gonadotrophins.

When managing a female athlete who presents with amenorrhea, it is inappropriate automatically to assume that she has exercise-associated amenorrhea. Ruling out other causes such as elevated prolactin and premature ovarian failure should also be considered.

In summary, menstrual disorders commonly occur among elite athletes. Patients should be counseled as to the potentially serious long-term consequences such as endometrial cancer and osteoporosis, depending on the severity of their menstrual dysfunction.

EXERCISE-ASSOCIATED AMENORRHEA

The pathogenesis of athletic amenorrhea is complex and multifactorial (Fig. 14.1). Amenorrhea, as defined by the International Olympic Committee, consists of one or fewer menstrual periods per year (Fagan 1998).

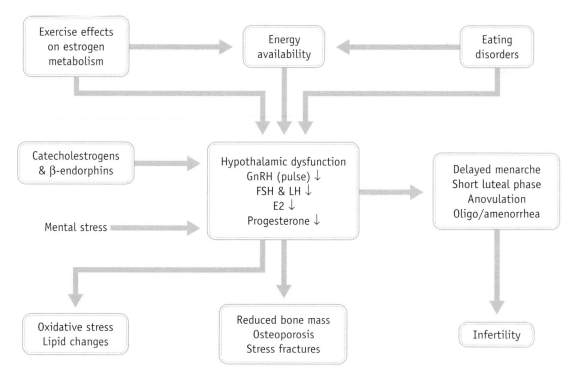

Figure 14.1 Pathogenesis of athletic amenorrhea.

The prevalence of amenorrhea in the general population ranges from 2 to 5%. Among athletes, amenorrhea is much more prevalent, ranging from 3.4 to 66% (West 1998). The incidence is higher in sports such as running and ballet (40–50%), and lower in sports such as swimming (12%) (Sanborn et al 1982, West 1998).

Intensity of training is positively correlated to frequency of amenorrhea among the runners, while this is not true among swimmers and cyclists. At the same level of intensity of training, 26% of runners and 12% of swimmers and cyclists will experience amenorrhea. Lower body weight in runners is associated with higher intensity of training. In contrast, body weight remains stable as intensity increases among cyclists and swimmers.

A recent study by Constantini & Warren (1995) looked at the hormone profile of swimmers. They reviewed the menstrual histories of 69 competitive swimmers and compared them with 279 age-matched controls. Age at menarche was significantly delayed among swimmers. Menstrual irregularities were reported by 82% of swimmers compared with 40% of controls. The authors concluded that swimmers are prone to delayed menarche and menstrual irregularities, but the associated hormonal profile differs significantly from the hypothalamic amenorrhea commonly described in ballet dancers and runners. These findings suggest that reproductive dysfunction in swimmers is distinct from that of other female athletes, the former due to mild hyperandrogenism and the latter secondary to hypoestrogenism.

Pathogenetic mechanisms of athletic amenorrhea

The estrogen fuel hypothesis (Fig. 14.2)

Estrogen metabolism in female athletes was studied by Snow et al (1989). They prospectively followed 10 elite oarswomen over a year of training (3 months each of low intensity, followed by high intensity and then low intensity again). Five of the women had regular menstrual cycles throughout the study period. During the period of high-intensity training, the other five women experienced disrupted menses which returned back to normal during the low-intensity phases. The extent of estradiol (E2) metabolized by 2-hydroxylase oxidation was evaluated by radiometric analysis. The results were compared with four non-athletic controls.

The oarswomen who experienced menstrual disturbances during high-intensity training were found to metabolize a significantly greater fraction of E2 by 2-hydroxylase oxidation (~48%) than did the oarswomen who sustained normal menses throughout the training year (38%). The extent of E2 metabolized by 2-hydroxylase oxidation did not differ between normal cycling athletes and controls. The intensity of training did not change the extent of 2-hydroxylase activity. Both groups of athletes became leaner during the high-intensity phase.

The authors suggested that the group with menstrual irregularity had a greater fraction of estrogen

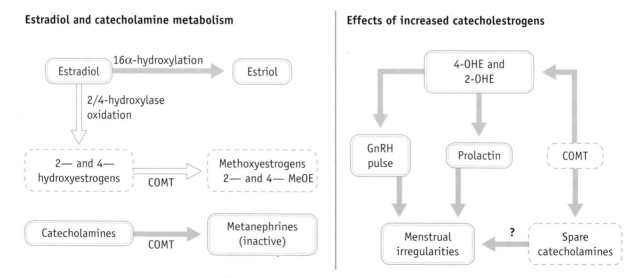

Figure 14.2 Estrogen metabolism in response to exercise – estrogen fuel hypothesis.

metabolites that are devoid of peripheral estrogen activity (increased catecholestrogens and decreased estriol), creating a hypoestrogenic state. The decrease in body fat during the high-intensity phase further limited peripherally active estrogen. During the high-intensity phase, the combination of decreased estrogen levels due to decreased body fat and decreased 16α-hydroxylation resulted in levels of estrogen low enough to disturb menstrual cycling. In summary, increased 2-hydroxylase oxidation is associated with oligomenorrhea during periods of high-intensity training and decreased body fat.

Multiple studies have confirmed the association between increased 2-hydroxylase oxidation and acute exercise and training. For example, Frisch et al (1992) showed a significant trend between increasing 2-hydroxylation of estradiol, yielding 2-hydroxyestrogen (2-OHE), and decreasing subcutaneous fat/total volume. They evaluated five athletes during low- and high-intensity training and four controls by MRI. Decreased body fat, common among athletes, and higher levels of 2-OHE were associated with anovulation and amenorrhea among the athletes.

Competition between catecholestrogens and catecholamines for COMT. The effect of estrogen metabolism on catecholamine metabolism was studied by De Cree et al (1997). The 2-hydroxylase oxidation pathway and catecholamine degradation pathway share the enzyme catechol-*O*-methyltransferase (COMT) (Fig. 14.2). The authors evaluated the effects of acute exercise and short-term intensive training on COMT activity. Blood samples were obtained from 15 previously untrained eumenorrheic women before and after a 5-day intensive training period, at rest, and during incremental exercise. COMT activity was determined in erythrocytes after incubation of blood lysate with primary catecholestrogens. A trend between increased COMT activity in estrogen metabolism and increased exercise intensity was observed. In contrast, incremental exercise did not significantly alter COMT activity. They found that COMT activity is increased by brief intensive training, but not by acute exercise. The authors speculated that an increase in COMT-catalyzed methylation of catecholestrogens may indicate that less COMT is available to degrade norepinephrine, thereby safeguarding fuel support in the form of catecholamines.

To further evaluate the role of COMT in estrogen metabolism, De Cree & Fujimori (1997) studied 4-methoxyestrogen (4-MeOE) formation in addition to 2-methoxyestrogen (2-MeOE) in response to exercise.

They assessed the effects of an incremental exercise test to exhaustion on six untrained, healthy eumenorrheic women. The study spanned three menstrual cycles, each with a specific level of exercise: control, moderate training, and heavy training. They looked at phase-specific plasma hormone levels, including the 2- and 4-hydroxyestrogens (2-OHE and 4-OHE) and the 2- and 4-methoxyestrogens (2-MeOE and 4-MeOE). During exercise, catecholamines, prolactin, estradiol, unconjugated and conjugated estrogens, 4-OHE and 4-MeOE increased. The increase of 4-OHE and 4-MeOE further supports the observation that, during exercise, COMT activity increases with increased catecholestrogen production. Whether this COMT activity is at the expense of catecholamines was not tested, because the authors were unable to measure the plasma metanephrines (degraded catecholamines). The authors suggest that changes in the peripheral levels of 4-OHE reflect changes in the intrahypothalamic and intrapituitary levels of 4-OHE, which may be of physiologic significance in mediating the GnRH pulsatility and prolactin secretion (Fig. 14.2).

Catecholestrogens and the menstrual cycle. The role of catecholestrogens and menstrual cycle regulation was studied by Villard et al (1987). They found that administration of 2-OHE antiserum to the third ventricle of cycling female rats prevented the preovulatory LH surge despite high peripheral 17β-estradiol. They concluded, in agreement with prior animal studies, that 2-OHE plays a role in the control of cycling LH release.

Russell et al (1984) followed 13 competitive swimmers over a 2-year period during which they trained at different intensities, and found distinct changes in five of the subjects' menstrual cycles that coincided with the level of exercise. Mean and median levels of LH, FSH, PRL, and 17β-estradiol were decreased, while catecholestrogens and β-endorphins were increased during strenuous training as compared with moderate training. The authors postulate that the significant difference between β-endorphins and catecholestrogens during strenuous training may serve as an explanation for oligomenorrhea in female athletes during periods of high-intensity training.

Subtle ovarian suppression in oligomenorrheic athletes

The role of exercise-induced production of β-endorphins was studied by Harber et al (1997). They measured β-endorphin concentrations in 10 eumenorrheic sedentary, 11 eumenorrheic trained, and 11 amenor-rheic trained women over one menstrual cycle or a 4-week period of time. Levels of β-endorphins were elevated in both groups of trained athletes compared with sedentary women but did not differ significantly between the trained groups. No significant differences in hormone levels were detected across the menstrual cycle. The trained eumenorrheic group had significantly lower luteal phase E2 and progesterone concentrations than the sedentary eumenorrheic group, although the low levels were still within the normal range for reproductive endocrine functions. Luteal phase abnormalities may be asymptomatic, since luteal shortening is usually matched by lengthening of follicular phase. The borderline levels of hormones in the luteal phase among female athletes who appear to have regular cycles may be suggestive of subtle ovarian suppression, possibly secondary to increased β-endorphin levels.

Exercise changes in circulating growth factors and leptins

The role of circulating nutritional hormones in exercise-associated amenorrhea has been reported in the recent scientific literature. Several molecules act primarily as nutritional hormones. Insulin, insulin-like growth factors (IGF) type I and II, their binding proteins, and leptins change their concentration in response to stress and vigorous exercise. Since members of the IGF system are present in brain, pituitary and ovarian tissue, they can regulate the reproductive hormones (GnRH, FSH and LH). Recently, leptins have been identified as humoral signals involved in the feedback to the reproductive axis about nutritional status. In response to leptins, the hypothalamic areas involved in energy homeostasis increase basal metabolism and decrease appetite (Kalra 1997).

The energy availability hypothesis

The role of energy availability during exercise is a popular theory explaining the association of exercise and menstrual irregularities (Box 14.1). In women, the appearance and maintenance of reproductive function rely heavily on the balance between nutrition and energy expenditure. Weight, body composition, fat distribution, eating behavior and exercise influence the hormonal patterns ultimately responsible for reproduction capability.

The role of diet and exercise in supplying and reducing energy, respectively, was studied by Loucks &

Box 14.1 Equations for the energy availability hypothesis

Low calorie intake combined with increased caloric expenditure results in an energy drain and amenorrhea (Loucks & Heath 1994, Loucks et al 1998)

Energy expenditure (EE) = resting metabolic rate + thermic effect of feeding + thermic effect of activity + work performed

Exercise EE = controlled EE during exercise − estimated EE

Energy availability = dietary intake − exercise EE

Heath (1994) and Loucks et al (1998). They studied LH pulse frequency in nine young, habitually sedentary, regularly menstruating women on days 8, 9, and 10 of two menstrual cycles after 4 days of intense exercise. The subjects were divided and dietary energy intake was controlled to set their energy availability to high or low (45 or 10 kcal/kg lean body mass per day, respectively) (Loucks et al 1998). Energy availability was defined as the net energy after subtracting exercise energy expenditure from dietary intake (Box 14.1). These subjects were compared with seven subjects from a previous study (Loucks & Heath 1994) with a similar energy availability control but without exercise. LH pulse frequency was reduced by 10% in the subjects who exercised with low energy availability. However, subjects with low energy availability and no exercise had an even larger decrease in LH pulse frequency (23%). The authors concluded that these results contradict the hypothesis that LH pulsatility is disrupted by exercise stress, and suggested that LH pulsatility in women depends on energy availability. Dietary restriction that does not meet the criteria of an eating disorder is common in women athletes. The limited caloric intake does not provide adequate fuel for exercise expenditure and may lead to athletic amenorrhea. This could be an adaptive response to conserve energy.

Mental stress

Psychological stress plays an important compounding role. Prospective studies have shown that women who had regular menses at the onset of their training continued to be regular even with the increased intensity of their training. However, when psychological stress (as the competition approaches) is added to the training, the regularity of the menstrual cycle may be affected.

Consequences of exercise-associated amenorrhea: the loss of estrogen protection

Infertility, deleterious lipid changes, and decreased bone mineral density are the most concerning consequences of athletic amenorrhea.

Reduced bone mass

Peak bone mass is achieved in early adulthood and is a major determinant of osteoporosis. Young athletes with low estrogen levels are at risk of losing bone density during a time when they should be storing bone. Athletes with amenorrhea show only partial recovery in bone density after restoration of normal menstrual cycles.

Cumming (1996) performed a retrospective study over a 24–30 month period to evaluate the efficacy of hormone replacement therapy (HRT). Sixteen women with exercise-associated amenorrhea underwent vertebral and femoral neck bone density measurements by dual-energy X-ray absorptiometry (DEXA) of more than 1.0 standard deviation below the mean. All were counseled on the use of HRT. Eight of these women continued HRT therapy for 2 years. The other eight subjects refused or quickly discontinued HRT treatment. There were no significant differences between the two groups prior to the study, including bone density. After 2 years, repeat DEXA scan showed a significant increase in vertebral and femoral neck bone density in the HRT group. In the women not taking HRT, there was a non-significant decrease in bone density at these sites.

Hergenroeder et al (1997) briefly commented on the increased rate of turnover in trabecular compared with cortical bone. Treatment by HRT had the earliest and most beneficial effects on trabecular bone.

Oxidative stress and lipid changes

During physical exercise, the production rate of reactive oxygen species is increased, and greater demand is placed on the body's defense systems to inactivate these substances. Increased oxidative stress can lead to destructive biological processes, including DNA and cellular membrane damage leading to cell and tissue injury or death and aging. Estrogens have been shown to inhibit LDL peroxidation by the reactive oxygen species *in vitro* and *in vivo*, and it has been suggested that this effect is involved in the protection against cardiovascular disease in premenopausal women. Amenorrheic athletes may be at risk of cardiovascular disease secondary to the lack of estrogen protection effect.

Ayres et al (1998) studied plasma and LDL oxidation parameters and creatine kinase activity in seven eumenorrheic and seven amenorrheic athletes before and after an acute bout of exercise. They found that the amenorrheic athletes had decreased mean plasma estradiol, higher baseline creatine kinase, increased oxysterol formation (a measure of LDL peroxidation) and a greater decrease in lag time of diene conjugation (a second measure of LDL oxidation) after exercise. They concluded that amenorrheic female athletes demonstrate an increased potential for lipid peroxidation after exercise which may put them at risk for cardiovascular disease. The higher creatine kinase was suggested to be secondary to increased muscle damage from the oxidative stress without estrogen protection.

CONTRACEPTION FOR THE ATHLETE

Young athletes who have contraceptive needs have a variety of choices: OCPs, intrauterine devices (IUDs), barrier methods such as diaphragms and condoms, and depot progesterone preparations.

OCPs have many advantages for this particular population of patients. First, OCPs help to prevent problems associated with irregular menses, a common concern for competitive athletes. Second, OCPs decrease the risk of ovarian cancer, endometrial cancer and ovarian cysts. The amount of menstrual bleeding is decreased in OCP users from an average of 35 mL/cycle to about 20 mL/month. This reduction in blood loss helps to prevent anemia and increases red blood cell count and iron content. Premenstrual syndrome incidence and dysmenorrhea (extreme menstrual pain) are decreased in women on the OCP. Third, athletes may use oral contraceptives to regulate and time their cycles so as not to coincide with the dates of major competitions. The rationale behind this practice is in question because there is conflicting evidence that the menstrual cycle affects athletic performances. For those who wish to practice artificial regulation of their cycles, they should skip the placebo week and start a new pack of pills every 21 days. A pseudopregnancy state is created and menses will not occur until cessation of the OCP when menstrual flow usually starts within 3–4 days. Evidence suggests that it is safe to go at least 5–6 months without menses using this protocol. In fact, this pseudopregnancy state, created by taking continuous OCPs, is sometimes employed as treatment for certain conditions such as endometriosis.

BREAST INJURIES

Breast injuries associated with athletic activity are rare. They may occur in sports with heavy contact such as basketball or in sports such as softball, field hockey or lacrosse where projectiles may cause breast trauma. Proper padding can minimize this risk of injury. Many athletes complain of breast pain while running or engaging in other high-impact exercises, especially during the premenstrual days. Special sports bras which give firmer support and limit breast motion are recommended. Extra support can also help to alleviate anxiety in patients who are concerned that high-impact exercise might accelerate breast sagging.

The treatment of breast injuries consists of basic soft tissue injury care. Most incidences involve bruising, which can be treated by rest, ice packs and pressure to avoid swelling. Another common breast complaint is irritation of the nipples from repetitive friction against clothing during running. This problem is solved with proper padding or even bandaging in severe situations. Athletes with breast implants risk implant rupture with trauma. Implants are not recommended for competitive athletes.

CHALLENGES TO UNDERSTANDING THE YOUNG FEMALE ATHLETE

All of the studies mentioned fall short of what is generally considered 'good science'. Studies using young athletes as subjects are limited by small numbers, selection group bias, and methodological differences. Few studies were designed as prospective randomized control studies. With these flaws in mind, the current literature should not be discounted. Current knowledge has greatly advanced since the mid-1970s, when this field was first studied. The complexity of exercise-associated menstrual irregularities is now well appreciated, although not fully understood. The critical reader should remain cognizant of the gaps in knowledge still present in the current explanations of the pathogenesis of athletic amenorrhea.

CONCLUSIONS

1. Competitive female athletes commonly experience menstrual irregularities secondary to a down regulation of the hypothalamic–pituitary–ovarian axis.
   — The estrogen fuel hypothesis states that during periods of exercise stress the metabolism of estrogen into catecholestrogens via COMT increases. This shift in metabolism serves to conserve catecholamines and maintain fuel for the activity.
   — The energy availability hypothesis contradicts the estrogen fuel hypothesis by stating that it is not exercise stress that affects LH pulse frequency, but rather it is the balance of caloric intake and exercise energy expenditure that determines LH pulse frequency. Decreased energy availability results in decreased LH pulse frequency, thereby providing fuel for activity at the expense of reproductive function.
2. Trained athletes who appear to have regular menstrual cycles may experience subtle ovarian suppression, resulting in a low-normal hormone profile, due to elevated β-endorphins and catecholestrogens.
3. The consequences of athletic amenorrhea are secondary to the loss of estrogen and include decreased bone density, increased oxidative stress and related lipid changes, and infertility. Athletes with normal levels of estrogen and low levels of progesterone are at increased risk for endometrial cancer.
4. Contraceptive choices include the OCP, which offers athletes the option to regulate the dates of menses to avoid conflicts with sporting events.
5. Breast injury, although rare, is a concern for female athletes. Proper padding and support lower the risk of trauma.
6. Current literature on the young female athlete is lacking statistical power. Future studies should include prospective, randomized, controlled, multicentered studies in order to achieve significant results.

REFERENCES

Ayres S, Baer J, Subbiah M T 1998 Exercise-induced increase in lipid peroxidation parameters in amenorrheic female athletes. Fertility & Sterility 69(1): 73–77

Constantini N W, Warren M P 1995 Menstrual dysfunction in swimmers: a distinct entity. Journal of Clinical Endocrinology and Metabolism 80: 2740–2744

Cumming D C 1996 Exercise-associated amenorrhea, low bone density, and estrogen replacement therapy. Archives of Internal Medicine 156(19): 2193–2195

De Cree C, Fujimori Y 1997 4-hydroxycatecholestrogen metabolism responses to exercise and training: possible implications for menstrual cycle irregularities and breast cancer. Fertility & Sterility 67(3): 505–516

De Cree C, Van Kranenburg G, Geurten P, Fujimuri Y, Keizer H A 1997 Exercise-induced changes in enzymatic O-methylation of catecholestrogens by erythrocytes of eumenorrheic women. Medicine and Science in Sports and Exercise 29(12): 1580–1587

Fagan K M 1998 Pharmacologic management of athletic amenorrhea. Clinics in Sports Medicine 17(2): 327–341

Frisch R E, Snow R, Gerard E L, Johnson L, Kennedy D, Barbieri R, Rosen B R 1992 Magnetic resonance imaging of body fat of athletes compared with controls, and the oxidative metabolism of estradiol. Metabolism 41: 191–193

Harber V J, Sutton J R, MacDougall J D, Woolever C A, Bhavnani B R 1997 Plasma concentrations of beta-endorphin in trained eumenorrheic and amenorrheic women. Fertility & Sterility 67(4): 648–653

Hergenroeder A C, O'Brian Smith E, Shypaiolo R, Jones L A, Klish W J, Ellis K 1997 Bone mineral changes in young women with hypothalamic amenorrhea treated with oral contraceptives, medroxyprogesterone, or placebo over 12 months. American Journal of Obstetrics and Gynecology 176(5): 1017–1026

Kalra S P 1997 Appetite and body weight regulation: Is it all in the brain? Neuron 19: 227–230

Loucks A B, Health E M 1994 Dietary restriction reduces luteinizing hormone (LH) pulse frequency during waking hours and increases LH pulse amplitude during sleep in young menstruating women. Journal of Clinical Endocrinology and Metabolism 78: 910–915

Loucks A B, Verdun M, Heath E M 1998 Low energy availability, not stress of exercise, alters LH pulsatility in exercising women. Journal of Applied Physiology 84(1): 37–46

Russell J B, Mitchell D E, Musey P I, Collins D C 1984 The role of beta-endorphins and catechol estrogens on the hypothalamic-pituitary axis in female athletes. Fertility & Sterility 42(5): 690–695

Sanborn C F, Albrecht B H, Wagner W W Jr 1987 Athletic amenorrhea: lack of association with body fat. Medicine and Science in Sports and Exercise 19: 207–212

Sanborn C F, Martin B J, Wagner W W Jr 1982 Is athletic amenorrhea specific to runners? American Journal of Obstetrics and Gynecology 143: 859–861

Snow R C, Barbieri R L, Frisch R E 1989 Estrogen 2-hydroxylase oxidation and menstrual function among elite oarswomen. Journal of Clinical Endocrinology and Metabolism 69: 369–376

Villard M F, Ladosky W, Janots D, Lenoir V, Adeline J, Kerdelhue B, Scholler R 1987 Inhibition of the preovulatory LH surge after a catecholestrogen (2-hydroxyestrone) antiserum injection in the third ventricle in cycling female rats. Neuroscience Letters 78(2): 187–192

Warren M P, Shangold M M 1997 Sports gynecology: problems and care of the athletic female. Blackwell Science, Malden, MA

West R V 1998 The female athlete. The triad of disordered eating, amenorrhea and osteoporosis. Sports Medicine 26: 63–71

15

Exercise in pregnancy

Bruno Arena   Nicola Maffulli

KEY POINTS

1. The level of exercise that may benefit, or indeed harm, pregnancy outcome depends on the individual concerned, and exercise programmes should therefore be adjusted accordingly.
2. The 'safe' level of exercise for a pregnant woman is governed by her level of training and general fitness, particularly her cardiovascular and respiratory reserves.
3. On current evidence, a programme of moderate exercise in the healthy mother allows her to enjoy a sense of well-being, is often associated with a shorter labour and a lower incidence of operative deliveries, and may help in the management of conditions such as diabetes and hypertension.
4. Working mothers who spend many hours standing are at significant risk of premature labour compared with sedentary controls, though the difference in birthweight appears to be less significant.

INTRODUCTION

Exercise in pregnancy is an important issue in sports medicine as it involves two subjects, mother and fetus, at the same time. As more and more women are engaged in the practice of sport to keep fit, often in the reproductive years, the decision to abandon a programme of regular exercise when pregnancy is confirmed should be based on objective and reliable information. Often, women may be advised by friends or by their doctors to adopt a more sedentary lifestyle when pregnant on the assumption that exercise may increase the risk of miscarriage or cause harm to the developing fetus. On other occasions, this decision may be taken by pregnant women themselves.

Not all sports have the same impact on pregnancy, and intensity and duration of exercise sessions are important variables to consider. A distinction should therefore be made between leisure exercise, such as moderate walking, biking or swimming, which generally involve aerobic work and cause limited increases in maternal heart rate and ventilatory frequency, and competitive sport, with frequent maximal or near-maximal performances when the aerobic-anaerobic threshold may be reached. Maternal level of training and general fitness, particularly respiratory and cardiovascular reserves, set the 'safe' level of exercise for a pregnant woman.

In pregnancies classified as 'at risk', discontinuation of exercise may be necessary, and it is important that the management of such cases is undertaken by expert medical personnel. Current evidence indicates that, in the absence of maternal cardiovascular or respiratory problems, a programme of moderate exercise allows the mother to enjoy a sense of well-being, is often associated with a shorter labour and a lower incidence of operative deliveries, and may help in the management of conditions such as diabetes and hypertension. The influence of regular maternal exercise on fetal development has been a matter of debate, as diversion of blood from the placenta to maternal muscles and other organs involved in the exercise is deemed by some authors to interfere with normal fetal growth. At present, a significant difference in birthweight between babies born to exercising mothers and sedentary controls has not been confirmed. Other studies evaluating mental and physical development of children born to exercising mothers also show encouraging data.

Finally, an important issue for its impact on pregnancy outcome is maternal physical activity in the workplace. Working mothers who spend many hours standing are at significant risk of premature labour in comparison with sedentary controls, while the difference in birthweight appears to be less significant. The quality of nutrition and the energy expenditure in caring for other children at home also deserve careful considerations.

PHYSIOLOGICAL CHANGES IN PREGNANCY

The increased hormonal production from the feto-placental unit during pregnancy produces significant changes of several maternal parameters. Oxygen consumption ($\dot{V}O_2$) increases, reaching its maximum at around 32 weeks. Ventilation, tidal volume, heart rate and stroke volume also show a gradual increase. Carbon dioxide output ($\dot{V}CO_2$) follows the same trend as $\dot{V}O_2$, and peripheral resistance decreases while circulating plasma volume increases, producing a drop in the haematocrit. Body temperature rises by about 0.5°C. Forced vital capacity remains relatively constant, while expiratory reserve decreases (Artal & Wiswell 1986, Spatling et al 1992).

EXERCISE AND THE MATERNAL RESPIRATORY SYSTEM

Carbon dioxide output at peak exercise is lower during pregnancy compared with the postpartum period (Lotgering et al 1995), and submaximal exercise produces higher ventilatory frequency, tidal volume and lactate levels than in non-pregnant controls. This response decreases gradually after delivery, but takes several weeks to return to the normal non-pregnant state. Fit women who continue to exercise regularly during pregnancy can engage in heavier physical activities compared with sedentary pregnant controls without causing fetal hypoxia: the immediate post-exercise recovery period can be somewhat more risky for the fetus, probably due to the fall in stroke volume (Webb et al 1994). Physical activity at moderately high altitudes can affect physical performance during pregnancy: a passive trip by aerial cableway in the third trimester to an altitude of 2200 m, which is equivalent to a drop in barometric pressure to 583 mmHg and a drop in atmospheric PO_2 of 18 mmHg, does not cause any change in maternal PO_2, respiratory rate, heart rate, systolic and diastolic blood pressure at rest (Baumann et al 1985), but $\dot{V}O_{2\,max}$ of lowlander pregnant women can be limited, although performance of submaximal exercise may be unaffected (Webb et al 1994). The choice of the type of sport practised by a pregnant woman is important, as not all disciplines have the same effect on the maternal respiratory system: immersion in water to the level of the xyphoid in pregnancy produces a decrease of maximal voluntary ventilation compared with rest on land or exercise in water (Berry et al 1989), and perceived maximal exertion is reached at a lower percentage $\dot{V}O_{2\,max}$ during swimming compared with cycling; peak CO_2 output, peak ventilation and lactic acid production are also lower during swimming than during cycling (Spinnewijn et al 1996).

The anaerobic threshold (AT) decreases in normal circumstances with advancing gestation, in proportion to increasing maternal body weight. The maternal heart rate at the AT also declines, but without close relation to maternal body weight. Maternal heart rate increases with more difficulty during exercise with advancing gestational age, and this has to be taken into account when the maximal heart rate is evaluated as an index of exercise intensity (Matsushita et al 1996). On the other hand, in recreational athletes who continue to exercise during pregnancy, albeit at a reduced intensity, there is an increase in the absolute AT, which persists up to 36–44 weeks postpartum. Weight and maximal heart rate remain unchanged (Clapp & Capeless 1991a).

The amount of oxygen required to complete a three-step graded workload treadmill exercise test decreases significantly by 6–15% starting from the first weeks of pregnancy, and, in women who continue a moderate-to high-intensity exercise regime, the oxygen requirement remains the same or is lower than before conception for the rest of the pregnancy and early postpartum. By contrast, in those who discontinue regular exercise, the oxygen requirement increases progressively by 2% a month with a peak at 37 weeks. The additional oxygen requirement caused by weight gain must be taken into account when net physical efficiency is evaluated (Clapp 1989). In fact, physical efficiency improves during normal pregnancy compared with the non-pregnant state, with an increase in the $\dot{V}O_{2\,max}$ and a lower production of lactate when the AT is exceeded (Kusche et al 1986). A significant increase in $\dot{V}O_2$ consumption during exercise is observed in late pregnancy compared with the postpartum period if measurements are taken at rest, during steady-state exercise on a bicycle ergometer and for 10 min during recovery. The oxygen debt produced by the exercise is also higher compared with that at 12 weeks postpartum (Pernoll et al 1975). Maximal transdiaphragmatic pressure remains unchanged when healthy women perform progressive cycle exercise tests at 33 and 12 weeks postpartum, and the higher tidal volume produces an increase in minute ventilation (Field et al 1991).

EXERCISE AND THE MATERNAL MUSCULOSKELETAL SYSTEM

Women who exercise during pregnancy complain less frequently of leg oedema, muscular cramps, fatigue and shortness of breath compared with sedentary pregnant controls (Horns et al 1996). Abdominal muscle function is affected by the structural adaptations that occur during pregnancy, particularly the increasing size of the uterus, and the ability to stabilize the pelvis against resistance decreases until about 8 weeks postpartum (Gilleard & Brown 1996). In addition, generalized ligament laxity occurs, in connection with increasing levels of relaxin, a peptide hormone of the insulin-like growth factor family, produced from the first weeks of pregnancy by the corpus luteum and the placenta. Knee cruciate ligament laxity is common, but exercise programmes employing minimal to moderate weight-bearing have not been shown to produce any significant knee instability (Dumas & Reid 1997).

About 10% of pregnant women develop severe low back pain that interferes with daily life activities, and the ability to perform sit-ups decreases significantly because of the inefficiency of the abdominal muscles (Fast et al 1990).

EXERCISE AND THE MATERNAL CARDIOVASCULAR SYSTEM

Exercise produces an increase in cardiac output: blood flow to muscles, myocardium and skin increases, while sympathetic vasoconstriction reduces the flow to organs and tissues not directly involved in the exercise. The response to exercise, although influenced by physiological conditions such as menstrual cycle and pregnancy, does not differ significantly from the one occurring in men (O'Toole 1989). The cardiac response to exercise in pregnancy (increased heart rate and stroke volume), which is greater than in non-pregnant controls, decreases by 2 months postpartum, but a longer period of time is required to return to non-pregnant conditions (Sady et al 1990). Activation of the sympathetic nervous system either at rest or during strenuous exercise is blunted in pregnancy, and the circulatory system is affected by the increased activity of the renin–angiotensin system (Eneroth-Grimfors et al 1988). Plasma noradrenaline, in particular, increases less significantly in pregnancy during standing and isometric exercise than in non-pregnant controls, while adrenaline response is less affected by pregnancy, with a linear correlation between heart rate and urinary excretion of adrenaline, both at rest and during exercise (Barron et al 1986).

Changes in submaximal exercise $\dot{V}O_2$ during pregnancy are dependent on the type of exercise: at the same workload, $\dot{V}O_2$ increases during weight-bearing exercise, but does not differ from postpartum values during weight-supported exercise. Exercise arterio-venous oxygen difference is lower during pregnancy than in the non-pregnant state, probably because the higher cardiac output is distributed to vascular districts not directly involved in the exercise. Perfusion of muscles would not increase significantly during exercise, and the increased cardiac output can therefore cover the requirements of blood flow to the uterus (Sady & Carpenter 1989).

Aerobic dancing at an intensity of about 65% of expected maximal heart rate in the third trimester produces a significant increase in blood pressure and an increase in heart rate that may continue for up to 20 min. Systolic peak velocity and flow volume in the femoral arteries increase significantly and the pulsatility index decreases. On the fetal side, the systolic peak velocity and the pulsatility index of the umbilical artery do not change significantly, but the fetal heart rate can increase in relation to maternal heart rate (Asakura et al 1994). When exercise in water is evaluated, immersion produces in normal pregnant women a decrease in vasopression production, which instead increases after exercise. Plasma renin activity decreases both during and after exercise. Atrial natriuretic peptide concentration increases after exercise in water, and affects the volume of urine produced (Asai et al 1994). In another study on exercise in water, immersion for 20 min at 30°C at 15, 25 and 35 weeks of pregnancy and 8–10 weeks postpartum produced a decrease in the resting heart rate by about 8 beats/min (bpm). Twenty minutes of bicycle ergometry to 60% $\dot{V}o_{2\,max}$ in water caused an increase in the heart rate lower than that produced by the same exercise on land in all stages of pregnancy (McMurray et al 1988). The positive effects of exercise in water have been confirmed in another study, where immersion for 20 min at 30°C in pregnancy followed by exercise to 60% $\dot{V}o_{2max}$ produced substantial diuresis and natriuresis without changes in osmolarity or serum sodium. Exercise in water during pregnancy can therefore be potentially beneficial to treat oedema without producing a decrease in plasma volume (Katz et al 1990).

Pregnancy is accompanied by specific electrocardiographic changes: T-wave inversion in V_2 is present both in early and late pregnancy more frequently, while Q waves in II, III and aVF are less common than in nonpregnant subjects. With bicycle exercise, the time to onset of maximum ST depression is significantly shorter during pregnancy (Veille et al 1996). In another study, a depression of ST segment was found in 12% of pregnant women undergoing a strenuous bicycle exercise who did not show any signs of ischaemia (van Doorn et al 1992). Knowledge of this helps in the correct evaluation of the electrocardiogram in pregnancy.

The systolic/diastolic (S/D) ratio measured in the uterine artery before and within 3 min after a submaximal stationary bicycle exercise in healthy women with singleton pregnancies between 16 and 28 weeks remains basically unchanged, suggesting that submaximal exercise does not compromise uterine artery blood flow in healthy, normal pregnant women (Moore et al 1988), and peak velocities and mean blood flow velocities in the femoral and carotid arteries and femoral vein of healthy pregnant women performing exercise tests in a sitting position on a bicycle ergometer with a workload of 100 watts for 3 min show an increase with no variation in the vessel diameter. The systolic and end-diastolic velocities in the femoral artery also increase, with a reversal of the post-systolic flow, which normally shows negative velocity at rest (Baumann et al 1989). An improvement in maternal circulation with exercise has been confirmed by other studies: a bicycle stress test in the third trimester by healthy pregnant women in a semi-supine position at 75 watts for 3 min shows a significant decrease of the resistant index (RI) of the maternal femoral artery (from 93 to 69%), a rise in maximum systolic velocity (from 73 to 194 cm/s), and a rise in maximum diastolic velocity (from 5 to 61 cm/s). In the maternal carotid artery and uteroplacental vessels these parameters remain basically unchanged. Fetal cardiotocograms remain within normal limits in all cases. These studies confirm that, provided placental function is normal, uteroplacental and fetoplacental circulations are not affected negatively by moderate physical exercise (Drack et al 1988). When the exercise intensity increases, there can be negative effects on uterine circulation: submaximal maternal exercise at approximately 75% $\dot{V}o_{2\,max}$ during the third trimester can cause a gradual increase in S/D ratio of the uterine artery with a maximum at 1 min of recovery. No change has been found in the S/D ratio of the umbilical artery, but the fetal heart rate can increase significantly (Erkkola et al 1992).

Maternal blood pressure response to exercise is not affected by pregnancy, and is inversely related to the individual capacity to perform isometric exercise. An isometric exercise in the form of a hand-grip test at 28 weeks was found to be useful in predicting which women were going to develop pregnancy-induced hypertension and pre-eclampsia. The test rated positive when the systolic blood pressure increased by 15 mmHg or more during isometric exercise, or decreased by 14 mmHg or more immediately after isometric exercise (Baker & Johnson 1994, Tomoda et al 1994).

EXERCISE AND THE FETOPLACENTAL UNIT

Exercise confined to early pregnancy increases the parenchymal component of the placenta, total vascular volume and surface area. Exercise taken throughout pregnancy increases these and other histomorphometric parameters associated with the rate of placental perfusion and transfer, with significant changes confined only to villi with a diameter of more than 80 μm (Bell et al 1995). Placental blood flow is lower in hypertensive, diabetic and cholestatic pregnancies compared with normal controls, but increases within a few minutes after a submaximal exercise. Conversely, in normal pregnancies, a short submaximal exercise has little effect on placental blood flow (Rauramo & Forss 1988). Even though it does not have significant effects on uterine artery perfusion, submaximal exercise can be associated with an increase in the fetal internal carotid artery mean velocity and a decrease in the cerebral resistance index, consistent with a slight fetal cerebral vasodilatation (Bonnin et al 1997). The S/D ratio of the umbilical artery close to the placental insertion site does not change significantly in the third trimester before and after a submaximal exercise bout at 85% of predicted maximum heart rate on a bicycle ergometer (Veille et al 1989). A lack of effect on the umbilical artery S/D ratio has also been found in growth-retarded fetuses with placental dysfunctions following graded walking on a treadmill with an upper limit of maternal heart rate of 150 bpm (Nabeshima et al 1997). Elevated erythropoietin levels in the fetal compartment (cord blood and amniotic fluid) are deemed to reflect fetal hypoxaemia, but erythropoietin levels obtained at the time of membrane rupture do not differ in women who exercise regularly until the onset of labour and non-exercising controls, confirming the absence of detrimental effects of regular maternal exercise on fetal oxygenation (Clapp 1995).

Moderate to heavy maternal exercise such as a bicycle exercise test reaching a median of 82% of maximal increase in maternal heart rate between 29 and 32 weeks can produce an increase of the fetal heart rate (FHR) for 30 min, and a reduction in the FHR variability for 20 min compared with pre-exercise parameters. Fetal body movements are also affected, showing a reduction following exercise which may last for up to 5 min (Manders et al 1997). A brief submaximal maternal exercise up to about 70% of maximal aerobic power (maternal heart rate not more than 148 bpm) can occasionally produce drops in FHR, while maximal exertion is generally followed by fetal bradycardia, probably due to inadequate fetal gas exchange (Carpenter et al 1988). FHR tends to increase during mild, moderate and strenuous maternal exercise in the majority of cases, with bradycardia occurring only sporadically. FHR variations during exercise are not directly correlated with gestational age, exercise intensity and maternal levels of circulating catecholamines (Artal et al 1986). When light maternal exercise is performed at an altitude of 2500 m, no significant FHR changes are recorded in normal pregnancies. The same probably cannot be recommended for women with 'high risk' pregnancies (Baumann & Huch 1986).

Fetal heart rate, cardiac size and fetal ventricular function do not change significantly 5 min after short-term moderate maternal exercise between 18 and 36 weeks of pregnancy (bicycle ergometer load test of 5 watts) in spite of a median maternal heart rate acceleration to 68% of the expected maximum heart rate (Sorensen & Borlum 1986). Furthermore, with maternal heart rate reaching, during a 15 min graded treadmill exercise, 168 bpm (84% training intensity), FHR increases significantly in only four out of 10 women (Nabeshima et al 1992). In this study, the baseline FHR has remained in the normal range (120–160 bpm) in the cases where training intensity was below 70% of expected maximal maternal heart rate.

Fetal breathing movements respond differently according to the type of exercise performed by the mother: they increase after dynamic work (bicycle exercise), remain unchanged after passive or static work (isometric muscle contraction), and decrease after maternal hyperventilation and hyperoxygenation. They appear to respond to environmental changes more promptly than fetal heart rate, and CO_2 has been confirmed to be a stimulator of breathing movements also in intrauterine life (Marsal et al 1979). Unlike breathing movements, which tend to decrease after 20 min of aerobic dance carried out at 35 weeks, fetal shoulder movements or kick response show no significant variation (Hatoum et al 1997). During immersion and exercise in water at 60% $\dot{V}O_{2\,max}$ in pregnancy, contrary to what occurs with exercise on land, FHR does not vary significantly and no uterine activity is recorded at either 25 or 35 weeks. Plasma volume expansion taking place with immersion might contribute to preserve the normal FHR (Katz et al 1988).

EXERCISE AND FETOMATERNAL METABOLIC CHANGES

— Blood glucose levels decrease more promptly and to lower values with exercise in pregnant women than in non-pregnant controls.
— Glucose tolerance normally decreases in pregnancy, but increases with exercise.
— Regular physical activity improves glucose tolerance in diabetic mothers.

— Regular exercise reduces total maternal weight gain and subcutaneous fat deposition towards the lower end of the normal range.
— Exercise in pregnancy produces an increase in urinary prostaglandins and thromboxane levels.
— The increase in plasma beta-endorphin levels associated with exercise tends to last longer in pregnant women compared to non-pregnant controls.

During exercise there is an increase in tissue uptake of glucose and insulin sensitivity. Serum adrenaline, noradrenaline, growth hormone, cortisol and glucagon increase with a breakdown of hepatic and muscular glycogen. Failure of this mechanism to take place can result in hypoglycaemia (Field 1989), and animal studies have shown that recurrent acute exercise during pregnancy can have detrimental effects on fetal development only if dietary glucose is severely restricted (Cobrin & Kooki 1995). Blood glucose levels of pregnant women decrease at a faster rate and to significantly lower values after 1 h of moderate-intensity exercise (55% $\dot{V}O_{2\,max}$) in the third trimester compared with non-pregnant controls. Insulin levels also decrease, and lactate levels are maintained at a lower level 15 min after exercise (Soultanakis et al 1996). Strenuous exercise produces an increase in mean values of [H^+], P_{CO_2} and total protein and a decrease in bicarbonate concentration in physically active pregnant women at a gestational age of 33 weeks, as well as in age-matched non-pregnant controls. At rest and during post-exercise recovery, pregnant women show significantly lower mean values of P_{CO_2} and total protein (Kemp et al 1997).

Glucose tolerance decreases during pregnancy as a consequence of increased peripheral insulin resistance, but physical exercise can improve both glucose tolerance and the insulin response to a glucose load (Young & Treadway 1992).

Pregnancy decreases the net cost of weight-dependent and weight-independent standard exercises when expressed per kg body weight (Prentice et al 1989) and causes a progressive increase in 24 h energy expenditure which is proportional to body weight and significant at 36 weeks of gestation (Heini et al 1992). It also reverses the hyperglycaemic response to intensive exercise that occurs in non-pregnant women in proportion to the intensity of the exercise. At 8 weeks, blood glucose increases only when exercise intensity exceeds 80% of maximum. At 15 weeks, this trend is even more marked, while by the 23rd week exercise determines a decrease in blood glucose. The change in glucose response occurring from the first trimester of pregnancy may be due to

decreased hepatic glucose release associated with increased peripheral glucose oxidation, which increases in the last part of pregnancy for the requirements of placenta and fetus (Clapp & Capeless 1991b).

Moderate exercise by insulin-dependent pregnant women to improve glucose tolerance is useful and does not cause any fetal or maternal complications (Bung et al 1991), while uptake of glucose by the fetus may be compromised following exercise only as a result of excessive glucose uptake by maternal skeletal muscles (Treadway & Young 1989). Twenty-four hour whole-body calorimetry measured before pregnancy and at 6, 12, 18, 30 and 36 weeks of gestation has shown a significant decrease of basal metabolic rate up to 24 weeks of gestation. At 36 weeks, basal metabolic rate increases by +8.6% to +35.4% relative to the baseline before pregnancy. Even if caloric intake is kept constant, body weight and fat increase progressively until delivery, but women who continue to exercise regularly accumulate less fat in the first and second trimesters and postpartum compared with non-exercising controls (Clapp & Little 1995, Dibblee & Graham 1983). Weight retention 1 year after delivery is higher in women who increase their caloric intake during and after pregnancy. There is a negative correlation between the degree of physical activity in the postpartum period and weight retention (Ohlin & Rossner 1994). Prenatal exercise is one of the most important parameters, in addition to pre-pregnancy weight, gestational weight gain and parity, in influencing postpartum weight gain (Boardley et al 1995).

Plasma ACTH, cortisol and glucose levels increase less markedly in response to a stressor event such as a treadmill exercise set at 90% $\dot{V}O_{2\,max}$ in lactating women between 7 and 18 weeks postpartum compared with non-lactating controls, suggesting that stress-responsive neurohormonal systems are somewhat less responsive in women who are breast-feeding (Altemus et al 1995). Exercise appears also to affect prostaglandin metabolism in pregnancy: pregnancy, in fact, is characterized by a 3.6- to 4.3-fold increase in urinary prostacyclin excretion with no significant change in thromboxane output, but, following 30 min of submaximal exercise, both prostacyclin and thromboxane excretion increase (Rauramo et al 1995).

An important issue regarding safety of exercise in pregnancy is the increase in body temperature. In animal models, exercise in hot conditions during the first trimester of pregnancy is associated with a significant increase of anomalies in fetal rats, particularly neural tube defects (Sasaki et al 1995), but this has not been confirmed in humans. Later in pregnancy, the intensity of the exercise performed is important.

High-intensity exercise, such as upright cycling for 15 min at 87.5 W (maternal heart rate 156 bpm), produces higher maternal temperature and FHR changes than a longer-duration lower-intensity exercise such as cycling for 30 min at 62.5 W (maternal heart rate 142 bpm). In either case, the temperature does not rise beyond 38°C, nor does it produce adverse FHR changes (O'Neill 1996).

Isometric exercise, such as a handgrip test in the third trimester of pregnancy, causes a significant increase in plasma corticotrophin and immunoreactive beta-endorphin concentrations in both normal and hypertensive pregnancies (Raisanen et al 1990). Women who exercise throughout pregnancy show higher plasma beta-endorphin levels compared with non-exercising controls throughout labour, and a reduced pain perception. Cortisol, growth hormone and prolactin levels are also lower during labour (Varrassi et al 1989). Mean basal concentration of corticotrophin is higher in women with pregnancy-induced hypertension compared with normal controls, while beta-endorphin concentration does not differ significantly. In response to a handgrip test, concentrations of both substances increase significantly in both groups. The increased basal concentration of corticotrophin in women with pregnancy-induced hypertension has been linked to increased circulating levels of corticotrophin-releasing hormone (Raisanen et al 1990). The secretion of beta-endorphins increases in response to exercise in both non-pregnant and pregnant women, but the response lasts longer in pregnant women (Rauramo et al 1986). Plasma beta-endorphin concentration is higher in women who undergo aerobic training on a bicycle ergometer during pregnancy compared with sedentary controls. This difference is present also during labour; pain perception is also reduced in patients who exercise compared with sedentary controls. Cortisol, human growth hormone and prolactin levels are lower during labour in exercise-conditioned patients (Varrassi et al 1989).

EXERCISE, LABOUR AND DELIVERY

— Women who exercise regularly during pregnancy have a lower incidence of 3rd and 4th degree tears.
— Onset of uterine contractions with exercise appears to be related more to the type of exercise performed than to its intensity.

Endurance training has been shown to have no harmful effects on labour or delivery in a group of Finnish elite athletes practising cross-country skiing, running, speed-skating or orienteering (Penttinen & Erkkola 1997). Women who practise sport regularly have a smaller incidence of third- and fourth-degree tears compared with sedentary controls (Klein et al 1997).

As to the influence of different sports on early miscarriage, in a prospective study on exercise performance before and during pregnancy in 47 recreational runners, 40 aerobic dancers and 28 physically active, fit controls, spontaneous abortion occurred on the whole in 19% of pregnancies. The rate of spontaneous abortion was 17% in runners, 18% in aerobic dancers, and 25% in the control group. One congenital abnormality was detected at term in each group (Clapp 1989). Contractions appear to depend more on the type of exercise than on the level of exertion. At equivalent levels of aerobic exercise, bicycle ergometry produces the onset of uterine contractions in 50% of sessions, treadmill running in 40%, and rowing ergometry in 0% (Durak et al 1990). Hypertensive pregnant women undergoing a short-term submaximal bicycle ergometer test are more prone to the onset of uterine contractions compared with normal women or women with other medical problems such as diabetes or intrahepatic cholestasis of pregnancy (Rauramo 1987).

Treadmill exercise for periods of 10 min in the second and third trimesters and postpartum increases uterine activity in 10 out of 14 women during exercise or recovery. FHR increases with exercise independently of uterine contractions and plasma noradrenaline levels (Cooper et al 1987).

Women who practise aerobic exercise during pregnancy tend to have a shorter second stage of labour and fewer obstetric complications than sedentary controls (Botkin & Driscoll 1991), and birthweight and neonatal Apgar scores remain unchanged.

The lack of negative effects of moderate exercise on uterine activity has been confirmed in a study on 102 healthy pregnant women between 25 and 38 weeks who showed no statistically significant difference in the number of contractions 1 h before and 1 h after gymnastics (Zahn & Raabe 1984). Women who perform regular leisure time physical activity during the first half of pregnancy also show a reduced risk of pre-eclampsia (relative risk [RR] = 0.67) and gestational hypertension (RR = 0.75), the reduction being greater the longer the average time spent in the leisure time physical activity (Marcoux et al 1989).

No association has been found between the frequency of uterine contractions and smoking, use of alcohol and coffee, or prolonged standing or lifting in low-risk pregnant women after 30 weeks of pregnancy. Uterine contractions appear to increase to a small degree only with climbing stairs and walking (Grisso et al 1992), and upper extremity exercise does not produce uterine contractions, which are instead stimulated by lower extremity exercise. The former therefore appears advisable in diabetic pregnant women when exercise is used in addition to insulin therapy for better control of hyperglycaemia (Jovanovic-Peterson & Peterson 1991).

Maternal exercise during labour, at an intensity approximately 60% of $\dot{V}O_{2\,max}$, decreases maternal pain perception (Artal et al 1993).

PHYSICAL ACTIVITY IN THE WORKPLACE AND PREGNANCY OUTCOME

Women employed in jobs that require intensive physical activity are at somewhat lower risk of developing pregnancy-induced hypertension compared with women employed in jobs entailing low levels of physical activity but standing for more than 8 h. Cleaning house for more than 7 h per week and looking after young children for more than 50 h per week are, by contrast, associated with a decreased risk (Eskenazi et al 1994).

Long working hours and fatigue seem to predispose to premature delivery, while work entailing lifting heavy weights or shiftwork affects fetal growth and duration of pregnancy (Armstrong et al 1989). A study carried out in 50 French factories showed a significant relationship between periods of rest due to 'sick leave' prescribed especially for fatigue, without any specific pathological cause, and a lower preterm birth rate (Mamelle et al 1989). Another study showed that mothers involved in heavy labour have a mean pregnancy weight gain of 3.3 ± 2.4 kg, independent of the weight of their offspring, compared with a weight gain of 5.9 ± 3.3 kg for the less active mothers (Tafari et al 1980).

Duration of rest in women involved in hard work during pregnancy has a strong influence on birthweight and length in newborn females, but to a lesser extent in newborn males, with a 7.5-fold decrease in the rate of low birthweight in girls when the duration of maternal rest is longer than 21 days. In boys, the rate of low birthweight does not change (Manshande et al 1987).

Increased observed/expected (O/E) ratio for late abortion has been found in operating room nurses, radiology technicians and agricultural and horticultural employees. The latter also show a significantly raised O/E ratio for stillbirths. The O/E ratio for stillbirth can approach 2, and the abortion ratio can increase by approximately 20% in women exposed to solvents (McDonald et al 1988). In another study on possible associations between structural fetal malformations and occupational exposure in 1475 mothers of malformed babies and an equal number of mothers of normal babies, a significant relationship was found between physical load and growth retardation. Mothers employed in jobs that entail occasional high physical workloads show more frequent pregnancy-induced hypertension, and women who have to stand for long hours because of their work show a higher risk of threatened abortion (Nurminen et al 1989).

Many studies have evaluated the effect of stressors, such as prolonged standing, physical exertion and long working weeks, on pregnancy. They suggest an influence on the duration of pregnancy (risk of premature delivery) rather than on birthweight (Marbury 1992). In a study on women who had delivered babies weighing 2500 g or less and controls with normal size babies, no association was found between the level of activity at work of the mother and delivery of a low birthweight baby (Meyer & Daling 1985).

EXERCISE AND THE NEONATE

Women doing more than four sessions of vigorous exercise weekly at 25 weeks of pregnancy tend to deliver babies whose mean birthweight is 315 g lower than that of babies of non-exercising controls. Participation in aerobic exercise during pregnancy does not adversely affect birthweight or other maternal and fetal parameters, and may render pregnancy generally more comfortable (Sternfeld et al 1995).

A study on 2743 pregnant women divided into five groups on the basis of daily energy expenditure showed that women in the medium energy expenditure group give birth to babies of higher weight than in the other groups, but that mean birthweight within each group remains within the normal range (Magann et al 1996).

Average birthweight and length of gestation do not differ significantly between women who continue to exercise during pregnancy and sedentary controls (Pivarnik 1994). In physically trained pregnant women, there appears to be no significant effect of maternal fitness on the state of the newborn at birth, while the short duration of labour in trained mothers reflects a more active role and higher fitness in all stages of labour (Wong & McKenzie 1987). When aerobic fitness is maintained during pregnancy, there is no increase in neonatal morbidity or obstetric complications, and mothers tend to experience a significant level of well-being (Kulpa et al 1987).

In a recent study comparing the offspring of 20 women who exercised during pregnancy and those of 20 controls, head circumference and fetal length at birth were similar, but babies of exercising women weighed less and had less fat. At 5 years of age, head circumference and height were similar, but the children of the women who exercised weighed less and had a lower sum of five site skinfolds. Motor, integrative and academic readiness skills were similar, but performance on the Wechsler scale and tests of oral language skill were significantly higher in children of exercising women (Clapp 1996).

PSYCHOLOGICAL ASPECTS OF EXERCISE IN PREGNANCY

Adolescent pregnant women participating in a 6-week aerobic exercise programme showed a significant decrease in depressive symptoms and an increase in total self-esteem, while those in the control sedentary group reported a significant increase in physical discomfort associated with pregnancy. Aerobic exercise programmes during pregnancy have been shown to reduce depressive symptoms and increase total self-esteem in adolescents compared with a non-exercising control group and can represent an important aspect of antenatal care in adolescents (Koniak-Griffin 1994).

CONCLUSIONS

The American College of Obstetricians and Gynecologists has recently published guidelines (ACOG Technical Bulletin 1994) on physical exercise in pregnancy, in which it stresses that, if there are no specific obstetric or medical contraindications, fit pregnant women can safely maintain the same level of fitness during pregnancy, although exercise schedules may have to be reduced.

Exercise taken during pregnancy by healthy women at a level that does not produce exhaustion does not cause any significant risk for the mother or baby. Caution must be recommended for mothers with pre-existing medical conditions or complications developing during pregnancy.

There are at present no conclusive data regarding the level of exercise that can cause a reduction of fetal weight at birth or, conversely, can definitely improve pregnancy outcome. Therefore, a programme of physical exercise in pregnancy will have to be adjusted individually.

REFERENCES

American College of Obstetricians and Gynecologists (ACOG) 1994 Exercise during pregnancy and the postpartum period. ACOG Technical Bulletin Number 189. International Journal of Obstetrics and Gynecology 45(1): 65–70

Altemus M, Deuster P A, Galiiven E, Carter C S, Gold P W 1995 Suppression of hypothalamic-pituitary-adrenal axis responses to stress in lactating women. Journal of Clinical Endocrinology and Metabolism 80(10): 2954–2959

Armstrong B G, Nolin A D, McDonald A D 1989 Work in pregnancy and birth weight for gestational age. British Journal of Industrial Medicine 46(3): 196–199

Artal R, Wiswell R (eds) 1986 Exercise in pregnancy. Williams & Wilkins, Baltimore

Artal R, Rutherford S, Romen Y, Kommula R K, Darey F J, Wiswell R A 1986 Fetal heart rate responses to maternal exercise. American Journal of Obstetrics and Gynecology 155(4): 729–733

Artal R, Khodiguian N, Paul R H 1993 Intrapartum fetal heart rate responses to maternal exercise. Case reports. Journal of Perinatal Medicine 21(6): 499–502

Asai M, Saegusa S, Yamada A, Suzuki M, Noguchi M, Niwa S, Nakanishi M 1994 Effects of exercise in water on maternal blood circulation. Nippon Sanka Fujinka Gakkai Zasshi 46(2): 109–114

Asakura H, Nakai A, Yamaguchi M, Koshino T, Araki T 1994 [Ultrasonographic blood flow velocimetry in maternal and umbilical arteries during maternal exercise]. Nippon Sanka Fujinka Gakkai Zasshi 46(4): 308–314

Baker P N, Johnson J R 1994 The use of the hand-grip test for predicting pregnancy-induced hypertension. European Journal of Obstetrics, Gynecology, and Reproductive Biology 56(3): 169–172

Barron W M, Mujais S K, Zinaman M, Bravo E L, Lindheimer M D 1986 Plasma catecholamine responses to physiologic stimuli in normal human pregnancy. American Journal of Obstetrics and Gynecology 154(1): 80–84

Baumann H, Huch R 1986 [Altitude exposure and staying at high altitude in pregnancy: effects on the mother and fetus]. Zentralbl Gynakologie 108(5): 889–899

Baumann H, Bung P, Fallenstein F, Huch A, Huch R 1985 Reaction of mother and fetus to physical stress at high altitude. Geburtshilfe Frauenheilkd 45(12): 869–876

Baumann H, Huch A, Huch R 1989 Doppler sonographic evaluation of exercise-induced blood flow velocity and waveform changes in fetal, uteroplacental and large maternal vessels of pregnant women. Journal of Perinatal Medicine 17(4): 279–287

Bell R J, Palma S M, Lumley J M 1995 The effect of vigorous exercise during pregnancy on birthweight. Australia and New Zealand Journal of Obstetrics and Gynaecology 35(1): 46–51

Berry M J, McMurray R G, Katz V L 1989 Pulmonary and ventilatory responses to pregnancy, immersion and exercise. Journal of Applied Physiology 66(2): 857–862

Boardley D J, Sargent R G, Coker A L, Hussey J R, Sharpe P A 1995 The relationship between diet, activity and other factors and postpartum weight change by race. Obstetrics & Gynecology 86(5): 834–838

Bonnin P, Bazzi-Grossin C, Ciraru-Vigneron N et al 1997 Evidence of fetal cerebral vasodilatation induced by submaximal maternal dynamic exercise in human pregnancy. Journal of Perinatal Medicine 25(1): 63–70

Botkin C, Driscoll C E 1991 Maternal aerobic exercise: newborn effects. Family Practice Research Journal 11(4): 387–393

Bung P, Artal R, Khodiguian N, Kjos S 1991 Exercise in gestational diabetes. An optional therapeutic approach? Diabetes 40(suppl 2): 182–185

Carpenter M W, Sady S P, Hoegsberg B et al 1988 Fetal heart rate response to maternal exertion. Journal of American Medical Association 259(20): 3006–3009

Clapp J F 3rd 1989 The effects of maternal exercise on early pregnancy outcome. American Journal of Obstetrics and Gynecology 161(6 Pt 1): 1453–1457

Clapp J F 3rd 1996 Morphometric and neurodevelopmental outcome at age five years of the offspring of women who continued to exercise regularly throughout pregnancy. Journal of Pediatrics 129(6): 856–863

Clapp J F 3rd, Capeless E 1991a The VO$_2$ max of recreational athletes before and after pregnancy. Medicine and Science in Sports and Exercise 23(10): 1128–1133

Clapp J F, Capeless E L 1991b The changing glycemic response to exercise during pregnancy. American Journal of Obstetrics and Gynecology 165(6 Pt 1): 1678–1683

Clapp J F 3rd, Little K D 1995 Effect of recreational exercise on pregnancy weight gain and subcutaneous fat deposition. Medicine and Science in Sports and Exercise 27(2): 170–177

Clapp J F 3rd, Little K D, Appleby-Wineberg S K, Widness J A 1995 The effect of regular maternal exercise on erythropoietin in cord blood and amniotic fluid. American Journal of Obstetrics and Gynecology 172(5): 1445–1451

Cobrin M, Koski K G 1995 Maternal dietary carbohydrate restriction and mild-to-moderate exercise during pregnancy modify aspects of fetal development in rats. Journal of Nutrition 125(6): 1617–1627

Cooper K A, Hunyor S N, Boyce E S, O'Neill M E, Frewin D B 1987 Fetal heart rate and maternal cardiovascular and catecholamine responses to dynamic exercise. Australian and New Zealand Journal of Obstetrics and Gynaecology 27(3): 220–223

Dibblee L, Graham T E 1983 A longitudinal study of changes in aerobic fitness, body composition, energy intake in primigravid patients. American Journal of Obstetrics and Gynecology 147(8): 908–914

Drack G, Kirkinen P, Baumann H, Muller R, Huch R 1988 [Doppler ultrasound studies before and following short-term maternal stress in late pregnancy]. Geburtshilfe Perinatologie 192(4): 173

Dumas G A, Reid J G 1997 Laxity of knee cruciate ligaments during pregnancy. Journal of Orthopedics Sport Physical Therapy 26(1): 2–6

Durak E P, Jovanovic-Peterson L, Peterson C M 1990 Comparative evaluation of uterine response to exercise on five aerobic machines. American Journal of Obstetrics and Gynecology 162(3): 754–756

Eneroth-Grimfors E, Bevegard S, Nilsson B A, Satterstrom G 1988 Effect of exercise on catecholamines and plasma renin activity in pregnant women. Acta Obstetrica et Gynaecologica Scandinavica 67(6): 519–523

Erkkola R U, Pirhonen J P, Kivijarvi A K 1992 Flow velocity waveforms in uterine and umbilical arteries during submaximal bicycle exercise in normal pregnancy. Obstetrics & Gynecology 79(4): 611–615

Eskenazi B, Fenster I, Wight S, English P, Windham G C, Swan S H 1994 Physical exertion as a risk factor for spontaneous abortion. Epidemiology 5(1): 6–13

Fast A, Weiss L, Ducommun E J, Medina E, Butler J G 1990 Low back pain in pregnancy. Abdominal muscles, sit-up performance and back pain. Spine 15(1): 28–30

Field J B 1989 Exercise and deficient carbohydrate storage and intake as causes of hypoglycemia. Endocrinology and Metabolism of North America 18(1): 155

Field S K, Bell S G, Cenaiko D F, Whitelow W A 1991 Relationship between inspiratory effort and breathlessness in pregnancy. Journal of Applied Physiology 71(5): 1897–1902

Gilleard W L, Brown J M 1994 Structure and function of the abdominal muscles in primigravid subjects during pregnancy and the immediate postbirth period. Physical Therapy 76(7): 750–762

Grisso J A, Main D M, Chiu G, Synder E S, Holmes J H 1992 Effects of physical activity and life-style factors on uterine contraction frequency. American Journal of Perinatology 9(5–6): 489–492

Hatoum N, Clapp J F 3rd, Newman M R, Dajani N, Amini S B 1997 Effects of maternal exercise on fetal activity in late gestation. Journal of Materno-Fetal Medicine 6(3): 134–139

Heini A, Schutz Y, Jequier E 1992 Twentyfour hour energy expenditure in pregnant and nonpregnant Gambian women, measured in a whole body indirect calorimeter. American Journal of Clinical Nutrition 55(6): 1078–1085

Horns P N, Ratcliffe L P, Leggett J C, Swanson M S 1996 Pregnancy outcomes among active and sedentary primiparous women. Journal of Obstetrics Gynecology and Neonatal Nursing 25(1): 49–54

Jovanovic-Peterson L, Peterson C M 1991 Is exercise safe or useful for gestational diabetic women? Diabetes 40 (suppl 2): 179–181

Katz V L, McMurray R, Berry M J, Cefalo R C 1988 Fetal and uterine responses to immersion and exercise. Obstetrics & Gynecology 72(2): 225–230

Katz V L, McMurray R, Berry M J, Cefalo R C, Bowman C 1990 Renal responses to immersion and exercise in pregnancy. American Journal of Perinatology 7(2): 118–121

Kemp J G, Greer F A, Wolfe L A 1997 Acid-base regulation after maximal exercise testing in late gestation. Journal of Applied Physiology 83(2): 644–651

Klein M C, Janssen P A, MacWilliam L, Kaczorowski J, Johnson B 1997 Determinants of vaginal-perineal integrity and pelvic floor functioning in childbirth. American Journal of Obstetrics and Gynecology 172(2): 403–410

Koniak-Griffin D 1994 Aerobic exercise, psychological well-being, and physical discomforts during adolescent pregnancy. Research in Nursing Health 17(4): 253–263

Kulpa P J, White B M, Visscher R 1987 Aerobic exercise in pregnancy. American Journal of Obstetrics and Gynecology 156(6): 1395–1403

Kusche M, Bolte A, Hollman W, Roemer D 1986 [Physical performance in pregnancy]. Geburtshilfe Frauenheilkd 46(3): 151–156

Lotgering F K, Struijk P C, van Doorn M B, Spinnewijn W E, Wallenburg H C 1995 Anaerobic threshold and respiratory compensation in pregnant women. Journal of Applied Physiology 78(5): 1772–1777

McDonald A D, McDonald J C, Armstrong B et al 1988 Fetal death and work in pregnancy. British Journal of Industrial Medicine 45(3): 148–157

McMurray R G, Katz V L, Berry M J, Cefalo R C 1988 Cardiovascular responses of pregnant women during aerobic exercise in water: a longitudinal study. International Journal of Sports Medicine 9(6): 443–447

Magann E F, Evans S F, Newnham J P 1996 Employment, exertion and pregnancy outcome: assessment by kilocalories expended each day. American Journal of Obstetrics and Gynecology 175(1): 182–187

Mamelle N, Bertucat I, Munoz F 1989 Pregnant women at work: rest periods to prevent preterm birth? Paediatrics and Perinatal Epidemiology 3(1): 19–28

Manders M A, Sonder C J, Mulper E J, Visser G H 1997 The effects of maternal exercise on fetal heart rate and movement patterns. Early Human Development 48(3): 237–247

Manshande J P, Eeckels R, Manshande-Desmet V, Vlietinck R 1987 Rest versus heavy work during the last weeks of pregnancy: influence on fetal growth. British Journal of Obstetrics and Gynaecology 94(11): 1059–1067

Marbury M C 1992 Relationship of ergonomic stressors to birthweight and gestational age. Scandinavian Journal of Work and Environmental Health 18(2): 73–83

Marcoux S, Brisson J, Fabia J 1989 The effect of leisure time physical activity on the risk of pre-eclampsia and gestational hypertension. Journal of Epidemiology and Community Health 43(2): 147–152

Marsal K, Gennser G, Lofgren O 1979 Effects on fetal breathing movements of maternal challenges. Cross-over study on dynamic work, passive movements, hyperventilation and hyperoxygenation. Acta Obstetrica et Gynecologica Scandinavica 58(4): 335–342

Matsushita M, Asai M, Saegusa S et al 1996 [Study on anaerobic threshold in normal pregnant women]. Nippon Sanka Fujinka Gakkai Zasshi 48(7): 495–500

Meyer B A, Daling J R 1985 Activity level of mother's usual occupation and low infant birth weight. Journal of Occupational Medicine 27(11): 841–847

Moore D H, Jarret J C 2nd, Bendick P J 1988 Exercise-induced changes in uterine artery blood flow, as measured by Doppler ultrasound, in pregnant subjects. American Journal of Perinatology 5(2): 94–97

Nabeshima Y, Sasaki J, Mesaki N, Sohda S, Kubo T 1997 Effect of maternal exercise on fetal umbilical artery waveforms: comparison of IUGR and AFD fetuses. Journal of Obstetric and Gynecologic Research 23(3): 255–259

Nabeshima Y, Souda S, Sasaki J, Mesaki N, Iwasaki H 1992 [Effect of maternal exercise with graded treadmill on fetal heart rate]. Nippon Sanka Fujinka Gakkai Zasshi 44(3): 323–328

Nurminen T, Lusa S, Ilmarinen J, Kurppa K 1989 Physical work load, fetal development and course of pregnancy. Scandinavian Journal of Work and Environment Health 15(6): 404–414

Ohlin A, Rossner S 1994 Trend in eating patterns, physical activity and socio-demographic factors in relation to postpartum body weight development. British Journal of Nutrition 71(4): 457–470

O'Neill M E 1996 Maternal rectal temperature and fetal heart rate responses to upright cycling in late pregnancy. British Journal of Sports Medicine 30(1): 32–35

O'Toole M L 1989 Gender differences in the cardiovascular response to exercise. Cardiovascular Clinics 19(3): 17–33

Penttinen J, Erkkola R 1997 Pregnancy in endurance athletes. Scandinavian Journal of Medicine and Science in Sports 7(4): 226–228

Pernoll M L, Metcalfe J, Kovach P A, Wachtel R, Dunham M J 1975 Ventilation during rest and exercise in pregnancy and postpartum. Respiratory Physiology 25(3): 295–310

Pivarnik J M 1994 Maternal exercise during pregnancy. Sports Medicine 18(4): 215–217

Prentice A M, Goldberg G R, Davies H L, Murgatroyd P R, Scott W 1989 Energy sparing adaptations in human pregnancy assessed by whole body calorimetry. British Journal of Nutrition 62(1): 5–22

Raisanen I, Salminen K, Laatikainen T 1990 Response of plasma immunoreactive beta-endorphin and corticotropin to isometric exercise in uncomplicated pregnancy and in pregnancy-induced hypertension. European Journal of Obstetrics Gynecology and Reproductive Biology 35(2–3): 119–124

Rauramo I 1987 Effect of short-term physical exercise on foetal heart rate and uterine activity in normal and abnormal pregnancies. Annales Chirurgiae et Gynaecologiae 76(5): 274–279

Rauramo I, Forss M 1988 Effect of exercise on maternal hemodynamics and placental blood flow in healthy women. Acta Obstetrica et Gynaecologica Scandinavica 67(1): 21–25

Rauramo I, Salminen K, Laatikainen T 1986 Release of beta-endorphin in response to physical exercise in non-pregnant women. Acta Obstetrica et Gynaecologica Scandinavica 65(6): 609–612

Rauramo I, Elmonen S, Viinikka L, Ylikorkala O 1995 Prostacyclin and thromboxane in pregnant and non-pregnant women in response to exercise. Obstetrics & Gynecology 85(6): 1027–1030

Sady S P, Carpenter M W 1989 Aerobic exercise during pregnancy. Special considerations. Sports Medicine 7(6): 357–375

Sady M A, Haydon B B, Sady S P, Carpenter M W, Thompson P D, Coustan D R 1990 Cardiovascular response to maximal cycle exercise during pregnancy and two and seven months postpartum. American Journal of Obstetrics and Gynecology 162(5): 1181–1185

Sasaki J, Yamaguchi A, Nabeshima Y, Shigemitsu S, Mesaki N, Kubo T 1995 Exercise at high temperature causes maternal hyperthermia and fetal anomalies in rats. Teratology 51(4): 233–236

Sorensen K E, Borlum K G 1986 Fetal heart function in response to short-term maternal exercise. British Journal of Obstetrics and Gynaecology 93(4): 310–313

Soultanakis H N, Artal R, Wiswell R A 1996 Prolonged exercise in pregnancy: glucose homeostasis, ventilatory and cardiovascular responses. Seminars in Perinatology 20(4): 315–327

Spatling L, Fallenstein F, Huch A, Huch R, Rooth G 1992 The variability of cardiopulmonary adaptation to pregnancy at rest and during exercise. British Journal of Obstetrics and Gynaecology 100(4): 398–399

Spinnewijn W E, Wallenburg H C, Struijk P C, Lotgering F K 1996 Peak ventilatory responses during cycling and swimming in pregnant and non-pregnant women. Journal of Applied Physiology 81(2): 738–742

Sternfeld B, Quesenberry C P Jr, Eskenazi B, Newman L A 1995 Exercise during pregnancy and pregnancy outcome. Medicine and Science in Sports and Exercise 27(5): 634–640

Tafari N, Naeye R L, Gobezie A 1980 Effects of maternal undernutrition and heavy physical work during pregnancy on birth weight. British Journal of Obstetrics and Gynaecology 87(3): 222–226

Tomoda S, Kitanaka T, Ogita S, Hidaka A 1994 Prediction of pregnancy-induced hypertension by isometric exercise. Asia and Oceania Journal of Obstetrics and Gynaecology 20(3): 249–255

Treadway J L, Young J C 1989 Decreased glucose uptake in the fetus after maximal exercise. Medicine and Science in Sports and Exercise 21(2): 140–145

van Doorn M B, Lotgering F K, Struijk P C, Pool J, Wallenburg H C 1992 American Journal of Obstetrics and Gynecology 166(3): 854–859

Varrassi G, Bazzano C, Edwards W T 1989 Effects of physical activity on maternal plasma beta-endorphin levels and perception of labour pain. American Journal of Obstetrics and Gynecology 160(3): 707–712

Veille J C, Bacevice A E, Wilson B, Janos J, Helerstein H K 1989 Umbilical artery waveform during bicycle exercise in normal pregnancy. Obstetrics & Gynecology 73(6): 957–960

Veille J C, Kitzman D W, Bacevice A E 1996 Effects of pregnancy on the electrocardiogram in healthy subjects during strenuous exercise. American Journal of Obstetrics and Gynecology 175(5): 1360–1364

Webb K A, Wolfe L A, McGrath M J 1994 Effects of acute and chronic maternal exercise on fetal heart rate. Journal of Applied Physiology 77(5): 2207–2213

Wong S C, McKenzie D C 1987 Cardiorespiratory fitness during pregnancy and its effect on outcome. International Journal of Sports Medicine 8(2): 79–83

Young J C, Treadway J L 1992 The effect of prior exercise on oral glucose tolerance in late gestational women. European Journal of Applied Physiology 64(5): 430–433

Zahn V, Raabe V 1984 [Effect of exercise during pregnancy on uterine contractions] Zentralbl Gynakologie 106(1): 33–39

16

Dance medicine

Margaret Wan Nar Wong
William Wing Kee To
Kai Ming Chan

KEY POINTS

1. Dance is a special form of performing art, which places high physical and psychological demands on dancers. The physical profile of dancers approaches that of athletes.
2. The incidence and prevalence of dance injuries among dancers of various disciplines are high.
3. Most dance injuries are overuse problems related to dance technique and repetitive loading. Over half of the injuries involve the lower extremities. Different dance forms have their own special patterns of injury.
4. A good knowledge of dance is essential for effective treatment prescription, development of a rehabilitation programme and preventive care planning.
5. Menstrual dysfunction occurs with varying frequency across the different disciplines of dance. The underlying hormonal disturbance is probably heterogeneous.
6. Dance injuries, menstrual dysfunction, psychological stress, eating disorder and osteoporosis are the major problems seen in dance medicine. There is an intricate interplay among these problems, the mechanism of which has yet to be evaluated.

INTRODUCTION

Dance is a special form of performing art, which uses body motions and an aesthetic form to express and communicate. The physical, intellectual and psychological demands of dancing are comparable to those of most strenuous sports. Both dancers and athletes are seeking perfection, both need to keep in shape and undertake repetitive practices before a performance, and both often suffer a great deal of mental stress. Dance movements require explosive power, sustained effort, and local and general endurance. The physical profile of dancers is more highly developed than that of unconditioned individuals, but less so than that of high-level endurance athletes. Female dancers suffer from the 'female athletic triad', characterized by eating disorders, amenorrhoea and osteoporosis, as do other elite sportswomen. Like gymnasts, dancers often start training at an early age, thus placing unique stresses on their musculoskeletal system during their period of growth and development. Years of dedication, perseverance and intense practice are required before one can achieve the status of an elite dancer.

The knowledge of medical problems of dancers has expanded greatly in the past two decades, and dance medicine is developing into a subspeciality in itself. A good understanding of these dancers' aspirations, the special requirements and demands placed on them, the etiology and mechanism of injury, their risk for other medical problems and their possible interrelationship is required before effective treatment, a suitable rehabilitation programme and preventive care can be offered by trained medical personnel.

DANCE INJURIES
Epidemiology

Most publications on prevalence or incidence of dance injuries are on ballet dancers. The injury rate ranges from 70 to 90% (Quirk 1984, Wong et al 1995), with an over 60% prevalence rate of various degrees of disability. Although most are minor injuries or overuse problems, because of the high physical demand on dancers the resultant functional disability in dancers is significant. Dance injuries constitute an important cause of class suspension or withdrawal in dance students, and may result in temporary unemployment, loss of salary, or even an end to a career of a professional dancer. The mental stress involved in coping with these injuries can never be accurately measured. Many dancers tend to continue to dance or return to full performance before adequate recovery and rehabilitation, thus perpetuating the problem.

The majority of dance injuries are overuse injuries, which develop slowly over time. Tendinopathies, strains and sprains are commonly seen. The mechanism of these injuries is related to the repetitive movements and loading. Insufficient warm-up, fatigue and technical error were cited as contributing factors to dance injuries in over 50% of cases (Wong et al 1995). Inappropriate or ill-maintained dance floors, an unconditioned body, and low environmental temperatures may also play a role. Recognition and diagnosis of these injuries are often delayed, as dancers tend to ignore and tolerate minor symptoms. Problems are often not brought to medical attention for fear of the need to suspend dancing. An average lag time of 2.2 days was reported before medical consultation for an injury, with 40% seen after a week or more (Wong et al 1995). Over half of the injuries involve the lower extremities, with foot and ankle injuries being the commonest. The distribution and type of injuries vary with the type and style of dance.

Ballet dance

Most of the scientific literature in dance medicine focuses on ballet. Ballet dance is a highly selective form of performing art. Since the first ballet class, a selective process continues to select the fittest survivor: those with the correct body type, right mental attitude and talent. Serious ballet training usually starts at around 8 years old. The physical and emotional demands on these growing children and the subsequent professional dancers are probably the most severe among all forms of dance. The need to dance *en pointe* (dancing on tip of toes) and the wearing of pointe shoes with the rigid toe box are unique to classical ballet. The practice of turnouts (extreme external rotation of the lower extremities) and *plié* (bending down with hips turned out), with repetitive jumps and landing, places special stress on the lower extremities. The feet suffer the heaviest toll: the thin practice slippers provide no protection at all, and dancing *en pointe* in pointe shoes with rigid toe box results in high pressure on the forefoot (Teitz et al 1985). It is therefore not surprising that over 60% of ballet injuries involve the lower extremity, with half of them in the foot and ankle (Quirk 1984, Reid et al 1987).

Ballet dancers display an impressive range of movement, well beyond the ability of the average person. This joint laxity and hypermobility are the result of both inherent laxity and painstaking training. A

Beighton Score of four or more indicating hypermobility has been found present in 9.5% of ballet dancers. However, hypermobile dancers suffer from significantly more injuries than non-hypermobile ones, making it a liability rather than asset (Klemp et al 1984).

Many ballet injuries, especially overuse injuries, are related to dance techniques. Problems are more commonly seen in those less conformed to the ideal body physique, as they attempt to perform what they are ill-equipped to do. The repetitive injury sustained may lead to eventual withdrawal from training and professional career, and is a manifestation of a process of Darwinian selection.

A perfect turnout requires 90° of hip external rotation on each side, which can be achieved by only a few dancers. Compensation occurs below the hip level. Excessive stress is therefore placed on the knees and the ankles, forcing abnormal rotational movements. 'Forcing the turnout' is seen when dancers plant their heels together first, placing the feet at 180° to each other, before fully extending the knees and hips. The initially flexed hips and knees allow more external rotation to occur. However, the final extension and 'screwing in' of the knees stress the medial collateral ligament and the medial meniscus. Forced turnout also causes excessive foot pronation, leading to tenosynovitis of the posterior tibial and flexor hallux longus tendons. A partial tear of the flexor hallux longus tendon behind the talus may result in stenosis and in the phenomenon of trigger toe.

Dancing *en pointe* requires extreme ankle plantarflexion and good muscular control. Ankle sprain is the commonest dance injury in ballet dancers. The extreme ankle movements required in ballet predispose to anterior and posterior ankle impingement syndromes. The use of pointe shoes and standing on tip-toes regularly cause problems like callosities, soft corns, hallux valgus, metatarsophalangeal degeneration and hammer toes.

Dancers often practise up to 25 h a week (Wong et al 1995), with the lower limbs under repetitive loading. Evidence of excessive stress was seen as cortical thickening in the first, second and third metatarsal shafts in 23 out of 28 ballet dancers in a radiographical survey of the Cincinnati Ballet Company (Schneider et al 1974). Stress fractures are seen in the lower limbs, in the femoral neck, tibia, lower fibula and, most commonly, the metatarsals. Prolonged amenorrhoea and heavy training schedules predispose ballet dancers to stress fractures. Dancers dancing more than 5 h/day have a significantly higher chance of sustaining a stress fracture. Bone scan is helpful in clinically suspicious cases with negative plain radiography.

Lower back pain and wrist problems are seen in male ballet dancers who have to lift and support female dancers during partnering.

Modern dance

Modern dance was born out of a desire to have a freer form of dance which allows a wider range of emotional expression than is afforded by the confines of classical ballet. The freedom from tights and shoes puts the lower extremity in danger of injuries. Modern dancers perform a lot of movements while sitting, kneeling or lying on the floor, sometimes even throwing themselves across the floor. 'Floor burns' (abrasion) occur due to friction and contusions between the lower extremity bony prominences and the floor. Dancing barefoot also predisposes to plantar callosities, fissures and lacerations. Modern dancers are also at risk of knee injuries from patellofemoral compression during floor work, as well as ligament or meniscal injuries during sudden twists and turns.

Break dance

Break dancing was in fashion in the early 1980s, but its popularity has waned. It is characterized by acrobatic, gymnastics-like movements with leaps and spins on the back or the head. 'Floor work' or 'foot work' refers to dancing on the floor with body supported by hands or arms. Copperman (1984) described two cases of alopecia related to head spin in break dancing, and named it 'alopecia breakdancia'. The 'break dance back syndrome' refers to an acute lower back pain associated with difficulty in flexion after break dancing (Norman & Grodin 1984). Swellings at the thoracolumbar spine area have been seen associated with back spins. Fractures of the spinous process and extremities, cervical injuries and even quadriplegia have been described. As opposed to the overuse nature in most other forms of dance, break dancing may cause serious acute life-threatening injuries.

Aerobic dance

Aerobic dance is often taken as a form of health exercise because of its great variability and ease of participation. The dance programme can vary widely in intensity and duration. The high-impact form involves bouncing, hopping and jumping movements that cause repetitive stress, especially on the lower extremity and spine. The high-impact nature of aerobic dance and the subsequent epidemic of lower limb injuries prompted examinations of the dance form, dance floor and footwear. The low-impact form is differentiated from the high-impact form by always having one foot in contact with the ground, with greater use of the upper body and bending movements, and it causes significantly fewer loading problems. In a study of 1233 aerobic dancers (Richie et al 1985), 43.3% of students and 75.9% of instructors reported having sustained an injury. The average incidence was estimated to be 1.01 injuries per 100 h of dancing. A carpeted concrete floor was associated with more injuries than a wood-over-airspace floor with or without carpet (Richie et al 1985).

Chinese dance

Literature on Chinese dancing is extremely scanty. Chinese dance uses the upper limbs and trunk more compared with ballet. It often involves a lot of back movements and extreme hyperextension of spine. Motions are often slow and fluid, and require sustained efforts in maintaining postures. Chinese dancers, when compared with ballerinas, have a significantly higher body mass index, lower incidence of menstrual dysfunction and fewer musculoskeletal injuries (To et al 1995). However, an average of 2.7 injuries/year is still recorded. Back injuries are more prevalent when compared with other disciplines (Wong et al 1995).

MANAGEMENT OF DANCE INJURIES

The medical personnel managing dance injuries have to be aware of the high physical demands placed on dancers, their aspirations and the mental stress they have to endure. The physician must be sympathetic to their desire to return to dancing as early as possible, and understand their tendency to perform beyond their capabilities. The aim of management is to make the correct diagnosis, identify contributing factors, rehabilitate the dancers, and, most important, prevent future recurrences. Knowledge of the specific requirements of different dance forms and their specific risks is most helpful.

Most dance injuries are minor or overuse injuries which can be managed conservatively. A special dance clinic significantly facilitates early effective management. A physiotherapist and an orthopaedic surgeon

with knowledge of and experience in treating dancers are indispensable assets to every dance school and company. The therapists, working with the orthopaedic surgeon, can initiate acute case treatment, communicate with teachers and choreographers on improving dance training and techniques, and design rehabilitation programmes for individual dancers.

In rehabilitating dancers, it is essential to remember to maintain range of motion and strength. The target range of motion and strength should be the dancer's own pre-morbid state (or beyond), instead of the average normal, as a full recovery to the average is inadequate for a dancer. Simple rest and suspension from dancing are counterproductive. Range of motion and strength should be maintained as far as possible throughout the recovery process by tailored graduated exercises. A limited range of motion and weakened extremity will predispose the dancer to a second injury even if the initial one has apparently healed. Surgery should be avoided as far as possible.

The ultimate aim of all management is prevention of further injury or recurrence. Correctable contributing or predisposing factors like faulty technique, suboptimal dance floor, overwork, etc., if identified, should be communicated to the teachers and choreographers for amendment. Intrinsic physical deficiencies may need specific strengthening and training, depending on the individual case.

OTHER MEDICAL PROBLEMS IN DANCERS

Menstrual dysfunction

While exercise amenorrhoea is a common problem for exercising women in general, menstrual dysfunction in dancers has been studied in detail as a separate entity. Dance exercises require a combination of endurance and slenderness to achieve a weight that is uniform with other dancers, that can be lifted, and that fits costumes and the vision of the choreographer (Williams & Speroff 1987). The combination of intense exercise, low body weight and body fat, dietary restriction, and the psychological stress of performance and training contributes to menstrual dysfunction in dancers.

Various types of menstrual dysfunction have been documented among dancers. Delayed menarche is one of the earliest manifestations in dancers who start their training before puberty (Frisch et al 1980). This phenomenon appears more common in ballet dancers than in other dance disciplines, as ballerinas often undergo extensive training from early childhood. In dancers with normal menarche, secondary amenorrhoea represents one extreme of menstrual dysfunction (Warren 1980), and a gradation of milder abnormalities, including variable cycle lengths from irregular ovulation, and hypomenorrhoea and irregular bleeding, are frequently seen. Delay in menarche and prolonged intervals of amenorrhoea that reflect prolonged hypo-oestrogenism may predispose ballet dancers to scoliosis and stress fractures (Warren et al 1986). The prevalence of scoliosis seems to rise with increasing age at menarche, and the incidence of secondary amenorrhoea is significantly higher among dancers with stress fractures.

The incidence of adolescent problems in other disciplines of dance remains significant, but probably not as high as in ballerinas. In a comparative survey of collegiate dance students across various disciplines, ballet dancers had a higher incidence of menstrual dysfunction and musculoskeletal injuries compared with classic Chinese dance, modern dance and musical theatre dance students, as well as a significantly lower body mass index (To et al 1995). The overall incidence of amenorrhoea was 13%, while that of oligomenorrhoea was 15%. Those who had amenorrhoea reported longer training hours per week when compared with eumenorrhoeic and oligomenorrhoeic students, and both oligomenorrhoeic and amenorrhoeic students had a lower body mass index and a higher incidence of musculoskeletal injuries and chronic orthopaedic problems compared with eumenorrhoeic ones. Thus, it was postulated that prolonged hypo-oestrogenism, apart from its association with osteoporosis, deformities and stress fractures, could also be associated with non-bony musculoskeletal injuries.

Body fat composition is known to have a significant impact on female reproductive function. It has been hypothesized that a critical percentage body fat weight of 17% is required for menarche, and that 22% of body fat is required for resumption of menses after secondary amenorrhoea resulting from weight loss (Frisch 1984). Menstrual dysfunction has been correlated with excessive slimness in ballerinas in various studies (Frisch et al 1980, Warren 1980). However, an absolute threshold of body fat might not be obvious in all studies, as a substantial increase in amenorrhoea might not be associated with significant changes in weight (Abraham et al 1982). A survey of collegiate dance students showed that, irrespective of their discipline, amenorrhoeic dancers had a significantly lower percentage of total body fat as compared with eumenorrhoeic dancers. Comparing the different dis-

ciplines, modern and theatre dancers had thicker skinfold in the upper limbs, classical Chinese dancers had thicker subscapular folds, and ballerinas had the thinnest abdominal folds. These differences probably reflect the differential development of muscle groups and fat deposition in the different dance disciplines (To et al 1997).

A longitudinal study of collegiate dance students with menstrual dysfunction found that a proportion of dancers who developed amenorrhoea at the end of the training period had higher mean basal plasma dehydroepiandrosterone sulphate (DHEA-S) levels even before the commencement of training, as compared with those who remained eumenorrhoeic at the end of the season (To et al 1998). A similar picture was found in female competitive swimmers who developed menstrual dysfunction; they had a hormonal profile suggestive of mild hyperandrogenism, very different from simple hypothalamic amenorrhoea (Constantini & Warren 1995). Whether such patterns are restricted to particular dance disciplines requires further study.

Eating disorders

The aesthetic requirement of dance often calls for a slim figure. The classical ballet dancer look comprises long legs, short trunk, long neck and a small head. The ideal form is generally thin, ranging from 10 to 20% below the ideal body weight for ballet dancers (Brooks-Gunn et al 1987). Professional ballet dancers often weigh 12–15% below their ideal body weight for height. In the quest for this ideal, dancers often use dieting as a means of maintaining their thinness. There is a high prevalence of poor eating habits and food faddism among dancers. In a study on adult female ballet dancers, the mean caloric intake was found to be 1358 cal. The incidences of vitamin (A, B and C) and mineral (iron, calcium and zinc) deficiency were over 40 and over 60%, respectively (Calabrese et al 1983).

Common associated problems include binge eating, bulimia, anaemia, menstrual disorders and osteopenia. Clinical anorexia nervosa appears rare among professional dancers due to the inevitable failure to maintain physical performance. In Hamilton et al's (1997) study, 15% of adolescent dancers demonstrated clinical eating disorders. These dancers were significantly more depressed, isolated, impulsive, emotionally disturbed and alienated from dance upon psychological testing. They also had less optimal physique and missed more classes due to injuries when compared with those without eating disorders

(Hamilton et al 1997). This illustrated the intricate interplay between eating disorder, psychological stress and injury. Dieting and nutritional deficiency contributed to delayed menarche, menstrual irregularities, hypo-oestrogenaemia and subsequent osteopenia.

Psychological problems

In a study of 61 sports, ballet was deemed the most physically and mentally demanding activity, surpassing gymnastics and figure skating (Nicholas 1975).

Dance training involves considerable repetition and practice of a single motion until it is perfected. It demands obedience, perseverance and total dedication to achieve the best. Only a minority of those who aspire to reach the top can eventually fulfil their career aspirations and become professional dancers. The performing arts world is highly competitive: 55% of the adolescent girls in the School of American Ballet dropped out over a 4-year training period with injuries and eating disorders (Hamilton et al 1997). Weight requirement is an important source of psychological stress. Dancers are often anxious to fit into the norms of dance and peer culture. Open criticism of injured dancers and pressure on them from teachers and choreographers to resume dancing before rehabilitation sometimes exacerbate the problem. Serious injuries or anticipated retirement in professional dancers were related to depression, substance abuse and suicidal ideation (Hamilton & Hamilton 1991).

The impact of psychological stress on menstrual dysfunction in dancers has been difficult to determine. Stress combined with weight loss has been clearly shown to induce menstrual dysfunction in athletes (Bullen et al 1985). However, pure psychological testing for stress scores often fail to show a difference between amenorrhoeic and eumenorrhoeic individuals (Loucks & Horvath 1984, To et al 1998).

Osteoporosis

Initial reports of osteoporosis in exercise-induced amenorrhoeic women were met with scepticism because of previous documented evidence of exercise as a stimulus for bone mineral deposition (Drinkwater et al 1984). Since the documentation of reduced bone mass in amenorrhoeic athletes (Cann et al 1984), there are now adequate data to establish osteoporosis as a real risk for women with long-term exercise amenorrhoea.

Ballet dancers are at special risk for osteopenia, due to low body weight, nutritional deficiency and menstrual disorders with resultant hypogonadism. Although dance as an exercise has a protective effect on bone mineral density, it may not be adequate to compensate for the loss. The net result of vigorous exercise, hypogonadism and low body weight in dancers may not be generalized osteopenia, but a differential effect depending on the amount of weight-bearing.

Recent bone mineral studies showed significantly higher bone mineral density in the lower extremities of professional female ballet dancers (Karlsson et al 1993). A study of 44 ballet dancers compared their bone mineral density with that of 18 amenorrhoeic anorexic girls and 23 normal controls. There was a significant increase in trochanteric bone mineral density and a decrease in other non-weight-bearing sites before correcting for body mass index (Young et al 1994). So far, however, a definite association between bone loss and stress fracture has not been demonstrated.

With the established risk of oesteoporosis, hypo-oestrogenic dancers should be treated with oestrogen-progestogen hormonal replacement therapy. Moreover, given the substantial evidence that menstrual dysfunction and its related sequelae are not unique to ballerinas, dancers from other disciplines suffering similar problems should be managed under identical protocols.

CONCLUSIONS

1. Dance is a special form of performing art, which places high physical and psychological demands on dancers. The early age at which intensive training starts poses special problems in these growing artists.

2. The incidence and prevalence of dance injuries among dancers of various disciplines are high, both in students and in professional dancers. These injuries, although usually mild, may cause significant disability in dancers who have extreme demands placed on them due to high performance levels. Secondary problems of deteriorated performance, temporary suspension, unemployment or even termination of a career place heavy psychological stress on dancers, which can, in turn, lead to other medical problems.

3. Most dance injuries are overuse problems related to dance techniques and repetitive loading. Over half of the injuries involve the lower extremities. Most of the available literature is on ballet dancers. Different dance forms have their own special pattern of injury. Deficiency in knowledge on disciplines other than ballet also needs to be addressed.

4. The medical personnel managing dance injuries have to be aware of the high physical demands placed on dancers, their aspirations and the mental stress they have to endure. The physician must be sympathetic to their desire to return to dancing as early as possible, and understand their tendency to perform beyond their capabilities. A special dance clinic will facilitate early effective management and amend predisposing factors, and devise rehabilitation programmes and preventive measures.

5. Menstrual dysfunction occurs with varying frequency across the different disciplines of dance. A significant amount of scientific literature is available, with specific emphasis on the menstrual disorders of dancers. However, no conclusions can be drawn as to the underlying hormonal disturbance, which is probably heterogeneous.

6. Dance injuries, menstrual dysfunction, psychological stress, eating disorders and osteoporosis are major problems seen in dancers. There is apparently an intricate interplay among these complex problems. Each is related to the other, but the exact mechanism and association have not been clearly defined as yet. More scientific work in this growing field is needed.

REFERENCES

Abraham S F, Beumont P J U, Fraser I S, Llewellyn-Jones D 1982 Body weight, exercise and menstrual status among ballet dancers in training. British Journal of Obstetrics and Gynaecology 89: 507–510

Brooks-Grunn J, Warren M P, Hamilton L H 1987 Relationship of eating disorders to amenorrhoea in ballet dancers. Medicine and Science in Sports and Exercise 19: 41–45

Bullen B A, Skrinar G S, Beitins I Z, von Mering G, Turnbull B A, McArthur J W 1985 Induction of menstrual disorders by strenuous exercises in untrained women. New England Journal of Medicine 312: 1349–1353

Calabrese L H, Kirkendall D T, Floyd M 1983 Menstrual abnormalities, nutritional pattern and body composition in female classical ballet dancers. Physical Sports Medicine 11: 86–98

Cann C E, Martin M C, Genant H K, Jaffe R B 1984 Decreased spinal mineral content in amenorrhoeic women. Journal of American Medical Association 251: 626–629

Constantini N W, Warren M P 1995 Menstrual dysfunction in swimmers: a distinct entity. Journal of Clinical Endocrinology and Metabolism 80: 2740–2744

Copperman S M 1984 Two new cases of alopecia (letter). Journal of American Medical Association 252(24): 3367

Drinkwater B L, Nilson K, Chesnut C H, Bremner W J, Shainholtz S, Southworth M B 1984 Bone mineral content of amenorrhoeic and eumenorrhoeic athletes. New England Journal of Medicine 311: 277–281

Frisch R E 1984 Body fat, puberty and fertility. Biology Review 59: 161–169

Frisch R E, Wyshak G, Vincent L 1980 Delayed menarche and amenorrhoea in ballet dancers. New England Journal of Medicine 303: 17–19

Hamilton L H, Hamilton W G 1991 Classical ballet: balancing the costs of artistry and athleticism. Medical Problems of Performing Artists 6: 39–44

Hamilton L H, Hamilton W G, Warren M P et al 1997 Factors contributing to the attribution rate in elite ballet students. Journal of Dance Medicine and Science 1: 131–138

Karlsson M K, Johnell O, Obrant K J 1993 Bone mineral density in professional ballet dancers. Bone and Mineral 21(3): 163–169

Klemp P, Stevens J E, Isaacs S 1984 A hypermobility study in ballet dancers. Journal of Rheumatology 11: 692–696

Loucks A B, Horvath S M 1984 Exercise induced stress response of amenorrhoeic and eumenorrhoeic runners. Journal of Clinical Endocrinology and Metabolism 59: 1109–1113

Nicholas J A 1975 Risk factors, sports medicine and the orthopaedic system: an overview. Journal of Sports Medicine 3: 243–259

Norman R A, Grodin M A 1984 Injuries from break dancing. American Family Physician 30(4): 109–112

Quirk R 1984 Injuries in classical ballet. Australian Family Physician 13(11): 802–804

Reid D C, Burnham R S, Saboe L A, Kushner S F 1987 Lower extremity flexibility patterns in classical ballet dancers and their correlation to lateral hip and knee injuries. American Journal of Sports Medicine 15(4): 347–352

Richie D H, Kelso S F, Belluci P A 1985 Aerobic dance injuries: a retrospective study of instructors and participants. Physician Sports Medicine 13: 130–140

Schneider H J, King A Y, Bronson J L, Miller E H 1974 Stress injuries and developmental change of lower extremities of ballet dancer. Radiology 113: 627–632

Teitz C C, Harrington R M, Wiley H 1985 Pressures on the foot in pointe shoes. Foot and Ankle 5(5): 216–221

To W W K, Wong M W N, Chan K M 1995 The effect of dance training on menstrual function in collegiate dancing students. Australian and New Zealand Journal of Obstetrics and Gynaecology 35: 304–309

To W W K, Wong M W N, Chan K M 1997 Association between body composition and menstrual dysfunction in collegiate dance students. Journal of Obstetrics and Gynaecological Research 23(6): 529–535

To W W K, Wong M W N, Lam I 1998 Risk factors for menstrual dysfunction in adolescent dance students. Proceedings of the 12th World Congress of Pediatric and Adolescent Gynecology, Helsinki, Finland

Warren M P 1980 The effects of exercise on pubertal progression and reproductive function in girls. Journal of Clinical Endocrinology and Metabolism 51: 1150–1154

Warren M P, Brooks-Grunn J, Hamilton L H, Warren L F, Hamilton W G 1986 Scoliosis and fractures in young ballet dancers: relation to delayed menarche and secondary amenorrhea. New England Journal of Medicine 314: 1348–1350

Williams S, Speroff L 1987 Dance and menstrual function. In: Ryan A J, Stevens R E (eds) Dance medicine – a comprehensive guide. Pluribus Press, Chicago, p 82–89

Wong M W N, To W W K, Chan K M 1995 Musculoskeletal injuries in different disciplines of dancing. Proceedings in Western Pacific Orthopaedic Association Congress, Hong Kong

Young N, Formica C, Szmukler G, Seeman E 1994 Bone density at weight bearing and non-weight bearing sites in ballet dancers: the effects of exercise, hypogonadism, and body weight. Journal of Clinical Endocrinology and Metabolism 78(2): 449–454

17

Nutritional requirements of female athletes

Peter S. W. Davies
Rebecca A. Abbott

KEY POINTS

1. Greater emphasis is being placed on the influence an athlete's diet has on health, fitness and performance.
2. Women are taking part in more organized and high-level sport than ever before.
3. The diet and nutritional status of female athletes, while having a potential effect on athletic performance, may also contribute to long-term health outcomes including reproductive health.
4. The energy requirement of female athletes is a fundamentally important aspect of their nutrition and nutritional status.
5. There is a growing consensus that a majority of female athletes are not meeting their nutritional requirements.

INTRODUCTION

Women are taking part in more organized and high-level sport than ever before. Not only are the numbers of women participating in high-level sport increasing, but the range of sports in which they are competing is also widening. Women's ice hockey, for example, became an Olympic event in 1996, and ultra-endurance events, such as the women's triathlon, were contested at Olympic level for the first time at the 2000 games in Sydney. As with their male counterparts, female athletes are striving to achieve maximal performance, and the margins between top-flight athletes are constantly narrowing. There can be no doubt that training regimes and methods are significantly improved in comparison with methods employed, say, 50 years ago, but athletes are also looking for other ways to improve and maximize performance. Areas such as sports psychology, for example, are burgeoning. However, more and more emphasis is being placed on the ability of the athletes' diet to affect and influence health, fitness and performance. The nutritional requirements of female athletes warrant special consideration, as not only will the diet and nutritional status potentially affect athletic performance, but they may also contribute to long-term health outcomes, including reproductive health.

Suggestions and recommendations for appropriate levels of intake of macronutrients, vitamins, minerals etc. that may enhance performance abound, and to discuss all such data is beyond the scope of this chapter. There is also a rapidly developing literature relating to the use of nutrients as ergogenic aids, with claims that supplementation with a number of vitamins, amino acids and other compounds can improve performance. This field of research warrants its own review, and will not be covered here. Nevertheless, there are some fundamentally important aspects of nutrition and nutritional status in the female athlete that should be considered. Foremost of these is the energy requirement of such individuals.

ENERGY REQUIREMENTS

Good data on energy requirements in female athletes are extremely sparse in the literature. Knowledge of the energy required to sustain the training programme of an individual athlete and to complete a competitive event is of major importance. While it is intuitive that the energy expenditure, and hence energy requirements of female athletes, will be greater than their more sedentary peers, the evaluation of those requirements has been notoriously difficult due to a number of factors.

Until recently, researchers have had to rely upon estimates of energy intake to assess the energy requirement of sporting populations. This approach relies on the fundamental premise that, when weight is stable, energy intake will be equivalent to energy expenditure, and will therefore represent the long-term energy requirements of the individual or group of individuals. If an individual is not weight stable, at any given time, the gain or loss of body weight can be taken into account relatively easily, and a revised estimate of energy expenditure can be calculated.

The methods of dietary assessment employed vary, but include 24-h recall, food frequency questionnaires, and 3- to 7-day weighed records. The choice of the appropriate method is often a compromise between accuracy and compliance, with the quicker, easier, 24-h recall, for example, yielding less accurate data than the time-consuming 7-day weighed record which many people fail to complete. Nevertheless, using a variety of different assessment tools, some interesting data relating to energy requirements in female athletes have been reported. For example, Fogelholm et al (1995) recorded energy intake in young adult female gymnasts and soccer players who kept a 7-day diet record. Mean energy intake in the gymnasts and soccer players was 1682 and 2143 kcal/day, respectively, which are very low figures particularly for the gymnasts. The data were also at odds with estimates of energy expenditure calculated from a 7-day activity diary that indicated that there was a 31% mismatch between intake and expenditure in the young female gymnasts. This level of negative energy balance, if sustained for any amount of time, would undoubtedly lead to weight loss, including loss of adipose and lean tissue, and would probably lead to menstrual disturbances including amenorrhoea.

The concept of low energy requirements in elite athletes, while intuitively difficult to accept, has been reported in a number of other studies. Steen et al (1995) reported that, in a group of 16 heavyweight rowers with a mean body weight of 69 kg, daily energy intake was 2632 kcal, which was reported as 'lower than expected given the training regime of these athletes'. The diet of many of the rowers, as assessed via a 5-day food record, was also reported to be suboptimal in carbohydrate intake, high in fat, and significantly deficient in intake of calcium, zinc and vitamins B_6 and B_{12}. Similar findings, i.e. low energy intakes and thus presumably low energy requirements, have been reported in a wide range of elite sporting populations. van Marken Lichtenbelt (1995) estimated that the mean energy intake of a group of 24 elite ballet dancers was only 1553 kcal/day, with a range of 720–2222 kcal/day. Other groups for whom suspiciously low energy intakes have been reported are highly trained endurance runners (Edwards et al 1993) and middle distance runners (Mulligan & Butterfield 1990).

Data reported in numerous other studies primarily designed to investigate the relationship between diet, athletic performance, and amenorrhoea and bone mineral content also support the hypothesis of a markedly reduced energy intake in female athletes. Some studies have reported energy intakes that are hard to believe. Rucinski (1989) studied 23 female figure skaters with an average age of 18 years training 4–5 h daily, 6 days a week. They also spent 2 h/day practising jazz and ballet dancing and working on other dance routines. It is therefore hard to accept that these athletes were able to support such a level of physical activity with their mean reported energy intake of 1174 kcal/day. To put this intake in context, the FAO/WHO/UNU (1985) recommendations for the energy requirement for a 1-year-old child is 1200 kcal/day! Taken at face value, not surprisingly, these data led Rucinski to conclude that intakes of important nutrients such as iron and calcium were about 50% of the then current recommended dietary allowances.

There are two possible mechanisms that could explain the seemingly very low energy intakes, and hence energy requirements, reported in many athletic groups (Fogelholm et al 1995). Previous estimates of energy requirements may have been erroneously high, or, alternatively, there is intentional or unintentional under-recording of food intake in many cases. It should be remembered that the tools available to estimate food (and hence energy) intake, i.e. 24-h recalls, food frequency questionnaires, 3-, 4- and 7-day food records, all rely on the subject accurately recalling or recording information relating to food intake. It has been proposed that there may be marked under-reporting in populations in whom body image or weight control is important. Prentice et al (1987) described the phenomenon of under-reporting in obese individuals a decade ago and there is more and more evidence emerging to indicate that many elite athletic groups, for whatever reason, significantly under-report energy intake. A number of studies indicate that under-reporting energy intake is more widespread in female than in male athletes. For example, Ludbrook & Clark (1992) studied a total of 23 long distance runners all of whom were running at least 70 km/week. The athletes were required to keep a 7-day diary of their activity each hour and a detailed diary relating to food intake. Estimated energy expenditure was then calculated using the activity diary and standard values for the energy costs of differing activities (McArdle et al 1986). There were important discrepancies between the calculated energy expenditure and intakes, amounting to 15% in the men but reaching an average of 40% in the female athletes. A difference of such magnitude in female athletes over a period of 7 days would lead to a weight loss of 0.75 kg for the athletes to be in energy balance (Ludbrook & Clark 1992). The actual change in body weight over the study period was 0.09 kg, thus

suggesting that either the estimated energy expenditure was too high or, more probably, the estimates of energy intake were too low.

Hill & Davies (1998) recently explored the phenomenon of under-reporting food intake, and hence energy intake, in a small group of elite ballet dancers, a population in whom weight control and body image have a high priority. Energy intake, on average, was found to be under-reported by 21% each day. A larger level of under-reporting was found by Edwards et al (1993) in a group of highly trained female endurance runners. When compared with measurements of total energy expenditure over a 7-day period, recorded intakes were approximately 31% lower. Of special interest in this study was that the difference between energy intake and energy expenditure was significantly negatively correlated with the measured body mass index of the athletes. Edwards et al (1993) tentatively suggested that these findings could indicate that larger female athletes are metabolically more efficient than their smaller peers. Nevertheless, further examination of the metabolic data collected in the study led to the final conclusion that the primary reason for the marked discrepancies between intake and expenditure was under-reporting, and that female athletes perceive that they are heavier than their peers and larger than some internal perception of the 'ideal' size or weight for optimal performance. Finally, it was suggested that many female athletes may be just as weight-conscious as obese individuals in whom under-reporting has been confirmed in a number of studies (Bandini et al 1990, Prentice et al 1986).

These new findings have become possible due to the use of the doubly labelled water technique for the non-invasive measurement of total energy expenditure. This technique (Davies, 1991) allows an individual's total energy expenditure to be calculated over a 10- to 14-day period without impinging on the lifestyle or activities of the subject. Energy expenditure is calculated via the measurement of the differential loss of two stable isotopes in urine samples following a loading dose of the isotopes. The production of a small daily urine sample is the only requirement of the subject, and thus there is little room for error to be introduced by lack of compliance. The use of this technique in small groups of elite athletes will give us a new understanding of something as fundamentally important in the nutritional requirements of elite athletes as energy requirements. It is vital that we accept the distinct possibility that previous data, indicating extremely low energy requirements, may be flawed due to subconscious under-reporting of food intake.

Adequate nutrition and food energy to sustain training programmes and athletic competition is a basic requirement. It is perhaps one of the most important nutritional considerations, and one about which, until quite recently, we knew very little.

ACCURACY AND VALIDITY OF NUTRITIONAL DATA

From the preceding discussion the question therefore arises as to how it might be possible to evaluate nutritional data collected from athletes and others to determine the accuracy and validity of those data. Only when we can discriminate between good and poor data will we be able to start to really investigate the nutritional intake and requirements of female athletes. If under-reporting was macronutrient-specific, e.g. if dietary fat intake was more often under-reported than, say, dietary protein, then the analysis of dietary data in this way might give an insight into their validity. Unfortunately, this does not seem to be the case, with an elegant study by Lissner & Lindroos (1994) indicating that percentage nutrient intakes, even in under-reported records, are within the range of values that one might expect. Lissner & Lindroos (1994) concluded that traditional dietary methods, which have formed the backbone of assessment in athletic groups, seem capable of measuring qualitative intake patterns but do not provide good quantitative data. This observation has yet to be specifically made in athletic groups, but it is likely that the same findings would emerge.

Doubly labelled water technique

Some studies have validated recorded intake data against independent measures of energy expenditure using the doubly labelled water technique. This type of study offers the best insight into the validity or otherwise of the dietary data collected from athletes. However, the doubly labelled water technique is expensive, due to the high cost of one of the stable isotopes, and its application is still limited to relatively few specialized centres. While some small studies in very homogenous groups will continue to yield important data in an economic manner, the technique does not currently lend itself to a more widespread evaluation of nutritional requirements. The technique may be used to focus on the nutritional requirements of young athletes (Davies et al 1997), in whom its cost is less restrictive.

Ratio of basal metabolic rate to energy intake

Nevertheless, there is one method that discriminates, to a large extent, between energy (and hence nutrient) intakes that are believable and those that are less likely. Using fundamental principles of energy physiology, Goldberg et al (1991) were able to calculate values for the ratio of an individual's energy intake to the basal metabolic rate (BMR) below which doubt would be cast on the validity of the energy intake data. BMR is usually the largest component of any one individual energy expenditure, and therefore a large part of energy intake must fuel that energy expenditure. Further energy is required for thermogenesis, growth and physical activity. To carry out essential daily tasks compatible with life, there is therefore a minimum amount of energy above that required to fuel the BMR that has to be provided on a daily basis from the diet. The absolute minimum energy requirement has been calculated as being equivalent to BMR × 1.27. This level of energy intake, however, although compatible with life, is not conducive with long-term health, and an energy intake of BMR × 1.35 is usually quoted as the lowest possible in free living individuals. A sedentary lifestyle would require an intake of approximately BMR × 1.55, and an individual who is habitually and frequently physically active might require an energy intake of BMR × 2.0.

Using this approach, Goldberg et al (1991) described two different cut-off values for the ratio of energy intake to BMR. The first cut-off can be used to answer the question: 'Can the reported energy intake possibly be representative of habitual intake?'. The second cut-off can be used to answer the question: 'Even if the reported energy intake could not be representative of habitual intake, could it be a valid estimate of the particular period over which it was measured, allowing for the known day-to-day and week-to-week variability, and without having to postulate any systematic reduction in energy intake which may have been caused by the measurement procedure?'.

The value for the first cut-off is relatively easy to define. Goldberg et al (1991) stated that: 'We contend that recorded energy intakes of below 1.35 × BMR either in individuals or in populations are most unlikely to represent habitual intake'. The second cut-off value is more difficult to determine, as it requires consideration of the day-to-day variation in energy intake. This second cut-off, often termed 'cut-off two', effectively allows the ratio of BMR to energy intake to be low but believable. Goldberg et al (1991) provided extensive tables that allow the appropriate cut-off

Table 17.1 Goldberg et al (1991) cut-offs for the ratio of recorded energy intake to basal metabolic rates with differing sample sizes and days of data collection. These data refer to 'cut-off two'

Sample size	Days of data collection				
	1	4	7	14	28
1	0.90	1.06	1.10	1.12	1.14
10	1.30	1.38	1.39	1.40	1.40
20	1.37	1.42	1.43	1.44	1.45
50	1.43	1.47	1.48	1.48	1.48
100	1.47	1.49	1.50	1.50	1.50
1000	1.52	1.53	1.53	1.53	1.53

value to be determined based upon the number of days of data collection and the number of subjects in the study. For example, in a study of 10 athletes over a period of 7 days, a BMR to energy intake ratio of greater than 1.39 needs to be achieved for the data to be believable. If 100 subjects had been studied over the same time period, the cut-off would be raised to 1.50. More examples of appropriate cut-offs are shown in Table 17.1. Goldberg et al (1991) also showed a method for calculating a cut-off value for a population if the habitual level of physical activity is known for that population. This additional information allows a more appropriate cut-off to be calculated as it provides data relating to the habitual level of energy expenditure that must be supported by the measured energy intakes.

BMR can either be measured using indirect calorimetry or it can be predicted with reasonable accuracy using the equations of Schofield (1985). The equations used to predict BMR in any individual from anthropometric measurements such as height and weight are currently under review, and new, more accurate algorithms will shortly be forthcoming which will probably supersede Schofield's equations.

This approach to checking the validity of energy intake data has been little used to date in studies of nutritional requirements in athletes, and, as previously stated, with a possible bias to under-recording being found especially in female athletes, the method should be employed more frequently. In those studies where the BMR/energy intake ratio has been calculated or can be retrospectively calculated from published data, some interesting findings emerge. For example, data from the ballet dancers studied by Van Marken Lichtenbelt et al (1995) yield a mean ratio of 1.16, clearly indicating that the energy intake data are not accurate or valid. Hill & Davies (1998) found a mean ratio of 1.44 in ballet dancers, again indicating that

under-recording had occurred in that particular cohort, as this ratio falls below Goldberg et al's second cut-off. The gymnasts and soccer players studied by Fogelholm et al (1995) produce mean ratios of 1.32 and 1.54, respectively, indicating that under-reporting had occurred in the gymnasts but not in the soccer players.

Clearly, to determine the level of nutrient intake that sustains and enhances performance in female athletes, one must be able to measure both the input and output sides of that relationship. Performance can be assessed in many ways, such as improvements in times in running and swimming. Also, key physiological variables such as maximal aerobic capacity and muscle strength and endurance can be assessed. The problem, as highlighted here, is obtaining good data on the input side of the equation. Unless we are able to monitor accurately the composition of the diet, it will be difficult, if not impossible, to evaluate the relationship between diet and performance, and the way in which manipulating the diet may affect performance. When we are confident that our nutritional data are sound, then we can earnestly begin to answer the question of nutritional requirements in all athletes, not least female athletes.

SPECIFIC NUTRITIONAL CONCERNS FOR FEMALE ATHLETES

There are certain nutritional concerns pertinent to female athletes which merit specific mention. Despite the uncertainty of the accuracy of dietary intake data to date, it is known that the prevalence of subclinical and clinical eating disorders are on the increase, and are higher than that seen in female non-athletes (Sundgot-Burgen 1993). This pattern of disordered eating, which includes low calorie intakes, subsequent weight loss, body fat loss and excessive exercise, has emerged due to increasing demands on athletes in many sports. In addition to the normal societal demands and pressure to be thin, there are also added pressures from coaches and trainers. Sports that are predominantly affected are those that have an aesthetic appeal or weight concern, such as gymnastics, figure skating, diving and long distance running. Johnson (1994) reported the incidence of disordered eating to be as high as 30–60% in some sports. This was supported recently by the results of a survey of the Norwegian national gymnastics team, 33% of whom were described as having an eating disorder (Sundgot-Burgen 1996). Despite all the gymnasts having body fat levels lower than that recommended as 'healthy', all restricted their calorie intake and were dissatisfied with either their body weight or shape. Athletes who limit their food intake to achieve their desired leanness, however, will also limit their intake of specific nutrients. Of greatest concern are calcium and iron.

Calcium intake

Calcium plays a key role in the integrity of the skeleton. Adequate intakes throughout childhood and adolescence are essential for optimal peak bone mass (PBM), which occurs between 20 and 30 years of age (Matkovic et al 1990, Wardlaw 1993). A high PBM is an important contributory factor in the prevention of osteoporosis later in life. Maintaining adequate calcium intakes beyond the time of PBM is also important in sustaining good skeletal health (Halioua & Anderson 1989), and therefore suboptimal intakes of calcium at any age are of potential concern. Recommended dietary intakes of calcium differ slightly from country to country, but mostly all fall within the range of 800–1200 mg/day for female adults and young adolescents (Department of Health 1991, NHMRC 1991, National Research Council 1989). However, a consensus statement by the US National Institute of Health on optimal calcium intakes concluded that the calcium intake for most age groups should be greater than the published *Recommended Dietary Allowances* (NIH 1994). They put forward recommendations of 1200–1500 mg/day for adolescents and young adults, and 1000 mg/day for those aged between 25 and 65.

However, such intake levels are not reached by the majority of women, let alone athletes. Chapman et al (1995) observed that over 40% of women between the ages of 25 and 85 had calcium intakes below 60% of the RDA. Calcium intakes in the range of 700–900 mg have been observed in numerous sports including female heavyweight rowers, figure skaters, speed skaters and gymnasts (Jonnalagadda et al 1998, Steen et al 1995, Webster & Barr 1995, Ziegler et al 1998). In particular, the study of speed skaters and gymnasts competing at provincial level or higher reported that 63 and 32%, respectively, failed to meet the Canadian RDA (Webster & Barr 1995). Although all studies acknowledged that there may have been some level of underreporting with the dietary assessment tools used, the consistent findings of low calcium amidst adequate intakes of other nutrients suggest that this is a valid cause for concern. The difficulty in being able to assess calcium status directly and the fact that chronic low levels of calcium intake exert their effect later in life only add to the necessity of ensuring that female athletes are aware of the potential long-term damage of inadequate calcium intake.

The reason for poor calcium intake amongst female athletes and non-athletes lies in the lack of knowledge about good calcium sources and a desire for leanness. It is a common misconception that all dairy sources of calcium are high in fat. With the widespread availability of skimmed milks and low-fat yoghurts and cheeses, there is no reason why ensuring adequate calcium intake means increasing fat intake. Indeed Karanja et al (1994) recently showed that it was possible, via nutritional counselling, for subjects to meet dietary intakes of 1500 mg/day over a 12-week period, whilst only increasing their fat intake from 66 to 69 g/day. Good sources of calcium are dairy products, fortified foods, such as those made with enriched flour, and fish with soft bones. The major sources of calcium and the amounts that they provide are shown in Table 17.2.

The use of calcium supplements to maintain calcium intake is on the increase, especially in female athletes (Sobal & Marquardt 1994). The evidence for how effective they are in preventing bone loss is not conclusive, although several studies have shown a beneficial effect on bone density (e.g. Lloyd et al 1993). Caution should be taken, however, since calcium affects iron absorption when the two are consumed together. Therefore, it is important for female athletes to take dietary advice when calcium supplementation is considered. The preferred method of achieving optimal calcium intake is through calcium-rich foods.

Iron intake

Iron is present in all cells of the body, and is primarily concerned with the transport of oxygen around the

Table 17.2 Major dietary sources of calcium and iron

Calcium[a]	mg/100 g	Iron[b]	mg/100 g
Low-fat milk	120	Breakfast cereal	5–10
Skimmed milk	130	Wholemeal bread	2.5
Natural yoghurt	180	Beef mince	3
Fruit yoghurt	160	Lamb chop	2
Ice-cream	140	Liver	8
Cheddar cheese	800	Sausage	1.5
Edam cheese	740	Egg (whole)	2
Cream cheese	100	Egg (yolk only)	6
Canned sardines	460	Spinach	1.5
Canned salmon	100	Lentils/pulses	2.5
Muesli	200	Peas	1.5
White bread	100	Peanuts	2.5

[a] USA RDA for calcium = 1200 mg/day.
[b] USA RDA for iron = 15 mg/day.

body and energy production. A lack of iron will therefore result in a reduced capacity for exercise. Iron deficiency is the most common nutritional disorder in the world, predominantly affecting children, adolescents and women. Female athletes are at an increased risk due to the combined effects of low calorie intakes, intense physical exercise, menstrual loss and poor nutritional knowledge. Inadequate dietary iron intakes have been reported in many studies, from rowers, gymnasts and long distance runners through to general athletes, defined as training a minimum of 6 h/week (Beals & Manore 1998, Pate et al 1993, Steen et al 1995, Ziegler et al 1999). As noted earlier, part of the difficulty with such studies is the validity of the dietary intake data. However, it is possible to get an indication of iron status through a combination of blood indices such as ferritin, transferrin saturation, haemoglobin and iron binding capacity.

Studies which have assessed iron status conclude that, although female athletes are more prone to iron deficiency than their male counterparts, they do not appear to be significantly more at risk than female non-athletes (Balaban et al 1989, Risser et al 1988). Indeed, in Risser et al's study of 100 varsity athletes, iron deficiency was found in 31%, and in 45% of their non-athletic colleagues. Nevertheless, this degree of deficiency is important to the athlete, as fatigue and impaired performance may result if left uncorrected. Studies on the effects of iron supplementation have shown that improvement in performance is dependent on the initial degree of iron depletion.

For those athletes with iron deficiency sufficient to cause anaemia, there is a consensus that iron supplements will improve work output and exercise performance (Clarkson 1991). The effect of iron supplements on those athletes with iron depletion, but not anaemia, is less clear. Although supplementation may improve iron status, several studies have found no improvement in performance (Klingshirn et al 1992, Newhouse et al 1989). Iron-deficient female distance runners who were supplemented for 8 weeks showed no improvement in their endurance capacity or $\dot{V}O_{2\,max}$ output, despite an improvement in their iron status (Klingshirn et al 1992). This has been confirmed with other athletes. Although iron supplementation may therefore not improve performance for such individuals, it may serve to protect them from further iron deficiency that could have detrimental effects.

It is nevertheless still widely recommended to meet iron requirements through the diet, and not through supplementation. The most important sources of iron are those which are not only rich in iron but also eaten in significant quantities, and from which iron is reasonably well absorbed. Haem iron found in meat is more readily absorbed than non-haem iron, found in cereals, vegetables and legumes. There are also nutrients in the diet that can promote or inhibit iron absorption. Most notable amongst these are vitamin C, which enhances iron absorption, and the phytates and polyphenols (found in tea, coffee, wheatbran), which inhibit absorption. Good sources of dietary iron and the amount of iron that they provide are shown in Table 17.2.

CONCLUSIONS

Although much research is still needed to determine the optimal diet for female athletes, there is a growing consensus that the majority of female athletes do not meet their nutritional requirements. The desire to be thin is one of their greatest problems. Low energy and nutrient intakes put the athlete at risk for eating disorders, amenorrhoea, low bone density and iron deficiency anaemia, which may not only impair their performance in the short term, but could impact on their long-term health. As the number of women participating in sport continues to grow, it is important that these issues are addressed.

REFERENCES

Balaban E P, Cox J V, Snell P, Vaughan R H, Frenkel E P 1989 The frequency of anaemia and iron deficiency in the runner. Medicine and Science in Sports and Exercise 21(6): 643–648

Bandini L, Schoeller D A, Dietz W H 1990 Energy expenditure in obese and non-obese adolescents. Pediatric Research 27: 198–203

Beals K A, Manore M M 1998 Nutritional status of female athletes with sub-clinical eating disorders. Journal of the American Dietetic Association 98: 419–425

Chapman K M, Chan M W, Clark C D 1995 Factors influencing dairy calcium intake in women. Journal of the American College of Nutrition 14: 336–341

Clarkson P M 1991 Minerals: exercise performance and supplementation in athletes. Journal of Sports Science 9: 91–116

Davies P S W 1991 Measurement of energy expenditure and body composition using stable isotopes. Developmental Physiopathology and Clinics 2(2): 95–110

Davies P S W, Feng J Y, Crisp J A, Day J M E, Laidlaw A, Chen J, Liu X P 1997 Total energy expenditure and physical activity in young Chinese gymnasts. Pediatric Exercise Science 9(3): 243–252

Department of Health 1991 Dietary reference values for food energy and nutrients for the United Kingdom (Report No. 41). HMSO, London

Edwards J E, Lideman A K, Mikesky A E, Stager J M 1993 Energy balance in highly trained female endurance runners. Medicine and Science in Sports and Exercise 25(12): 1398–1404

FAO/WHO/UNU 1985 Energy and protein requirements. Technical Report Series 724. World Health Organization, Geneva

Fogelhom G M, Kukkonen-Harjula T K, Taipale S A, Sievanen H T, Oja P, Vuori I M 1995 Resting metabolic rate and energy intake in female gymnasts, figure skaters and soccer players. International Journal of Sport Nutrition 16: 551–556

Goldberg G R, Black A E, Jebb S A, Cole T J, Murgatroyd P R, Coward W A, Prentice A M 1991 Critical evaluation of energy intake data using fundamental principles of energy physiology: 1. Derivation of cut-off limits to identify under recording. European Journal of Clinical Nutrition 45: 569–581

Halioua L, Anderson J J B 1989 Lifetime calcium intake and physical activity habits: independent and combined effects on the radial bone of healthy pre-menopausal Caucasian women. American Journal of Clinical Nutrition 49: 534–541

Hill R J, Davies P S W 1998 Energy intake and energy expenditure in classical ballet dancers. Proceedings of the Nutrition Society of Australia 22: 172

Johnson M D 1994 Disordered eating in active and athletic women. Clinics in Sports Medicine 13: 355–369

Jonnalagadda S S, Benardot D, Nelson M 1998 Energy and nutrient intakes of the United States national women's artistic gymnastics team. International Journal of Sports Nutrition 8: 331–344

Karanja N, Morris C D, Rufolo P, Snyder G, Illingworth D R, McCarron D A 1994 Impact of increasing calcium in the diet on nutrient consumption, plasma lipids and lipoproteins in humans. American Journal of Clinical Nutrition 59: 900–907

Klingshirn L A, Pate R R, Bourque S P, Davis J M, Sargent R G 1992 Effect of iron supplementation on endurance capacity in iron-depleted female runners. Medicine and Science in Sports and Exercise 7: 819–824

Lissner L, Lindroos A K 1994 Is dietary under reporting macronutrient specific? European Journal of Clinical Nutrition 48: 453–454

Lloyd T, Andon M B, Rollings N et al 1993 Calcium supplementation and bone mineral density in adolescent girls. Journal of the American Medical Association 270: 841–844

Ludbrook C, Clark D 1992 Energy expenditure and nutrient intake in long distance runners. Nutrition Research 12: 689–699

Matkovic V, Fontana D, Tominac C, Goel P, Chesnut C H 1990 Factors that influence peak bone mass formation: a study of calcium balance and inheritance of bone mass in adolescents. American Journal of Clinical Nutrition 52: 878–887

McArdle W D, Katch, F I, Katch V L 1986 Exercise physiology: energy nutrition and human performance, 2nd edn. Lea and Febiger, Philadelphia, PA

Mulligan K, Butterfield G E 1990 Discrepancies between energy intake and expenditure in physically active women. British Journal of Nutrition 64: 23–36

National Health and Medical Research Council (NHMRC) 1991 Recommended dietary intakes for use in Australia. NHMRC, Canberra

National Institutes of Health 1994 Optimal calcium intake. NIH Consensus Statement, June 6–8. NIH, Bethesda, MD

National Research Council 1989 Recommended dietary allowances, 10th edn. National Academy Press, Washington

Newhouse I J, Clement D B, Taunton J E, McKenzie D C 1989 The effects of prelatent/latent iron deficiency on physical work capacity. Medicine and Science in Sports and Exercise 21: 263–268

Pate R R, Miller B J, Davis J M, Slentz C A, Klingshirn C A 1993 Iron status of female runners. International Journal of Sports Nutrition 3(2): 222–231

Prentice A M, Black A E, Coward W A, Davies H L, Goldberg G R 1986 High levels of energy expenditure in obese women. British Medical Journal 292: 983–987

Risser W L, Lee E J, Poindexter H B, West M S, Pivarnik I M, Risser J M H, Hickson J F 1988 Iron deficiency in female athletes: its prevalence and impact on performance. Medicine and Science in Sports and Exercise 20: 116

Rucinski A 1989 Relationship of body image and dietary intake of competitive ice skaters. Journal of the American Dietetics Association 89: 98–100

Schofield W N 1985 Predicting basal metabolic rate, new standards and review of previous work. Human Nutrition. Clinical Nutrition 39C (suppl 1): 5–41

Sobal J, Marquardt L F 1994 Vitamin/mineral supplement use among athletes: a review of the literature. International Journal of Sports Nutrition 4: 320–324

Steen S N, Mayer K, Brownell K D, Wadden T A 1995 Dietary intake of female collegiate heavyweight rowers. International Journal of Sports Nutrition 5: 225–231

Sundgot-Borgen J 1993 Prevalence of eating disorders in elite female athletes. International Journal of Sports Nutrition 3: 29–40

Sundgot-Borgen J 1996 Eating disorders, energy intake, training volume and menstrual function in high level modern rhythmic gymnasts. International Journal of Sports Nutrition 6: 100–109

van Marken Lichtenbelt W, Fogelholm M, Ottenheijm R, Westerterp K R 1995 Physical activity, body composition and bone density in ballet dancers. British Journal of Nutrition 74: 439–451

Wardlaw G M 1993 Putting osteoporosis in perspective. Journal of the American Dietetic Association 93: 1000–1006

Webster B L, Barr S I 1995 Calcium intakes of adolescent female gymnasts and speed skaters: lack of association with dieting behaviour. International Journal of Sports Nutrition 5: 2–12

Ziegler P, Hensley S, Roepke J B, Whitaker S H, Craig B W, Drewnowski A 1998 Eating attitudes and energy intakes of female skaters. Medicine and Science in Sports and Exercise 30(4): 583–586

Ziegler P J, Nelson J A, Jonnalagadde S S 1999 Nutritional and physiological status of US national figure skaters. International Journal of Sports Nutrition 9(4): 354–360

18

Female athlete triad

Constance M. Lebrun

KEY POINTS

1. Physical activity is to be encouraged for girls and women of all ages.
2. Societal preoccupations with body shape and composition, as well as sport-specific demands, may precipitate disordered eating patterns in susceptible female athletes.
3. Disordered eating may cause many health problems, including amenorrhea, or lack of menstrual cycles.
4. Although many physical and psychological stressors contribute to menstrual dysfunction, the major underlying factor is an energy deficit (insufficient energy intake for the needs of the exercising female).
5. Amenorrhea results in a hypoestrogenic state, which can have adverse effects on bone density, leading to premature osteoporosis.
6. The 'female athlete triad' of disordered eating, amenorrhea and osteoporosis should be identified and treated as early as possible, but ideally should be prevented by proper education of those caring for athletes, and sound training and nutritional practices.

INTRODUCTION

In general, regular physical activity provides significant health benefits for both males and females, and should therefore be encouraged for all ages. A small proportion of susceptible individuals may, however, develop medical problems which stem primarily from intrinsic and extrinsic pressures to achieve or maintain an unrealistically low body weight. This is most prevalent in sports where low body weight is deemed an essential part of athletic success, whether for performance or for appearance purposes, but no sport is completely immune.

The term 'female athlete triad' was initially coined in 1992, at a special consensus conference in Washington DC organized by the Task Force on Women's Issues of the American College of Sports Medicine (Yeager et al 1993). This organization has also recently published a position stand (American College of Sports Medicine 1997) on this important topic. The female athlete triad describes a syndrome of three distinct, yet often interrelated medical entities that can occur in physically active girls and women: disordered eating, osteoporosis and amenorrhea. Young women and girls who present with any one of the triad disorders are at risk and should be screened for the others. This chapter will discuss in further detail these medical problems, outline diagnostic criteria, and suggest strategies for treatment and prevention.

DEFINITIONS
Disordered eating

Disordered eating refers to a spectrum of eating patterns that can range from simple preoccupation with weight and diet all the way through to the frank eating disorders of anorexia nervosa and bulimia nervosa. The latter have specific criteria as set down by the American Psychiatric Association (DSM-IV) (1994). These are outlined in Box 18.1, and must *all* be satisfied in order to correctly make the diagnosis. Self-report questionnaires such as the Eating Disorder Inventory (EDI) or Eating Attitudes Test (EAT) can be used for initial screening purposes, but, because of the issues of denial as well as 'faked responses', a clinical interview by a qualified health care practitioner is essential.

The 1994 version of the *Diagnostic and Statistical Manual* differs from the previously published DSM-IIIR document in the inclusion of two subtypes for anorexia (restricting type and binge-eating/purging type) and bulimia (purging type and non-purging type). In addition, a category called 'eating disorders otherwise not specified' captures the patient population that does not meet the other criteria. With this classification system, patients can be more accurately identified.

In reality, athletes in particular may only have certain features of the disease. There is currently debate in the literature as to whether or not these women actually have a different disorder altogether. Psychological profiles of athletes and anorexics are similar in some features such as high achievement orientation, obsessive-compulsive tendencies and perfectionism. To some extent, these characteristics are necessary for athletic success. One author (Sundgot-Borgen 1993) has proposed a different classification called 'anorexia athletica' (Box 18.2), while others have suggested more clearly defined criteria for identifying the athlete with a subclinical eating disorder (Beals & Manore 1994).

Regardless of the classification system used, there appears to be a continuum of disordered eating behaviors. At any point along the gamut, there can be significant implications for the athlete's health, including short- and long-term morbidity, decreased performance, menstrual abnormalities and even death.

Amenorrhea

Amenorrhea is defined as either primary or secondary. In primary amenorrhea, a girl has not yet begun to menstruate by the age of 16, or develop secondary sexual characteristics by the age of 14. Secondary amenorrhea refers to the cessation of menstrual cycles for at least 3 months, or less than three cycles per year, in a woman who has already attained menarche. There can be many different medical causes of amenorrhea that must be excluded before making the diagnosis of exercise-associated amenorrhea.

This form of amenorrhea is hypothalamic in origin, and can evolve through several stages (Loucks et al 1992). In practice, many athletic women may develop menstrual dysfunction during times of intense training or weight loss, and revert to a more normal pattern during the rest of the year. Oligomenorrhea refers to cycles at intervals greater than 35 days, or less than six cycles per year. Luteal phase deficiency is a shortening of the luteal phase to less than 10 days. Individuals with anovulatory cycles may actually have regular menstrual bleeding, but levels of estrogen and progesterone are inadequate because ovulation does not occur. Decreased levels of the female hormones estrogen and progesterone are similar to those in menopause, and can lead to premature osteoporosis, among other problems.

Osteoporosis

Osteoporosis is 'a disease characterized by low bone mass and microarchitectural deterioration of bone

<table>
<tr><td>

Box 18.1 DSM-IV diagnostic criteria for eating disorders. (Reprinted with permission from the Diagnostic and Statistical Manual of Mental Disorders, 4th edn. Copyright 1994 American Psychiatric Association)

307.1 Anorexia nervosa
A. Refusal to maintain body weight at or above a minimally normal weight for age and height (e.g. weight loss leading to maintenance of body weight less than 85% of that expected; or failure to make expected weight gain during period of growth, leading to body weight less than 85% of that expected).
B. Intense fear of gaining weight or becoming fat, even though underweight.
C. Disturbance in the way in which one's body weight or shape is experienced, undue influence of body weight or shape on self-evaluation, or denial of the seriousness of the current low body weight.
D. In post-menarchal females, amenorrhea, i.e. the absence of at least three consecutive menstrual cycles.

Specify type
Restricting type. During the episode of anorexia nervosa, the person does not regularly engage in binge eating or purging behavior (i.e. self-induced vomiting or the misuse of laxatives or diuretics).
Binge eating/purging type. During this episode of anorexia nervosa, the person regularly engages in binge eating or purging behavior (as defined above).

307.51 Bulimia nervosa
A. Recurrent episodes of binge eating, characterized by both of the following:
   (1) eating in a discrete period of time (e.g. within any 2-h period), an amount of food that is definitely larger than most people would eat during a similar period of time and under similar circumstances
   (2) a sense of lack of control over eating during the episode (e.g. a feeling that one cannot stop eating or control what or how much one is eating).
B. Recurrent inappropriate compensatory behavior in order to prevent weight gain, such as self-induced vomiting; misuse of laxatives, diuretics, enemas, or other medications; fasting; or excessive exercise.
C. The binge eating and inappropriate compensatory behaviors both occur, on average, at least twice a week for 3 months.
D. Self-evaluation is unduly influenced by body shape and weight.
E. The disturbance does not occur exclusively during episodes of anorexia nervosa.

Specify type
Purging type. The person regularly engages in self-induced vomiting or the misuse of laxatives or diuretics.
Non-purging type. The person uses other inappropriate compensatory behavior, such as fasting or excessive exercise, but does not regularly engage in self-induced vomiting or misuse of laxatives or diuretics, or enemas.

307.50 Eating disorders not otherwise specified
The 'eating disorders not otherwise specified' category is for disorders of eating that do not meet the criteria for any specific eating disorder. Examples include:
1. For females, all of the criteria for anorexia nervosa are met except that the individual has regular menses.
2. All of the criteria for anorexia nervosa are met except that, despite significant weight loss, the individual's current weight is in the normal range.
3. All of the criteria for anorexia nervosa are met except that the binge eating and inappropriate compensatory mechanisms occur at a frequency of less than twice a week or for a duration of less than 3 months.
4. The regular use of inappropriate compensatory behavior by an individual of normal body weight after eating a small amount of food (e.g. self-induced vomiting after the consumption of two cookies).
5. Repeatedly chewing and spitting out, but not swallowing, large amounts of food.
6. Binge-eating disorder: recurrent episodes of binge eating in the absence of the regular use of inappropriate compensatory behaviors characteristic of bulimia nervosa (see Appendix B in DSM-IV for suggested research criteria).

</td></tr>
</table>

tissues leading to enhanced skeletal fragility and increased risk of fracture' (Kanis et al 1994). The World Health Organization (WHO) has further developed a standardized classification scheme:

- Normal – bone mineral density (BMD) that is no more than 1 standard deviation (SD) below the mean of young adults
- Osteopenia – BMD between 1 and 2.5 SD below the mean of young adults
- Osteoporosis – BMD more than 2.5 SD below the mean of young adults
- Severe osteoporosis – BMD more than 2.5 SD below the mean of young adults plus one or more fragility fractures.

The principal cause of premenopausal osteoporosis in active women is decreased production of ovarian hormones and hypoestrogenemia secondary to hypothalamic amenorrhea. In women who severely restrict

> **Box 18.2** Diagnostic criteria for 'anorexia athletica' (After Sundgot-Borgen 1994)
>
> - Weight loss (>5% of expected body weight)   +
> - Delayed puberty[a]   (+)
> - Menstrual dysfunction[b]   (+)
> - Gastrointestinal complaints   +
> - Absence of medical illness or affective
>   disorder explaining the weight reduction   +
> - Distorted body image   (+)
> - Excessive fear of becoming obese   +
> - Restriction of food (<1200 kcal/day)   +
> - Use of purging methods[c]   (+)
> - Binging   (+)
> - Compulsive exercise   (+)
>
> *Note*: +, absolute criteria; (+), relative criteria.
> [a] No menstrual bleeding at age 16 (primary amenorrhea).
> [b] Primary amenorrhea, secondary amenorrhea, oligomenorrhea.
> [c] Self-induced vomiting, laxatives, and diuretics.

their food intake (specifically milk products which they may perceive to be high in fat), the amount of dietary calcium may also be inadequate.

PREVALENCE OF THE TRIAD DISORDERS

The true prevalence of the triad disorders in the female athlete population has not yet been accurately determined. In part, this is due to the relatively recent identification of the interaction between these entities. There is also a great degree of denial, especially in terms of reporting disordered eating. It is important to remember that these problems are not limited strictly to elite athletes, but can also occur in girls and women active in a wide range of physical activities. The underlying driving force is generally an unhealthy preoccupation with body size, shape and composition. This is frequently initiated by societal mores and 'ideals', but reinforced by unrealistic expectations of coaches, judges, parents and athletes.

Approximately 0.5–1% of the general population have anorexia nervosa, and 1–4% have bulimia according to DSM-IV criteria. The reported prevalence in some studies of athletes is at least that high, if not higher. Pathological methods of weight control are common in many sports, and may be 'learned' from peers (Rosen & Hough 1988).

Between 2 and 5% of women of reproductive age can experience secondary amenorrhea, and studies have reported menstrual dysfunction in between 1 and 44% of athletic women. Whether through conscious restriction of food or through excessive exercise, a young woman may reach a point of 'energy drain', where energy expenditure exceeds available energy input. The reproductive system senses this, and effectively shuts down ovulation as a protective mechanism. The subsequent decrease in hormone production leads to osteoporosis and the other medical problems.

Factors that seem to play a role include training factors, nutrition, body composition changes, hormonal changes with exercise, stress and reproductive immaturity. Suppression of gonadotrophin-releasing hormone (GnRH) from the hypothalamus leads to reduced surges of luteinizing hormone (LH). Endorphins, catecholamines and other neuropeptides such as melatonin may also play a role.

A diet low in protein, fat or calories also seems to be more common in these women. There is a high incidence of amenorrhea in vegetarians. This may be due to increased dietary fiber intake, interfering with the reabsorption of estrogens. In addition, plant lignins and isoflavones have weak estrogenic activity and may compete with estradiol for binding sites, or reduce the biological activity of estradiol (Benson et al 1996).

In general, regular weight-bearing physical activity has a protective effect on bone (Taaffe et al 1997). However, if amenorrhea or even the more subtle forms of menstrual dysfunction ensue, some of these beneficial effects may be lost. Decreased bone mass has been linked to amenorrhea since 1984 (Cann et al 1984). This occurs at both axial and appendicular sites (Myburgh et al 1993). Both current and past menstrual status are thought to be important in terms of bone mineral density (Drinkwater et al 1990). Restoration of normal menstrual cycles and/or hormonal replacement can help, but will not completely reverse bone loss (Cumming 1996, Drinkwater et al 1986, Hergenroeder 1995). Lack of cost-effective screening tools means that the true incidence of osteoporosis is unknown. Myburgh et al (1990) found that athletes with stress fractures were more likely to have low bone density, lower dietary calcium intake, current menstrual irregularities and lower oral contraceptive use.

MORBIDITY AND MORTALITY

The eating disorders in particular can cause substantial morbidity in terms of depletion of muscle glycogen stores and loss of muscle mass, dehydration and electrolyte imbalance, bradycardia and other cardiac arrhythmias, hypoglycemia, anemia, depression, and amenorrhea. Inadequate nutrient intake deprives the body of the necessary energy to perform an event, including carbohydrate for glycogen replacement, protein for tissue building and repair, and micronutrients for normal metabolism and maintenance of body homeostasis.

Binging and purging behaviors can lead to chronic gastrointestinal problems such as esophagitis, esophageal bleeding, tears of the gastroesophageal junction from vomiting, or abnormal bowel tone due to laxative abuse etc. These will decrease, rather than increase, athletic performance. Up to an 18% mortality rate (due to suicide as well as cardiac arrhythmias) has been reported for untreated anorexia and bulimia (see Putukian 1995 for further references).

The biggest health risk from amenorrhea is the premature loss of bone density, which may result in early osteoporosis. Other concerns include loss of the cardioprotective effect of estrogen on lipids and vessel walls, and possibly a change in the incidence of reproductive cancers (breast, ovary, endometrium), due to a reduction in the number of ovulatory cycles that a woman has throughout her lifetime. Many young women think that amenorrhea is a desirable end-point of training, when in reality it reflects maladaptation and suggests a serious stress to the system.

Women with premature osteoporosis may incur stress fractures and other musculoskeletal injuries during their training years, but the biggest concern is the occurrence of fractures of the wrist, spine and hip at a much earlier age than usual. Hip fractures, in particular, are frequently the 'beginning of the end' for older women. They result in a loss of independence, a high mortality rate and heavy financial costs, both to the individual and to society. Over 50% of patients with a hip fracture require institutionalization and there is a 5–20% mortality rate during the first year.

PRECIPITATING FACTORS

An underlying preoccupation with body size, shape and composition often underlies the triad disorders. A misconception that losing weight will enhance performance is often (and sometimes inadvertently) precipitated or reinforced by comments from coaches, parents and judges. Sports with subjective scoring systems (such as gymnastics, figure skating, diving) and endurance sports emphasizing a low body weight (distance running, cycling, cross-country skiing) are

particularly at risk. The former group also tend to favor a prepubertal body habitus for success, because of the relative ease of carrying out some of the complicated maneuvers. Dancers are also at increased risk. Other sports, such as volleyball, swimming, and cheerleading, which are associated with clothing styles that reveal body contour, may also precipitate disordered eating patterns. Dietary restriction is very common in sports that require specific weight categories for participation (such as the martial arts or rowing). In sports such as wrestling, similar problems can also be seen in male athletes. Cyclical weight changes in these young men also have significant implications for their health and bone density, although this area has not been as extensively researched.

Psychosocial factors, family problems, and other life stressors may also contribute. Often, traumatic events, such as an injury, loss of a coach or even extensive dieting, can be trigger factors for more chronic problems (Sundgot-Borgen 1994).

DIAGNOSTIC CLUES

Decreased athletic performance may be the first clue to disordered eating patterns. There is often a 'honeymoon period' where the athlete initially receives positive feedback for her weight loss, but eventually the other physical problems lead to a decrement in performance. Suspicious behaviors, such as excessive dieting or self-criticism, depression and volatile moods, excessive exercise outside of normal practice hours, preoccupation with food, food hoarding, frequent bathroom visits after meals, smell of vomitus, or not wanting to eat with the team may not be completely diagnostic, but should arouse suspicions. Other possible signs and symptoms include muscle cramps, headaches, dizziness, weakness, numbness or tingling in limbs from electrolyte disorders or renal dysfunction, and loss or thinning of hair.

Florid anorexia nervosa can be recognized by the cachectic thin emaciated body habitus, although patients will often wear baggy, layered clothing in an attempt to disguise their disease (Fig. 18.1). Other signs of starvation include fine 'lanugo hair' on the face or trunk, a yellowish color to the skin from hypercarotenemia, cold and cyanosed extremities and sometime peripheral edema and hypotension.

Patients with bulimia are not as easily distinguished. They may be of less than average, normal, or higher than normal weight. Telling physical findings include oral ulcerations, erosion of the enamel on the back of the teeth from recurrent regurgitation of acidic

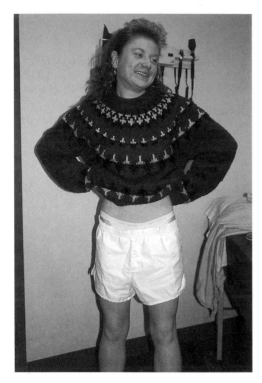

Figure 18.1 Florid anorexia nervosa can be recognized by the cachectic thin emaciated body habitus, although patients will often wear baggy, layered clothing in an attempt to disguise their disease.

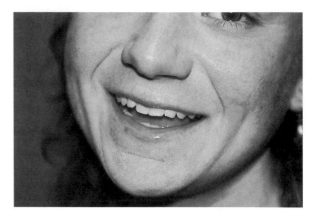

Figure 18.2 Erosion of the enamel on the teeth from recurrent regurgitation of acidic stomach contents.

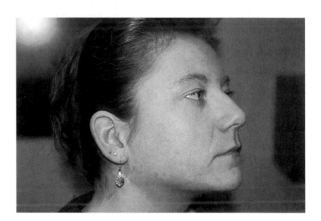

Figure 18.3 Parotid gland enlargement or 'chipmunk cheeks' in a bulimic patient.

stomach contents (Fig. 18.2), or enlarged parotid glands or 'chipmunk cheeks' (Fig. 18.3). They may present with sores or calluses on the knuckles or back of the hand from vomiting (Russell's sign). Many bulimics, however, learn to vomit spontaneously and almost silently. The only clue may be the feet pointing towards, rather than away from, the toilet in the cubicle.

Athletes with any type of menstrual dysfunction should also be questioned about their nutrition and a history of stress fractures. By extension, any athlete presenting with a stress fracture also needs to be asked about her menstrual history.

LABORATORY TESTS

There is no specific diagnostic laboratory test, but some blood and urine tests may be helpful, including complete blood count (CBC) and sedimentation rate, electrolytes, liver and kidney function. Depending upon the pathology, these may show hypokalemia, hypernatremia (or hyponatremia from too much water

ingestion), hypomagnesemia, or hypocalcemia. Laxative abusers frequently have a metabolic acidosis, while vomiters may have a metabolic alkalosis. A urinalysis with a high pH may suggest an eating disorder. It is extremely important to rule out any other underlying diseases that may present with some of the same signs and symptoms.

Electrocardiograms frequently show sinus bradycardia, and other conduction defects such as prolonged QT waves, low or inverted T waves or low-voltage complexes.

Osteoporosis is not seen on normal radiographs until 20–30% of bone density is lost. Modifiable risk factors that have been identified for osteoporosis include sedentary lifestyle, excessive tobacco, caffeine and alcohol use, thinness, and estrogen deficiency or premature menopause. However, these only predict about 70% of osteoporosis. Both estrogen therapy and exercise have been shown to prevent bone loss in post-menopausal women. In younger women with menstrual dysfunction, weight-bearing exercise may not be sufficient to offset the effect of decreased estrogen levels.

The initial presentation of osteoporosis in this population may be recurrent stress fractures, or fractures from minimal trauma. Bone density screening is not universally recommended, but should be considered for an athlete with multiple risk factors, including disordered eating, vegetarians, low daily calorie intake, high caffeine or protein, low calcium, and history of lactose intolerance. The best test is dual-energy X-ray absorptiometry (DEXA). With a cost between $100 and $200, it is the most accurate, and also gives information on body composition. A radiation dosage of 2–25 mrem compares favorably with 30 mrem from a routine chest X-ray, and is less than the natural annual radiation from the environment.

The use of calcaneal ultrasound measurements for screening purposes shows some promise. There is good correlation with future risk of hip fracture. These measurements also provide information on bone quality and architecture, which may be as, if not more, important. Evidence is generally supportive for a positive effect of physical activity on bone mineral accretion during growth (Barr & McKay 1998). High-impact sports are protective for bone mineral density, particularly if initiated before puberty, as growing bone has a greater response to load than mature bone (Grimston et al 1993). The Lanyon hypothesis postulates that infrequently repeated strains experienced during unusual activities are more likely to stimulate modeling and remodeling than are frequently repeated strains encountered during normal activity (Lanyon 1989). Residual osteogenic effects are likely maintained into adulthood, especially with continuing activity.

TREATMENT

The coach or trainer with best rapport can approach the athlete in a private confidential setting, with a caring supportive attitude. A team approach is necessary, involving the athlete, her family, the coach, a primary care physician, a registered nutritionist and a psychologist or other mental health provider. Associated emotional disorders including depression must also be addressed, preferably by a clinician familiar with eating disorders. Arrangements for follow-up and ongoing therapy are essential, particularly after the cessation of sporting activity.

The team physician is a critical part of the care-giving team, checking for other medical disorders, and providing treatment guidelines. Practice and competition only need to be limited if there is evidence that performance is compromised, or the athlete's health is at risk. These athletes often develop a decrease in basal metabolic rate (BMR) of up to 35% as their system attempts to compensate for a reduced energy intake. This makes it even more difficult to re-establish healthy eating patterns. Athletes may need to be hospitalized if more than 35% of ideal body weight has been lost, or if there is significant dehydration or electrolyte abnormalities. Fluoxetine in doses of 20–60 mg/day has been used successfully in some cases to treat bulimic behavior.

Menstrual dysfunction can initially be managed by a decrease in exercise or training of 10–20%, a slight increase in weight (2–3%) or better nutrition. Energy intakes of 1800–2200 kcal are generally recommended for sedentary females, with an additional 800–1200 kcal allotted for exercising females (i.e. 2600–3300 kcal daily or 47–60 kcal/kg per day). Extremely competitive athletes may have even greater needs. The addition of resistance training will help to promote muscle gain and improved bone density.

Therapy may also include hormone replacement, if the amenorrhea lasts more than 6 months (2 years in adolescents). Estrogen 0.625 mg/day, in combination with progesterone, may be prescribed (Cumming 1996), but frequently low-dose oral contraceptives are the most convenient form of administration (Hergenroeder 1995). These can be safely used in young women over the age of 16, or 2 years post-puberty (American Academy of Pediatrics 1989). Depo-Provera (depot medroxyprogesterone), which is used for birth control (one intramuscular injection every 3 months), may actually decrease bone density by inducing amenorrhea and subsequent hypoestrogenemia. Repeat measurements of bone density are indicated for follow-up of therapy at intervals not greater than every 6 months.

PREVENTION

Sports medicine professionals must be sensitive to early warning signs to detect and recognize the triad disorders. The preparticipation physical examination offers a perfect opportunity to discuss and further investigate any menstrual changes, weight changes, disordered eating patterns and associated medical problems, and stress fractures. A supplemental health history for female athletes is useful for screening purposes (Box 18.3). Physicians and trainers, in particular, are in a non-threatening position, and can be advocates for the athlete's health.

Coaches and other individuals involved with performance should be cognizant of training principles that are medically and psychologically sound. They should refrain from linking body composition measurements with performance. In addition, they should have a basic knowledge of nutrition and growth and development of young athletes. A referral network of other professionals can help with nutritional counseling and evaluation, and management of medical conditions, as well as mental health.

It is critical for parents to avoid pressuring their daughters into dieting and losing weight. They should be supportive of medical interventions and cooperative. Sports administrators and sport governing bodies have a responsibility to recognize and help prevent the triad disorders.

Nutritional counseling should include meeting recommended daily allowances, matching caloric intake with output and obtaining important vitamins and minerals through common food sources. Women with the triad disorders require 1000–1500 mg/day of elemental calcium. Calcium-rich non-dairy foods include leafy green vegetables such as collards, beets, turnips, kale, mustard greens, spinach, broccoli; fish and shellfish (canned sardines, canned salmon, oysters, shrimp); nuts and seeds (almonds, peanuts, sunflower seeds); and others (soybeans, dry beans, tofu, molasses).

Menstrual dysfunction should be recognized and treated early. Athletes and individuals involved in their support network must be educated about normal menstrual cycles and attainment of maximal bone density. Bone density starts to increase after the onset of puberty, and reaches 90% of peak bone mass by the end of the second decade. It is determined by both genetic and environmental factors. Maintenance of bone mass requires adequate dietary calcium and exercise, as well as normal blood levels of sex hormones following puberty.

Box 18.3 Supplementary health history questionnaire for the female athlete (After Johnson 1992)

1. How old were you when you had your first menstrual period?
2. How often do you have a period?
3. How long do your periods last?
4. How many periods have you had this year?
5. When was your last period?
6. Do you ever have trouble with heavy bleeding?
7. Do you have questions about tampon use?
8. Do you ever experience cramps during your period? If so, how do you treat them?
9. Are you currently on birth control pills or hormones? Previously? What type? For how long? Any side-effects?
10. Do you have any unusual discharge from your vagina?
11. When was your last pelvic examination?
12. Have you ever had an abnormal Pap smear?
13. How many urinary tract infections (bladder or kidney) have you had?
14. Have you ever been treated for anemia?
15. How many meals do you eat each day? How many snacks?
16. What have you eaten in the last 24 h?
17. Are there certain food groups that you refuse to eat (meat, breads, etc.)?
18. Have you ever been on a diet?
19. What is your present weight?
20. Are you happy with this weight? If not, what would you like to weigh?
21. Have you ever tried to lose weight by vomiting? Using laxatives? Diuretics? Diet pills?
22. Have you ever been diagnosed as having an eating disorder?
23. Do you have questions about healthy ways to control your weight?
24. How often do you drink alcohol?
25. How often do you use drugs? Smoke cigarettes?
26. Do you wear your seat belt when in a car?
27. Do you wear a helmet when you bike?
28. Do you have any questions about health or personal issues?

CONCLUSIONS

The problems of the female athlete triad – disordered eating, amenorrhea and osteoporosis – are seen in some active girls and women, but are certainly not a reason to discourage participation in regular physical activity. Increasing knowledge and research about these entities, as well as preventive strategies, will reduce the incidence of the triad disorders. Further large-scale studies to determine the prevalence of clinical and subclinical eating disorders in female athletes are needed. It is important to identify sports with the highest risk, as well as predisposing psychological factors. The rate of progression of subclinical eating disorders to frank anorexia or bulimia is not known. Long-term health consequences (including psychological disturbances, physiological adaptations and effects on general well-being) must be further explored.

REFERENCES

American Academy of Pediatrics. Committee on Sports Medicine 1989 Amenorrhea in adolescent athletes. Pediatrics 84(2): 394–395

American College of Sports Medicine 1997 Position stand: The Female Athlete Triad. Medicine and Science in Sports and Exercise 29(5): i–ix

American Psychiatric Association 1994 Diagnostic and statistical manual of mental disorders, DSM-IV, 4th edn. American Psychiatric Association, Washington, DC

Barr S I, McKay H A 1998 Nutrition, exercise, and bone status in youth. International Journal of Sport Nutrition 8: 124–142

Beals K A, Manore M M 1994 The prevalence and consequences of subclinical eating disorders in female athletes. International Journal of Sport Nutrition 4: 175–195

Benson J E, Engelbert-Fenton K A, Eisenman P A 1996 Nutritional aspects of amenorrhea in the female athlete triad. International Journal of Sport Nutrition 6: 134–145

Cann C E, Martin M C, Genant H K, Jaffe R B 1984 Decreased spinal mineral content in amenorrheic women. Journal of the American Medical Association 251: 626–629

Cumming D C 1996 Exercise-associated amenorrhea, low bone density and estrogen replacement therapy. Archives of Internal Medicine 156: 2193–2195

Drinkwater B L, Nilson K, Ott S, Chesnut III C H 1986 Bone mineral density after resumption of menses in amenorrheic athletes. Journal of the American Medical Association 256: 380–382

Drinkwater B L, Buremner B, Chesnut III C H 1990 Menstrual history as a determinant of current bone density in young athletes. Journal of the American Medical Association 263: 545–548

Grimston S K, Willows N D, Hanley D A 1993 Mechanical loading regime and its relationship to bone mineral density in children. Medicine and Science in Sports and Exercise 25(11): 1203–1210

Hergenroeder A C 1995 Bone mineralization, hypothalamic amenorrhea, and sex steroid therapy in female adolescents and young adults. Journal of Pediatrics 126(5 part 1): 683–689

Johnson M D 1992 Tailoring the preparticipation exam to female athletes. Physician and Sports Medicine 20(7): 61–72

Kanis J A, Melton III J, Christiansen C, Johnston C C, Kaltaev N 1994 The diagnosis of osteoporosis. Journal of Bone and Mineral Research 9: 1137–1141

Lanyon L E 1989 Bone loading, exercise and the control of bone mass: the physiological basis for the prevention of osteoporosis. Bone 6: 19–21

Loucks A B, Vaitukaitis J, Cameron J L, Rogol A D, Skrinar G, Warren M 1992 The reproductive system and exercise in women. Medicine and Science in Sports and Exercise 24: S288–293

Myburgh K D, Hutchins J, Fataar A B, Hough S F, Noakes T D 1990 Low bone density is an etiologic factor for stress fractures in athletes. Annals of Internal Medicine 113: 754–759

Myburgh K H, Bachrach L K, Lewis B, Kent K, Marcus R 1993 Bone mineral density at axial and appendicular sites in amenorrheic athletes. Medicine and Science in Sports and Exercise 25: 1197–1202

Putukian M 1995 Female athlete triad. Sports Medicine and Arthroscopy Review 3: 295–307

Rosen L W, Hough D O 1988 Pathogenic weight-control behaviors of female college gymnasts. The Physician and Sportsmedicine 16(9): 140–144

Sundgot-Borgen J 1993 Prevalence of eating disorders in female elite athletes. International Journal of Sport Nutrition 3: 39–40

Sundgot-Borgen J 1994 Risk and trigger factors for the development of eating disorders in female elite athletes. Medicine and Science in Sports and Exercise 26(4): 414–418

Taaffe D R, Robinson T, Snow C M, Marcus R 1997 High-impact exercise promotes bone gain in well-trained female athletes. Journal of Bone and Mineral Research 12(2): 255–260

Yeager K K, Agostini R, Nattiv A, Drinkwater B 1993 The female athlete triad: disordered eating, amenorrhea, osteoporosis. Medicine and Science in Sports and Exercise 25: 775–777

FURTHER READING

Ryan J 1995 Little girls in pretty boxes: the making and breaking of elite gymnasts and figure skaters. Warner Books, New York

Staeger J M, Wigglesworth J K, Hatler L K 1990 Interpreting the relationship between age of menarche and prepubertal training. Medicine and Science in Sports and Exercise 22: 54–58

Tofler I R, Katz Stryer B, Micheli L J, Herman L R 1996 Physical and emotional problems of elite female gymnasts. New England Journal of Medicine 335(4): 281–283

19

Physiological aspects of dance

Yiannis Koutedakis

KEY POINTS

1. Dance performance depends, among other features, on many technical, environmental, medical, psychological, nutritional and physiological attributes – these last constituting physical fitness.
2. Physical fitness depends on the ability to work under aerobic and anaerobic conditions, and on the capacity to develop high levels of muscle tension (i.e. strength) at high rates (i.e. power).
3. Certain aspects of physical fitness are often neglected in the dance profession, and conventional dance exercises alone are not sufficient to enhance physical fitness in male and female dancers.
4. Assessment of a dancer's physiological characteristics can help to quantify overall levels of physical fitness, and assist in the improvement of training techniques and the deployment of injury-prevention strategies.
5. Any changes in the traditional training of dancers must be made with caution, taking care not to affect the aesthetic content by the adoption of new training techniques.

INTRODUCTION

If one considers the three main 'theatre arts' (i.e. dancing, acting and singing), the 20th century could be seen by future generations as the century of dance, in the same way that the 19th century has been associated with opera, and the 18th century with the art of theatrical acting. Despite its recent advances, dance did develop rapidly in the 17th century, where fine posture was perceived as a physical reflection of high moral standing.

Dance, and in particular dance performance, is not a single act. Rather, it is a continuum of different but interrelated components which can satisfy the artistic, mental and physical aspirations of those involved. Specifically, dance performance depends, *inter alia*, on many technical, environmental, medical, psychological, nutritional and *physiological* attributes. The latter constitute *physical fitness*.

Physical fitness may be defined as *'the individual's ability to meet the demands of a specific physical task'*, and relates principally to muscle and its function (Koutedakis & Sharp 1999). Laboratory monitoring can detect areas of weakness that require special attention. Fitness depends upon the ability of individuals to work under *aerobic* and *anaerobic* conditions, and upon their capacity to develop high levels of muscle tension (i.e. *strength*), at high rates (i.e. *power*). *Body composition* and *joint mobility-muscle flexibility* are also important components of physical fitness. Regardless of the performance level, the dancers' talent, form of dance, gender or age, all dancers have to use some or all of these fitness attributes during their daily practice, and uniquely combine them with artistic creativity and expression.

As for many sports, dance has been part of the history of human culture and development through the centuries. However, unlike sport, there are surprisingly few published data on the extent that fitness can affect dance performance and other measurable factors such as injury. This is partly related to the fact that a proportion of the dance community mistakenly perceives science and art to be intrinsically opposed. Also, a variety of myths regarding certain physiological functions still condition the attitude of many master teachers and elite schools. In this chapter, some of these myths will be dispelled. At the same time, parallels will be drawn between dancers and athletes with respect to key physiological components of physical fitness.

AEROBIC FITNESS

Aerobic fitness has been closely linked to cardiovascular (or cardiorespiratory) function. *The ability to consume large volumes of oxygen during exhaustive physical effort* has been associated with the limits of human endurance. The term *maximal oxygen intake* ($\dot{V}O_{2\,max}$) has been introduced to represent the greatest utilization of oxygen during exercise. Age, sex and training state can affect $\dot{V}O_{2\,max}$ levels (Åstrand & Rodahl 1986). Thus, while the untrained, 20-year-old men and women have $\dot{V}O_{2\,max}$ of approximately 44 and 38 mL/kg per min, respectively (Table 19.1), trained distance runners may demonstrate values in excess of 85 and 75 mL/kg per min, respectively.

As with most other physiological components of fitness, the majority of the existing data on aerobic fitness in dancers have been derived from ballet. For instance, it has been found that $\dot{V}O_{2\,max}$ levels in elite ballet dancers are about 48 and 44 mL/kg per min, respectively, for men and women (Cohen et al 1982a). The same authors also noted that cardiac responses to ballet class work represented exercise of only low to moderate intensity. Yet, peak *heart rates* during ballet stage performances can be as high as 94% of the maximum age-predicted heart rate, although this may occur for a short duration only (Cohen et al 1982b). Given that a certain exercise intensity is required to enhance aerobic capabilities (i.e. aerobic endurance activities should last 15–50 min at an intensity which results in heart rates higher than 60% of age-predicted maximum), it becomes clear that ballet activities do not noticeably improve aerobic fitness.

Rimmer et al (1994), who studied male and female dance majors involved in rehearsals for an upcoming stage production of *Sleeping Beauty*, suggested that ballet dancers only achieve a moderate aerobic training effect. The relatively small improvements seen in aerobic fitness in professional dancers may be a

Table 19.1 Maximal oxygen intake ($\dot{V}O_{2\,max}$) values obtained from British dancers and untrained individuals

Form of dance/gender	Age	$\dot{V}O_{2\,max}$ (mL/kg per min)
Contemporary[a]		
Males	26.6	55.7
Females	27.1	43.5
Ballet[a]		
Males	25.8	53.2
Females	25.9	39.1
Dance students[a]		
Males	23.0	49.4
Females	21.3	46.0
NSCD[b]		
Males	20.2	54.9
Females	19.4	43.8
Untrained		
Males	25.0	44.0
Females	25.0	38.0

[a] From Brinson & Dick (1996).
[b] Northern School of Contemporary Dance, unpublished data, 1997.

function of the duration and frequency of participation, and may not be related to the intensity of dance classes (Kirkendall & Calabrese 1983). However, when dance routines elicit the required intensities for optimal aerobic work, significant improvements have been found in selected aerobic components such as $\dot{V}O_{2\,max}$ and *minute ventilation* (Galanti et al 1993).

Although the work by Galanti et al (1993) was conducted on jazz dancers, there is no reason to believe that, under similar conditions, a different result would be obtained in other forms of dance. Indeed, preliminary data have indicated that appropriate extracurricular exercise programmes are beneficial to both cardiovascular function and health in female ballet students (Dowson et al 1997).

Contemporary dancers generally show higher $\dot{V}O_{2\,max}$ values than ballet dancers (Chmelar et al 1988, Kirkendall & Calabrese 1983; Table 19.1). Whether this is the result of traditional training or due to selection procedures remains to be seen. Another interesting observation is that, at least in ballet, students demonstrate higher $\dot{V}O_{2\,max}$ values than their professional counterparts (Clarkson et al 1985, Dahlström et al 1996; Table 19.1). Due to often varying methodological procedures, it is difficult to draw conclusions by simply comparing data from different projects. However, given that the data which appear in Table 19.1 were obtained by the same investigator (i.e. the author of this chapter) using identical procedures, such observations deserve further study. Also in ballet dance, the levels of most aerobic components have not significantly changed during the course of the last 10–15 years (Cohen et al 1982a, Rimmer et al 1994).

ANAEROBIC FITNESS

Anaerobic fitness is *the ability to produce energy for muscular contraction via processes that do not require oxygen.* It applies to dance activities of short duration, but high intensity (e.g. leaps, jumps and turns). It is also synonymous with *anaerobic muscular endurance* (or local muscular endurance) which, in turn, may be seen as the opposite to *muscular fatigue*.

Anaerobic aspects are the least studied fitness attribute, both in dance and in sport, mainly because it is too difficult to partition what is aerobic and what is anaerobic in terms of mid-length (10–60 s) bursts of energy. However, the application of the *Wingate* anaerobic test and measurements of *lactate* levels provide useful information.

Only a few reports have been published where the Wingate test has been utilized to assess the anaerobic

Table 19.2 Average values for peak power (PP), mean power (MP) and time to peak power (T – PP) obtained from British elite sportsmen and women and dancers. (From Brinson & Dick 1996, with permission of Galouste Gulbenkian Foundation)

Activity/gender	PP (watts)	MP (watts)	T – PP (s)
Rowing			
Males	1140	880	5.1
Females	690	595	6.3
Gymnastics			
Males	790	690	6.0
Females	580	500	7.0
Dance (contemporary)			
Males	740	580	7.4
Females	465	359	8.3
Dance (ballet)			
Males	680	580	9.0
Females	410	329	8.3
Dance (students)			
Males	650	510	7.1
Females	477	374	8.5

fitness in dancers. One of the most recent is by Brinson & Dick (1996) (Table 19.2). From this table it is clear that the dancers show lower peak and mean power outputs and are generally slower in reaching peak powers (i.e. are less 'explosive') than the athletes. Within the dance community, contemporary male and female dancers demonstrate greater anaerobic capabilities than their colleagues participating in ballet, which is in line with the observations made earlier on aerobic fitness. The fact that a significant number of contemporary dancers have an athletic background (e.g. gymnastics, diving, athletics) may explain this difference.

The values which correspond to the British dance students (Table 19.2) are slightly lower than the equivalent reported from the USA (Rimmer et al 1994). These authors found peak power to be 725 and 503 W, respectively, in men and women, with mean power outputs of 568 and 372 W, respectively. This difference may be due to the fact that the British students were, on average, 5 years younger than their American counterparts.

Lactic acid is a product of the anaerobic energy production and is often measured in blood samples taken from a fingertip or ear lobe. Again, limited information exists on this physiological fitness variable in relation to dance. Findings focus on ballet and include the following:

● Ballet dancers achieve a moderate anaerobic training effect (Rimmer et al 1994).

• While a normal ballet class may elicit a mean lactic acid concentration of 3 mM in females, a solo part of choreographed dance may increase these levels to 10 mM (Schantz & Åstrand 1984).

• Professional female ballet dancers demonstrate lower lactic acid levels 4 min after the completion of a Wingate test than are demonstrated by professional contemporary dancers or dance students (Chmelar et al 1988, Dahlström et al 1996).

Given that lactic acid levels are inversely related to the proportion of slow-twitch fibres in the active muscle (Steinacker 1993), together with the fact that a high proportion of type I fibres have been found in male and female ballet dancers (Dahlström et al 1997), the lower lactic acid levels seen in these dancers, compared with those practising other forms of dance, may thus be tentatively explained. It is difficult, however, to explain the higher values found in dance students compared with professionals.

One of the widely held beliefs in dance is that muscular soreness is caused by the presence of high levels of lactic acid. In fact, muscle soreness is related more to the type of exercise (e.g. jumps and rebounds) than to lactic acid levels. Lactic acid is over 50% back to resting levels approximately 30 min after the end of exercise, and back to normal after about 1 h, especially when active 'cool-down' procedures replace complete rest (Koutedakis & Sharp 1985).

MUSCLE STRENGTH (AND POWER)

Background

Muscle strength *is the ability to overcome external resistance, or to counter external forces, by using muscle.* Although muscle strength has been part of the athlete's preparation since classical Greece, it has never been treated as an ingredient for success in dance. This is partly related to the scientifically unfounded fear that strength and strength training would disable dancers' flexibility, destroy their artistic prospects, and drag them away from the aesthetic standards of the profession.

There are no published reports that support such 'fears'. In contrast, questions often debated, such as 'When should a young dancer attempt pointe?' may become less subject to a teacher's intuition if knowledge on muscle strength and the ability of ligaments to sustain the load of the whole body is available before this technique is attempted (Micheli et al 1984).

Strength levels and strength training in dancers

Dancers generally show lower strength values than those of athletes (Kirkendall & Calabrese 1983). Within the dance world, contemporary male and female dancers are stronger than their counterparts in ballet, and in many cases contemporary dancers can easily compare in strength with some athletes (Table 19.3). Ballerinas appear to have the least muscular strength, normally demonstrating only 77% of the weight-predicted strength norms (Reid 1988). Also, and contrary to the common belief that one side of the body is stronger than the other, strength measurements in male and female dancers revealed no differences between left and right legs (Westblad et al 1995). In a recent study, designed to test whether different modes of activity and forms of preparation affect certain basic strength and muscle contractile characteristics, no significant differences were found between professional dancers, Olympic bob-sleighers, Olympic rowers and non-athletes (Koutedakis et al 1998).

Does dance alone promote strength enhancements? This was investigated by examining the effects of a 3-month supplemental strength-training programme on handgrip and arm/upper body strength in professional male ballet dancers (Koutedakis et al 1996). It

Table 19.3 Typical peak strength values for the muscles involved in knee extension (i.e. quadriceps) and knee flexion (i.e. hamstrings) in athletes and dancers[a]

Activity/gender	Knee extension (N m)	Knee flexion (N m)
Rowers		
Males	350	165
Females	212	89
Sprinters		
Males	330	220
Females	160	110
Squash		
Males	280	136
Females	168	79
Runners (long distance)		
Males	220	120
Females	160	85
Dancers (contemporary)		
Males	196	94
Females	133	68
Dancers (ballet)		
Males	181	89
Females	118	59

[a] All data (from Brinson & Dick 1996, Koutedakis 1994) were collected using isokinetic dynamometers in the concentric mode and at an angular velocity of 60°/s.

was confirmed that dance alone does not improve muscle strength in professional dancers, and that appropriate strength training, in addition to normal dance commitments, does lead to improvements in arm/upper body strength. These findings support previous research on male and female dancers (Groer & Fallon 1993, Stalder et al 1990), in which supplementary strength training contributed to improvements in leg strength, endurance and speed, without interfering with the dancers' artistic qualities.

Strength levels and injuries in dancers

Overwork, unsuitable floors, difficult choreography and insufficient warm-up are among the factors that may contribute to dance injuries. The possible link between strength levels and injuries in dancers has also been debated. A recent study revealed that the lower the thigh strength, the greater the degree of lower body injury in both male and female dancers (Koutedakis et al 1997a). The same authors also noticed that the female dancers were relatively weaker and sustained more severe injuries than their male counterparts. It was suggested that the introduction of supplementary strength training might circumvent such problems and provide a relatively cost-effective way of reducing injuries in dancers.

Although often overlooked, another factor associated with injuries in active individuals, including dancers, is the simultaneous presence of strong and weak muscles in the same limb. This was indeed the main finding of a study, the results of which appear in Figure 19.1. It was shown that the lower the ratio between hamstrings and quadriceps (knee Fl/Ext_{rat}) – or the weaker the hamstrings compared with the quadriceps – the worse the degree of injury, and that specific hamstring strength training can lead to reduced low back problems. It is interesting to note in Figure 19.1 that similar patterns in low back injuries were found in both rowers and dancers, possibly indicating a common basis of their physical and physiological functions regardless of the type of activity.

Power

Muscle power is the explosive aspect of strength (often called 'fast strength'). It is the functional application of both speed and strength, and is a key component in many human movements. Indeed, dance routines where jumping is required can only be performed successfully if dancers have sufficiently high levels of muscular power. However, as in the cases of aerobic and anaerobic fitness and strength, power is not likely to improve beyond certain levels using conventional dance exercises alone (Rimmer et al 1994), although both explosive strength and mechanical power in leg muscles have been found to be good in dance (ballet) trained boys (Pekkarinen et al 1989).

BODY COMPOSITION

Body composition may simply be defined as *the ratio of fat to fat-free weight* and is often expressed as *percentage*

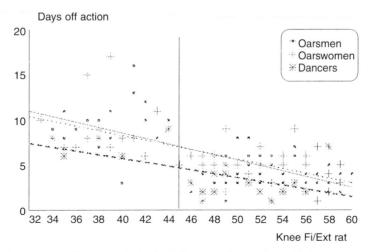

Figure 19.1 Trends between days off serious physical activity due to low back injuries for dancers and rowers. (From Koutedakis et al 1997b, with permission of Georg Thieme Verlag.)

body fat. Appropriate active body weight coupled with the right levels of body fat are essential items for optimizing physical performance. This not only applies to activities involving specific weight categories, but also to activities where carrying excess body mass (i.e. fat) is detrimental to performance.

Table 19.4 shows the sex, age, body weight and percentage body fat of various dancers and sports persons. In dance, body composition has been viewed primarily in the context of ballet, where typical body fat values for females range from 16 to 18% (Clarkson et al 1985, van Marken Lichtenbelt et al 1995). The equivalent values in male ballet dancers range from 5 to 15% (Hergenroeder et al 1991, Koutedakis et al 1996, Sawyer-Morse et al 1989). However, results obtained from ballet dancers may not be applicable to other dancers, as ballet dancers appear to be among the leanest (Pacy et al 1996).

Dancers do not demonstrate the lowest body fat values among active individuals (Table 19.4). This is despite attempts by sections of the profession to comply with the well-established 'aesthetic' standards which dominate traditional dance education. Also, considering the well-established link between lean body weight (or fat-free weight) and physical performance, preliminary research has shown comparable lean body weights in dancers and untrained control subjects (van Marken Lichtenbelt et al 1995).

Professional dancers and elite athletes appear to have constant body composition values throughout their careers. In fact, lean body weight in accomplished female ballet dancers can be adequately estimated from body weight alone, thanks to the homogeneity of body size and body composition in female ballet dancers at this level (Hergenroeder et al 1993). If body fat changes do emerge in professional dancers, they are relatively small and have little or no effect on the actual dance performance. Such changes, though, would threaten the 'aesthetic balance' which dancers faithfully observe.

MUSCLE FLEXIBILITY AND JOINT MOBILITY

Dance is an expressive art that relies on human movement for communication. As levels of communication increase and greater precision and purity of movement are required, modern dancers are constantly confronted with new movement expectations and choreographic demands. Therefore, optimal levels of muscle flexibility and joint mobility (MFJM) become key determinants of dance performance, given that such levels are normally associated with greater versatility of movement. The term MFJM refers to the individual's ability to move a joint through the required range of motion without undue stress to the involved musculotendinous unit. Good MFJM usually indicates that there are no adhesions or abnormalities in or around the joint and that there are no serious anatomical or muscular limitations.

MFJM has been the main physical fitness component that dancers have regularly sought to improve, and it is certainly an asset for selection as a future dancer (Nilsson et al 1993). However, while it is well established that inadequate MFJM detrimentally affects the quality of dance, it is not clear yet whether poor MFJM contributes to certain dance-related injuries, or whether MFJM exercises will guarantee a reduction of the severity or number of injuries in dancers and other active individuals. When MFJM levels were considered in rowers and dancers, no relationships were found between these levels and the frequency and

Table 19.4 Typical percentages of body fat (BF), age and weight in selected physically active men and women

Activity/gender	Age (years)	Weight (kg)	BF (%)
Dancers (ballet)			
Males	26.0	64	10
Females	25.0	52	17
Dancers (contemporary)			
Males	27.2	72	12
Females	26.3	59	20
Gymnasts			
Females	15.2	45.3	13.4
Middle distance runners			
Males	25.7	62.9	7.3
Females	24.1	52.8	14.8
Sprinters			
Females	21.6	60.7	18.1
Ice dancers			
Females	19.3	52.1	22.0
Squash players			
Females	18.4	62.1	24.7
Sprinters			
Males	23.4	82.3	9.1
Hockey players			
Males	27.8	75.6	12.3
Road cyclists			
Males	20.0	68.9	8.7
Lightweight rowers			
Males	24.3	70.3	6.7
Rugby players			
Males	20.6	64.4	21.0
Nordic skiers			
Males	25.8	73.6	8.2

Data on athletes are from Koutedakis (1994).
Data on dancers are from Brinson & Dick (1996).

severity of lower back injuries in physically active individuals (Koutedakis et al 1997b).

Although dancers spend a considerable amount of time throughout their career in MFJM exercises, there is little information on deconditioning rates and on the effects of periods of reduced physical activity in maintaining satisfactory levels of MFJM. A controversial set of data appeared recently where 3–5 weeks of summer holiday – during which very little physical work was reported – caused no changes in MFJM, and in some cases revealed unexpected increases, in professional ballet dancers (Koutedakis et al 1999). It was hypothesized that the increased amount of work done prior to holiday triggered a 'burn-out' effect, which may explain these controversial findings.

CONCLUSIONS

While aesthetic goals are of the utmost importance, dancers remain subject to the same unyielding physical laws as athletes. Assessment of physiological characteristics of dancers can help to quantify overall levels of fitness. This knowledge will then assist dancers and their teachers to improve training techniques, to employ effective injury-prevention strategies, and to determine better standards of health and physical conditioning.

To this day, physiological aspects of dance have been viewed primarily in the context of ballet. Certain aspects of physical fitness are often neglected by dance professionals, and conventional dance exercises alone are not sufficient to promote enhanced fitness in male and female dancers. Training to elevate standards of fitness, especially strength, may help in coping with the increased number of musculoskeletal injuries. However, any change in the traditional training of dancers must be approached cautiously, and great care must be taken to ensure that the aesthetic content is not affected by new training techniques. Further scientific research on the physical and physiological aspects of all forms of dance is required.

REFERENCES

Åstrand P-O, Rodahl K 1986 Textbook of work physiology: physiological bases of exercise, 3rd edn. McGraw-Hill, Singapore

Brinson P, Dick F 1996 Fit to dance? Galouste Gulbenkian Foundation, London

Chmelar R D, Schultz B B, Ruhling R O et al 1988 A physiological profile comparing levels and styles of female dancers. The Physician and Sportsmedicine 16(7): 87–96

Clarkson P M, Freedson P S, Keller B et al 1985 Maximal oxygen uptake, nutritional patterns, and body composition of adolescent female ballet dancers. Research Quarterly for Exercise and Sport 56(2): 180–184

Cohen J L, Segal K R, Witriol I et al 1982a Cardiorespiratory responses to ballet exercise and the $\dot{V}O_{2\,max}$ of elite ballet dancers. Medicine and Science in Sports and Exercise 14: 212–217

Cohen J L, Segal K R, McArdle W D 1982b Heart rate response to ballet stage performance. The Physician and Sportsmedicine 10(11): 120, 122, 125–133

Dahlström M, Inasio J, Jansson E, Kaijser L 1996 Physical fitness and physical effort in dancers: a comparison of four major dance styles. Impulse 4: 193–209

Dahlström M, Esbjörnsson Liljedahl M, Gierup J et al 1997 High proportion of type I fibres in thigh muscle of young dancers. Acta Physiologica Scandinavica 160: 49–55

Dowson A, Evans A, Randolph C et al 1997 The effects of an exercise programme on fitness levels and health in female ballet students. Paper presented at the 7th Annual Meeting of the International Association for Dance Medicine & Science, Tring, England

Galanti M L A, Holland G J, Shafranski P et al 1993 Physiological effects of training for jazz dance performance. Journal of Strength and Conditioning Research 7(4): 206–210

Groer S, Fallon F 1993 Supplemental conditioning among ballet dancers: preliminary findings. Medical Problems of Performing Artists 12: 25–28

Hergenroeder A C, Fiorotto M L, Klish W J 1991 Body composition in ballet dancers measured by total body electrical conductivity. Medicine and Science in Sports and Exercise 23: 528–533

Hergenroeder A C, Brown B, Klish W J 1993 Anthropometric measurements and estimating body composition in ballet dancers. Medicine and Science in Sports and Exercise 25(1): 145–150

Kirkendall D T, Calabrese L H 1983 Physiological aspects of dance. Clinics in Sports Medicine 2(3): 525–537

Koutedakis Y 1994 The physiology of fitness. In: The runner's guide. Collins Willow, London

Koutedakis Y, Sharp N C C 1985 Lactic acid removal and heart rate frequencies during recovery after strenuous rowing exercise. British Journal of Sports Medicine 19(4): 199–202

Koutedakis Y, Sharp N C C 1999 The fit and healthy dancer. Wiley, Chichester

Koutedakis Y, Cross V, Sharp N C C 1996 The effects of strength training in male ballet dancers. Impulse 4: 210–219

Koutedakis Y, Khalouha M, Pacy P J et al 1997a Thigh peak torques and lower-body injuries in dancers. Journal of Dance Medicine and Science 1: 12–15

Koutedakis Y, Frischnecht R, Murphy M 1997b Knee flexion to extension peak torque ratios and low-back injuries in highly active individuals. International Journal of Sports Medicine 18: 290–295

Koutedakis Y, Agrawal A, Sharp N C C 1998 Isokinetic characteristics of knee flexors and extensors in male dancers, Olympic oarsmen, Olympic bob-sleighers and non-athletes. Journal of Dance Medicine and Science 2(2): 63–67

Koutedakis Y, Myszkewycz L, Soulas D et al 1999 The effects of rest and subsequent training on selected physiological parameters in professional female classic dancers. International Journal of Sports Medicine 20: 379–383

Micheli L J, Gillespie W J, Walaszek A 1984 Physiological profiles of female professional ballerinas. Clinics in Sports Medicine 3(1): 199–209

Nilsson C, Wykman A, Leanderson J 1993 Spinal sagittal mobility and joint laxity in young ballet dancers. Knee Surgery, Sports Traumatology, Arthroscopy 1(4): 206–208

Pacy P J, Khalouha M, Koutedakis Y 1996 Body composition, weight control and nutrition in dancers. Dance Research 14: 93–105

Pekkarinen H, Litmanen H, Mahlamaki S 1989 Physiological profiles of young boys training in ballet. British Journal of Sports Medicine 23(4): 245–249

Reid D C 1988 Prevention of hip and knee injuries in ballet dancers. Sports Medicine 6(5): 295–307

Rimmer J H, Danielle J, Plowman S A 1994 Physiological characteristics of trained dancers and intensity level of ballet class and rehearsal. Impulse 2(2): 97–105

Sawyer-Morse M K, Smolik T, Mobley C, Saegert M 1989 Nutrition beliefs, practices, and perceptions of young dancers. Journal of Adolescent Health Care 10: 200–202

Schantz P G, Åstrand P-O 1984 Physiological characteristics of classical ballet. Medicine and Science in Sports and Exercise 16(5): 472–476

Stalder M A, Noble B J, Wilkinson J G 1990 The effects of supplemental weight training for ballet dancers. Journal of Applied Sport Science Research 4: 95–102

Steinacker J M 1993 Physiological aspects of training in rowing. International Journal of Sports Medicine 14: S3–10

van Marken Lichtenbelt W D, Fogelholm M, Ottenheijm R, Westerterp K R 1995 Physical activity, body composition and bone density in ballet dancers. British Journal of Nutrition 74: 439–451

Westblad P, Tsai-Fellander L, Johansson C 1995 Eccentric and concentric knee extensor muscle performance in professional ballet dancers. Clinical Journal of Sport Medicine 5(1): 48–52

20

Aspects in the rehabilitation of the injured classical ballet dancer

Aileen Kelly

KEY POINTS

1. A model for dance injury rehabilitation has been pioneered at the Royal Ballet in which a communicating team of practitioners caters for the rehabilitative needs of the injured dancer.
2. An understanding of how the dancer functions in the unique world of dance is necessary to rehabilitate the injured dancer back to the demands of this environment.
3. Dancers have a special relationship with pain.
4. The physiotherapist is ideally placed as a key worker in dance injury rehabilitation.
5. The rehabilitation process combines both physical and psychological input.
6. Research and education are necessary in order to change attitudes within the dance world towards health care, injury prevention and rehabilitation.

INTRODUCTION

The classical ballet dancer is, in effect, both an elite artist and an athlete, and these two aspects are inextricably linked to produce a performing artist. For the professional dancer, the body is the performing instrument, and any injury to it has both physical and psychological consequences. Dance, by its very nature, is physical, and inevitably injuries will occur. The incidence of injuries among ballet dancers in the UK is high, 83% of dancers reporting injury in a 12-month period (Brinson & Dick 1996). The world of dance places unique demands upon the dancer.

Whether through the process of natural selection – 'the Darwinism of dance' – or through long and vigorous training, usually from a young age, dancers exhibit specific differences that could be viewed as adaptations for the art form. These include anatomical differences, e.g. flexibility patterns (Reid et al 1988) and alignment (Woodhall et al 1995), physiological differences, e.g. body fat (Hamilton et al 1988), and neurological differences, e.g. vestibular habituation (Hood 1970) and a loss of reflexes (Goode & van Hoven 1982). Injuries in ballet are 'sports specific', and, with clinical exposure to dance injuries, recognized patterns of dysfunction become apparent. The rehabilitation of the injured dancer is, in essence, the restoration of function with minimal risk of re-injury on return to performance, encompassing both physical and psychological needs of the individual. Since discussion of all aspects of this process is beyond the scope of this chapter, only those issues appearing as key points above will be explored.

THE TEAM APPROACH – BACKGROUND

When injured, dancers often consult a variety of practitioners in search of the 'miracle cure'. A single therapist cannot give total care to the injured dancer, and it is rare for a single therapist to be seen in isolation. The individual needs of the injured are multifaceted, and indeed change over the rehabilitation period. Therefore, the rehabilitation of dance injuries requires an approach that accommodates these needs.

A model of care

Since 1990, a model of care has been pioneered at the Royal Ballet, where the dancer's needs are paramount during the rehabilitation process. This model has been adopted to ensure continuation of care through full rehabilitation. The on-site team comprises two chartered physiotherapists, a psychologist, a body conditioning instructor, a ballet coach and a masseur, together with an orthopaedic surgeon at an off-site clinic. There is a regular chiropody clinic and input from a dietician/nutritionist with lectures and individual consultations. Many areas of expertise are drawn upon, including physiotherapy, medicine, psychology and sports science, together with the art of dance and ballet. The physiotherapist is commonly the first point of contact, and, when indicated, refers and liaises with other rehabilitation team members. The priority given to each injury by the physiotherapist will dictate the referral to the appropriate practitioner. In practice, financial and time constraints can limit this access. This approach ensures optimal recovery without delay and reduces the risk of re-injury on return to performance. This model has taken time to build and be accepted by both dancers and management, but allows science to meet with art. A key aspect in the success of this approach is the mutual respect and understanding of each member's role (Tajet-Foxell & Booth 1996), as well as good communication between the practitioners.

Communication

A weekly meeting attended by all the on-site team members provides a forum to review the progress of the individual dancer's rehabilitation, to share information and an opportunity to discuss, modify and redirect goals for individual programmes. In practice, there are daily updates between individual practitioners. Following the team meeting, a written report on all injured dancers is compiled by the physiotherapist, and a further meeting takes place with management. This two-way communication process ensures an understanding by management of a dancer's workload at different stages of rehabilitation, and from management their requirements for rehearsals and performance schedules. Communication between both parties is important for goal-setting for the rehabilitation team, and useful for prognostic purposes for management in terms of casting for present and future performances. This meeting with management also provides an important opportunity to discuss aetiology of injuries and to raise injury prevention issues. The team approach requires both good communication and consistent effort on the part of all members, and when working well, it provides an integrated service for the rehabilitation of injured dancers and a cost-effective use of on-site facilities.

THE DANCER'S WORLD

There is an overlap between the worlds of ballet and sport, as both groups undergo rigorous training from an early age, depend on the body functioning at optimal level for performance, and have careers that are unusually short. Injury can mean an end to a career, and the transition out can be traumatic. The culture of the ballet world and that of the sports world, however, are quite different. Dancers view themselves as artists first and foremost. It is only relatively recently that they have acknowledged and begun to view themselves as elite athletes as well.

Success for the dancer is not objectively measured as in competitive sport. It is usually more subjectively appraised, in the public domain, with feedback from the audience and the media. It is appraised by the individual via feedback from peers, teachers and coaches, or by the artistic director with further casting in roles which provide greater challenges and opportunities to perform, which in turn may lead to promotion within the hierarchy of the company.

The professional ballet dancer's world can be insular. A 6-day week begins with daily class, followed by long rehearsals throughout the day, and several evening performances per week. A long season often involves touring away from the home base, and as a consequence dancers spend long periods of time working, travelling and living in close proximity to each other, and often this world provides their only social life and support structures.

Injury – the dancer's perspective

Reaction to injury, as well as when and how dancers report pain/injury, has implications for the therapist planning the rehabilitation process. From the dancer's perspective, any time away from dancing can mean loss of physical fitness, loss of performances and roles, withdrawal from the dance world environment, loss of confidence and possible loss of earnings. The time at which an injury strikes has implications for the roles currently being performed and rehearsed, and the roles due to be rehearsed and performed, and must therefore affect advancement in the dancer's career. The psychological effects of injury for dancers, as in sports, can have implications for the process and outcome of rehabilitation (Brinson & Dick 1997, Tajet-Foxell 1997). Factors such as personality, social support structures, coping strategies and attentional styles are important (Nideffer 1989). The physiotherapist needs to be aware of the importance placed upon the injury by the individual dancer at that time, in that particular week, or in that particular season. By recognizing the dancer's verbal and non-verbal cues, the therapist can adjust the rehabilitation approach and, when necessary, refer to the psychologist.

Injury – management's perspective

From management's perspective, an injury means loss of a dancer in a role, unexpected changes in the casting and extra rehearsals for another dancer(s), all of which have financial implications. To reduce the internal tensions that may arise, the Royal Ballet has adopted a policy whereby injuries are quickly reported to management. This enables management to instigate contingency plans for forthcoming performances as early as possible. Unfortunately, within the wider dance world there is a prevailing belief and attitude, despite all dance research to the contrary, that suspects the injured dancer of malingering. The dancer undergoing treatment invariably becomes labelled 'injured', but also risks being labelled 'unreliable', 'always injured' or 'weak'. This negative labelling is not only dangerous for the self-esteem and confidence of the rehabilitating dancer, but also for motivation. Negative labelling can seriously damage a dancer struggling to come to terms with a difficult injury.

One approach that has been adopted is to view rehabilitation as a positive learning experience: as a time of education for the prevention of further injury. Also, the dancer can use the time away from dance as an opportunity to work on weak areas of the body, on technique, and flexibility, strength and coordination etc. This positive approach towards injury rehabilitation requires a shift in attitude and mindset for both dancers and management. It has led to wider access to physiotherapy, massage, dance coaching and the use of body control facilities. Dancers attending any rehabilitation team practitioner are viewed positively, as taking care of themselves.

DANCERS AND PAIN

The assessment of dance injuries invariably involves the assessment of pain. Since ballet dancers are renowned for dancing through pain, assessment can sometimes be difficult. As one dancer commented: 'Dancers know pain – dancers live in pain'. A study by Tajet-Foxell & Rose (1995) found that dancers, when compared with non-dancers, displayed a higher pain threshold and a higher pain tolerance. They suggest that the most likely explanation is that dancers are exposed to physical training, which gives them a familiarity with the interface between physical activity and pain experience. That in turn may give them the perception of some degree of control over the pain. It is not known whether these findings are acquired or inherent. In an unpublished study involving vocational school ballet students and non-dance students, Briggs (1997) found that differences were apparent even at a young age for pain threshold and sensitivity. Both pain threshold and pain tolerance increase with age.

Time lapse in reporting pain

One characteristic in the pattern of reporting injury among ballet dancers is the time lapse between the reported onset of pain and the time of seeking assistance. Goertzen et al (1989) found that ballet dancers often ignored injuries. Briggs (1997) suggested that ballet students perceived the ability of being able to perform in pain as normal, and, from her interviews with student dancers, there appears to be a certain amount of acceptance of pain as a normal part of ballet life. Despite higher pain threshold and pain tolerance, dancers felt pain more acutely than non-dancers (Tajet-Foxell & Rose 1995). Furthermore, dance students perceived pain more intensely than non-dancers, and yet did not seem frightened by it (Briggs 1997). In clinical practice, this may explain why dancers can characteristically pinpoint the injured tissue and recall in vivid detail the onset and progression of the injury. Likewise, it may explain the time lapse before reporting an injury. The clinical implication is that dancers' behaviour may be influenced by discussing their beliefs and knowledge of pain. Tajet-Foxell & Rose (1995) called for the need to discuss, in the training of young dancers, 'the meaning of pain, the importance of acknowledging pain, and of learning how to respond to it'. In practice, this requires the physiotherapist to have a role in educating young dancers with respect to pain.

Reporting injury

Another phenomenon which occurs with regularity is the dancer who presents with an injury that, on assessment, is found to be secondary to a primary injury for which the body has adapted. Typically, only when the severity of the pain or dysfunction, from either injury, reaches a level that affects performance does the dancer seek assistance. Thus, it may be the dysfunction rather than the pain severity that spurs the dancer to report. The dancer makes the decision to report against a backdrop of the attitude to health care and injury previously outlined. In a study by Brinson & Dick (1996), company dancers perceived a strong managerial pressure to perform while injured, and, in addition, management exploited the dancers' fear of what might happen if they refused to perform. This study high-

lights the importance of communication between the dancer, management and the rehabilitation team to ensure early intervention for injury management.

At the Royal Ballet, the dancer is encouraged to seek help as soon as an injury occurs. When a dancer is deemed unable to dance, the injury is discussed with the appropriate member of staff. The dancer is also encouraged to discuss the injury with the member of staff. However, understandably, many are reluctant to do so.

PHYSIOTHERAPIST – KEY WORKER

Compared to medical, paramedical and alternative practitioners, physiotherapists are the most popular practitioners consulted by dancers (Bowling 1989, Brinson & Dick 1996). The physiotherapist will assess each injury and, in conjunction with the dancer and other members of the team, tailor a rehabilitation programme. The physiotherapist needs to empathize and have good communication skills. Interestingly, Tajet-Foxell (1994) found that dancers rated communication skills higher than technical skills as qualities needed by a dance physiotherapist. The aim of physiotherapeutic intervention is to restore the *mobility, flexibility, strength, stamina, speed, coordination* and *self-confidence* of the dancer.

On-site physiotherapist

The challenge for the physiotherapist is to provide the best environment to prevent delayed healing of an injury. The company physiotherapist needs to have a knowledge of classical ballet technique, the company's current repertory, and the demands of individual roles on the body of the injured dancer to tailor a rehabilitation programme. One may gain this in-depth knowledge by being on-site.

The on-site physiotherapist will benefit dance injury rehabilitation by having knowledge of:

- the individual dancer's body, either through pre-season screening or previous injury history
- the company's repertory and will therefore have insight into the demands placed upon the individual dancer
- previous experience of how an individual dancer may react to an injury
- the current demands of training, rehearsal and the performance schedule
- possible reasons why a dancer reports or fails to report an injury
- the pressures, policies and politics of the company.

With this knowledge, the physiotherapist can plan for the individual needs of the dancer and help to ensure an injury-free return to full performance.

The dance physiotherapist has a multiplicity of roles. Hall (1989) noted similar findings among physiotherapists working with elite athletes at Olympic level. The dance physiotherapist, like the sports physiotherapist, must possess a certain personality and flexibility in order to tolerate a constantly fluctuating environment in terms of attitude, behaviour and sense of values (Wright 1979).

REHABILITATION – REST AND WORKLOAD

The immediate assessment of an injury and subsequent rehabilitation often involve the consideration of past, present and future workloads of the dancer. Rehabilitation will usually require a period of rest, something that dancers are not keen to accept. The idea of relative rest as opposed to complete rest was introduced at the Royal Ballet and called 'selective rest'. This allows the dancer to continue dancing in some capacity in class/rehearsal, for example, working without pointe shoes, or avoiding jumping sequences to reduce active work. Decisions regarding 'selective rest' often have to be taken by the physiotherapist in consultation with the dancer and management. The team will decide the appropriate workload in order to enable full recovery.

Psychology

Injury affects the dancer psychologically as well as physically, and it may take significantly longer to recover from the psychological damage than from the physical damage. In an ideal situation, a psychologist should be part of the support team involved in the rehabilitation from the onset throughout the various stages of the recovery. The contribution and importance of the psychologist have been well documented within the sport context (Butler 1997). A model described by sport psychology will be similar in content to a model applied to dance. Such a model deals with issues of the effects of anxiety, pain perception, memory trace, self-esteem, confidence, motivation, concentration, emotional dysfunction and coping, as well as issues related to optimizing potential and facilitating elite physical/technical performance. Recognizing the fundamental importance of psychological factors has a long way to go in the dance world in comparison with the sport world, where such practice is part of elite performance.

Body conditioning

In the initial stages of rehabilitation, the dancer will start exercises for maintenance of the non-injured areas of the body and, as healing allows, specific exercises for the injured area. This aspect of rehabilitation is known as 'body control', and the Royal Ballet uses exercises in body control developed by Joseph Pilates in the 1930s. This approach has been adopted by the dancing fraternity, with each teacher adapting and developing the exercises. The core elements of *body control* are that of relaxation, concentration, coordination, alignment, breathing, flowing movements, centring and stamina (Robinson & Thomson 1997). It appears that, with repetition of movement patterns at submaximal voluntary contraction under direct cortical control, there is improvement in precise muscle group action, symmetry of movement, stabilization of the body part and postural alignment. Many of the exercises, performed on a floor mat and on specially designed equipment, replicate ballet-specific patterns of movement. The body conditioning instructor has an expert eye, and gives verbal and tactile input to correct classical technique, ensure control of spinal alignment, and encourage trunk stability, symmetry of movement and balance. Although some research has appeared in the literature (Fitt et al 1993, McLain et al 1997), further research needs to be undertaken to ascertain its effectiveness. Cardiovascular training and specific upper and lower body strength training programmes are incorporated into the rehabilitation programme as the injury allows.

Coaching

Taking daily class is the core training for the classical ballet dancer. All elements of ballet class need to be addressed in rehabilitation and this is referred to as 'coaching' at the Royal Ballet. It exposes the recovering dancer to the full spectrum of balletic movement necessary for the safe return to class (Kelly 1994). Coaching requires an experienced ballet teacher, whose input tailors the needs of the dancer at each session. The emphasis is on early identification of faulty movement patterns to correct technique. It begins with supported work at the barre in a weight-bearing position, and progresses to free-standing movement known as 'adage'. Coaching progresses from simple exercise to the increasingly complex, faster sequences of steps. It advances to turns of increasing difficulty and from small to big jumps. Coaching introduces rhythm and musicality and increases confidence in performance.

The dancer then moves from coaching into company class, to rehearsals and then, ultimately, to performance on stage.

Re-injury

Occasionally, the dancer may be re-injured during the rehabilitation period. Often this occurs at a transition period, e.g. at the transition between returning to class and rehearsal (i.e. at the first rehearsal period post-injury) or between rehearsal and the first performance period post-injury. This may be related to:

- a dramatic increase in workload
- high expectations by both the dancer and management
- the dancer feeling vulnerable, anxious and under pressure
- the rehabilitation not addressing all the parameters of fitness and psychological preparation for return to ballet.

During transition periods, communication between the rehabilitation team and rehearsal staff is important to ensure an appropriate increase in workload. This has resulted in an adjustment to the typical working practices at the Royal Ballet. For example, dancers could work in soft flat ballet shoes as opposed to pointe shoes, could mark out steps rather than rehearse with full effort, limit their jumping and reduce the number of repetitions. The benefits of these new working practices far outweigh any drawbacks. More importantly, they have prompted the instigation of specific training for parameters of fitness necessary for classical ballet.

THE FUTURE FOR DANCE REHABILITATION

Dance rehabilitation is now a major division of dance medicine, a branch of performing arts medicine, and is still in its infancy in the UK. Because of the similar physical nature of dance and sport, research in sports medicine can often transfer directly to dance medicine. Ballet, however, is steeped in tradition, and any changes in the methods and practices of training are not easy to bring about. Brinson & Dick (1996) found that dancers thought management should do more with respect to injury management, while management felt this was the dancers' responsibility. Clearly there is a need for education on both sides. Dancers require empowerment, and need to be encouraged to be actively responsible for maintaining their own healthy bodies and not to be the passive recipients of treatment. Management has to accept responsibility for their employees in terms of promoting injury prevention and providing adequate rehabilitation facilities. Only education regarding the multiple factors involved in dance injury will produce changes in attitude. Attitude towards health care and injury and rehabilitation in the ballet world has changed, and must continue to change. The dance physiotherapist is in the forefront of education of both dancer and management. If education is insufficient, outside influences, in particular the threat of litigation, may enforce change. One way of facilitating change may be the creation of an objective outside body, a dance council that could provide a forum for discussion, education and research. This could set minimum standards for dance training and health care facilities. The high number of injuries has emotional and financial costs to the dancer and company alike that cannot be ignored. In the classical ballet world, the Royal Ballet Company has been pioneering in its attitude and provision of injury care.

CONCLUSIONS

1. A multidisciplinary team can best provide for the needs of the injured dancer. This model of care has been successfully adopted by the Royal Ballet Company, London, UK.
2. An understanding of the demands and attitudes of the dance world is essential in order to plan and manage the rehabilitation of the injured dancer.
3. There is a need for education regarding pain from the very earliest training of classical ballet dancers.
4. An on-site dance physiotherapist has multiple roles and is ideally placed for the rehabilitation of the injured dancer.
5. The level of rest, workload and risk of re-injury, together with psychological aspects, need to be addressed in rehabilitation.
6. Further research and education are necessary to achieve improvements in the rehabilitation of the injured dancer.

Acknowledgements

The author wishes to thank Britt Tajet-Foxell for her helpful comments on this chapter and for her support and friendship over the last decade. She would also like to thank all the members of the healthcare team, with special thanks to Monica Mason and Sir Anthony Dowell. The cooperation and assistance of all the dancers of the Royal Ballet during research projects has been greatly appreciated.

REFERENCES

Bowling A 1989 Injuries to dancers: prevalence, treatment, & perceptions of causes. British Medical Journal 298: 731–734

Briggs J 1997 Pain threshold and pain tolerance in adolescent ballet students. Unpublished MSc Thesis, Manchester Metropolitan University, Division of Sport Science, Alsager Campus, Alsager, Cheshire, UK

Brinson P, Dick F 1996 Fit to dance? The Report of the National Inquiry into Dancer's Health & Injury. Galouste Gulbenkian Foundation, UK

Butler R J (ed) 1997 Sport pyschology in performance. Butterworth Heinemann, Oxford

Fitt S, Sturman J, McLain-Smith S 1994 Effects of Pilates-based conditioning on strength, alignment, and range of motion in university ballet and modern dance majors. Kinesiology and Medicine for Dance 16(1): 36–51

Goertzen M, Ringelband R, Schulitz K P 1989 Injuries and damage due to excessive loading in classical ballet. Sportorthopadie 127: 98–107

Goode D H, van Hoven J 1982 Loss of patellar and Achilles tendon reflexes in classical ballet dancers. Archives of Neurology 79: 323

Hall J 1989 The role of chartered physiotherapists in Olympic sports. Physiotherapy 75(12): 686–690

Hamilton L H, Brooks-Gunn J, Warren M P, Hamilton W G 1988 The role of selectivity in the pathogenesis of eating problems in ballet dancers. Medicine and Science in Sports and Exercise 20(6): 560–565

Hood J D 1970 The clinical significance of vestibular habituation. Advances in Oto-Rhino-Laryngology 17: 149–157

Kelly A 1994 Rehabilitation – the classical ballet dancer. Sportcare Journal 1(3): 30–31

McLain S, Carter C L, Abel J 1997 The effect of a conditioning and alignment program on the measurement of supine jump height and pelvic alignment when using the current concepts reformer. Journal of Dance Medicine and Science 1(4): 149–154

Nideffer R M 1989 Psychological aspects of sports injuries: issues in prevention and treatment. International Journal of Sports Psychology 20: 241–255

Reid D C, Burnham R S, Saboe L A, Kushner S F 1988 Lower extremity flexibility patterns in classical ballet dancers and their co-relation to lateral hip and knee injuries. Physiotherapy in Sport 11(1): 4–7

Robinson L, Thomson G 1997 Body control the Pilates way. Boxtree, UK

Tajet-Foxell B 1994 The role of the physiotherapist in ballet and football. Unpublished MSc Thesis, University of Hertfordshire, Hatfield, Herts, UK

Tajet-Foxell B 1997 The management of ballet injuries. Performing Arts Medicine News: 7–10

Tajet-Foxell B, Booth L 1996 An 'equal expertise' approach to rehabilitation of athletes. Physiotherapy 82(4): 686–689

Tajet-Foxell B, Rose F D 1995 Pain and pain tolerance in professional ballet dancers. British Journal of Sports Medicine 29(1): 31–34

Woodhall A M, Maltrud K, Mello B L 1995 Alignment of the human body in standing. European Journal of Applied Physiology and Occupational Physiology 54(1): 109–115

Wright D 1979 Prevention of injuries in sport. Physiotherapy 65(4): 114–119

21

Faulty alignment and posture perpetuating musculoskeletal problems

Jenny McConnell

KEY POINTS

1. It would appear that some individuals are very prone to musculoskeletal problems, while others are not, and that faulty alignment and posture may help to perpetuate such problems.
2. It has been claimed that musculoskeletal pain syndromes are seldom caused by isolated precipitating events, but are the consequences of habitual imbalances in the movement system, and that poor neuromotor function contributes to various postural anomalies.
3. There are not many objective criteria for establishing what is normal posture, and this shortage has created difficulties for physiotherapists in determining appropriate management strategies for multifactorial chronic problems.
4. Treatment should be directed towards minimizing the patient's symptoms, improving the flexibility of hypomobile structures and improving the dynamic control of hypermobile segments.
5. Individuals with faulty alignment must continue to maintain the dynamic control over the hypermobile segments for the rest of their athletic career, if they want to remain symptom-free in their sport.

INTRODUCTION

It seems unjust that some athletes rarely have injuries, whereas others are plagued by musculoskeletal problems, even though they stretch, warm up and appear to do the 'right things' pre-training and in competition. These oft-injured athletes are a challenge for the sports medical team who try desperately to keep them competing. This raises the question as to why some individuals are so prone to problems and others not at all. Is it the amount or intensity of training, the age of the athlete, the genetic characteristics or a combination of many factors? Many studies have tried to correlate faulty posture and musculoskeletal pain and/or injury without much success (Pope et al 1985, Sward et al 1990). In an effort to correlate postural characteristics with musculoskeletal conditions, investigators have often examined only one or two factors in isolation, such as forward head posture to headache and joint hypermobility to anterior knee pain, rather than hypothesizing that many musculoskeletal problems may be multifactorial. It has been claimed that musculoskeletal pain syndromes are seldom caused by isolated precipitating events, but are the consequences of habitual imbalances in the movement system, and that poor neuromotor function contributes to various postural anomalies (Janda 1988, S A Sahrmann, unpublished work, 1990).

Posture was defined in 1947 by the American Academy of Orthopaedic Surgeons as the:

relative management of the parts of the body. Good posture is that state of muscular and skeletal balance which protects the supporting structures of the body against injury or progressive deformity irrespective of attitude (erect, lying, squatting, stooping) in which these structures are working or resting. Under such conditions, the muscles will function most efficiently and the optimum positions are afforded for the thoracic and abdominal organs. Poor posture is a faulty relationship of the various parts of the body which produces increased strain on the supporting structures and in which there is less efficient balance of the body over its base of support.

To date, however, objective criteria for normal posture are not in abundance and some criteria, particularly in dynamic situations, are quite contradictory (Adams & Hutton 1985, Andersson et al 1977, Dolan et al 1988, During et al 1985). The shortage of readily pertinent information for physiotherapists has resulted in difficulties in determining the appropriate management strategies for multifactorial chronic problems such as patellofemoral pain, supraspinatus tendinitis and low back pain. This chapter will examine the multifactorial nature of musculoskeletal problems and the relationship between alignment, posture and musculoskeletal conditions, addressing static and dynamic assessment as well as intervention strategies.

ASSESSMENT

As the cause of the symptoms of many musculoskeletal problems is often quite remote from the site of the symptoms, management of the problem can be difficult. Identification of the structure(s) causing the symptoms requires a methodical approach during the examination of a patient. The initial part of the examination of the patient involves obtaining a detailed history, so a differential diagnosis can be proposed. The diagnosis is later confirmed or modified by the physical findings. In the history, the clinician needs to elicit the area of symptoms, which may be pain, pins and needles, numbness, swelling and/or weakness; the type of activity precipitating the symptoms; the history of the onset of the symptoms; and the behaviour of the symptoms. This gives an indication of the structure involved and the likely diagnosis. For example, a patient presenting with intense low back and leg pain with some numbness in the foot 3 days after lifting some suitcases up the stairs, and finding that sitting, coughing and straining increase the symptoms, would be provisionally diagnosed with a nerve root irritation or even compression due to a disc bulge. Further testing, both physical and radiographic (MRI or CT scan) would confirm the diagnosis. In this situation, the therapist can be fairly confident about the structures involved and direct treatment accordingly. Similarly, if a patient playing netball lands, pivots, hears a pop and feels a tearing sensation in the knee, with immediate swelling in the joint, this would give the therapist a strong index of suspicion that the anterior cruciate ligament was ruptured. Again, this can be confirmed with a physical and radiological examination.

However, if the symptoms have a more chronic and recurrent nature, then management becomes more challenging (see the more complex case study in Box 21.1). In this situation, to address the problem adequately, the therapist needs to consider not just where the pain is coming from, but what is causing it. For example, is it due to:

- an increased sensitivity of structures in the vicinity of the problem
- hypomobility, i.e. a lack of flexibility of the joint structures, neural, fascial and muscle tissues
- hypermobility/instability demonstrating a lack of passive and/or dynamic control

---

Box 21.1 Case study: multidirectional instability of the shoulder – a complex management issue

A 19-year-old elite female volleyball player presented with right shoulder pain, which radiated slightly into the deltoid region. The pain had been gradual in onset and worsened as her frequency of training and playing increased. Her symptoms were of 12 months' duration. She had undergone thermal capsular shrinkage surgery 6 months previously, and, although initially there was some improvement in the pain, as soon as she tried to go back to volleyball, the symptoms returned. At the time of the examination, she was experiencing pain when brushing her hair, but she was playing some volleyball matches as she was the star player of the team. On examination, she had an arc of pain from 60° to 120° of abduction, pain on resisted external rotation testing and in the empty can position. On ligamentous testing, she had a positive containment test as well as increased laxity in the sulcus and posterior drawer tests. She also exhibited laxity on ligamentous testing of the left shoulder. Following the examination, a diagnosis of impingement due to a multidirectional instability was made.

- centrally generated/maintained sensitivity
- a combination of two or more of the factors above?

In the case study in Box 21.1, it is apparent that not only is there some local sensitivity of structures, but there is also passive instability contributing to the problem locally. Analysis of the volleyball serve of this individual revealed extremely poor trunk and pelvic stabilization, so generalized strength training of the shoulder musculature would not improve the patient's symptoms, as the reason for the shoulder instability had not been addressed. It is not adequate to focus on the shoulder complex alone, as the overhead or throwing athlete must be able to transfer energy generated from the lower extremity and the ground through the spine to the upper extremity (Young et al 1996). Rehabilitation must optimize the energy transfer. During the throwing motion, for example, the shoulder goes from a close pack position to one of humeral abduction and maximal external rotation which places the powerful internal rotator muscles (latissimus dorsi and pectoralis major) on stretch. An explosive transition from maximal external to internal rotation ensues as the combined efforts of the trunk and internal rotator muscles result in a peak angular velocity of 7000°/s. The transfer of energy from the gluteus maximus to the latissimus dorsi occurs through the thoracolumbar fascia. The thoracolumbar fascia is a multilayered structure – the superficial fibres emerge from the latissimus dorsi above and the gluteus maximus below, giving it connections to both the upper and lower extremities. The gluteus maximus of the throwing side causes a push-off force, whereas the gluteus maximus on the opposite side acts as a stabilizer of the pelvis. The lumbar spine needs to remain stable during overhead activities. During wind-up, the lumbar lordosis needs to be controlled by eccentrically contracting the abdominals, so the thrower does not lock out too early, resulting in a decrease of shoulder external rotation.

The appropriately timed and coordinated activation of muscles influencing spinal motion reduces the need for the shoulder muscles to act as prime movers of the arm. Inefficiency of the throwing motion results in a loss of force imparted to the shoulder so the shoulder musculature has to generate more tension to maintain the kinetic energy. The asymptomatic elite overhead athlete utilizes the larger trunk muscles for force generation so the prime movers are not the cuff muscles which are deactivated during arm acceleration (except for subscapularis) (Perry & Glousman 1990). In fact, it has been shown that isokinetic shoulder muscle strength has little bearing on throwing velocity (Bartlet et al 1989). Although the internal/external rotator strength in pitchers compared with non-pitchers was shown to be greater, the tests were performed at one-twentieth the velocity (Brown et al 1988). The shoulder muscles should therefore be trained for stability and endurance (low load, high repetitions), particularly if the ligamentous integrity of the joint is poor. If the thrower has a multidirectional instability, initial muscle training should be directed at the posterior deltoid muscle to improve the centring of the humeral head in the glenoid fossa, as training to the rotator cuff may result in a downward displacement of the humeral head, thus initially increasing the instability. As soon as the athlete is able to control the humeral head position, rotator cuff muscle training should be incorporated into the rehabilitation programme.

Training of the rotator cuff musculature at 90° should concentrate on endurance. This is due to the fact that at 90°, where the space between the humeral head and the acromion process is at a premium, and the deltoid is now providing a compressive force on the joint rather than a vertical humeral displacement as it does earlier in the range, a maximal contraction will increase the size of the rotator cuff tendons and may compromise their function. Biofeedback should be used so that the timing of the muscles is assessed and the appropriate motor pattern can be retrained. If the athlete has dynamic control over the unstable shoulder joint, the motion segment will no longer be unstable. For efficient transfer of energy from the lower extremity to the upper extremity, the abdominal, spine extensor and gluteus medius muscles should be trained to improve the stability of the pelvis and trunk. Additionally, to maximize the explosive force generation, the gluteus maximus and latissimus dorsi need to be trained for strength and power (higher load, low repetitions).

Resolution of symptoms alone should not be the goal of rehabilitation, as the symptoms will only recur. Improving the efficiency of the overhead motion perhaps with some technique modification should be the ultimate direction of the management of the patient with multidirectional instability. Interestingly, the causative factors of the athlete's shoulder instability (Box 21.1) were not apparent until the volleyball serve was analysed. In many instances, the therapist can glean a great deal of information about the relative contribution of structures to the patient's symptoms by observing the physical alignment and examining the effect of this alignment on dynamic activities.

Physical examination – observation

At the beginning of most assessment forms, there is a section labelled observation. Often the significance of the observation and what the therapist is trying to observe are lost. If the patient presents with an overuse problem in the lower extremity, the therapist needs to examine the lower limb alignment and determine the effect this has on the patient's gait – walking and running. The underlying causative factors can then be identified, allowing the appropriate treatment to be implemented.

The therapist can start at the feet and move up the lower limb, or at the pelvis and move down the limb. From the front, the therapist can observe the femoral position, which is easier to see when the patient has the feet together. A position of internal rotation of the femur is a common finding in many athletes with overuse injuries. This femoral position has been associated with patellofemoral pain, chronic low back pain, iliotibial friction syndrome and trochanteric bursitis. The internal rotation of the femur is usually associated with a tight iliotibial band (ITB) and poor functioning of the posterior gluteus medius muscle. This gives rise to instability of the pelvis, causing an increase in the dynamic Q angle and an increase in mobility of a specific lumbar segment.

Moving down the leg to the knee, the therapist can observe the bulk of the different heads of the quadri-

ceps muscle, the tightness of the ITB attachment and any swelling or puffiness about the knees. An enlarged fat pad, for example, is indicative that the patient is standing in hyperextension or with the knee in a 'locked back' position. From this, the clinician can infer that the quadriceps control, particularly eccentric control, in inner range (0–20° flexion) will be poor. The position of the tibia relative to the femur (valgus/ varus) is noted and the presence or absence of torsion of the tibia is determined, as these bony malalignments can affect the way the foot hits the ground.

At the foot, the clinician palpates the talus on the medial and lateral sides to check for symmetry. In relaxed standing, there should be equal amounts of talus palpable on both the medial and lateral sides. This is the mid-position of the subtalar joint. If the talus is more prominent medially, then the patient's subtalar joint is pronated. The position of the talus from the front is correlated with the position of the calcaneum from behind. If the talus is prominent medially, the calcaneum should be sitting everted. If the calcaneum is sitting straight or inverted then the clinician can infer that the patient has a stiff subtalar joint and will pronate not at heel strike but at midstance, thus exhibiting a midfoot collapse. Some patients may have an asymmetrical amount of pronation of one foot relative to the other. The pronation may be increased in one foot for many reasons – for example, the patient may have shifted away from the painful side causing the foot to pronate; the pronated foot may be compensating for a longer leg; the femur may be more internally rotated on that side; or the intrinsic foot structure may dictate the difference. The therapist needs to determine why there is a difference, as the management will vary accordingly.

Further along the foot, the great toe and first metatarsal are examined for callus formation as well as position. If the patient has callus on the medial aspect of the first metatarsal or the great toe, or has a hallux valgus, then the therapist will expect the patient to have an unstable push-off in gait. This patient will therefore lose some of the efficiency of push-off in a mediolateral direction. Further indications of an unstable push-off are increased activity in the long toe extensors, which is often associated with a flattening of the transverse arch of the foot.

From the side, the clinician can check pelvic and lumbar spine position, to determine whether the pelvis has an anterior or a posterior tilt, or whether the patient has a 'sway back' posture. A 'sway back' posture is one where the pelvis is displaced forward of the shoulders. The amount of extension of the knees, confirming the presence of hyperextension or a 'locked back' position, can also be seen from the side.

From behind, the level of the posterior superior iliac spine (PSIS) is checked, to determine any leg length discrepancies, gluteal bulk is assessed and the position of the calcaneum is observed. When investigating gluteal bulk, the therapist is interested in any asymmetry of bulk; for example, if the gluteus medius bulk is decreased on the right, the therapist should expect that when the patient is weight-bearing on the right, the pelvis will drop on the left. However, if the patient is standing with the feet wider than the pelvis and the gluteus medius bulk is diminished on the right, the patient will trunk side flex to the right more than the left. This patient exhibits a 'swaggery' gait. After observing a patient's alignment, the clinician will have a reasonable idea of the athlete's dynamic picture. Any deviations from what is anticipated give a great deal of information about the muscle control of the activity.

Dynamic examination

The aim of the dynamic examination is primarily to reproduce the patient's symptoms so the clinician has an objective reassessment activity to evaluate the effectiveness of the treatment. Additionally, the effect of muscle action on the limb mechanics can be evaluated. The first dynamic activity examined is walking. For example, if an individual stands in hyperextension of the knees, the quadriceps will not function well in inner range due to lack of practice, so the initial shock absorption at heel strike will be minimal. Initial shock absorption occurs with knee flexion of 10–15°, because the foot is supinated when the heel first strikes the ground. As soon as the heel hits the ground, the foot rapidly pronates, so if that same individual has a stiff subtalar joint, shock absorption must come from higher up in the body, in this case the pelvis. This patient will demonstrate a pelvic instability, which, depending on the tilt of the pelvis, will cause an increase in either pelvic and ultimately trunk rotation or lateral flexion.

If the pelvis is anteriorly tilted, then the patient will exhibit an increase in pelvic rotation when walking, because that individual has a lack of hip extension and external rotation. If the pelvis is posteriorly tilted, the patient will present with a Trendelenburg gait, indicating weak gluteal musculature. The individual with a sway back posture walks with a combination of increased tilt and rotation. The optimal amount of pelvic movement is reported to be 10° for rotation, 4° for lateral tilt and 7° for anteroposterior tilt (Perry 1992). If there is any increase in any of these pelvic movements, there will be an associated increase of a particular segment in the lumbar spine. It has been established that excessive movement, particularly in rotation, is a contributory factor to disc injury and the torsional forces may irrevocably damage fibres of the annulus fibrosus (Farfan et al 1970, Hickey & Huskins 1980). Therefore, an excessive amount of movement about the lumbar spine because of limited hip movement and control, in combination with poor abdominal support, seems to be a significant factor in the development of low back pain.

The initial response, when evaluating a patient with abnormal pelvic motion, is to give that patient pelvic stability work to control the excessive motion. However, if this is the case, the patient, who is not shock-absorbing at the knee or the foot, and now no longer shock-absorbing at the pelvis, must absorp shock even higher up, perhaps at the cervical spine – is this a potential cause of whiplash? If stabilization work is given to a patient, the therapist must make sure the patient has some scope for movement elsewhere, so asking the patient to walk with the knees slightly flexed will improve the shock absorption and decrease the need for the excessive movement at the pelvis.

At midstance the subtalar joint should be resupinating so it is in a neutral position. This occurs due to the action of the tibialis posterior muscle, which distributes the body weight among the lateral four metatarsal heads, thus controlling the amount of internal rotation of the leg at midstance (Basmajian & De Luca (1985). The tibialis posterior effectively raises the base of the first metatarsal so that it is higher than the cuboid. This enables the peroneus longus to act more efficiently in stabilizing the first metatarsal in preparation for heel-off. The peroneus longus and the tibialis posterior work synergistically to provide the stability at midstance. If a person's foot is maintained in a pronated position, as is the case of a plantarflexed first ray, the cuboid is higher than the base of the first metatarsal, which reduces the efficiency of the peroneus longus muscle (Root et al 1977). The position and control over the midfoot can be a contributing factor for athletes presenting with shin pain. These athletes generally exhibit a stiff subtalar joint and a more mobile midfoot. One of three things may happen to cause the shin pain:

- The tibialis anterior contracts to resupinate the foot as the tibialis posterior is so elongated that it is unable to contract. The tibialis anterior, which is active on heel strike to control the rate of foot slap, is an antagonist to the peroneus longus, so is generally not as active in midstance, to allow the peroneus longus to work more efficiently. Prolonged activation of the tibialis anterior will cause fatigue of the muscle, which ultimately will cause a failure of the tibialis anterior to control foot motion at heel strike, and increase the impact pressure on the bone. This gives rise to anterior compartment problems.

• The peroneus longus contracts in an elongated position, causing further pronation and instability at toe-off. This often results in lateral shin pain or possibly a stress fracture of the fibula.

• The tibialis posterior is unable to shorten effectively to control the midfoot position, so the activity in the flexor hallucis longus muscle, which is greatest at midstance to position and stabilize the great toe in preparation for push-off (Basmajian & De Luca 1985), increases further to compensate for the lack of stability of the forefoot. The resultant posterior compartment pain is common in ballet dancers.

During the last half of stance, the calcaneus inverts 2° before heel-off, which increases the rigidity of the foot. Concurrently, the hip should be externally rotating. At this time the abductor hallucis and flexor digitorum brevis are most active. The gastrocnemius and soleus begin to contract before the heel is lifted from the ground; the activity stops before the great toe leaves the ground, so they have a supportive rather than a propulsive function.

Propulsion begins with heel lift and concludes with toe-off. At the time of toe-off, the calcaneus is everted 4–6°. Before and during toe-off, the quadriceps and sometimes the hamstrings reach another (but smaller) peak of activity. The middle part of gluteus maximus has a peak of activity just before to just after toe-off (Basmajian & De Luca 1985). All the fibres of gluteus maximus show small peaks of activity at heel strike and near the end of swing.

The anterior part of the gluteus medius muscle exhibits a moderate amount of activity at heel strike, which persists through to midstance. There is also a brief burst at toe-off and another just before heel contact. The posterior fibres are rather similar in activity. The gluteus minimus acts biphasically, unlike the gluteus medius, which is triphasic. It is active at heel contact to 40% of stance and again at midswing. Tensor fasciae latae is also biphasic in action, with a peak during early stance to midstance and another short smaller peak during toe-off. If the tensor is tight, it will cause an anterior rotation of the ilium in the final stages of stance phase (Lyons et al 1983).

If the patient's symptoms have not been provoked in walking, then evaluation of more stressful activities such as stair climbing are performed. If the symptoms are still not provoked, then squat, one leg squat, jumping and hopping may be examined and used as a reassessment activity. With athletes, however, these clinical tests may not be strenuous enough to reproduce their symptoms, as it may be longer duration activities, such as running 15 km, that provoke them. In this situation, fatigue is an issue, so muscle control will be poor. The clinician can therefore be quite justified in evaluating the control of the one leg squat to determine the effect of treatment outcome.

MEASUREMENT OF OUTCOME

As most patients are concerned about their pain, a baseline measurement of the severity of pain at rest and during activity can be recorded on a visual analogue scale (Zussman 1986). This can be used to monitor initial treatment outcome and treatment effectiveness on a treatment-to-treatment basis. Physiotherapists may use this information to determine if there is a pattern emerging for particular conditions, which may help them to refine treatment techniques.

To document whether there has been a change in function, objective measurements are required. Physiotherapists can quantify range of affected movements with a measuring device such as a goniometer, spondylometer or tape measure. They can also assess muscle performance by measuring torque output, using an isokinetic device such as a KINCOM or a Cybex, and/or by examining the timing of muscle contraction, using ultrasonography and/or electromyography (EMG) biofeedback. The value of EMG biofeedback for rehabilitation is being challenged in the literature, particularly with regards to the management of patellofemoral pain. The literature is confused about the issue of timing and intensity of the vastus medialis oblique (VMO) and the vastus lateralis (VL) in symptomatic and asymptomatic individuals. There is an assumption that a person with patellofemoral symptoms was, at one time when not symptomatic, like an asymptomatic. Much as we can say that apples and oranges are round pieces of fruit, yet as we know that is where the similarity ends. Thus, with a patellofemoral sufferer, the factors that cause the patellofemoral symptoms, such as internal femoral rotation, excessive pronation or increased Q angle, have always been present, but the condition may not yet have manifested itself because the muscle control is adequate. Perhaps the excessive subluxer requires a greater ratio of VMO:VL activity, whereas the laterally tilted patella requires an earlier timing of the VMO relative to the VL.

The issue of VMO and VL timing is still controversial. Voight & Weider (1991) found that the reflex response time of the VMO was earlier than the VL in an asymptomatic group, but in a symptomatic patellofemoral group there was a reversal of the pattern. These findings were recently confirmed by Witvrouw et al (1996), but curiously these investigators found that there was a shorter reflex response time in the patellofemoral group relative to the control group. Dynamically this issue has been supported by the work of Koh et al (1991), who examined isokinetic knee extension at 250°/s, following hamstring preactivation, finding that the VMO activated 5.6 ms earlier than VL. Even though this finding was statistically significant, these authors questioned the functional relevance. The above findings are at odds, however, with the findings of other investigators (Gilleard et al 1998, Karst & Willett 1995, Powers et al 1997) who found that the VMO did not fire earlier than the VL in the asymptomatic group, and that the VMO was not delayed in the symptomatic group. Because of this lack of change in the firing pattern, some of the investigators have concluded that general quadriceps strengthening alone is required in the rehabilitation of patellofemoral pain. However, it has been found that taping the patella of patellofemoral pain sufferers causes an earlier activation of the VMO and a delayed activation of the VL, particularly on stair descent (Gilleard et al 1998). Perhaps it could be surmised that the VMO of the patellofemoral pain sufferers needs to fire earlier to overcome the abnormal tracking forces. Perhaps the ability to selectively fire the VMO is a learned skill rather than an innate ability, much like one would train the abductor hallucis or, for that matter, individually isolate one frontalis to elevate one eyebrow and not the other. Training should therefore further enhance this ability.

Although the early literature suggested there was a difference in the ratio of the VMO and the VL activity, with the VL activity being greater than the VMO (Mariani & Caruso 1979), recent literature has not supported this contention. The early literature did not normalize the EMG data. Normalization involves obtaining a ratio of the recorded muscle activity and muscle activity from the maximal voluntary contraction (MVC), which then enables you to compare the ratio of one muscle relative to its maximal with another muscle relative to its maximal. For example, if the recorded VMO is 20 µV and the maximum is 100 µv, and the measured VL is 40 µV and the maximum is 200 µV, then the ratio of VMO:VL is 1:1. There has been some discussion that normalization is affected by the presence of pain, which will mask differences, as there may be error in the MVC which may appear in the error of the recorded EMG (Souza & Gross 1991).

There has also been some debate about the reliability of the maximal contraction throwing some concern on the normalization process. Howard & Enoka (1991) found that there was considerable variation in the MVC of the VL EMG, even though the force exerted by the leg remained constant. Yang & Winter (1983) found that the averaged rectified EMG had a coefficient of variation (SD/mean) of 9.1% in one day and 16.4% between days. Where does this leave the clinician and what is the best method of facilitating recovery in a patient with patellofemoral pain? This issue is addressed in the section concerned with muscle training (p. 214).

Interestingly, timing and magnitude of muscle contraction have been shown to be significant factors in the presence of low back pain. When examining the role of the transversus abdominis muscle in trunk stabilization, Hodges & Richardson (1996) found that the muscle preceded the activation of the prime mover in patients without low back pain when individuals were performing rapid arm movements in a randomly assigned direction, whereas transversus abdominis activated after the prime mover in individuals with low back pain. Size of muscle has been found to be a factor in acute low back pain. The multifidis muscle atrophies at the level of the acute low back pain, and even though the symptoms disappear, the muscle size does not change (Hides 1995), suggesting that failure to specifically train the multifidis contributes to the recurrences seen in low back pain sufferers. To assist clinicians in their ability to assess and train the trunk-stabilizing muscles, Richardson et al (1992) developed a pressure transducer (Chattanooga Australia, Pressure Biofeedback) which monitors changes in pressure in the spine and a support surface (plinth, chair or wall) during stabilization exercises. The use of the biofeedback device has enhanced patient precision and control during stabilization exercises for the lumbar and cervical spines.

Dynamic segmental alignment, particularly during an athletic pursuit, can be recorded objectively to help the physiotherapist determine any dysfunctional elements in the activity and to provide an objective measure of change. Numerous techniques of varying capability and cost as well as suitability are available (Winter 1982). A relatively cost-effective method is the use of a videotape, markers on identifiable bony landmarks and a digitizer. A software program to compute angular displacements, velocities and accelerations of the segments of interest make the kinematic analysis less arduous for the clinician. Analysis of patients' movements and the response of their symptoms to movement will determine the treatment approach of the patient with a musculoskeletal disorder. The broad principles of treatment for most musculoskeletal problems are relatively straightforward. It is the execution of the treatment that can sometimes be difficult.

TREATMENT

Treatment should be directed towards:

- minimizing the patient's symptoms
- obtaining an optimal loading of the joint
- improving the dynamic control of a hypermobile segment
- improving the flexibility of hypomobile structures – whether it be joint, muscle, neural or fascial tissue.

Minimizing a patient's symptoms – unloading painful structures

When the patient has a great deal of pain or the symptoms are easily aggravated by treatment, it is often difficult for the therapist to achieve much change in the initial treatments and to maintain a lasting treatment effect. If the therapist is able to minimize the patient's symptoms by at least 50% before addressing the causative factors, there will be a greater and faster treatment effect. Reduction in the patient's symptoms can be achieved by unloading or shortening the soft tissues. The principle of unloading is based on the premise that inflamed soft tissue does not respond well to stretch. For example, if a patient presents with a sprained medial collateral ligament, applying a valgus stress to the knee will aggravate the condition, whereas a varus stress will decrease the symptoms. The same principle applies for patients with an inflamed fat pad, an irritated iliotibial band or a pes anserinus bursitis. The inflamed tissue needs to be shortened or unloaded. To unload an inflamed fat pad, for example, a 'V' tape is placed below the fat pad, with the point of the 'V' at the tibial tubercle coming wide to the medial and lateral joint lines. As the tape is being pulled towards the joint line, the skin is lifted towards the patella, thus shortening the fat pad (Fig. 21.1). The case study in Box 21.2 highlights the importance of an accurate assessment and the subsequent unloading of the appropriate soft tissues.

Box 21.2 Case study: inferior patellar pain – a diagnostic dilemma

A 14-year-old freestyle swimmer competing at state level had been experiencing infrapatellar pain for the past six months. The pain, which was localised to the region underneath the patellar tendon, was aggravated when tumble turning and occasionally when swimming with a more vigorous kick. The knee sometimes would become puffy inferiorly. It had reached the stage where she was no longer able to compete at swim meets because the knee had become so painful, and it was even troubling her at school when she was climbing stairs. The swimmer had been receiving treatment, which consisted of 250 straight leg raises per day and no breaststroke in her training regime. Even though the girl diligently pursued the suggested treatment, it seemed to be exacerbating her symptoms as she could only swim twice a week as any more than that meant her knee would ache all day at school.

On examination, the pain was reproduced as the knee of the symptomatic weight-bearing leg was extending, going up the stairs. Passively, the symptoms were reproduced by an extension overpressure of the tibiofemoral joint. The compromised structure was the fat pad which was being irritated by the inferior pole of the patella being pulled posteriorly during end-range extension manoeuvres of the knee (McConnell 1991). The fat pad was unloaded with tape and the patient was given a specific training programme for the posterior fibres of gluteus medius and the vastus medialis oblique. The patient's symptoms were dramatically reduced and she was able to return to swimming. It was not the breaststroke action that was exacerbating her symptoms, as is commonly the case with young swimmers. It was the forceful extension of the knee during the tumble turn and the rapid kicking which impinged the fat pad initially, so technique modification was required to minimize the symptom recurrence. This involved improving the gluteal contraction, so that stroke acceleration was not relying solely on a forceful end-range contraction from the quadriceps.

The differential diagnoses in this case study are patellofemoral pain, patellar tendinopathy, Osgood–Schlatter disease, Sinding–Larsen–Johansson syndrome and fat pad irritation. Fat pad irritation is confirmed as the diagnosis because pain is reproduced on extension overpressure and the fat pad is inflamed; neither the inferior pole nor the tibial tubercle were tender, thus excluding Osgood–Schlatter disease and Sinding–Larsen–Johansson syndrome. The clinician must be aware that any locking back of the knee will further irritate the inflamed fat pad, so straight leg raise manoeuvres are totally inappropriate.

Unloading the inflamed soft tissues for a patient with chronic low back and leg symptoms can also be

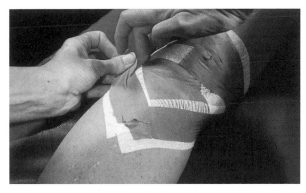

Figure 21.1 Unloading the fat pad. Tape can be used to decrease the tension in an inflamed fat pad by taping from the tibial tubercle to the joint line on the medial and lateral sides. While the tape is being applied, the skin is lifted towards the patella, to shorten it. The aim is to achieve an orange peel look to the skin, so in effect the fat pad looks fatter.

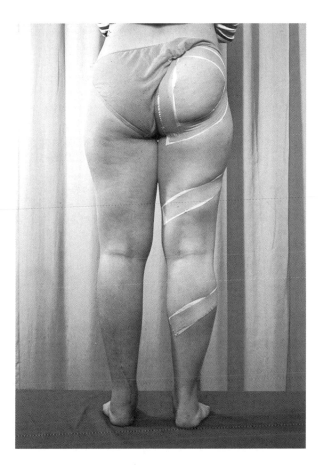

extremely effective, causing an immediate relief of symptoms. First, the buttock can be unloaded, then tape is applied on a diagonal halfway down the femur following the involved dermatome, and again in the same manner on the tibia until the symptoms have significantly diminished (Fig. 21.2). The direction of the diagonal depends on the patient's symptoms. Initially, the symptoms may increase distally as the tension is reduced from the proximal segment and relatively increased in the distal segment. Once the tissues have been unloaded, the patient may continue most training without an increase in symptoms and the therapist can treat the condition more effectively.

Optimal loading of a joint

Optimal loading of a joint can be accomplished, to some extent, by increasing the surface area of contact of the joint, because, although pressure is proportional to the force, it is inversely proportional to the area (Merriam 1980). If the physiotherapist can optimize the surface area of contact of a joint during treatment, then the force through the joint is distributed over a wider area, so the pressure per unit area will decrease. There should be a corresponding decrease in the pain. An example of how optimization of joint contact area can be promoted is given below using the patello-femoral joint. The relevant anatomy and biomechanics of the joint is reviewed to help explain the rationale behind the method of optimization.

The functions of the patella are to link the divergent quadriceps muscle to a common tendon; to increase the extensor moment of the quadriceps muscle; to protect

Figure 21.2 Unloading inflamed soft tissue in chronic low back and leg pain. Tape is applied to buttock and down the leg: first along the gluteal fold, lifting the soft tissue towards the spine; then parallel to the natal cleft, lifting the soft tissue up; and finally from the greater trochanter to the sacrum. Two other pieces of tape are applied down the leg diagonally across the relevant dermatome, one on the thigh and the other on the tibia. The skin is lifted towards the buttock when this tape is applied. The direction of taping is dependent on symptom response, i.e. the tape should immediately decrease the symptoms, so if taping in one direction increases the symptoms, then taping in the opposite direction should decrease the symptoms.

the tendon from compressive stress; and to minimize stress concentration by transmitting forces evenly to the underlying bone (Ahmed et al 1983, Huberti & Hayes 1984, Huberti et al 1984, Matthews et al 1977, Reilly & Martens 1972). Like all lower limb joints, the patello-femoral joint handles compressive stress by maximizing its surface area of contact (Goodfellow et al 1976, Hungerford & Barry 1979). With increasing knee flexion, when the compressive force increases (from 0.5 × body weight for level walking, to 7–8 × body weight for squatting) (Ahmed et al 1983, Matthews et al 1977, Reilly & Martens 1972), a greater proportion of the patellar surface is in contact with the femur (Fujikawa et al 1983, Goodfellow et al 1976, Hungerford & Barry 1979, Matthews et al 1977, Radin 1979).

The position of the patella relative to the trochlea of the femur is, to a large extent, controlled by the surrounding soft tissues (Matthews et al 1977). Patients with patellofemoral symptoms, however, demonstrate a failure of the intricate balance of the soft tissue structures. The imbalance, due to various biomechanical faults, alters the distribution of the load to the undersurface of the patella which ultimately produces pain (Fulkerson & Hungerford 1990, Goodfellow et al 1976, Gresalmer & McConnell 1998, Matthews et al 1977). A major objective in treatment is to realign the patella with the trochlea of the femur so that the patella is parallel to the femur in the frontal and the sagittal planes, and the patella is midway between the two condyles when the knee is flexed to 20° (Fulkerson & Hungerford 1990, Gresalmer & McConnell 1998). Maintaining the patella in this position reduces pain immediately, enabling patients to perform previously painful activities without pain.

As the patellofemoral joint is essentially a soft tissue joint, the position of the patella can be changed by stretching the tight lateral retinacular structures and by changing the activation pattern of the VMO muscle. Stretching adaptively shortened retinacular tissues can be achieved by a sustained low load to facilitate a permanent elongation of the tissues, utilizing the creep phenomenon, which occurs in viscoelastic material when a constant low load is applied (Herbert 1993, Hooley et al 1980, Taylor et al 1990). If a constant force is applied to a collagenous structure for a prolonged period, further movement is detected. The movement is small and imperceptible. It appears to be due to the gradual rearrangement of collagen fibres, proteoglycans and water in the ligament, disc or capsule being stressed. Creep manifests itself over a period of time that may vary from several seconds to several days. It is probably most effective between 1 and 72 h (Herbert

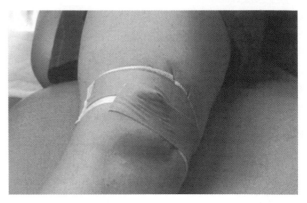

Figure 21.3 Taping more than one patellar component. The components taped and the amount of tape required depend on the symptom response.

1993, Hooley et al 1980, Taylor et al 1990). After this period, biomechanical adaptation comes into play, so that permanent plastic deformation of tissues occurs.

Taping the patella into an improved alignment should provide a relatively constant low load to the shortened retinacular tissue. The new patellar position should always decrease the patient's symptoms immediately. More than one component may need to be corrected (Fig. 21.3). The effect of each piece of tape on the patient's symptoms should be evaluated. Figure 21.4 demonstrates the effect of tape on a patella during MRI testing of an elite track athlete diagnosed with patellar tendinopathy.

- the patella without tape – notice the lateral tilt of the patella and the increased signal (whiteness) in the fat pad suggestive of inflammation.
- the patella is corrected with tape correction of a lateral tilt, glide and unload of the fat pad. It is now less tilted and the tendon appears healthier and plumper and the area of inflammation in the fat pad is less obvious.

Effects of tape

It has been fairly well established that taping the patella relieves pain (Bockrath et al 1993, Cerny 1995, Cushnaghan et al 1994, Gilleard et al 1998, Powers et al 1997), but the mechanism of the effect is still being debated in the literature. It has been found that taping the patella of symptomatic individuals such that the pain is decreased by 50% results in an earlier activation of the VMO relative to the VL on both step up and step down. Stepping down in particular caused an 8.3° differential between the VMO and VL, as not only was

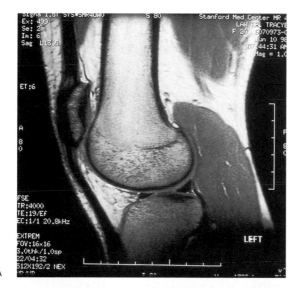

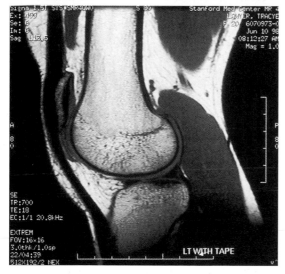

Figure 21.4 This demonstrates the effect of tape on a patella during MRI testing of an elite track athlete diagnosed with patellar tendonitis. A: The patella without tape – notice the lateral tilt of the patella, the stringiness of the patellar tendon and the increased signal (area of white) in the fat pad, suggestive of oedema. B: The patella is corrected with tape correcting a lateral tilt and glide and unload of the fat pad – it is now less tilted and the tendon appears healthier and plumper and the area of inflammation in the fat pad is less obvious.

the VMO activating earlier than the pre-taped condition, but the VL was significantly delayed in the taped condition (Gilleard et al 1998). However, in a study by Cerny (1995), where all subjects had a medial tilt and internal rotation of the inferior pole taping, there was

no change in activation pattern of the VMO and VL when the subjects were taped. But patellar taping has been associated with increases in loading response knee flexion as well as increases in quadriceps muscle torque. When the quadriceps torque of symptomatic army personnel was evaluated in taped, braced and control conditions, it was found that the taping group generated both higher concentric and eccentric torque than both the control and braced groups. The braced group did perform better than the control group in the eccentric situation. This increase in muscle torque did not correlate with pain reduction (Conway et al 1992).

Even in an osteoarthritic group, taping the patellofemoral joint in a medial direction has a significant effect on pain. Fourteen patients with a mean age of 70 years and radiographic evidence of tibiofemoral and patellofemoral osteoarthritis participated in a single-blind, blind observer randomized crossover trial of three different forms of taping – neutral, lateral and medial. Patients were not told which tape was thought likely to be effective. The knee pain was recorded with a 10 cm visual analogue scale before and 1 h after tape application. The tape was kept on for 4 days and overall pain on each of the 4 days was recorded in a diary. After this time, the patients removed the tape and were asked to score the change in symptoms in the treated knee compared with before taping. After a 3-day interval the procedure was repeated for the second tape position, and following a further 4 days of tape application and another 3-day interval, they entered the final arm of the study. At the end of the study, the assessor recorded which week of treatment each patient had preferred. Medial patellar taping was significantly better than lateral or neutral taping for pain scores, symptom change and patient preference. In this elderly osteoarthritic group, medial patellar taping resulted in a 25% reduction in knee pain (Cushnaghan et al 1994).

The tape is only necessary while the muscle is being trained – in this case the VMO, the only dynamic medial stabilizer of the patellofemoral joint. However, unless the dynamic control of the joint is maintained, the patient's symptoms could recur.

Improving the dynamic control

Long-term promotion of optimal joint loading requires analysis of the contribution of each of the surrounding muscles to the mobility and stability of the joint during various activities, i.e. ensuring balanced muscle activation patterns. Although the contribution of each of the muscles participating in a specific activity can be highly variable, some patterns of movement may not be as desirable because they are more likely to cause musculoskeletal problems, particularly when the demand on the segment changes (Gresalmer & McConnell 1998, Pope et al 1985, Sward et al 1990, Watson & Trott 1991). For example, individuals with internally rotated femurs lose flexibility in their tensor fascia latae, which shortens the iliotibial band, causing a lateral tracking of the patella and an increase in length of the VMO (Fulkerson & Hungerford 1990, Gresalmer & McConnell 1998, Jull 1986). When these individuals commence an aerobics programme, increase their running routine or rekindle their interest in snow skiing, they are more susceptible to experiencing patellofemoral pain (Gresalmer & McConnell 1998). Individuals with a forward head posture are another example. The upper cervical flexors elongate and lose their stabilizing ability, so these individuals are more susceptible to cervical headaches (Kendall & Kendall 1968, Watson & Trott 1991).

Watson & Trott (1991) investigated the association of cervical headache, natural head posture and function of the upper cervical flexor muscles for isometric strength and endurance, measuring two groups of females – a 'headache' group, consisting of individuals who experienced more than one headache per month, and a 'non-headache' group, consisting of subjects who experienced no cervical spine pain or headaches. They found that the headache group, when compared with the non-headache group, demonstrated a forward head posture and significantly less isometric strength and endurance capacity of the upper cervical flexor muscles. In the headache group, these muscles fatigued in 50% of the time taken by the same muscles in the non-headache group. The lack of upper cervical muscle endurance in the headache group was found to be significantly ($P <0.01$) related to forward head posture. Watson & Trott (1991) concluded that their results have considerable clinical significance in the areas of prevention and management of headache.

Physiotherapists need to restore the balance of the synergists around the joint by specific muscle training before commencing a strengthening programme, otherwise a poor pattern of recruitment will be reinforced and may actually be harmful (Addison & Schultz 1980, Sinaki & Mikkelson 1984). For example, it has been found that patients with low back pain have greater weakness in their trunk extensors than in their trunk flexors. Many back pain patients are routinely given sit-up exercises to increase abdominal strength, but these exercises may have a potentially harmful effect on patients with low back pain. It has been shown that intradiscal pressure in sit-up exercises far exceeds the forces in sitting and is equal to those in forward bend holding 20 kg (Nachemson & Elfstrom 1970). If the patient has been advised to avoid bending, lifting or sitting, it does not seem logical to create similar or greater intradiscal pressures during 'therapeutic' exercise. Through-range abdominal exercises have also been found to be inadvisable for postmenopausal spinal osteoporotic women. A study by Sinaki & Mikkelson (1984), which followed, for 1–7 years, four groups of osteoporotic women performing different spinal exercise regimes, demonstrated an increased incidence of spinal fractures in the through-range abdominal exercise group compared with the control group, and a significantly increased incidence in fractures compared with the isometric extension group.

However, it is the lack of endurance capacity of the stabilizing muscles that is more of a challenge to the therapist, because it requires low-load, high-repetition training, which can be difficult for a patient to maintain. The stabilizing muscles function predominantly at 20–30% of the MVC, so that they can provide the subtle adjustments and control required to enhance performance. Exercises (training) given to the patient should be aiming to correct any neuromuscular imbalances, so training initially is a motor skill acquisition rather than a strengthening procedure. Specific exercises for stabilizing muscles must therefore be carefully supervised by the therapist, so the appropriate muscles are recruited during the exercise. If there has been habitual disuse of muscles, activation will be difficult. Feedback to the patient must be precise to achieve the desired outcome (Carr & Shepherd 1982).

Specificity of training

Before examining the issue of exercise prescription for a patient, some discussion on the different philosophies of strength training is required. The traditional strengthening view holds that strength gained in non-specific muscle training can be harnessed for use in performance – i.e. the engine (muscles) is built in the strength training room; learning how to turn the engine on (neural control) is acquired on the field (Sale & MacDougall 1981). Strength is therefore increased by utilizing the overload principle, meaning exercising to at least 60% of maximal (Grabiner et al 1994). A more recent interpretation of how to facilitate strength is based on the premise that the engine (muscles) and how it is turned on (neural control) should both be built in the strength training room (Sale & MacDougall 1981). Training should therefore simulate movement in terms of anatomical movement pattern, velocity, type and force of contraction. Thus, with training, the neuromuscular system will tend to become better at generating tension for actions that resemble the muscle actions employed in training, but not necessarily for actions that are dissimilar to those used in training. For example, training of the scapular and glenohumeral stabilizers – the lower trapezius and the rotator cuff muscles – for a swimmer who has shoulder impingement pain during freestyle should be given in the prone position. However, training for a tennis player with shoulder impingement pain would be inappropriate in the prone position as the muscle control is required in a weight-bearing position – the position in which tennis is played. Training requires the appropriate synergistic patterning of the muscles. Strength gains are not observed when a trained muscle is acting in a different functional position to the one where the training occurred, as different muscle synergies are required (Grabiner et al 1994, Nyland et al 1994, Sale & MacDougall 1981). Figure 21.5 depicts a 22-year-old netball player training her lower trapezius muscle to minimize her shoulder pain, using a dual-channel biofeedback. Tape has been used to reposition the humeral head and minimize her symptoms.

This also applies when considering the training for lower extremity problems. The evidence from the literature suggests that closed-chain exercise, i.e. when the foot is on the ground, is the preferred method of training for patients with patellofemoral problems, because not only has muscle training been found to be specific to limb position, but closed kinetic training has been shown to improve patellar congruence. In a group of patients with lateral patellar compression syndrome, it was found that open-chain isometric quadriceps exercise resulted in more lateral patellar tilt and glide from 0° to 20° on CT scan, whereas closed-chain exercise demonstrated improved congruence from 0° to 20° (Doucette & Child 1996).

EMG biofeedback has been found to hasten the rehabilitation process (Ingersoll & Knight 1991). It was found that after 3 weeks of EMG biofeedback training to the VMO in healthy females, the patella moved medially and posteriorly during a quadriceps contraction as measured on a tangential X-ray, improving the congruence angle and 're-establishing the fit' of the patella in the trochlea. However, after 3 weeks of daily, progressive resisted quadriceps exercises in another group of healthy females, the patella demonstrated an increased lateral glide and a posterior rotation. A 170% increase in quadriceps strength was recorded but there was a deterioration of the patellar tracking in the asymptomatic individuals who were in the non-specific quadriceps-strengthening group. This study indicates that it is possible to selectively train the VMO to have an effect on the patellar position. Therefore, to train the VMO appropriately, an understanding of the function and the anatomy of the muscle is necessary.

The vastus medialis consists of two parts – the longus, whose fibres are oriented 15–18° medially to the frontal plane, and the obliquus, whose fibres are oriented 50–55° medially in the frontal plane (Lieb & Perry 1968). The vastus medialis longus acts with the rest of the quadriceps to extend the knee. The vastus medialis oblique has no function in extending the knee. In fact, Lieb & Perry (1968) found that in cadaver specimens, when weight was applied only to the VMO, the femur fractured before any extension occurred. They found that the vastus medialis oblique was active throughout the entire range of extension and was responsible for realigning the patella medially. The VMO is the only dynamic medial stabilizer. The muscle arises from the tendon of the adductor magnus (Bose et al 1980) and is supplied in most cases by a separate branch of the femoral nerve (Thiranagama 1990), so it should be possible to activate it independently of the rest of the quadriceps (Basmajian & De Luca 1985).

To facilitate a VMO contraction, it has been suggested that the adduction of the thigh, rather than extension of the knee, is emphasized (Hanten & Schulties 1990, Hodges & Richardson 1993, Rice et al 1995). Weight-bearing activities should be commenced early in rehabilitation to improve the muscle activation for functional activities. Small-range knee flexion and extension movements (the first 30°) in walk stance

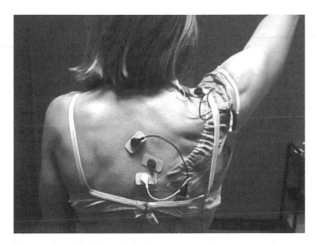

Figure 21.5 Training of the lower trapezius muscle using a dual-channel biofeedback in a 22-year-old netball player. Tape has been used to reposition the humeral head and minimize the symptoms.

position, with the VMO constantly active, would be a suitable starting position, provided the patient is relatively pain-free during this activity. This position simulates the motion of the knee during the stance phase of walking, and is also the position where VMO recruitment is poor. A reversal of the VMO activity pattern in patients with patellofemoral pain has been demonstrated by Petschnig et al (1991), where more VMO activity relative to vastus lateralis occurred at 90° than at 20°. In asymptomatic individuals, more activity was recorded at 20°, so it was concluded that this was because the VMO had to centralize the patella against the lateralizing forces of the screw home mechanism (Petschnig et al 1991). Training causes changes within the nervous system that allow an individual to better coordinate the activation of muscle groups.

Marked changes in muscle activation patterns can occur during adolescence as a result of rapid growth. At this time, soft tissue adaptation lags behind growth of long bones, so individuals who have grown rapidly have difficulties not only with tight soft tissues, but also with control of their limbs, as the muscles are attempting to control a longer lever. The intensity and timing of the muscle synergies are often significantly altered, so motor performance deteriorates and the individual is prone to injury. These individuals have often been very athletic in their pre-teens and are consequently very popular at school. Their sporting prowess deteriorates with their rapid growth, which often causes a plummeting of their popularity. This can cause further frustration as, not only are they not performing in their sport, but their self-esteem is taking a battering. These individuals require particular understanding and direction from the health care practitioner. They must be shown the appropriate stretches and muscle training for their sport and relevant injury. The case studies in Boxes 21.3 and 21.4 highlight the importance of this.

Improving the flexibility of hypomobile structures

Hypomobility often occurs in areas quite remote from the site of the symptoms, so the patient has to compensate for the lack of movement by abnormally increasing the mobility elsewhere, often at the site of the symptoms. When considering shoulder problems, the therapist must examine the mobility of the thoracic and lumbar spine regions. Although shoulder movement has traditionally been described as a rhythmical combination of scapulothoracic and glenohumeral movement, shoulder mobility is affected by a decrease in thoracic extensibility as well as an increase in tho-

---

> **Box 21.3** Case study: growth, training and musculoskeletal pain
>
> A 15-year-old schoolgirl who commenced competitive fencing 6 months ago presented with low lumbar pain after her training regime increased. The pain was localized to the right side of the low lumbar region. Her range of motion was as follows: flexion to floor; extenstion a quarter of full range and painful; and lateral flexion and rotation both painful and restricted to the right. Her walking revealed a lack of pelvic control, with an increase in pelvic rotation to the right when the left leg was forward, indicating that the right hip lacked extension and external rotation. She exhibited an increase in mobility in the low lumbar area around the L4–L5 level. On examination, she had a full, pain-free SLR (90°), her thoracic spine was stiff and her anterior hip joint structures were tight on the right. Her low lumbar spine was tender on palpation, but if this area alone was the focus of treatment she would experience a return of her symptoms as soon as she commenced fencing again.

> **Box 21.4** Case study: structure at fault – not at site of symptoms
>
> A 19-year-old university student presented with right shoulder pain which was only experienced at the top of the tennis serve. The pain only occurred if she increased the pace of the serve. The shoulder had full pain-free motion; no symptoms were reproduced on shoulder testing, although the external rotation range improved after the containment test. When he was asked to demonstrate the first serve it became clear that it was lack of flexibility in the latissimus dorsi and thoracolumbar fascia, and stiffness in the lumbar and thoracic spines that were limiting his range of motion. Mobilizing the glenohumeral joint – the site of her symptoms – would be an inappropriate and ineffective treatment. Treatment must therefore aim to improve both the control of the hypermobile areas and the flexibility of the hypomobile areas to minimize the possibility of symptom recurrence.

---

racic kyphosis (Bowling et al 1986, Crawford & Jull 1991, Norkin & Levangie 1983). Bilateral shoulder flexion induces spinal extension, while unilateral shoulder flexion is accompanied by contralateral lateral flexion of the spine (Crawford & Jull 1991).

An increased thoracic kyphosis may limit shoulder flexion in one of two ways. Limited movement may be due to a lack of the thoracic spine's contribution to motion, or to an associated lack of scapulothoracic movement. An increased thoracic kyphosis is said to abduct the scapula and this can result in proximal shoulder girdle muscle imbalance (Ayub 1987). A downward rotated and protracted scapula could result in premature abutment of the humerus on the acromion and a reduced range of total shoulder flexion (Pope et al 1985). A downward and protracted scapula will also increase the resting length of some of the scapular stabilizers, such as the lower trapezius muscle, which acts with the serratus anterior and upper trapezius to rotate the scapula in an upward direction to increase shoulder girdle stability past 90° (Perry 1983). A decrease in activity of an elongated lower trapezius will alter the balance in the scapular force couple and often result in an increase in the onset and amount of upper trapezius activity. This results in a completely altered arm elevation pattern and may further predispose the individual to an impingement problem. A shoulder assessment is incomplete if the therapist has not examined the mobility of the thoracic spine. It is preferable if this examination is performed in sitting, so the mobility of the spine is not constrained by the treatment table. The sitting position also allows greater treatment options, e.g. the latissimus dorsi may be placed on stretch before the spine is mobilized (Fig. 21.6), or a straight leg raise may be added to increase the tension on the neural and fascial structures (this technique would be contraindicated if the patient had an acute lumbar disc problem). The flexibility of motion segments in the lumbar spine may be improved by an active passive manoeuvre in side-lying with the hips flexed to 90° and the lower legs straight (Fig. 21.7). The patient is instructed to push the buttock back into the therapist's arm, while the therapist resists the movement. After holding the contraction, the patient is

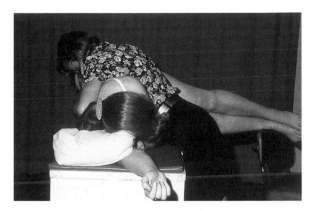

Figure 21.7 Improving the mobility of the neural, fascial and lumbar motion segments. This is performed in side-lying with the hips flexed to 90° and the lower legs straight.

asked to relax, at which time the therapist further flexes the lumbar spine. This is repeated several times.

Neural tissue can, after injury or because of rapid growth, become less extensible so that it inherently does not elongate sufficiently or it becomes adhered to an interface structure (Breig 1978, Butler 1991). A structure may be an anatomical one, such as a bone, ligament or muscle, or a pathological interface such as an osteophyte or oedema (Breig 1978, Butler 1991). C6, T6 and L4 are the approximate locations where there is minimal neural elongation relative to the interface structure (bone), so the neural tissue often becomes tethered in one or more of these regions. The lack of mobility can be a source of, or contribute to, an individual's symptoms. Similarly, at the posterior knee and the anterior elbow region, the neural tissue is relatively constrained due to the surrounding soft tissue and again more susceptible to injury and symptoms (Breig 1978). Lack of mobility of the neural tissue will interfere with smooth coordinated movement, especially when the neural tissue is put on stretch – such as the sciatic nerve and its branches when driving a car, or the median nerve when reaching to get something from the back seat of the car. Previous injury to another structure resulting in inflammation and scarring may mean that the nervous system loses its flexibility and is susceptible to giving symptoms in a region of the body remote from the original injury (Breig 1978, Butler 1991). For example, a previous Colles' fracture may cause a scarring of the median nerve. The loss of mobility of the median nerve can lead to restriction in range and pain in the shoulder or the cervical spine, and possibly even in the other arm, long after the fracture has healed. The case study in Box 21.5 illustrates a neural component to the patient's symptoms.

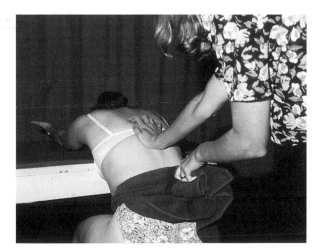

Figure 21.6 Mobilization of the thoracic spine in sitting with latissimus dorsi on stretch.

Box 21.5 Case study: neural tissue – a potent source of symptoms

A 21-year-old netball player presented with left inferior patellar pain, just medial to the patellar tendon. Twelve months previously, she had undergone an arthroscopic anterior cruciate ligament reconstruction, using the middle third of her patellar tendon. Rehabilitation progressed fairly well until 6 months ago when she was preparing to return to her sport. She then developed pain in the patellar tendon region, and was diagnosed as having patellar tendinitis. For 6 months, she rested from sport and treatment was directed at minimizing the tendinitis symptoms. This did not alleviate her pain. She could not run or jump without the pain becoming quite severe. She was now complaining of some stiffness in her mid-thoracic region. On examination, her pain was reproduced on squatting and jumping. She localized the pain to just medial to the patellar tendon. On palpation, distal to the arthroscope portal, there was a thickened, tender area. When the patient was examined in the prone position, her symptoms were reproduced by flexing the knee (90°) and externally rotating her tibia. Palpation of her thoracic spine, specifically T6 and T7, in this position increased her symptoms further. On further questioning, the patient volunteered that the lateral aspect of the knee had a slightly altered sensation.

The symptoms in this case were probably due to a scarring of the infrapatellar branch of the saphenous nerve as a result of the arthroscopy. Treatment was aimed at freeing the nerve. This was done locally at the site, by flexing the knee and externally rotating the tibia and stretching the soft tissue around the medial knee, and also from the site of the proximal tethering in the spine, by mobilizing the thoracic spine while the peripheral nerve was in the stretch position.

Although lack of mobility of an area often contributes to a patient's symptoms, it is not always passive limitation of range which causes dynamic hypomobility. For example, a hyperextended or locked-back knee in stance phase of gait will diminish the patient's shock-absorbing capability at the knee and increase the amount of instability at the pelvis. The knee has the range, but not the muscle control, for the loaded knee flexion. This results in a suboptimal gait pattern which places increased stress on other parts of the body. Pathological gait may therefore be viewed as an attempt to preserve as low a level of energy consumption as possible by exaggerated motions at the unaffected levels. There are six major determinants of gait that have been identified as being essential for the smooth 'translation of the body requiring the least expenditure of energy' (Saunders et al 1953):

- pelvic rotation
- pelvic tilt
- knee flexion
- hip flexion
- knee and ankle interaction
- lateral pelvic displacement.

When a person loses one of the determinants, compensation is reasonably effective, but loss of more than one component results in a less energy-efficient, more abnormal gait pattern. Loss of the control at the knee, however, proves to be the most costly (Saunders et al 1953). For the patient with insufficient knee flexion at stance, controlled practice of small-range flexion and extension movements in weight-bearing, followed by pelvic control work, would be required.

CONCLUSIONS

Faulty alignment and posture perpetuate many of the musculoskeletal problems seen in the athlete. The challenge for the clinician is to determine the factors contributing to the patient's symptoms. A comprehensive problem analysis is required, which involves examining the athlete's static alignment and dynamic activities, including the movements involved in the particular sport. An understanding of the sport and the effect the patient's alignment may have on the performance of that sport may help to minimize the many overuse and recurrent injuries seen in some athletes. Treatment should be directed towards minimizing the patient's symptoms, improving the flexibility of hypomobile structures – whether it be joint, muscle, neural or fascial tissue – and improving the dynamic control of hypermobile segments. Training must therefore be specific to limb position, joint angle and contraction type and force. As with all training, its success or failure depends on the amount of practice. The training must be simple, requiring minimal equipment so it is readily accessible to the individual and can be practised frequently. Individuals with faulty alignment must continue to maintain the dynamic control over the hypermobile segments for the rest of their athletic career, if they want to remain symptom-free in their sport.

REFERENCES

Adams M, Hutton W 1985 The effect of posture on the lumbar spine. Journal of Bone and Joint Surgery 67B: 629–635

Addison R, Schultz A 1980 Trunk strengths in patients seeking hospitalisation for chronic low back disorders, Spine 5(6): 539–544

Ahmed A M, Burke D L, Yu A 1983 In-vitro measurement of static pressure distribution in synovial joints – part II: retropatellar surface. Journal of Biomedical Engineering 105: 226–236

Andersson G B T, Ortengen R, Nachemson A 1977 Intradiscal pressure, intra-abdominal pressure and myoelectric back activity related to posture and loading. Clinical Orthopaedics 129: 156–164

Ayub E 1987 Posture and the upper quarter. In: Donatelli R (ed) Physical therapy of the shoulder. Churchill Livingstone, New York

Bartlet L, Storey M, Simons B 1989 Measurement of upper extremity torque production and its relation to throwing speed in the competitive athlete. American Journal of Sports Medicine 17(1): 89–91

Basmajian J V, De Luca C J 1985 Muscles alive. Williams & Wilkins, Baltimore

Bockrath K, Wooden C, Worrell T, Ingersoll C, Farr J 1993 Effects of patella taping on patella position and perceived pain. Medicine Science in Sports and Exercise 25(9): 989–992

Bose K, Kanagasuntherum R, Osman M 1980 Vastus medialis oblique: an anatomical and physiologic study. Orthopaedics 3: 880–883

Bowling R W, Rockar P A, Erhard R 1986 Examination of the shoulder complex. Physical Therapy 66(12): 1866–1877

Breig A 1978 Abnormal mechanical tension in the central nervous system. Almqvist & Wiksell, Stockholm

Brown L P, Niehues S L, Harrah A, Yavorsky P, Hirshman H P 1988 Upper extremity range of motion and isokinetic strength of the internal and external shoulder rotators in major league baseball players. American Journal of Sports Medicine 16(6): 577–585

Buff H, Jones L C, Hungerford D S 1988 Experimental determination of forces transmitted through the patellofemoral joint. Journal of Biomechanics 21(1): 17–23

Butler D S 1991 Mobilisation of the nervous system. Churchill Livingstone, London

Carr J, Shepherd R 1982 A motor relearning programme for stroke. Heinemann, London

Cerny K 1995 Vastus medialis oblique/vastus lateralis muscle activity ratios for selected exercises in persons with and without patellofemoral pain syndrome. Physical Therapy 75(8): 672–683

Conway A, Malone T, Conway P 1992 Patellar alignment/tracking alteration: effect on force output and perceived pain. Isokinetics and Exercise Science 2(1): 9–17

Crawford H J, Jull G A 1991 The influence of thoracic form and movement on range of shoulder flexion. In: Proceedings of the MPAA 7th Biennial Conference, Blue Mountains, New South Wales, Australia, p 154–159

Cushnaghan J, McCarthy R, Dieppe P 1994 The effect of taping the patella on pain in the osteoarthritic patient. British Medical Journal 308: 753–755

Dolan P, Adams M, Hutton W 1988 Commonly adopted postures and their effect on the lumbar spine. Spine 13(2): 197–201

Doucette S, Child D 1996 The effect of open and closed chain exercise and knee joint position on patellar tracking in lateral patellar compression syndrome. Journal of Orthopaedic and Sports Physical Therapy 23(2): 104–110

During J, Goudfrooij H, Keessen W, Crowe A 1985 Towards standards for posture. Postural characteristics of the lower back system in normal and pathological conditions. Spine 10(1): 88–87

Farfan H F, Cossette J W, Robertson G H, Wells V, Kraus H 1970 The effects of torsion on the lumbar intervertebral joints: the role of torsion in the production of disc degeneration. Journal of Bone and Joint Surgery 52A: 468–497

Fujikawa K, Seedhom B, Wright V 1983 Biomechanics of the patellofemoral joint. Part 1: a study of the patellofemoral compartment and movement of the patella. Engineering in Medicine 12(1): 3–11

Fulkerson J, Hungerford D 1990 Disorders of the patellofemoral joint, 2nd edn. Williams & Wilkins, Baltimore

Gilleard W, McConnell J, Parsons D 1998 The effect of patellar taping on the onset of vastus medialis obliquus and vastus lateralis muscle activity in persons with patellofemoral pain. Physical Therapy 78(1): 25–32

Goodfellow J, Hungerford D, Zindel M 1976 Patellofemoral joint mechanics & pathology, 1 & 2. Journal of Bone and Joint Surgery 58B(3): 287–299

Grabiner M, Koh T, Dragnich L 1994 Neuromechanics of the patellofemoral joint. Medicine and Science in Sports Exercise 26(1): 10–21

Gresalmer R, McConnell J 1998 The patella: a team approach. Aspen, MD

Hanten W, Schulties S S 1990 Exercise effect on electromyographic activity of the vastus medialis oblique and the vastus lateralis muscles. Physical Therapy 70: 561–565

Herbert R 1993 Preventing and treating stiff joints. In: Crosbie J, McConnell J (eds) Key issues in musculoskeletal physiotherapy. Butterworth-Heinemann, Oxford

Hickey D S, Huskins D W L 1980 Relation between the structure of the annulus fibrosus and the function and failure of the intervertebral disc. Spine 5: 100–116

Hides J A 1995 Multifidus inhibition in acute low back pain: recovery is not spontaneous. MPAA Conference Proceedings, 9th Biennial Conference of the MPAA, Gold Coast, Queensland, p 57–60

Hodges P, Richardson C A 1993 The influence of isometric hip adduction on quadriceps femoris activity. Scandinavian Journal of Rehabilitation Medicine 25: 57–62

Hodges P W, Richardson C A 1996 Inefficient muscular stabilization of the lumbar spine associated with low back pain. Spine 21(22): 2640–2649

Hooley C, McCrum N, Cohen R 1980 The visco-elastic deformation of the tendon. Journal of Biomechanics 13: 521

Howard J, Enoka R 1991 Maximum bilateral contractions are modified by neurally mediated interlimb effects. Journal of Applied Physiology 70: 306–316

Huberti H, Hayes W 1984 Patellofemoral contact pressures. Journal of Bone and Joint Surgery 66A(5): 715–724

Huberti H H, Hayes W C, Stone J L, Shybut G T 1984 Force ratios in the quadriceps tendon and ligamentum patellae. Journal of Orthopaedic Research 2(1): 49–54

Hungerford D S, Barry M 1979 Biomechanics of the patello-femoral joint. Clinical Orthopaedics and Related Research 144: 9–15

Ingersoll C, Knight K 1991 Patellar location changes following EMG biofeedback or progressive resistive exercises. Medicine and Science in Sports and Exercise 23(10): 1122–1127

Janda V 1988 Muscle and cervicogenic pain syndromes. In: Grant E R (ed) Physical therapy of the cervical and thoracic spine. Clinics in Physical Therapy 17. Churchill Livingstone, New York, ch 9

Jull G A 1986 Headaches of cervical origin. In: Grant E R (ed) Physical therapy of the cervical and thoracic spine. Clinics in Physical Therapy 17. Churchill Livingstone, New York, ch 11

Karst G, Willett G 1995 Onset timing of electromyographic activity in the vastus medialis oblique and vastus lateralis muscles in subjects with and without patellofemoral pain syndrome. Physical Therapy 75(9): 813–822

Kendall H O, Kendall F P 1968 Developing and maintaining good posture. Physical Therapy 48(4): 319–326

Koh T, Grabiner M, DeSwart R 1991 In vivo tracking of the human patella. Journal of Biomechanics 25(6): 637–643

Lieb F, Perry J 1968 Quadriceps function. Journal of Bone and Joint Surgery 50A(8): 1535–1548

Lyons K, Perry J, Gronley J, Barnes L, Antonelli D 1983 Timing and relative intensity of hip extensor and abductor muscle action during level and stair ambulation. Physical Therapy 63: 1597–1605

Mariani P, Caruso I 1979 An electromyographic investigation of subluxation of the patella. Journal of Bone and Joint Surgery 61: 169–171

Matthews L, Sonstegard D, Henke J 1977 Load bearing characteristics of the patellofemoral joint. Acta Orthopaedica Scandinavica 48: 511–516

McConnell J 1991 Fat pad irritation – a mistaken patellar tendonitis. Sport Health 9(4): 7–9

Merriam J L 1980 Engineering mechanics, vol 1. Statics. John Wiley, New York

Nachemson A L, Elfstrom G 1970 Intravital dynamic pressure measurements in lumbar discs. A study of common movements, maneuvers and exercises. Scandinavian Journal of Rehabilitation Medicine 1(suppl): 1–40

Norkin C, Levangie P 1983 Joint structure & function. F A Davis, Philadelphia

Nyland J, Brosky T, Currier D, Nitz A, Caborn D 1994 Review of the afferent neural system of the knee and its contribution to motor learning. Journal of Orthopaedic and Sports Physical Therapy 19(1): 2–11

Perry J, Glousman R 1990 Biomechanics of throwing. In: Nicholas J A, Hershman E B (eds) The upper extremity in sports medicine. St Louis, Mosby, p 725–750

Perry J 1992 Gait analysis. Slack Inc., McGraw-Hill, New Jersey

Perry J 1983 Shoulder anatomy and biomechanics. Clinics in Sports Medicine 2(2): 247–270

Petschnig R, Baron R, Engel A, Chomiak J, Ammer K 1991 Objectivation of the effects of knee problems on vastus medialis and vastus lateralis with EMG and dynamometry. PMR 2(2): 50–54

Pope M H, Bevins T, Wilder D G, Frymoyer J W 1985 The relationship between anthropometric, postural, muscular and mobility characteristics of males aged 18–55. Spine 10(7): 644–648

Powers C, Landel R, Sosnick T, Kirby J, Mengel K, Cheney A, Perry J 1997 The effects of patellar taping on stride characteristics and joint motion in subjects with patellofemoral pain. Journal of Orthopaedic and Sports Physical Therapy 26(6): 286–291

Radin E 1979 A rational approach to treatment of patellofemoral pain. Clinical Orthopedics and Related Research 144: 107–109

Reilly D, Martens M 1972 Experimental analyses of the quadriceps muscle force and patellofemoral joint reaction force for various activities. Acta Orthopaedica Scandinavica 43: 126–137

Rice M, Bennett G, Ruhling R 1995 Comparison of two exercises on VMO and VL EMG activity and force production. Isokinetics & Eokinetics & Exercise Sports Science 5: 61–67

Richardson C, Jull G, Toppenberg R, Comerford M 1992 Techniques for active lumbar stabilisation for spinal protection: a pilot study. Australian Journal of Physiotherapy 38(2): 105–114

Root M, Orien W, Weed J 1977 Clinical biomechanics, vol II. Clinical Biomechanics, Los Angeles

Sale D, MacDougall D 1981 Specificity of strength training: a review for coach and athlete. Canadian Journal of Applied Sports Sciences 6(2): 87–92

Saunders J, Inman V, Eberhart H 1953 The major determinants in normal and pathological gait. Journal of Bone and Joint Surgery 35A: 543–558

Sinaki M, Mikkelson B A 1984 Post menopausal osteoporosis: flexion versus extension exercises. Archives of Physical Medicine and Rehabilitation 65: 593–596

Souza D, Gross M 1991 Comparison of vastus medialis obliquus:vastus lateralis muscle integrated electro-myographic ratios between healthy subjects and patients with patellofemoral pain. Physical Therapy 71: 310–320

Sward L, Erikson B, Peterson L 1990 Anthropometric characteristics, passive hip flexion and spinal mobility in relation to back pain in athletes. Spine 15(5): 376–382

Taylor D, Dalton J, Seaber A 1990 Visco-elastic properties of muscle-tendon units. The biomechanical effect of stretching. American Journal of Sports Medicine 18: 300

Thiranagama R 1990 The nerve supply of the human vastus medialis muscle. Journal of Anatomy 170: 193–198

Voight M, Weider D 1991 Comparative reflex response times of the vastus medialis and the vastus lateralis in normal subjects and subjects with extensor mechanism dysfunction. American Journal of Sports Medicine 10: 131–137

Watson D H, Trott P H 1991 Cervical headache: an investigation of natural head posture and upper cervical flexor muscle performance. Proceedings of the MPAA 7th Biennial Conference, Blue Mountains, NSW, Australia

Winter D A 1982 Camera speeds for normal and pathological gait analysis. Medical and Biological Engineering and Computing 20: 407–412

Witvrouw E, Sneyers C, Lysens R, Jonck L, Victor J 1996 Comparative reflex response times of vastus medialis obliquus and vastus lateralis in normal subjects and subjects with patellofemoral pain syndrome. Journal Orthopaedic Sports Physical Therapy 24(3): 160–166

Yang J, Winter D 1983 Electromyography reliability in maximal contractions and submaximal isometric contractions. Archives of Physical Medicine and Rehabilitation 64: 417–420

Young J, Herring S, Press J, Casazza B 1996 The influence of the spine on the shoulder in the throwing athlete. Journal of Back and Musculoskeletal Rehabilitation 7: 5–17

Zussman M 1986 The absolute visual analogue scale as a measure of pain intensity. The Australian Journal of Physiotherapy 32(4): 244–246

Ageing and master athletes

22

Bone metabolism in ageing

Susan A. New   David M. Reid

KEY POINTS

1. Osteoporotic fractures occur in almost 1 in 3 white women and consume over £940 million of exchequer funds per annum.
2. Bone mass is under strong genetic control and reaches a peak in the third decade of life.
3. Age-related bone loss occurs in both sexes, but with a substantial increased rate of loss in the immediately postmenopausal years in women.
4. A complex interaction of genetic, hormonal, endocrine and environmental factors controls both attainment of peak bone mass and rates of loss, with genetic factors predominating in early life and environmental influences being greater in later years.
5. Strategies to prevent osteoporotic fractures need to be developed to maximize peak bone mass, reduce rates of perimenopausal bone loss and maintain bone mass in later years.
6. In addition to the benefits to skeletal health of stopping smoking and reducing excessive alcohol intake, weight-bearing exercise and nutritional supplementation may be particularly valuable in the young and elderly.

INTRODUCTION

Predisposition to poor bone health resulting in osteoporotic fracture is a major public health problem, the impact of which can be measured not only from the huge financial strain it places on health care resources, but also by the enormous suffering it causes to susceptible individuals. Furthermore, with the increasing life expectancy, the future health and economic impact of this condition is likely to be phenomenal.

Adult bone health is governed principally by two factors: firstly, the maximum attainment of peak bone mass, and secondly, by the rate of bone loss which occurs with ageing. Both aspects are determined by a combination of, and interaction between, genetic, hormonal, endocrine, nutritional and mechanical factors. Although genetic factors are believed to account for up to 75% of the variation in bone mass, modifiable factors such as nutrition and physical activity do have a role to play in the development of young adult bone health and the prevention of osteoporosis in later life.

OSTEOPOROSIS

Definition

The first description of osteoporosis appeared in France around 1820 by Lobstein, a pathologist, who defined it as 'deteriorated human bone'. He took the definition from the Greek element *osteon* and added 'porous' to it, thus osteoporosis literally means 'porous bone'. It was only in the 1940s however, that a more rigorous definition was applied by Albright, who described osteoporosis as 'a decreased production of osteoid by the osteoblast', and noted that the disorder was not one of abnormalities of 'calcium-phosphorus metabolism but of tissue metabolism' (Albright 1941). The last two decades have seen an enormous expansion in osteoporosis research, which has been mirrored by much debate as to its correct definition (Box 22.1). The more recent definition shifts the focus of attention from reduced bone mass alone to that of bone fragility, and reflects the growing recognition that bone weakness is related to poor structural quality as well as decreased bone mass.

However, the clinical significance of osteoporosis does not relate to bone mineral loss but to the associated fractures, affecting particularly the proximal femur (hip fractures), the spine (fractures of the vertebral body) and the distal radius (Colles' fracture). However, since prevention of fracture is much easier than treatment, osteoporosis has been defined on the basis of bone mineral measurements, as bone mineral density (BMD) is a major risk factor. Four general diagnostic categories in relation to the definition of

Box 22.1 Definitions of osteoporosis

'An age related disorder characterised by a reduced bone mass and an increase in susceptibility to fracture in the absence of other recognisable causes of bone loss.'
(*Consensus Development Conference 1984, 1987*)

'A disorder characterised by increased skeletal fragility due to decreased bone mass and to microarchitectural deterioration of bone tissue.'
(*Consensus Development Conference 1991, 1993, 1996*)

Table 22.1 Four general diagnostic categories for osteoporosis (WHO 1994)

Category	Definition
Normal	BMD or BMC no more than 1 SD below the mean for young adults
Low bone mass (osteopenia)	Value for BMD or BMC more than 1 SD below the young adult mean but not less than 2.5 SD below this value
Osteoporosis	Value for BMD or BMC 2.5 SD or more below the young adult mean
Severe osteoporosis (established osteoporosis)	Value for BMD or BMC more than 2.5 SD below the young adult mean in the presence of one or more fragility fractures

BMD, bone mass density; BMC, bone mineral; SD, standard deviation.

osteoporosis have been established (WHO 1994) (Table 22.1). Although problems still exist with the use of these categories, such as differences according to site and technique of measurement, equipment and reference population, the values provide universal standards for identifying populations who may be 'at risk' of future fracture.

Epidemiology

It is estimated that about 1.7 million hip fractures occurred worldwide in 1990 and lifetime risks are 17.5% in women and 6.0% in men (Cooper 1993). Approximately 50 000 hip fractures are believed to occur in British women each year. Vertebral fractures are more difficult to define since they tend to be asymptomatic, and perhaps only one-third come to clinical attention. However, recent UK data suggest that lifetime risks are 15.6% in women and 5.0% in men (Cooper 1993). Between the ages of 60 and 90 years, the occurrence of vertebral fractures rises 20-fold, and estimations of the annual number occurring in England and Wales range from 70 000 to 140 000, although clinically presenting fractures may occur in 40 000 women in the UK each year. The lifetime risk of a wrist fracture is 16% for women and 2.5% for men, and it is estimated that 50 000 distal forearm fractures occur in British women each year (Cooper 1993).

Implications for public health

Of all osteoporotic fractures, hip fractures most seriously affect mortality rates and are believed to be associated with an overall reduction in survival of 10–20%. Hip fractures are also the major contributor to the morbid burden posed by osteoporotic fractures in general. Fractures of the hip, spine and forearm result in affected women becoming more dependent in basic activities of daily living, with up to one-third of hip fracture victims becoming totally dependent and over half being unable to walk independently.

The economic costs of osteoporosis are difficult to assess since they include hospital care (both in- and outpatient), loss of working days, long-term nursing homes costs and medication. However, annual costs to the exchequer have recently been estimated at nearly £750 million for women alone, and around £942 million if the costs of treating male fractures are included (Dolan & Torgerson 1998).

As life expectancy in the developed world increases, the number of elderly individuals will also rise. The current figure of 323 million individuals over the age of 65 years is expected to be nearer 1555 million by 2050. Such demographic changes alone are likely to be paralleled by increases in the number of hip fractures from 1.66 million in 1990 to 6.26 million in 2050 (WHO 1994).

PATHOGENESIS OF OSTEOPOROSIS

Reduced bone mass is a major determinant of osteoporotic fractures, and results from either a reduced amount of bone attained at skeletal maturity or subsequent age-related bone loss. Attainment of peak bone mass is the most important variable before bone loss begins, but the rate of loss becomes increasingly important in later life. The adult skeleton is composed of two types of bone: cortical or compact (approximately 80%), which predominates in the shafts of the long bones; and cancellous or trabecular (approximately 20%), which is the major constituent of bones in the axial skeleton.

It is important to note that the bones differ in several aspects, including three-dimensional structure, surface-to-volume ratio and remodelling activity. Cancellous bone is more sensitive to changes in bone resorption, as its turnover is between three and 10 times more rapid than that of cortical bone (Compston 1990). The lumbar spine is estimated to contain approximately 66% of cancellous bone, and the femoral neck a combination of cortical and cancellous bone approximating 75 and 25%, respectively. In the forearm, the distal radius contains approximately 30% cancellous bone, with approximately 75% of cancellous bone at the ultradistal radial site.

Changes in bone mass with ageing

Peak bone mass

Throughout early childhood, bone mass increases linearly with skeletal growth. A rapid increase in density occurs during puberty, by as much as 40%, but is known to vary according to skeletal site. Bone density continues to increase for several years after the cessation of growth, until maximum bone mass is achieved. This is known as peak bone mass, and the age at which it is attained is believed to be during the third decade, although it is recognized to vary between the sexes and according to skeletal site.

Peak bone mass is known to be influenced by a combination of genetic (which would explain the familial clustering that tends to occur with osteoporosis), mechanical, nutritional and hormonal factors. Genetic influences are believed to account for 75% of the variation in peak bone mass, and environmental factors a further 25% (Flicker et al 1995).

Aged-related bone loss

Following attainment of peak bone mass, a gradual loss of bone occurs with ageing, which results in an increased risk of osteoporotic fracture. There is some controversy, however, as to when bone loss begins, the rate at which it occurs and the influence of the menopause upon bone loss rate.

In women, bone loss before the menopause is small (<1% per annum), accelerating in the immediate 5-year postmenopausal period to 1–2% per annum at most sites (WHO 1994).

Normal bone remodelling sequence

To maintain its integrity and mechanical strength, the adult skeleton is continually undergoing a process known as 'bone remodelling'. To enable this process to occur, a section of old bone is removed by a discrete series of cellular processes and is replaced by newly formed bone matrix which is subsequently mineralized. The surface area of cancellous bone is greater than that of cortical bone, even though it occupies only 20% of skeletal mass in the healthy adult skeleton. This higher surface-to-volume ratio causes remodelling disorders to affect cancellous sites earlier. Indeed, bone remodelling is known to occur at an annual rate of 25% in cancellous bone, but at only 2–3% in cortical bone (Dempster & Lindsay 1993).

A schematic representation of the bone remodelling sequence is shown in Figure 22.1. The sequence begins with bone resorbing cells (osteoclasts) migrating to, or differentiating at, the specific location on the bone surface to excavate a resorption cavity. This stage is known as activation. At completion, osteoclasts disappear and are replaced by bone-forming cells (osteoblasts) to fill in the resorption cavity. This is known as the reversal phase, where resorption switches to formation. The entire group of cells involved in the 'activation', 'resorption', 'reversal' and 'formation' process comprises a 'bone remodelling unit'. This sequence of events allows repair of bone and is one of the mechanisms involved for preserving bone mass and its architecture. In the healthy adult skeleton, the rate of bone resorption equals the rate of bone formation, a mechanism known as 'coupling', where no net loss of bone occurs.

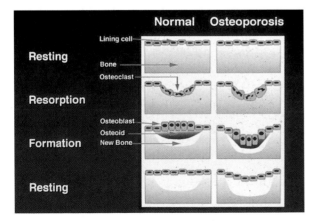

Figure 22.1 Schematic representation of the bone remodelling sequence.

Bone loss is greatest in the cancellous-rich axial skeleton during the early menopause years, which helps to explain the earlier occurrence of vertebral fractures compared with hip fractures. However, there is evidence to suggest that the rate of spinal bone loss slows by the age of 75 years.

Variations in rates of bone loss have also been shown to occur among women. There is some suggestion that 25–30% of the population are 'fast bone losers', and thus are particularly vulnerable to osteoporotic fractures in later life, although it may be that actual rates become equal when measured over a longer period of time.

Mechanisms of bone loss in osteoporosis

Mechanisms of bone loss in relation to the bone remodelling unit are complex, but there is now some agreement that loss is caused by an 'uncoupling' of bone formation from the previous resorption, meaning that the amount of bone formed is less than that resorbed, and is due to either increased bone resorption or decreased formation. Within the bone remodelling unit, this process is irreversible. There is also some evidence to suggest that an increase in the number of bone remodelling units on the bone surface will lead to an increase in the number of resorption cavities, and in turn increased bone loss.

The increased bone turnover in postmenopausal women is largely due to oestrogen deficiency. As the oestrogen concentration falls, osteoclasts become hyperactive (Dempster & Lindsay 1993). There is also some evidence to suggest that menopausal bone loss is due to a decrease in the functional capacity of osteoblasts, although the exact mechanisms remain largely unexplained.

The bone remodelling changes which occur with bone loss result in increased cortical porosity, decreased cortical width and reduced trabecular connectedness. This rapid disruption of the microarchitecture, as well as trabecular thinning, accounts for the increased incidence of crush fractures of the vertebrae and bone fragility at other sites.

Factors which affect bone loss

Several factors are responsible for age-related bone loss. Those that have been identified predominately affect bone turnover. Clearly premature oestrogen deficiency is one of the main factors leading to early menopausal bone loss. A reduction in parathyroid hormone secretion with age also occurs, leading to a reduction in 1,25-hydroxyvitamin D concentrations and, in turn, reducing calcium absorption. There is further evidence to suggest that the effects of oestrogen may be mediated by changes in the concentration of systemic and local factors such as calcitonin, interleukin-1 and -6, transforming growth factors (TGFB), prostaglandin E2, tumour necrosis factor, insulin-like growth factors I and II and nitric oxide (Ralston 1997). Oestrogen deficiency may cause excessive production of these, which in turn leads to enhanced osteoclast recruitment and accelerated bone loss.

GENETIC INFLUENCES ON BONE MASS

There is now much evidence for a strong genetic influence on adult bone density. This helps to explain the familial clustering which occurs with osteoporosis. Although no studies to date have shown that daughters of patients with vertebral or hip fractures are likely to fracture more frequently when compared with the general population, the importance of familial history has been inferred from studies of bone mass in identical and non-identical twins and in mother and daughter pairs. At the DNA level, recent studies have shown bone mass to be associated with polymorphisms of the vitamin D receptor gene (Morrison et al 1994), oestrogen receptor gene, and, more recently, the collagen I alpha 1 gene (Grant et al 1996), although consistency among populations has not yet been established. Further research work is required but there is some evidence to suggest that the effect of dietary calcium on bone mass is influenced by vitamin D receptor gene alleles. This would lend support to the view that dietary advice could be most usefully targeted at those individuals with genetic predisposition to either attainment of a low peak bone mass or increased perimenopausal bone loss.

MODIFIABLE RISK FACTORS FOR OSTEOPOROSIS

Lifestyle factors

A summary of risk factors for osteoporosis is shown in Box 22.2.

Body weight

There is much evidence suggesting a positive association between body weight and bone mass in pre-, peri-, and postmenopausal women. Recent data also

---

> **Box 22.2** Risk factors for osteoporosis
>
> *Lifestyle*
> - Smoking
> - Excess alcohol
> - Lack of weight-bearing exercise
> - Dietary deficiencies (see text)
>
> *Medical*
> - Low body weight
> - Hyperthyroidism
> - Hyperparathyroidism
> - Cushing's syndrome
> - Exogenous corticosteroid prescription

---

suggest that weight is protective against bone loss. Furthermore, data suggest that body weight is possibly more strongly related to postmenopausal bone loss than to the achievement of higher peak bone mass.

Several factors may explain the positive association between body weight and bone mass. These include increases in mechanical strain on the skeleton and increased peripheral oestrogen production. Adipose tissues are a likely site for the production of oestrogen from the adrenal precursors, and this mechanism is particularly important in the postmenopausal period.

Smoking

Evidence for the effect of smoking on bone mass and risk of fracture is conflicting. Smoking is often cited as a risk factor for osteoporosis, and there are several studies demonstrating that peri- and postmenopausal women who smoke have a greater risk and higher incidence of hip, vertebral and forearm fracture than nonsmokers, as well as having lower bone mass. However, some studies have found no association. A recent meta-analysis on the effects of smoking and fracture risk indicated that the deleterious effect of smoking on fracture events was more pronounced in older women than in either premenopausal or early postmenopausal women (Law & Hackshaw 1997), perhaps in part explained by a tendency to lower body weight in older smokers. Furthermore, there is some evidence in the literature to suggest that smokers have an earlier menopause than non-smokers.

Physical activity

General

More than a century ago, the German scientist Julius Woolf stated the theory which is now called Woolf's law: 'bone accommodates the forces applied to it by altering its amount and distribution of mass'. More recently, this concept has been refined to a general theory of bone mass regulation, known as the mechanostat model (Frost 1987). However, the mechanism whereby mechanical loading affects bone remains to be clarified, although the cells previously considered to be effete osteoblasts – osteocytes – may be important.

Without weight-bearing exercise, as in prolonged bed rest, loss of gravitational influences in space flight and prolonged saturation diving, bone loss will occur in the axial and appendicular skeleton. There is evidence supporting a positive relationship between physical activity, physical fitness, and muscle strength and bone mass at the wrist (in tennis players), lumbar spine and femoral neck sites, the latter specifically in runners.

Influence on postmenopausal bone loss

Studies investigating the influence of physical activity on postmenopausal women, and in particular its effects on bone loss, are conflicting. There is some evidence that physical activity can play a role in prevention of bone loss at and around the menopause, but exercise cannot entirely compensate for the decreased endogenous oestrogen levels during this time.

Exercise and risk of fracture

Very few data are available on the relationship between exercise and fracture. Lau et al (1988) reported a significantly decreased relative risk of hip fracture in individuals who undertook regular walking activities, while, in a parallel study, Cooper et al (1988) noted that increased daily activity was a protective factor against hip fracture in both sexes.

In summary, results are conflicting, but there is some evidence of a beneficial effect of exercise on bone mass. High loading exercise programmes appear to be more effective than low-intensity, long-duration exercises such as walking. Exercise may be of benefit in the prevention of osteoporosis, not only by increasing bone mass but also by increasing muscle strength, coordination, flexibility and balance, thus reducing the propensity to falls. However, the effect is likely to be small in most circumstances.

Nutritional factors

General

The influence of nutrient intake on bone health is still largely undefined. Whilst the importance of calcium intake in maximizing peak bone mass development and reducing peri- and postmenopausal bone loss has received considerable attention in the literature, few studies have examined the effects of other nutrients on bone health. A diet chronically low in calcium is likely to be deficient in a number of other important micronutrients (Reid & New 1997). As a consequence, the role that dietary intake has to play on development and maintenance of bone health requires considerably more research before any substantial conclusions can be drawn. Recent data certainly suggest that other micronutrients (such as potassium, trace elements and antioxidant vitamins) may be important to adult bone health (New et al 1997, 2000).

Calcium

Calcium is the most important mineral constituent of the skeleton, with approximately 1 kg present by the time we reach adulthood. Consequently, the role of calcium intake in the regulation of bone mass and its metabolism has been the centre of much controversy and, while there is now some agreement that calcium does have a positive influence on bone health, the debates have been intense and continue.

Relationship of calcium intake to bone loss. As shown in Table 22.2, virtually all published studies show little or no effect of dietary or supplementary calcium during the 5 years immediately following the menopause. Elders et al (1991) showed that supplementation with 1000 and 2000 mg/day of elemental calcium retarded bone loss in the first year of supplementation by reducing bone turnover, but did not prevent its loss in the second year. In women who were less than 5 years postmenopause, bone loss was rapid

Table 22.2 Calcium and bone health in peri- and early postmenopausal women: intervention studies

Authors	n	Age (years)	TSM (years)	Effect of calcium[a]
Aloia et al (1994)	101	52	3–6	Positive
Elders et al (1991)	248	49	1.2	Negative/ no change
Dawson-Hughes et al (1990)	67	54	<5	No change
Ettinger et al (1987)	73	51	<3	No change
Riis et al (1987)	36	49	<3	Positive
Nilas et al (1984)	103	—	<3	No change

TSM, time since menopause in years.
[a] Ca effect – overall effect of Ca supplementation.

Table 22.3 Calcium and bone health in late post-menopausal women: intervention studies

Authors	n	Age (years)	TSM (years)	Effect of calcium[a]
Dawson-Hughes et al (1995)	169	60	>5	Positive
Prince et al (1995)	168	63	>10	Positive
Reid et al (1995)	78	58	9	Positive
Reid et al (1993)	122	58	9	Positive
Nelson et al (1991)	36	60	11	Positive
Dawson-Hughes et al (1990)	67	—	>5	Positive

TSM, time since menopause in years.
[a] Ca effect–effect of Ca supplementation.

and not affected by a supplement of 500 mg/day of calcium (Dawson-Hughes et al 1990). In women who had been postmenopausal for 6 years or more, bone loss was significantly reduced with a daily intake of calcium of less than 400 mg. Further studies have shown that calcium supplementation reduces bone loss in older postmenopausal women (Table 22.3).

Vitamin D

Vitamin D can either be obtained from food or synthesized within the body by a process initiated by the action of ultraviolet light on the skin. 1,25-Vitamin D (calcitriol) is the active form of the vitamin, and 25-hydroxyvitamin D (D_3) is the principal storage and best clinical indicator of vitamin D status. The effect of vitamin D and its metabolites on bone is highly complex. It stimulates matrix formation and bone maturation, enhances osteoclastic activity, and may influence differentiation of bone cell precursors. Together with parathyroid hormone (PTH) and calcium, it regulates calcium and phosphorus metabolism, and promotes calcium absorption from the gut and kidney tubules. A deficiency of vitamin D reduces calcium absorption and increases PTH excretion, thereby stimulating osteoclastic activity and increasing bone loss.

There is now increasing evidence that vitamin D levels fall with age, vary with the season, being lower in the winter, and are inversely related to PTH, which itself has a seasonal variation.

Supplementation of 25(OH)D improves calcium absorption, lowers PTH levels and reduces wintertime bone loss in postmenopausal women (Dawson-

Hughes et al 1991), while menopausal bone loss is also inversely related to dietary intake of vitamin D.

Patients with hip fractures also have reduced vitamin D levels. Attempts to investigate the effect of vitamin D supplementation on prevention of hip fractures have been made, but with conflicting results. In a 4-year study by Heikinheimo et al (1992), substantial reductions in fractures of elderly Finns given a single injection of vitamin D (150 000–300 000 IU) were observed. In a study of 3270 institutionalized elderly supplemented with vitamin D plus calcium, a significantly reduced bone loss and fracture rate were demonstrated in the first year of treatment (Chapuy et al 1992). However, no differences were seen in Dutch elderly free-living patients supplemented with vitamin D (without calcium) (Lips 1995).

In summary, the abnormalities developing in the vitamin D endocrine system with increasing age make the elderly a vulnerable group. However, there is still uncertainty as to who will benefit from supplementation, what form and dosage of vitamin D are required, and whether additional calcium is needed.

STRATEGIES TO IMPROVE BONE HEALTH

While the genetic component certainly has a major role to play in the pathogenesis of osteoporosis, it has not yet been fully established which gene polymorphism is most crucial to adult bone health. Early indications were for the vitamin D receptor, but research has shown a lack of consistency among populations. Oestrogen receptor and collagen I alpha 1 gene polymorphisms provide exciting prospects, but there may be many more and further research is required (Ralston 1997).

Clearly hormonal and endocrine factors play an important role in bone health maintenance. In addition, physical activity has a positive influence on both, maximizing peak bone mass and reducing perimenopausal bone loss, but more population-based studies are required. More research is also needed on adolescent females engaged in high-intensity activities, who may be at an increased risk of osteoporosis in later life, due mainly to the high incidence of amenorrhoea and extremely low body weight.

On the nutritional front, our knowledge is limited due to the lack of consideration by scientists of nutrients other than calcium as potentially essential ingredients for optimum bone health. There are now some good data to show that high calcium intake is important to peak bone mass development and more studies are required, especially in the adolescent years, to see whether the effect is greatest with milk and milk products or with calcium supplementation alone (Cadogan et al 1997). There are consistent data showing an effect of increased calcium intake in women who are greater than 5 years postmenopause, but further work is required in women in the perimenopausal years and in men, as well as on its effectiveness in reducing fracture rates in the elderly. The effect of other micronutrients on perimenopausal bone loss requires substantially more attention (New 1999).

On a final note, if dietary manipulation is to be proved an effective preventive strategy, wider population-based lifestyle intervention studies are required, targeted possibly at those individuals who are genetically more susceptible to develop osteoporosis in later life.

CONCLUSIONS

1. Adult bone health is determined by genetic and environmental influences on peak bone mass, the genetic influences being strongly predominant in most studies. Maintenance of the skeleton has great importance in the prevention of fractures in later life, which may occur in as many as 1 in 3 women over the age of 65 years.

2. Increased rates of bone loss occur during the menopause and in the immediate postmenopausal period, with increasing bone resorption being the predominating influence, rather than a decrease in bone formation. However, the additional genetic and environmental factors which influence the hormonal control of bone loss require further research.

3. At present, it is considered that genetic factors influence bone health primarily by pre-programming peak bone mass, but future research may indicate that they also play an independent role in fracture occurrence and response of the skeleton to environmental and therapeutic influences.

4. There is a subtle interaction between hormonal and endocrine factors at all ages, with oestrogen being the predominant hormone in adolescence, early adult life and in the perimenopausal period. In the elderly, vitamin D becomes more prominent with its influences on parathyroid hormone and calcium metabolism.

5. Physical activity has a positive effect on bone health in children and may be a moderately strong influence on peak bone mass. While there is some role of exercise in the prevention of bone loss in later life, this may be relatively minor, although immobilization is a very important factor, inducing rapid and excessive bone loss.

6. Nutritional influences on peak bone mass and subsequent loss rates have concentrated on calcium and to a lesser extent vitamin D. Intake of calcium-containing foods in the young may have a positive influence on peak bone mass, but fruit and fibre may also have a positive effect. Supplementation of large doses of both calcium and vitamin D may reduce fracture rates in the elderly and perhaps in the late postmenopausal years. However, the influence of other micronutrients on the attainment of peak bone mass and subsequent loss, particularly potassium, magnesium, zinc and vitamin K, requires further study.

REFERENCES

Albright F 1941 Postmenopausal osteoporosis: its clinical features. Journal of the American Medical Association 116: 2465–2474

Aloia J F, Vaswani A, Yeh J K, Ross P L, Flaster E, Dilmanian F A 1994 Ca supplementation with and without hormone replacement therapy to prevent postmenopausal bone loss. Annals of Internal Medicine 120: 97–103

Cadogan J, Eastell R, Jones N, Barker M E 1997 Milk intake and bone mineral acquisition in adolescent girls: randomised, controlled intervention trial. British Medical Journal 315: 1255–1260

Chapuy M C, Arlot M E, Dubeouf F et al 1992 Vitamin D and calcium to prevent hip fractures in elderly women. New England Journal of Medicine 327: 1637–1642

Compston J E 1990 Osteoporosis. Clinical Endocrinology 33: 653–682

Consensus Development Conference 1991 Prophylaxis and treatment of osteoporosis. American Journal of Medicine 90: 107–110

Cooper C 1993 Epidemiology and public health impact of osteoporosis. In: Reid D M (ed) Baillière's clinical rheumatology. Baillière Tindall, London, p 459–477

Cooper C, Barker D J P, Wickham C 1988 Physical activity, muscle strength and calcium intake in fracture of the proximal femur in Britain. British Medical Journal 297: 1443–1446

Dawson-Hughes B 1995 Calcium supplementation and postmenopausal bone loss. American Journal of Clinical Nutrition 62: 740–745

Dawson-Hughes B, Dallal G E, Krall E A, Sadowski L, Sahyoun N, Tannenbaum S 1990 A controlled trial of the effect of Ca supplementation on bone density in postmenopausal women. New England Journal of Medicine 323: 878–883

Dawson-Hughes B, Dallal G E, Krall E A, Harris S, Sokoll L J, Falconer G 1991 Effect of vitamin D supplementation on wintertime and overall bone loss in healthy postmenopausal women. Annals of Internal Medicine 115: 505–512

Dempster D W, Lindsay R 1993 Pathogenesis of osteoporosis. The Lancet 341: 797–805

Dolan P, Torgerson D J 1998 The costs of treating osteoporotic fractures in the United Kingdom female population. Osteoporosis International 8: 611–617

Elders P J, Lips P, Netelenbos J C et al 1991 Ca supplementation reduces vertebral bone loss in postmenopausal women: a controlled trial in 248 women between 46 and 55 years of age. Journal of Clinical Endocrinology and Metabolism 73: 533–540

Ettinger B, Genant H K, Cann C E 1987 Postmenopausal bone loss is prevented by treatment with low-dosage oestrogen with calcium. Annals of Internal Medicine 106: 40–45

Flicker L, Hopper J L, Rodgers L, Kaymakci B, Green R M, Wark J D 1995 Bone density in the elderly: a twin study. Journal of Bone and Mineral Research 10: 1607–1613

Frost H M 1987 The mechanostat: a proposed pathogenic mechanism of osteoporosis and the bone mass effects of mechanical and non-mechanical agents. Bone and Mineral 2: 73–85

Grant S F A, Reid D M, Blake G, Herd R, Fogelman I, Ralston S H 1996 Reduced bone density and osteoporotive fracture associated with polymorphic Sp binding in collagen type Iα 1 gene. Nature Genetics 14: 203–205

Heikinheimo R J, Inkovaara J A, Harju E J et al 1992 Annual injection of vitamin D and fractures of aged bone. Calcified Tissue International 51: 105–110

Kanis J A, Pitt F A 1992 Epidemiology of osteoporosis. Bone 13: S7–15

Lau E, Donnan S, Barker D J P, Cooper C 1988 Physical activity and calcium intake of the proximal femur in Hong Kong. British Medical Journal 297: 1441–1443

Law M R, Hackshaw A K 1997 A meta-analysis of cigarette smoking, bone mineral density and risk of hip fracture: recognition of a major effect. British Medical Journal 315: 841–846

Lips P 1995 The effect of vitamin D supplementation in the elderly. Nutritional Aspects of Osteoporosis '94 Serono Symposia Publications. Raven Press, Rome, Italy, p 311–317

Morrison N A, Qi J C, Tokita A, Kelly L, Eisman J A 1994 Prediction of bone density from vitamin D receptor alleles. Nature 367: 284–287

Nelson M E, Fisher E C, Avraham Dilmanian F A, Dallal G E, Evans W J 1991 A 1-year walking program and increased dietary calcium in postmenopausal women: effects on bone. American Journal of Clinical Nutrition 53: 1304–1311

New S A 1999 Bone health: the role of micronutrients. Micronutrients in health and disease. British Medical Bulletin 55(3): 619–633

New S A, Bolton-Smith C, Grubb D A, Reid D M 1997 Nutritional influences on bone mineral density: a cross-sectional study in pre-menopausal women. American Journal of Clinical Nutrition 65: 1831–1839

New S A, Robins S P, Martin J C et al 2000 Nutritional influences on bone metabolism – further evidence of a positive link between fruit & vegetable consumption and bone health. American Journal of Clinical Nutrition 71: 142–151

Nilas L, Christiansen C, Rodbro P 1984 Calcium supplementation and postmenopausal bone loss. British Journal of Medicine 289: 1103–1106

Prince R P, Devine A, Dick I, Criddle A, Kerr D, Kent N, Price R, Randell A 1995 The effects of Ca supplementation (milk powder or tablets) and exercise on bone density in postmenopausal women. Journal of Bone and Mineral Research 10: 1068–1075

Ralston S H 1997 Osteoporosis (review). British Medical Journal 315: 469–672

Reid D M, New S A 1997 Nutritional influences on bone mass: a review. Proceedings of the Nutrition Society 56: 977–987

Reid I R, Ames R W, Evans M C, Gamble G D, Sharpe S J 1995 Long term effects of Ca supplementation on bone loss and fractures in postmenopausal women: a randomised controlled trial. American Journal of Medicine 98: 331–335

Reid I R, Ames R W, Evans R C, Gamble G D, Sharpe S J 1993 Effect of Ca supplementation on bone loss in postmenopausal women. New England Journal of Medicine 328: 460–464

Riis B, Thomsen K, Christiansen C 1987 Does Ca supplementation prevent postmenopausal bone loss? New England Journal of Medicine 316: 173–177

World Health Organization 1994 Assessment of fracture risk and its application to screening for osteoporosis. Technical Series Report 843. WHO, Geneva

FURTHER READING

Reid D M (ed) 1993 Baillière's clinical rheumatology. Osteoporosis. Baillière Tindall, London

Burckhardt P, Dawson-Hughes B, Heaney R P (eds) 1997 Nutritional aspects of osteoporosis. Proceedings of the 3rd International Symposium, Lausanne, Switzerland, May

Burckhardt P, Dawson-Hughes B, Heaney R P (eds) 2000 Nutritional aspects of osteoporosis. Proceedings of the 4th International Symposium, Lausanne, Switzerland, May

Stevenson J C, Lindsay R (eds) 1998 Osteoporosis. Chapman & Hall Medical, London

23

Musculoskeletal and functional changes following lower limb amputation: implications for exercise prescription

Anthony W. Parker
Jarrod D. Meerkin

KEY POINTS

1. The majority of lower limb amputations are performed secondary to ischaemic vascular disease.
2. The vast majority of amputations are performed on the over-60s, but younger amputees, who generally lose their limbs as a result of motor accident trauma or malignant bone tumour, present longer-term rehabilitation problems.
3. Lower limb amputation is associated with decreases in muscle size, muscle strength and bone mineral density of the residual limb.
4. Elderly amputees often present with other age-related problems that have important implications for function, physical fitness and exercise prescription.
5. Exercise to restore and maintain muscular function and to optimize functional status must be prescribed individually, taking account of, among other things, the patient's health, physical fitness, previous exercise history and socioeconomic status.

INTRODUCTION

The vast majority of lower limb amputations are performed secondary to ischaemic vascular disease, with transtibial (TT) outnumbering transfemoral (TF) amputations by 3 to 1 (Treweek & Condie 1998). Seventy-eight per cent of amputations are performed on patients over 60, and elderly individuals undergoing amputation of the lower limb for peripheral vascular disease (PVD) account for the majority of patients requiring rehabilitation services. Younger amputees most frequently lose their limbs as a result of motor accident trauma or malignant bone tumour and, although a minority, present longer-term rehabilitation problems.

Approximately 80% of the population over 65 years have at least one comorbidity, with arthritis (40%), impaired hearing and/or vision (20–30%), diabetes (10–15%), cardiovascular disease (15–20%) and cognitive disorders (<5%) being the most common (Leonard 1994). In addition, there are other age-related disorders that can result in alterations in muscle strength, cardiorespiratory endurance, flexibility, balance and coordination, thus making it difficult or impossible for the elderly amputee to continue to function independently. Consequently, amputees present with their own set of problems, which are often compounded by others associated with the elderly, such as reductions in muscular strength and endurance, decreased flexibility and limited mobility. Thus, PVD and age-related degenerative changes are not only important factors that distinguish the elderly amputee from the younger person with lower limb loss, but ones that, in themselves, have important consequences for physical fitness and exercise prescription. Exercise prescription is an individualized process that takes into consideration the patient's health, physical fitness, previous exercise history, socioeconomic status, motivation and amount of social support. These issues are particularly important for the amputee, as, without an appropriate exercise management plan, the chances of attaining success, in terms of achieving long-term physical fitness goals and optimal patient compliance and satisfaction, will be greatly reduced.

This chapter describes the changes which occur in musculoskeletal structures and their functional implications following lower limb amputation. This will provide the background for suggestions with respect to the prescription of activity for this population with the aim of minimizing disability associated with loss of a limb.

MUSCULOSKELETAL CHANGES FOLLOWING LOWER LIMB LOSS

A major goal of amputation surgery is to retain a functional stump which minimizes muscular atrophy following surgery. The achievement of this goal will depend on the reasons for the amputation and the opportunity to implement both short- and longer-term rehabilitation programmes. Victims of trauma often present with significant complications, which make retention of normal muscle function difficult, particularly for TF amputees where previously biarticular muscles are converted to a monoarticular function. Amputation of vascular origin may present with additional complications often affecting the contralateral limb, which may limit opportunities for rehabilitation. Irrespective of the cause of amputation, all patients will experience periods of immobilization and constraints with respect to regaining functional independence. For TF amputees, an important determinant of future muscle function is the surgical technique used to secure the resected muscles of the hip. There are no biomechanical data to indicate the most appropriate surgical technique required for efficient use of the residual limb in terms of muscle function and force development.

Following surgery, functional restoration will be determined by short- and longer-term rehabilitation procedures, the success of which will be influenced by factors such as age, previous condition, adherence and commitment to activity, and financial and social support. In the immediate postoperative period, the residual limb is bandaged and immobilized for a period of 7–14 days. Knowledge of the extent of muscular atrophy in lower limb amputees during this period is limited. However, evidence of the effects of immobilization in non-amputees suggests that the inactivity and immobilization associated with amputation are a major factor in muscle atrophy (Fig. 23.1).

Cross-sectional studies of longer-term amputees have shown significant muscle atrophy in the residual limb in comparison with the sound limb. These studies have generally measured the cross-sectional area (CSA) of the thigh or leg, and knowledge of the effects on individual muscles is more limited. In TT amputees, computed tomography (CT) showed that the CSA of the residual thigh was 86% of that of the sound thigh at the same level. There was also greater atrophy present in the quadriceps compared with the hamstrings (Renstrom et al 1983a).

Similar atrophy has been demonstrated for longer-term (average 9.4 years post-amputation) TF amputees aged 38 years (Jaegers et al 1995). Atrophy was calculated as the difference between the muscle volumes of the sound and residual hip muscles, determined from three-dimensional reconstructions of two-dimensional MR images. There was a 0–30% decrease in the volume

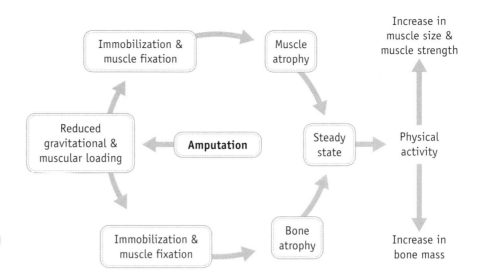

Figure 23.1 Sequence of events leading to muscle and bone adaptation following amputation.

of the intact muscles of the residual limb, but the previously biarticular muscles showed a greater atrophy of 40–60%. The degree of atrophy in each amputee was significantly related to the length of the residual limb, which highlights the functional importance of retaining as long a stump as possible. Using similar techniques, we have shown similar losses in volume and CSA of the hip musculature of TF amputees 16 years post-amputation (Meerkin & Parker 1999a).

Transfemoral amputees experience greater atrophy in hip musculature, with 20–30% reductions in the volumes of rectus femoris and biceps femoris, and 10–20% differences in psoas major, adductor longus, gluteus medius and gluteus maximus in comparison with TT amputees (Meerkin & Parker 1999a). These differences reflect the more extensive surgical reconstruction of the biarticular muscles of the TF amputee, and the consequent alteration of the biomechanical loading patterns that occurs.

Evidence of atrophic changes following amputation is confined to longer-term amputees, and there is little longitudinal data on the extent of these changes over time and the influence of any intervention (Fig. 23.2). A recent case study involving a 19-year-old TF amputee showed considerable atrophy 4 months postoperatively, with the previously biarticular muscles at the hip showing a muscle volume 47% smaller than that of the sound limb. The intact muscles demonstrated decreases up to 30% (Meerkin & Parker 1999b). Muscle atrophy continued to show marginal increases up to 10 months post-amputation before stabilizing and reaching a level consistent with that of longer-

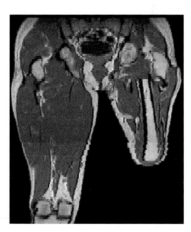

Figure 23.2 MRI showing a coronal section of the sound and residual thighs of a transfemoral amputee.

term amputees. In an examination of the CSA of four TT amputees over 30 weeks (Lilja et al 1998), a rapid decrease occurred (range 8–20%) in total CSA of the residual limb and of tibialis anterior between the second and sixth weeks. A more moderate decrease was found up to the 30th week, and triceps surae showed a similar response in the earlier period but increased in area by the 30th week. The different responses of individual muscles reflect the specific mechanical loading associated with each muscle, and indicate the complexity of neuromuscular interactions that occur following amputation.

The residual femur of the lower limb amputee is prone to bone demineralization well in advance of the bone loss that occurs as a normal consequence of ageing. The structure and composition of bone are influenced by the strains resulting from mechanical loading, and the more significant alterations to these parameters occur in situations of disuse and reduced loading. As shown in Figure 23.1, such decreases occur following amputation as a result of immobilization and reduced activity levels. In addition, there is decreased muscular loading on the bone, and an absence of direct loading on the femur imposed by the design of the prosthesis. In contrast, there may be increased loading on the contralateral limb structures as the sound limb bears a greater proportion of the load during gait. This increased loading is reflected in the maintenance of normal levels of bone mineral density (BMD), and in some cases accounts for the increased incidence of osteoarthritis in affected joints.

Bone densitometry studies of lower limb amputees are limited, but confirm the radiographical evidence of disuse atrophy in the residual femur. The BMD of the residual femoral neck of 48-year-old TF amputees was significantly reduced (32.7% decrease) when compared with their contralateral femur (Rush et al 1994). Bone mineral density of the L2–L4 vertebrae and femoral neck of the sound limb was similar to that of the control group. A recent retrospective analysis of British male war veterans with lower limb amputation indicated that TF amputees had greater bone loss than TT amputees (Kulkarni et al 1998). The greater use of the amputated leg by the TT group and the more normal muscle and biomechanical loading patterns may have contributed to maintenance of BMD levels. Similar results were demonstrated in an investigation of the BMD of eight long-term TF and eight TT amputees (Meerkin & Parker 1999a). The TF group showed a 30% reduction in BMD of the residual femoral neck, while there was no difference between the residual and sound femoral necks of the TT group.

Transtibial amputees retain the insertions of the hip musculature, which may allow for the normal transmission of compressive and tensile loading of the residual femur. No differences were found in BMD of the vertebral sites in the two experimental and control groups. The rate of bone loss following TF amputation occurs rapidly, and BMD has been shown to be 38.4% lower in the residual femur than in the sound femur at 4 months post-amputation (Meerkin & Parker 1999b). Further loss in the residual femoral neck (44.8%) occurred during months 4–7 post-amputation, following which relative stability was achieved (42.1%), with BMD levels similar to those of longer-term amputees (Meerkin & Parker, 1999a, Rush et al, 1994). As BMD is an important predictor of bone strength, any reductions in bone mass may increase the risk of fracture for the elderly amputee as a result of falling. Falls may result from the reduced stability experienced by amputees and altered gait mechanics, which may impose greater loads on the sound limb.

FUNCTIONAL CONSEQUENCES OF LOWER LIMB LOSS

Atrophy of the musculature of lower limb amputees limits their capacity to generate torque and to propel the prosthetic unit effectively without undue fatigue. The functional significance of such changes will depend on the level of amputation, the extent of surgical intervention, the length of immobilization, and the efficacy of rehabilitation procedures. The strength of the residual hip musculature of TF amputees is lower than that of the sound limb, and there is a relationship between strength loss and residual limb length (Jaegers 1993). For example, amputations in the distal third of the femur were associated with a torque reduction of 20–40%, while loss of two-thirds of the femur was associated with a torque reduction of 70–80%. Hip abductor torque of TF amputees increases with progressive hip adduction (Ryser et al 1988), which suggests that greater control and strength may be achieved if fitted with a socket that allows the residual limb to be pulled into adduction. The strength deficit found in the residual hip musculature of TF amputees may occur because of the difficulties faced by the surgeon when attempting to preserve as much of the length of the residual limb as possible and attaching resected muscles to optimize functional outcomes.

Not surprisingly, the major deficits in muscular strength of TT amputees are found at the knees, whereas the hip musculature shows similar values to those of the sound limb (Meerkin & Parker 1999a). Isometric and isokinetic knee flexor and extensor strength in the residual limb of TT amputees is significantly reduced (Renstrom et al 1983b). However, implementation of appropriate rehabilitation procedures may compensate for the initial deficits in strength, and improvements of up to 80% in knee extensor torque have been achieved following isokinetic strength training (Klingenstierna et al 1990). Such strength gains from resistance training are also critical to the maintenance of posture and gait and to general mobility. In addition, improvements in these functions will enhance amputees' compliance with their prosthesis and help to prevent secondary injury from compensatory overload of sound structures.

The aesthetic and mechanical efficiency characteristics of amputee gait are essentially a function of the anatomical and functional deficits outlined earlier, the limitations of the prosthesis prescribed, and the ability of the amputee to use the prosthesis. The complexity of amputee gait makes it difficult to account for the influence of each of these factors, but the combined effects of decreased muscle mass, strength, flexibility and cardiovascular fitness make ambulation extremely difficult for the young amputee and even more challenging for the elderly amputee. As such, walking aids are regularly prescribed to improve stability, decrease the amount of muscle activity required, and reduce the load on the weight-bearing joints. The elderly amputee walks at a reduced velocity primarily to compensate for the increased energy requirements of prosthetic ambulation, which occur as a result of a number of factors, both intrinsic and extrinsic to the amputee (Jaegers 1993).

Degenerative joint changes and associated pain may further compound this loss of mobility in the elderly amputee. The incidence of osteoarthritis is higher in elderly individuals with unilateral lower limb loss, with 83.3% showing radiographic evidence of degenerative joint disease compared with only 50% of elderly non-amputees (Lemaire & Fisher 1994). The mechanism responsible is most likely a combination of an increase in activity of the muscles of the non-amputated limb, to maintain stability, and an increase in the vertical knee ground reaction force that occurs during gait. In TF amputees, loadings through the prosthetic and sound limbs were approximately 40 and 60% of body weight, respectively (Lord & Smith 1984). In TT amputees, peak vertical force in the residual limb was reduced when compared with the sound limb (Powers et al 1994). Exercise programmes that place excessive loading through the sound hips and knees of lower limb amputees may exacerbate any predisposed problems associated with osteoarthritis.

A comprehensive review (Ward & Myers 1995) of the exercise performance of lower limb amputees found that TT amputees expend 9–33% more energy than able-bodied subjects when walking at the same speed. Elderly vascular TT amputees may exhibit greater energy expenditure and choose to ambulate at slower speeds than traumatic amputees. TF amputees expend 37–100% more energy than able-bodied amputees. As such, the development of the aerobic component of an exercise programme for lower limb amputees must take into account the increased metabolic cost of ambulation.

SPECIAL CONSIDERATIONS FOR ELDERLY INDIVIDUALS

The disability associated with amputation is further exacerbated for the elderly amputee by the morphological and functional changes that occur with increasing age. In particular, problems of prolonged inactivity prior to amputation and lowered functional fitness may complicate the rehabilitation process and limit compliance with the prosthesis and functional independence. Lower limb amputation in the elderly is associated with significant mortality and deterioration in function and living status. In a study of the functional independence of elderly amputees, 55% had decreased capacity and were often required to use a wheelchair and spend extended periods of time confined to bed (Frykberg et al 1998).

There is limited research to confirm the degree and extent of musculoskeletal and cardiovascular problems in the elderly amputee. Although not extensive, most research has involved younger subjects who have undergone lower limb amputation due to trauma. Thus, the complicating factors of ageing and, in most cases, peripheral vascular insufficiency, which distinguish the older from the younger amputee, have not been considered. Both ageing, with its association with increased comorbidity and degenerative changes in connective tissue, and contralateral limb vascular dysfunction have themselves been associated with lowered functional status and altered exercise response.

The incidence of chronic disease is considerably higher in the elderly, and is an important consideration when designing and implementing individualized rehabilitation programmes. For example, unilateral lower limb amputation as a result of vascular complications may occur in the presence of similar, though less severe, problems in the contralateral limb. This situation may have an adverse effect on the patient's functional status and is a common factor in the increased inactivity associated with this population.

The prevalence of severe coronary artery disease and associated cardiac complications in patients with severe peripheral vascular disease may be as high as 50% (Cutler 1986), and these patients need appropriate exercise testing before engaging in exercise training programmes. Ninety-three per cent of elderly amputees present with at least one associated problem such as coronary heart disease, hypertension, diabetes mellitus or a history of stroke. As such, their rehabilitation is not only concerned with mobility, but also designed to optimize medical outcomes by including and implementing ongoing assessment procedures to monitor cardiac status and general health risk. Exercise that promotes muscle hypertrophy and improvements in strength may be necessary as soon as the lower limb amputee is pain-free and can tolerate a greater intensity and frequency of activity. Consideration must also be given to the loads generated by the activity, as the osteopenia at the residual femoral neck may continue to worsen as the amputee ages. High-impact activities would not be appropriate for elderly amputees or for those amputees known to be at risk, such as postmenopausal women.

EXERCISE PRESCRIPTION FOR INDIVIDUALS WITH LOWER LIMB LOSS

As indicated earlier, the fitness of lower limb amputees is generally lower than that of able-bodied individuals of a similar age. At any given velocity, amputees have a higher rate of energy expenditure, reach their anaerobic threshold (AT) at slower walking speeds, and exhibit higher heart rates (HR) than do able-bodied individuals walking at the same speed (Czerniecki 1996). Fitness is further compromised in vascular amputees and in those with more proximal amputations. Deficits of 36.2 and 18.3% have been reported for peak $\dot{V}o_2$ and peak HR following a bout of one-legged cycling by lower limb amputees (Chin et al 1997). A study of young trauma-related amputees demonstrated an abnormal cardiovascular response during wheelchair ergometry (Kurdibaylo 1994), with significant increases in blood pressure and a decrease in stroke volume (SV). These adverse haemodynamic responses to exercise may reduce the exercise capacity of both young and elderly lower limb amputees. Muscle fatigue and pain were frequently cited as common reasons for termination of the exercise. However, despite these difficulties, modest improvements in cardiovascular function at submaximal exercise intensities were shown following the training period (Davidoff et al 1992).

Arm ergometry and one-legged cycling have been found to be safe and effective modes for testing and prescription of both young and elderly lower limb amputees (Chin et al 1997, Davidoff et al 1992). The strong correlation ($r = 0.82$) between peak $\dot{V}o_2$ and AT suggests that AT may be a suitable indicator of fitness and may be useful in the determination of exercise intensity for amputees. The sensitivity of AT at comparatively low exercise intensities enhances its potential for safe use with amputees with more limited exercise capacity. For example, arm ergometry performed at an initial intensity of 50% HR reserve for 15 min, five times per week, reduced submaximal HR and increased the duration of exercise and the maximum work output by 29.4 and 37.4%, respectively (Davidoff et al 1992). Box 23.1 provides some suggestions for appropriate cardiovascular training of lower limb amputees.

Implementation of resistance training following post-surgical immobilization has been associated with improvements in strength (Kegel et al 1981) and cardiovascular function (Kurdibaylo 1994). A 2-month period of strength training of young amputees increased SV and cardiac output by 26.6 and 27.7%, respectively, after a bout of submaximal wheelchair ergometry. There was an additional increase in working capacity and peak $\dot{V}o_2$, but these improve-

---

Box 23.1 Guidelines for cardiovascular training of lower limb amputees

Type	Frequency
Swimming	Maintenance – 3 days/week
Walking	Improvement – 5–7 days/week
Hydrotherapy	
Cycling	
Arm ergometry	

Intensity	Duration
50–85% maximum HR	15–60 min (depending on fitness level)
or	or
at a level set by AT	interval training
or other scale	

- Use standard exercises principles
- Determine exercise intensity from submaximal anaerobic threshold or use a simple Borg/pain/claudication scale rather than setting intensity relative to $\dot{V}o_{2\,max}$
- Interval training in the initial phases of exercise training may help to increase total exercise time
- Initiate exercise at a low intensity to avoid central and/or peripheral fatigue
- Condition both the residual and sound limbs to prevent muscle imbalance
- High repetitive loading of the prosthetic socket during cycling or running may cause pressure sores and/or skin irritation
- Avoid unaccustomed loading of the prosthetic socket as this may cause skin breakdown and injury
- If the amputee has a good residuum and good socket fit, bilateral activity such as walking may be recommended

ments may also be peripheral adaptations such as increased muscle strength and endurance resulting from the strength programme.

For TF amputees, resistance training which emphasizes the hip flexors and extensors of the residual limb may help to optimize gait efficiency (Jaegers 1993). Isokinetic dynamometers can be easily adapted to amputees, and their velocity can be adjusted to reduce the demands on the cardiovascular system, which is particularly important in elderly vascular amputees to avoid complications. Incorporation of resistance training exercises of the contralateral limb and trunk and upper limb musculature is also important to prevent muscle asymmetry and to improve postural stability. Strengthening of the upper limb musculature is necessary as most elderly amputees lack the upper limb strength to successfully use a wheelchair or other supportive devices such as crutches and walkers. Resistance training programmes must be progressive and must involve changes in volume and intensity, while always considering the cardiovascular condition of the lower limb amputee (Box 23.2).

Resistance training may compensate the loss of BMD associated with TF amputation. The maintenance of and/or improvement in BMD in those who participate in resistance training activities have been demonstrated in both young (Virvidakis et al 1990) and older individuals (Sinaki et al 1996). While such effects have not been investigated in amputees, the increase in strength and improvement in muscle coordination are also important for postural stability and the avoidance of fracture resulting from falls.

LIMITATIONS AND IMPLICATIONS

The lack of exercise intervention studies involving amputees limits precise definition of the most appropriate mode, duration, frequency and intensity of exercise for this population. Exercise for the lower limb amputee should involve the entire body without undue stress on the joints, and the intensity should be sufficient both to delay the onset of peripheral muscle fatigue and to provide adequate stress to the cardiovascular system. Exercises such as swimming or combinations of arm and leg ergometry may provide a sufficient conditioning effect. The intensity may be based on AT, and the exercises performed in 5-min training blocks for 15 min/day, 5 days each week.

Reduced flexibility due to contractures, immobility or connective tissue changes presents a problem for both elderly and younger amputees. Consequently, it is essential to incorporate activities and exercises which involve maintenance of full motion of proximal joints, with particular attention to the hip abductors and extensors, and the knee extensors.

In the acute phase of rehabilitation, emphasis is placed on the prevention of contractures and on the enhancement of mobility skills of daily living, while increasing muscle strength and endurance. Following this early period of clinical rehabilitation, amputees are trained in the use of assistive devices such as walking aids and wheelchairs. They are also retrained in making transfers and maintaining personal hygiene, so as to maximize their independence and enable them to live at home. Ideally, prior to discharge, amputees should be able to transfer from the wheelchair, demonstrate the proposed exercise programme, perform essential activities of daily living independently and, if possible, safely ambulate short distances independently with a walker or crutches. Opportunities for advice and supervision of activity programmes are more limited when the amputee returns home or is institutionalized. On their return home, many amputees believe that the loss of a limb restricts them from participating in recreational activities, and many fail to reach acceptable levels of fitness and functional capacity.

Box 23.2 Guidelines for resistance training of lower limb amputees

Type	Frequency
Machine weights	Two to three sessions/week
Free weights	Eight exercises
Therabands	One to three sets/exercise
	Eight to 15 repetitions/set

Intensity	Duration
60–80% 1 RM	–

- Upper body exercises as for an able-bodied individual
- Machine weights to increase loads on the lower limbs and safety
- Free weights for improvement of lower limb proprioception
- Unilateral and bilateral exercises, e.g. squats (Smith machine), single and/or double leg press
- Abdominal and low back exercises
- Hip stabilization exercises for mediolateral stability of the pelvis during stance
- Exercises that maintain and promote a full range of movement
- Avoid isometric exercises for those with peripheral vascular disease and/or hypertension

CONCLUSIONS

1. Lower limb amputation is associated with a decrease in muscle size, muscle strength and BMD of the residual limb.
2. The atrophic changes of the residual musculature are probably responsible for any decrements in muscular function and, together with the design of the prosthesis, influence the aesthetic, mechanical and physiological efficiency of amputee movement and gait.
3. The severity of the changes in morphology and function is influenced by the level of amputation, surgical fixation and the altered loading environment.
4. For the elderly amputee, these problems may be compounded by the high incidence of coronary heart disease along with other conditions such as PVD, diabetes mellitus, hypertension and osteoarthritis.
5. The prescription of aerobic and resistance exercise following amputation may help to restore and maintain muscular function and optimize the functional status of the lower limb amputee.
6. More longitudinal research is required to determine the morphological and functional consequences of amputation from the period beginning immediately post-amputation to the time when stability in the measures occurs. Such information may be applied to the design of appropriate interventions and to establish the most effective mode, frequency and intensity of activity for this population.

REFERENCES

Chin T, Sawamura S, Fujita H et al 1997 The efficacy of the one-leg cycling test for determining the anaerobic threshold (AT) of lower limb amputees. Prosthetics and Orthotics International 21: 141–146

Cutler B 1986 Prevention of cardiac complications in peripheral vascular surgery. Surgical Clinics of North America 66: 281–292

Czerniecki J M 1996 Rehabilitation in limb deficiency – 1: gait and motion analysis. Archives of Physical Medicine and Rehabilitation 77: S3–8

Davidoff G N, Lampman R M, Westbury L, Deron J, Finestone H M, Islam S 1992 Exercise testing and training of dysvascular amputees: safety and efficacy of arm ergometry. Archives of Physical Medicine and Rehabilitation 73: 334–338

Frykberg R G, Arora S, Pomposelli F B, LoGerfo F 1998 Functional outcome in the elderly following lower extremity amputation. Journal of Foot and Ankle Surgery 37: 181–185

Jaegers S M H J 1993 The morphology and functions of the muscles around the hip joint after a unilateral transfemoral amputation. PhD thesis, Proefschrift Groningen, Nederlands

Jaegers S M H J, Arendzen J H, de Jongh H J 1995 Changes in the hip muscles after an above-knee amputation: an anatomical study based on magnetic resonance imaging. Clinical Orthopaedics and Related Research 319: 276–284

Kegel B, Burgess E M, Starr T M, Daly W K 1981 Effects of isometric muscle training on residual limb volume, strength and gait of below-knee amputees. Physical Therapy 61: 1419–1426

Klingenstierna U, Renstrom P, Grimby G, Morelli B 1990 Isokinetic strength training in below-knee amputees. Scandinavian Journal of Rehabilitation Medicine 22: 39–43

Kulkarni J, Adams J, Thomas E, Silman A 1998 Association between amputation arthritis and osteopenia in British male war veterans with major lower limb amputations. Clinical Rehabilitation 12: 348–353

Kurdibaylo S F 1994 Cardiorespiratory status and movement capabilities in adults with limb amputation. Journal of Rehabilitation Research 31: 222–235

Lemaire E D, Fisher F R 1994 Osteoarthritis and elderly amputee gait. Archives of Physical Medicine and Rehabilitation 75: 1094–1099

Leonard J A Jr 1994 The elderly amputee. In: Felsenthal G, Garrison S J, Steinberg F U (eds) Rehabilitation of the aging and elderly patient. Williams & Wilkins, Baltimore, p 397–406

Lilja M, Hoffmann P, Oberg T 1998 Morphological changes during early transtibial prosthetic fitting. Prosthetics and Orthotics International 22: 115–122

Lord M, Smith D M 1984 Foot loading in amputee stance. Prosthetics and Orthotics International 8: 159–164

Meerkin J D, Parker A W 1999a Musculo-skeletal changes in lower limb amputees. Conference Proceedings of the Fifth IOC World Congress on Sports Sciences, 31 October– 5 November, Sydney, Australia

Meerkin J D, Parker A W 1999b Musculo-skeletal changes following a recent traumatic transfemoral amputation: a case study. Conference Proceedings of the Fifth IOC World Congress on Sports Sciences, 31 October– 5 November, Sydney, Australia

Powers C M, Torburn L, Perry J, Ayyappa E 1994 Influences of prosthetic foot design on sound limb loading in adults with unilateral below-knee amputations. Archives of Physical Medicine and Rehabilitation 75: 825–829

Renstrom P, Grimby G, Morelli B, Palmertz B 1983a Thigh muscle atrophy in below-knee amputees. Scandinavian Journal of Rehabilitation Medicine 15: 150–162

Renstrom P, Grimby G, Larsson E 1983b Thigh muscle strength in below-knee amputees. Scandinavian Journal of Rehabilitation Medicine 15: 163–173

Rush P J, Wong J S-W, Kirsh J, Devlin M 1994 Osteopenia in patients with above knee amputation. Archives of Physical Medicine and Rehabilitation 75: 112–115

Ryser D K, Erickson R P, Cahalan T 1988 Isometric and isokinetic hip abductor strength in persons with above-knee amputation. Archives of Physical Medicine and Rehabilitation 69: 840–845

Sinaki M, Wahner H W, Bergstralh E J et al 1996 Three year controlled randomised trial of the effect of dose-specified loading and strengthening exercises on bone mineral density of spine and femur in nonathletic physically active women. Bone 19: 233–244

Treweek S P, Condie M E 1998 Three measures of functional outcome for lower limb amputees: a retrospective review. Prosthetics and Orthotics International 22: 178–185

Virvidakis K, Georgiou E, Korkotsidis A, Ntalles K, Proukakis C 1990 Bone mineral content of junior competitive weightlifters. International Journal of Sports Medicine 11: 224–246

Ward K H, Myers M C 1995 Exercise performance of lower extremity amputees. Sports Medicine 20: 207–214

24

Exercise and cardiovascular health

Domhnall MacAuley

KEY POINTS

1. There is strong epidemiological evidence of a cardiovascular benefit to be gained from physical activity.
2. Inactivity is as important a risk factor for cardiovascular disease as the conventional risk factors of hypertension, smoking and elevated cholesterol.
3. Physical activity has a beneficial effect on lipids, lipoproteins and plasma fibrinogen, and there is a reduced risk of developing hypertension.
4. There is, however, a statistically increased likelihood of death while exercising.
5. The most common cause of sudden death in older people during exercise is coronary artery disease, although other less common causes include anomalous coronary artery, cardiomyopathies, cerebrovascular events and aortic dissection.
6. We should each be physically active, above the baseline activity level of daily living, to an equivalent calorie expenditure of 1000 kcal/week (4200 kJ), which equates to 30–40 min of moderate physical activity on 5–7 days/week.

INTRODUCTION

The are clear cardiovascular benefits to be gained from physical activity. There is also the paradox, however, that, although those who are active have lower all-cause and cardiovascular mortality, there is a statistically increased likelihood of death while exercising. For the middle-aged or older person, the commonest cause of sudden death during exercise is ischaemic heart disease, the very condition one is trying to prevent. Balancing the risks and benefits of physical activity to cardiovascular health is a major challenge as we encourage people to become active yet wish to avoid sudden cardiac death.

There is well validated epidemiological evidence of a lower death rate from myocardial infarction in those who are physically active. There are improvements in lipoprotein profile (Stefamick & Wood 1994) so that exercise is associated with lower levels of total cholesterol and triglycerides and raised HDL cholesterol. Further benefits are seen in the relationship with hypertension and with insulin resistance, which is particularly important as insulin resistance is the central factor associated with high blood pressure, glucose intolerance, hyperlipidaemia and obesity in Syndrome X. Exercise helps to reduce blood pressure (Van Baak 1998) and increases insulin sensitivity. There are also beneficial effects on blood clotting (MacAuley et al 1996) and it may aid weight loss (Blair 1993). Well documented physiological changes include a reduction in heart rate and an increase in end-diastolic volume.

The evidence of benefit from physical activity is of such magnitude that physical inactivity is considered to be as important a risk factor for cardiovascular disease as the conventional risk factors of hypertension, smoking and elevated cholesterol (American Heart Association Committee on Exercise 1992). Even more striking is the fact that the inverse relationship between physical activity, physical fitness and cardiovascular disease persists after adjustment for possible confounding variables and also that these benefits are seen in many different populations.

PHYSICAL ACTIVITY, PHYSICAL FITNESS AND CARDIOVASCULAR DISEASE

Much of the evidence for the beneficial effect of physical activity is from population studies of middle-aged men. In 1953, Morris et al compared the relative health and mortality of bus drivers with conductors, and those of postmen with their more sedentary office counterparts. They found that drivers of London's double-decker buses were more likely to die suddenly from coronary thrombosis than were conductors, and that government clerks suffered more often from rapidly fatal cardiac infarction than did postmen.

Although subsequent studies introduced information on confounding variables, demonstrating that the drivers were taller and heavier with higher cholesterol values (Oliver 1967), this was the first major epidemiological study of physical activity and heart disease. Later, they demonstrated that ischaemic myocardial fibrosis was more common in men with light occupations than in those with active and heavy occupations (Morris & Crawford 1958). In the Whitehall Study (Morris et al 1973), 16 882 male executive grade civil servants aged 40–64 years recorded their activities over a weekend. The relative risk of developing coronary disease in those who were vigorously physically active was about one-third of the value in those who were not. Morris et al followed this cohort of middle-aged civil service office workers for 8.5 years and found that men who had engaged in vigorous sports during the initial survey in 1968–70 had an incidence of coronary heart disease less than half that of their colleagues who recorded no vigorous exercise (Morris et al 1980). Further work (Morris et al 1990) confirmed a protective effect only in those who took part in vigorous exercise (again defined as energy expenditure of 7.5 kcal/min).

Similar evidence began to appear in the United States where Paffenbarger & Hale (1975) studied cardiovascular disease among cargo handlers, a group of very active of dock workers. Their high level of work activity was associated with a lower death rate and a lower incidence of sudden death. Paffenbarger et al (1984) also studied Harvard alumni and found that the risk of first heart attack was inversely related to the energy expenditure in adult life, so that the risk of first heart attack was 64% higher in men who expended less than 2000 kcal/week in leisure time physical activity. An important finding of this study was that current level of physical activity was the factor that demonstrated the protective effect and that exercise had to be continued to maintain this benefit. Those who had been sedentary as students but who became more physically active then gained low-risk status and the exercise benefit was independent of other lifestyle elements, including smoking, obesity, weight gain, hypertension and family history. In a follow-up study, Paffenbarger et al (1986) showed that not only did physical activity have a protective effect against coronary artery disease, but that deaths from all causes were significantly lower. For example, death rates were one-quarter to one-third lower among those expending 2000 kcal/week or more in leisure time physical activity, a level which corresponds to 5 h of brisk walking (7 km/h) or 3.5 h of running (9 km/h) per week. Mortality rates were significantly lower among the physically active, irrespective of the effect of hypertension, cigarette smoking, obesity or family history.

The beneficial effects of exercise were also documented in the Framingham Heart Study (Kannel et al 1986), where cardiovascular mortality and morbidity were inversely related to physical activity; it was also found that moderate activity may be sufficient for cardiovascular health. One of the methodological problems in cohort studies is that most examine the relationship between physical activity at baseline and long-term outcomes, but people change and baseline physical activity may not reflect long-term habits. A recent study (Kaplan et al 1996) demonstrated that taking into account changes in physical activity over the period of the study showed a stronger protective effect than when these changes were not considered, and that changes in other risk factors did not eliminate the protective effect of physical activity.

In their review of the beneficial relationship between physical activity and cardiovascular disease, Powell et al (1987) compiled a list of 121 articles representing at least 54 studies. To quantify the benefits of exercise, they selected only those studies that conformed to very strict criteria where incident cases could be separated from prevalence cases, and incidence rates, relative rates, odds ratios, mortality ratios or a regression analysis were possible. Forty-three studies met the selection criteria, and among these were 36 cohort studies, three mortality studies and four case–control studies, with information provided primarily about American and European working men. Using Bradford Hill's (1965) criteria, that associations should be consistent, strong, appropriately sequenced, graded, plausible, coherent and supported by experimental evidence, they reviewed the studies discussing bias, including confounding variables such as age, sex, blood pressure, smoking status and total serum cholesterol. They concluded that the inverse association between physical activity and incidence of coronary heart disease was observed consistently, especially in the better designed studies, was biologically graded, plausible and in keeping with existing knowledge and thus inversely and causally related to the incidence of coronary heart disease.

A subsequent meta-analysis by Berlin & Colditz (1990) confirmed the increased risk associated with inactivity in a sedentary population, concluding that physical inactivity was a risk factor for coronary heart disease of equal standing to the classical risk factors. There was a dose–response relationship between activity level and coronary heart disease, and although the studies used different measures of outcome, such as coronary heart disease incidence or death, myocardial infarction (MI) with or without sudden death, angina and congestive heart failure, the association between lack of physical activity and increased risk of coronary heart disease was consistent. The relative risk for both coronary heart disease and coronary heart disease death was 1.8, and higher-quality studies tended to show a higher relative risk. If the effect of exercise had been to reduce the severity of the event only, there would be a high relative risk for coronary heart disease rather than the reduced overall coronary heart disease incidence that was found. They concluded that lack of physical activity was a potentially modifiable risk factor that should receive greater emphasis.

THE ENERGY THRESHOLD

Morris et al (1973) believed that a minimum of 30 min of vigorous physical activity per day at an intensity of 7.5 kcal/min was needed for a reduction in cardiovascular mortality, equivalent to 225 kcal/day or 1575 kcal/week. Paffenbarger et al (1986) found a consistent gradient towards a lower death rate, from less than 500 to more than 2000 kcal energy expenditure per week, and that above 2000 kcal there was little additional improvement. In some studies (e.g. Magnus et al 1979), it was found that moderate exercise such as walking, cycling and gardening reduced risk and no improvement was gained by additional vigorous exercise, and that as little as 20 min of walking per day was satisfactory (Shapiro et al 1969). Others (e.g. Haskell 1986) believed that a threshold of 150 kcal/day of leisure time moderate energy expenditure was required to decrease coronary heart disease risk (for 7 days = 1050 kcal) and that mortality was reduced in those who expended greater than 1000 kcal/week in leisure time physical activity, equivalent to 30 min of moderate intensity activity (see also Slattery et al 1989).

The evidence for a continuous protective effect with increasing expenditure is growing (Ekelund et al 1988), as is the evidence that even moderate physical activity may offer some benefit (Blair et al 1989). It appears, therefore, that there is a gradient of risk across activity or fitness levels and that moderate levels of activity or fitness are associated with important and clinically significant reductions in risk (Blair et al 1992).

PHYSICAL FITNESS AND CARDIOVASCULAR DISEASE

Physical activity and physical fitness are not the same thing, but are often used interchangeably when discussing the cardiovascular benefits of exercise. Many studies look at patterns of physical activity using questionnaires, but few measure fitness and there are even fewer cohort studies which have related physical fitness, as determined by $\dot{V}O_{2\,max}$, to subsequent risk of heart attack. Of those that have studied physical fitness and cardiovascular disease, however, all have suggested a favourable long-term trend.

The difference between physical activity and physical fitness was explored by Sobolski et al (1987), who concluded that fitness level and not physical activity pattern was the independent protective factor and showed that physical activity was not always correlated with cardiovascular fitness, which was mostly determined by genetic factors. These findings have been confirmed by others (Ekelund et al 1988, Peters et al 1983, Sandvik et al 1993). The inverse relationship between physical fitness and cardiovascular mortality remains after adjustment for possible confounding factors (Blair & Kohl 1989, Blair et al 1995). While most of the early research was carried out in men, a recent large study of 40 417 postmenopausal women found that those who exercise regularly live longer than those who do not. The risk of death in follow-up decreased with the quantity of exercise taken, and those who exercised moderately only once per week had a 22% lower risk of death (Kushi et al 1997).

Recent evidence also shows that there is an inverse gradient of mortality rates in both men and women, so that those who are most active have the lower death rates (Blair et al 1996). One of the most interesting features of this high-quality cohort study was the inclusion of other cardiovascular risk factors and the ability to compare the relative importance of the different risk factors. For example, the relative risks of all-cause mortality due to low fitness (1.52) and cigarette smoking (1.65) were similar in men and women (2). This suggests that becoming fit would have a similar effect on mortality as stopping smoking. The corresponding relative risk in men for blood pressure and cholesterol was 1.3. A further important finding in this study was the protective effect of cardiorespiratory fitness against other risk factors in combination. Those in the high-fitness group with multiple risk factors had lower death rates than those in the low fitness group who had no other risk factors. This paper carries a very important message for the physician who is encouraging patients to exercise: even if subjects had risk factors including smoking, elevated blood pressure, raised cholesterol, obesity or a family history of heart disease, or a combination of these, they would all benefit from being physically active. Therefore, physicians should encourage all sedentary patients to become more physically active and improve cardiorespiratory fitness (Paffenbarger et al 1993).

LIPIDS AND LIPOPROTEINS

The benefits of physical activity may be mediated through changes in lipids and lipoproteins (MacAuley 1993), although it has also been shown that this association is reduced after adjustment for covariates (Superko 1991). In a meta-analysis of 66 training studies, however, the average exercising subject was found to have a reduction in total cholesterol, triglyceride and LDL cholesterol, with an increase in HDL cholesterol. The strength of association between physical activity and lipoproteins, especially HDL cholesterol, seen in cross-sectional, case–control and, to a lesser extent, intervention studies has not been seen in population studies (MacAuley et al 1996), and the differences in lipid levels seen across populations are much less than the differences seen between trained athletes and controls. The relationship may be mediated by apolipoproteins, the peptide components of the various lipoproteins which act as membrane receptor sites and cofactors for enzymes in lipoprotein metabolism. Patients with coronary artery disease have significantly lower apoAI, and apoAI and apoAII which are discriminants in atherosclerosis. It may be that apoAI is more important than HDL cholesterol in the development of coronary artery disease. ApoB is the apolipoprotein associated with LDL cholesterol. In cross-sectional studies comparing active and less active people and in training studies, there is a relationship with physical activity although there are inconsistencies in this relationship (Durstine & Haskell 1994). The changes in lipids and lipoproteins associated with physical activity do not appear to be seen in relation to physical fitness (MacAuley et al 1997). While poor physical fitness remains a strong independent predictor of coronary mortality, there is a lack of strength and consistency in the relationship between physical fitness, lipids and apolipoproteins, which suggests that the beneficial effect of physical fitness may be mediated through an alternative pathway.

HYPERTENSION

Epidemiological studies have shown a reduced risk of developing hypertension in those who are physically active (Gordon et al 1990, Montoye et al 1972). A meta-analysis of 25 longitudinal studies (Hagberg 1988) confirms the benefits of aerobic exercise in lowering elevated systolic and diastolic blood pressures. There is an inverse relationship between vigorous sports participation and hypertension (Paffenbarger et al 1991), and this relationship is independent of age, BMI and fasting plasma insulin levels (Reaven et al 1991). Those with low levels of physical fitness have a relative risk of 1.52 for the development of hypertension when compared with highly fit subjects (Blair et al 1984). In a controlled trial in those with high-normal blood pressure at baseline, an intervention which included exercise reduces the risk of developing hypertension (Stamler et al 1989), and can lower systolic blood pressure by 11 mmHg and diastolic blood pressure by 8 mmHg in those with mild to moderate hypertension (Hagberg 1988). Not everyone is in agreement with this, and a critical appraisal of Hagberg's meta-analysis pointed out the wide variability in outcome between the selected studies and suggested that the blood pressure-lowering effects may be at least partly dependent on gender, BMI, intensity of exercise, duration of training and initial blood pressure. Those who appear to benefit most are women, those with higher initial diastolic blood pressure, and those who exercise at low intensity and make a long-term commitment to exercise. While in general there is a negative relationship between activity and blood pressure, the MRFIT (Leon et al 1987) and British Regional Heart Study (Shaper & Wannamethee 1991) suggested a J-shaped curve. There are also guidelines for exercise prescription in hypertension (American College of Sports Medicine 1993).

FIBRINOGEN

Plasma fibrinogen is a well documented risk factor for cardiovascular disease (Kannel et al 1987, Wilhelmsen et al 1984) and there is evidence from cross-sectional and intervention studies of a relationship between physical activity and fibrinogen. Lower levels of fibrinogen associated with exercise may be a further factor in the reduction in deaths from cardiovascular disease in those who are most active. Cross-sectional population studies have shown lower fibrinogen levels in the most active groups in the Whitehall Civil Servants Study (Morris et al 1990), the Gothenburg Study (Rosengren et al 1990), the Caerphilly Prospective Heart Disease Study (Elwood et al 1993), the Scottish Heart Health Study (Lee et al 1990) in men aged 40–59 years, and in the ARIC study. In the Caerphilly Prospective Heart Disease Study (Folson et al 1991), fibrinogen was reduced by 0.24 g/L in the

most active tertile, and in the MRC study (Connelly et al 1992), those who were vigorously active had lower fibrinogen levels, even after adjustment for age, smoking, alcohol, body mass index and occupation. They believed that a relationship between physical activity and fibrinogen may help to explain the protective effects of physical activity, and in support of this hypothesis, pointed out that in Morris & Crawford's (1958) Necropsy Study there was no difference in the extent of coronary artery atheroma between those previously in occupations involving light, medium or heavy physical activity, but that there was a gradient of occlusion and large healed infarcts with physical activity at work. Ernst (1993) reviewed the relationship between physical activity and fibrinogen levels in longitudinal studies and found evidence of a reduction of about 0.4 g/L with physical activity, which would correspond to a substantial decrease in the risk of coronary heart disease. The strength of association is such that a 0.1 g/L difference in fibrinogen should correspond to a risk reduction of 15% (Meade et al 1986).

PHYSICAL ACTIVITY AND SUDDEN CARDIAC DEATH

On the debit side of the physical activity and health equation is the incidence of sudden cardiac death during exercise. Sudden death does occur, and physical activity may be the precipitating factor. The most common cause of sudden death in older people during exercise is coronary artery disease, although other less common causes include anomalous coronary artery, cardiomyopathies, cerebrovascular events and aortic dissection (Northcote & Ballantyne 1983, Ragosta et al 1984, Thompson et al 1994). The incidence of sudden cardiac death in exercise is 5.4 deaths per 100 000 or a rate of 1 death for every 18 000 men (Siscovick et al 1984, Thompson 1996). In Rhode Island there was an incidence of 1 death per 15 000 previously healthy joggers (Thompson et al 1982) and, interestingly, the relative risk of sudden death in joggers was seven times higher than in other activities. Physical activity may therefore be the trigger for myocardial infarction (Tofler et al 1996). In a study of 60 sudden deaths (59 men, one women) in squash (Northcote et al 1986), the cause of death was coronary artery disease in 51, valvular heart disease in four, cardiac arrhythmia in two, and hypertrophic cardiomyopathy in one, with two non-cardiac deaths. Some of these deaths could possibly have been avoided, because, of these, 45 had reported prodromal symptoms. Other studies show similar findings: coronary heart disease was the most common cause of death in a study of British soldiers (Lynch 1980); and of 21 sudden deaths in rugby football players and referees, 18 were due to coronary heart disease (Opie 1975). From this study, the estimated risk of sudden death was 1 in every 50 000 rugby playing hours and 1 in every 3000 referee hours. Such were the findings of Northcote's group, whose work on squash-related deaths is cited above, that they believe it is unwise to begin playing squash after the age of 40 years (Northcote et al 1983).

Physical activity has also been implicated as a trigger to myocardial infarction in the Multicentre Investigation of Limitation of Infarct Size study (MILIS), where 14% stated that they had recently undertaken moderate physical activity and 9% stated that they had been vigorously physically active (Tofler et al 1990). It is virtually impossible to identify control data, so one cannot calculate relative risk, but it seems likely that exercise was the trigger. The Myocardial Infarction Onset Study (MIOS) attempted to introduce a control group. In this study, 4.4% of those suffering a myocardial infarction reported heavy exertion within an hour of their infarction (Mittleman et al 1993), but they pointed out that it was unaccustomed heavy exertion that provoked the incident. A high level of general physical activity reduced the risk, so that the relative risk of suffering a myocardial infarction dropped from 107 among sedentary people to 2.4 in those who were active on five or more occasions per week.

In most cases, the cause of death is atherosclerotic plaque rupture and acute coronary artery occlusion, but there are a number of postulated means by which physical activity could trigger infarction. A recent review suggested three possible mechanisms (Tofler et al 1996). First, as suggested above, a sudden increase in blood flow may disrupt an atherosclerotic plaque; secondly, with prior endothelial disease, exercise may cause a vasoconstriction rather than a dilatation; or thirdly, in patients with coronary artery disease, the infarction may occur because of platelet activation, a reduced fibrinolytic response and reduced prostacyclin release (Khann et al 1975, Mehta et al 1983). In previously symptomatic patients, or those with known coronary heart disease, pathological changes do not suggest coronary artery occlusion or an acute myocardial infarction, and the most likely cause is ventricular fibrillation.

The risk of myocardial infarction is always greatest in the morning, so one may suggest that physical activity should be avoided in the morning, but evidence from post-coronary rehabilitation programmes suggests that this is not necessarily the case, and there is no evidence to confirm a greater risk for those who exercised in the morning in comparison with those attending in the afternoon (Murray et al 1993). In most cases, it is impossible to avoid sudden and unaccustomed exercise, but in any case, the absolute risk of such an event is low. The risk in cardiac patients is 1:60 000, compared with a risk of 1:565 000 per person-hour of vigorous activity (American Heart Association 1994).

Based on current evidence of the risk of sudden cardiac death during exercise, we can make some suggestions to those undertaking an exercise programme, and those who give advice on exercise. Participants should be advised about the relative risk, their individual risk, and the benefits of exercise. They should be advised about the type, intensity and pattern of exercise that would be most suitable. Those in a high-risk group should be advised about the importance of an appropriate warm-up, that exercise should be of moderate intensity, that they should also perform an appropriate warm-down and that they must seek medical advice if they have symptoms. Above all, they should avoid sudden vigorous unaccustomed exercise.

Since most sudden cardiac deaths in adults are related to coronary artery disease, it would seem reasonable to explore the possibility of screening asymptomatic adults prior to undertaking an exercise programme. A review of studies of screening programmes suggests that they are expensive and ineffective (Thompson 1996). The exercise stress test is insufficiently sensitive to detect those at risk, and at the same time has an unacceptably high false-positive rate. Surprisingly, a high-risk strategy is also limited. Furthermore, in a study of ambulatory electrocardiography (ECG) in squash players, it was not possible to identify those who would develop arrhythmia by history, examination or exercise electrocardiography (Northcote et al 1983).

The American College of Sports Medicine recommends selective screening of those at high risk, however, and in this group they include men over 40 years of age, women over 50 years of age, and individuals with more than one coronary risk factor. In addition, those with known coronary heart disease should undergo exercise testing before undertaking a vigorous exercise programme.

CURRENT LEVELS OF ACTIVITY

Levels of population physical activity throughout the Western world are low (MacAuley 1994). Stephens et al (1985) reviewed a number of surveys in the

United States and Canada and found that the young and those of high socioeconomic status were more active during leisure time. Overall, 20% were regularly vigorously active, 40% were active to a moderate level and 40% were sedentary, and the difference between the sexes was greater when the definition of the level of activity was most rigorous. Similarly, a national risk factor prevalence study in Australia (Bauman & Owen 1991) classified 32% as inactive, 54% as moderately active and 15% as aerobic. A further study (Owen & Bauman 1992) showed that those who were inactive were more likely to be older, less well educated and to have lower incomes. The *Allied Dunbar National Fitness Survey* (Sports Council 1992) in England was the most comprehensive study of activity fitness and related lifestyle in the British Isles. Overall, they concluded that 7 out of every 10 men, and 8 out of 10 women fell below the age-appropriate activity level necessary to achieve a health benefit, and that 1 in 6 were relatively sedentary. The proportion who were inactive increased with age and the proportion of the population who were vigorously active on a regular basis declined with age. Similar results were found in the Northern Ireland Health and Activity Survey (MacAuley et al 1994), so that after adjusting for possible confounding factors (such as age, BMI, alcohol intake, smoking, education, social class, diet, family history and religion), males aged 35–54 years were only half (0.48 times) as likely to be moderately active as those aged 16–34 years.

EXERCISE PRESCRIPTION

Having established that there is convincing evidence of a beneficial effect both directly on deaths from cardiovascular disease and on the risk factors associated with cardiovascular disease, and accepting that, although there is some risk, it is low, we can now explore how we can increase the population level of physical activity. Evidence for the benefits of exercise in cardiovascular disease have been integrated into public health policy and there have been a number of major position statements and policy statements issued by the ACSM and Surgeon General in the United States. The current exercise prescription for cardiovascular health is that we should each be physically active, above the baseline activity level of daily living, to an equivalent calorie expenditure of 1000 kcal/week (4200 kJ). This equates to 30–40 min of moderate physical activity on 5–7 days/week. Such guidelines seek to find a balance between the benefits to be gained from physical activity and the risks of

such activity. In addition, this prescription does not insist that the activities be of a sporting nature and accepts that the energy expenditure in many activities is equivalent. Exercise is generic and can include a wide variety of sport and leisure activities. One can achieve the exercise targets from an aggregate of many different activities, ranging from the traditional aerobic-type exercise such as running, swimming, cycling and rowing, to other sports such as recreational tennis, football and golf, and even to non-sporting activities around the home such as gardening or washing the car. Even more exciting is the suggestion that exercise need not be continuous and that the benefits can be accrued from a number of shorter bursts of activity rather than a single longer period (De Busk et al 1990).

It is important, however, for the individual doctor to appreciate that these are population guidelines and not an individual prescription. Those individuals who are fit, active and healthy should aim for a greater energy expenditure, while those who may be disabled or in whom this level of exercise would be a risk should seek more modest targets. The evidence supporting the benefits of exercise are dose-related, and the population guidelines are a pragmatic attempt to find general guidelines.

CONCLUSIONS

There is strong epidemiological evidence of the cardiovascular benefit to be gained from physical activity and the inverse relationship between physical activity, physical fitness and cardiovascular disease persists after adjustment for possible confounding variables. Inactivity is now considered to be as important a risk factor for cardiovascular disease as the conventional risk factors of hypertension, smoking and elevated cholesterol. There is evidence of a continuous protective effect with a greater reduction in risk with increasing expenditure and a gradient of risk across activity or fitness levels. Moderate levels of activity or fitness are, however, associated with important and clinically significant reductions in risk, so that exercise need not necessarily be vigorous to achieve some health benefit.

The cardiovascular benefits of exercise may be mediated through changes in risk factors. There are documented changes in lipids and lipoproteins with physical activity, although the effect is reduced after adjustment for covariates. There is also evidence from cross-sectional and intervention studies of a relationship between physical activity and fibrinogen. Moreover, those who are physically active are at reduced risk of developing hypertension.

There is, however, notwithstanding the overall cardiovascular benefits of an active lifestyle, a statistically increased likelihood of death while exercising, although the absolute risk of such an event is low. The most common cause of sudden exercise-related death in older people is coronary artery disease. The precipitating event is atherosclerotic plaque rupture and acute coronary artery occlusion, and physical activity may be the precipitating factor.

Those who wish to undertake an exercise programme should be advised about the type, intensity and pattern of exercise that would be most suitable. All participants should be advised about the importance of an appropriate warm-up, that exercise should be of moderate intensity, that they should also perform an appropriate warm-down and that they must seek medical advice if they have symptoms. High-risk participants, in particular, should avoid sudden vigorous unaccustomed exercise. The generic advice is that we should all be physically active, above the baseline activity level of daily living, to an equivalent calorie expenditure of 1000 kcal/week (4200 kJ). These guidelines are adopted by many population programmes and the cumulative energy expenditure equates to 30–40 min of moderate physical activity on 5–7 days/week. These exercise targets can be achieved from participation in many different activities including traditional aerobic-type exercise such as running, swimming, cycling and rowing. But the targets may also be achieved from other sports, such as recreational tennis, football and golf, and even non-sporting activities around the home, such as gardening or washing the car. Recent evidence suggests that exercise need not be continuous and that the benefits can be accrued from a number of shorter bursts of activity rather than a single longer period. Physical activity need not be of sporting nature and energy expenditure may be achieved in many ways.

Population guidelines may not be appropriate for every individual and personalized advice may be more appropriate depending on each person's current level of activity and risk profile. Those who are fit, active and healthy should aim for a greater energy expenditure, while less active individuals and those at high risk should seek more modest targets.

REFERENCES

American Heart Association 1994 Medical/scientific statement. Cardiac rehabilitation programmes. Circulation 90: 1602–1610

American Heart Association Committee on Exercise 1992 Circulation 86: 340–344

Bauman A, Owen N 1991 Habitual physical activity and cardiovascular risk factors. Medical Journal of Australia 154(1): 22–28

Berlin J A, Colditz A 1990 A meta-analysis of physical activity in the prevention of coronary heart disease. American Journal of Epidemiology 132(4): 612–627

Blair S N 1993 Evidence for the success of exercise in weight loss and control. Annals of Internal Medicine 119: 702–706

Blair S N, Goodyear N N, Gibbons L W, Cooper K H 1984 Physical fitness and incidence of hypertension in healthy normotensive men and women. Journal of the American Medical Association 252(4): 487–490

Blair S N, Kampert J B, Kohl H W III, Barlow C E, Macera C A, Paffenbarger R S, Gibbons L W 1996 Influences of cardiorespiratory fitness and other precursors on cardiovascular disease and all cause mortality in men and women. Journal of the American Medical Association 276(3): 205–210

Blair S N, Kohl H W, Barlow C E, Paffenbarger R S Jr, Gibbons L W, Macera C A 1995 Physical fitness and all cause mortality. Journal of the American Medical Association 273: 1093–1098

Blair S N, Kohl H W, Gordon N F, Paffenbarger R S 1992 How much physical activity is good for health? Annual Review of Public Health 13: 99–126

Blair S N, Kohl H W, Paffenbarger R S, Clark D G, Cooper K H, Gibbons L W 1989 Physical fitness and all cause mortality: A prospective study of healthy men and women. Journal of the American Medical Association 262(17): 2395–2401

Connelly J B, Cooper J A, Meade T W 1992 Strenuous exercise, plasma fibrinogen, and factor VII activity. British Heart Journal 67: 351–354

DeBusk R F, Stenestrand U, Sheehan M, Haskell W L 1990 Training effects of long versus short bouts of exercise in healthy subjects. American Journal of Cardiology 65: 1010–1013

Durstine J L, Haskell W L 1994 Effects of exercise training on plasma lipids and lipoproteins. In: Holloszy J O (ed) Exercise and sports science reviews. Williams and Wilkins, Baltimore, p 477–521

Ekelund L G, Haskell W L, Johnson J L et al 1988 Physical fitness as a predictor of cardiovascular mortality in asymptomatic North American men. The Lipids Research Clinics Mortality follow up study. New England Journal of Medicine 319: 1379–1384

Elwood P C, Yarnell J W G, Pickering J, Fehily A M, O'Brien J R 1993 Exercise, fibrinogen, and other risk factors for ischaemic heart disease: Caerphilly Prospective Heart Disease Study. British Heart Journal 69: 183–187

Ernst E 1993 Regular exercise reduces fibrinogen levels: a review of longitudinal studies. British Journal of Sports Medicine 27(3): 175–176

Folson A R, Wu K K, Davis C E, Conlan M G, Sorlie P D, Szklo M 1991 Population correlates of plasma fibrinogen and factor VII, putative cardiovascular risk factors. Atherosclerosis 91: 191–205

Gordon N F, Scott C B, Wilkinson W J, Duncan J J, Blair S N 1990 Exercise and mild essential hypertension. Recommendations for adults. Sports Medicine 10: 390–404

Hagberg J M 1988 Exercise, fitness and hypertension. In: Bouchard C, Shepherd R J, Stephens T, Sutton J, McPherson B (eds) Exercise, fitness and health. A consensus of current knowledge. Human Kinetics, Champaign, IL, p 455–466

Haskell W L 1986 The influence of exercise training on plasma lipids and lipoproteins in health and disease. Acta Medica Scandinavica 711: 25–37

Hill A B 1965 The environment and disease: association or causation. Proceedings of the Royal Society of Medicine 58: 295–300

Kannel W B, Belanger A, D'Agostino R, Israel I 1986 Physical activity and physical demand on the job and risk of cardiovascular disease and death: The Framingham Study. American Heart Journal 112(4): 820–825

Kannel W B, Wolf P A, Castelli W P, D'Agostino R B 1987 Fibrinogen and risk of cardiovascular disease. The Framingham Study. Journal of the American Medical Association 258: 1183

Kaplan G A, Strawbridge W J, Cohen R D, Hungerford L R 1996 Natural history of leisure time physical activity and its correlates: associations with mortality from all causes and cardiovascular disease over 28 years. American Journal of Epidemiology 144: 793–797

Khann P K, Seth H N, Balasubramanian V, Hoon R S 1975 Effect of submaximal exercise on fibrinolytic activity in ischaemic heart disease. British Medical Journal ii: 910–912

Kushi L H, Fee R M, Folson A R, Mink P J, Anderson K E, Sellers T A 1997 Physical and mortality in postmenopausal women. Journal of the American Medical Association 27: 1287–1292

Lee A J, Smith W C S, Lowe G D O, Tunstall-Pedoe H 1990 Plasma fibrinogen and coronary risk factors: The Scottish Heart Health Study. Journal of Clinical Epidemiology 9: 913–919

Leon A S, Connett J, Jacobs D R, Rauramaa R 1987 Leisure time physical activity levels and the risk of coronary heart disease and death. The multiple risk factor intervention trial. Journal of the American Medical Association 258: 2388–2395

Lynch P 1980 Soldiers, sport and sudden death. Lancet I: 1235–1237

MacAuley D 1993 Exercise, cardiovascular disease and lipids. British Journal of Clinical Practice 47: 323–327

MacAuley D 1994 A descriptive epidemiology of physical activity from a Northern Ireland perspective. Irish Journal of Medical Science 163(5): 228–233

MacAuley D, McCrum E E, Stott G et al 1997 Physical fitness, lipids and apolipoproteins in the Northern Ireland Health and Activity Survey. Medicine and Science in Sports and Exercise 29(9): 1187–1191

MacAuley D, McCrum E E, Stott G, Evans A E, Boreham C A G, Trinnick T 1994 The Northern Ireland Health and Activity Survey. HMSO, London

MacAuley D, McCrum E E, Stott G, Evans A E, Trinnick T T, Sweeney K, Boreham C A G 1996a Physical activity, physical fitness, blood pressure, and fibrinogen in the Northern Ireland Health and Activity Survey. Journal of Epidemiology and Community Health 50(3): 258–263

MacAuley D, McCrum E E, Stott G, Evans A E, Trinnick T T, Sweeney K, Boreham C A G 1996b Physical activity, physical fitness, lipids, apolipoproteins, and Lp(a) in the Northern Ireland Health and Activity Survey. Medicine and Science in Sports Exercise 28(6): 720–737

Magnus K, Matroos A, Strackee J 1979 Walking, cycling, or gardening with or without seasonal interpretation in relation to acute coronary events. American Journal of Epidemiology 110: 724–733

Meade T W, Mellows S, Brozovic M et al 1986 Haemostatic function and ischaemic heart disease: principal results of the Northwick Park Heart Study. Lancet 2: 533

Mehta J, Mehta P, Horalek C 1983 The significance of platelet vessel wall prostaglandin equilibrium during exercise induced stress. American Heart Journal 105: 895–900

Mittleman M A, Maclure M, Tofler G H, Sherwood J B, Goldberg R J, Muller J E 1993 Triggering of acute myocardial infarction by heavy physical exertion. Protection against triggering by regular exertion. Determinants of the Myocardial Infarction Onset Study Investigators. New England Journal of Medicine 329: 1677–1683

Montoye H J, Mentzer H L, Keller J B 1972 Habitual activity and blood pressure. Medicine and Science in Sports Exercise 4: 175–181

Morris J N, Chave S P W, Adam C, Sirey C, Epstein I, Sheehan D S 1973 Vigorous exercise in leisure time and the incidence of coronary heart disease. Lancet i: 333–339

Morris J N, Clayton D G, Everitt M G, Semmence A M, Burgess E H 1990 Exercise in leisure time: coronary attacks and death rates. British Heart Journal 63: 325–334

Morris J N, Crawford M D 1958 Coronary heart disease and physical activity at work. Evidence of a national necropsy survey. British Medical Journal ii: 1485–1496

Morris J N, Everitt M G, Pollard R, Chave S P W, Semmence A M 1980 Vigorous exercise in leisure time: protection against coronary heart disease. Lancet ii: 1207–1210

Morris J N, Heady J A, Rafle P A B, Roberts C G, Parks J W 1953 Coronary heart disease and physical activity at work. Lancet ii: 1053–1057, 1111–1120

Murray P M, Herrington D M, Pettus C W, Miller H S, Cantwell J D, Little W C 1993 Should patients with heart disease exercise in the morning or afternoon? Archives of Internal Medicine 153: 833–836

Northcote R J, Ballantyne D 1983 Sudden cardiac death in sport. British Medical Journal 287: 1357–1359

Northcote R J, Flannigan C, Ballantyne D 1986 Sudden death and vigorous exercise – a study of 60 deaths associated with squash. British Heart Journal 55(2): 198–203

Northcote R J, MacFarlane P, Ballantyne D 1983 Ambulatory electrocardiography in squash players. British Heart Journal 50: 372–377

Oliver R M 1967 Physique and serum lipids of young London busmen in relation to ischaemic heart disease. British Journal of Industrial Medicine 24: 181–188

Opie L K 1975 Sudden death and sport. Lancet I: 263–266

Owen N, Bauman A 1992 The descriptive epidemiology of a sedentary lifestyle in adult Australians. International Journal of Epidemiology 21(2): 305–310

Paffenbarger R S Jr, Hyde R T, Wing A L, Lee L M, Jung D L, Kampert J B 1993 The association of changes in physical activity level and other lifestyle characteristics with mortality in men. New England Journal of Medicine 328: 538–545

Paffenbarger R S, Hale W E 1975 Work activity and coronary heart mortality. New England Journal of Medicine 292: 545–550

Paffenbarger R S, Hyde R T, Wing A L, Hsieh C C 1986 Physical activity, all cause mortality, and longevity of college alumni. New England Journal of Medicine 314: 605–613

Paffenbarger R S, Hyde R T, Wing A L, Hsieh C C 1991 Physical activity and hypertension: an epidemiological review. Annals of Medicine 23: 319–327

Paffenbarger R S, Hyde R T, Wing A L, Steinmetz C H 1984 A natural history of athleticism and cardiovascular disease. Journal of the American Medical Association 252(4): 491–495

Peters R K, Cady L D, Bischoff D P, Bernstein L, Pike M C 1983 Physical fitness and subsequent myocardial infarction in healthy workers. Journal of the American Medical Association 249(2): 3052–3056

Powell K E, Thompson P D, Casperson C J, Kendricks J S 1987 Physical activity and the incidence of coronary heart disease. Annual Review of Public Health 8: 253–287

Ragosta M, Crabtree J, Sturner W Q, Thompson P D 1984 Death during recreational exercise in the state of Rhode Island. Medicine and Science in Sports Exercise 16: 339–342

Reaven P D, Barrett-Connor E, Edelstein S 1991 Relationship between leisure time physical activity and blood pressure in older women. Circulation 83: 559–565

Rosengren A, Wilhelmsen L, Welin T, Tsipogianni A, Teger-Nilsson A C, Wedel H 1990 Social influences and cardiovascular risk factors as determinants of plasma fibrinogen concentration in a general population sample of middle aged men. British Medical Journal 300: 634–638

Sandvik L, Erikssen J, Thaulow E, Erikssen G, Mundal R, Rodhal K 1993 Physical fitness as a predictor of mortality among healthy middle aged Norwegian men. New England Journal of Medicine 328(8): 533–538

Shaper A G, Wannamethee G 1991 Physical activity and ischaemic heart disease in middle aged British men. British Heart Journal 66: 384–394

Shapiro S, Weinblaff E, Franck C W et al 1969 Incidence of coronary heart disease in population insured for medical care (HIP): myocardial infarction, angina pectoris and possible myocardial infarction. American Journal of Public Health 59(suppl 2): 1–101

Siscovick D S, Weiss N S, Fletcher R H, Lasky T 1984 The incidence of primary cardiac arrest during vigorous exercise. New England Journal of Medicine 311: 874–877

Slattery M L, Jacobs D R, Nichaman M Z 1989 Leisure time physical activity and coronary heart disease death: The US Railroad Study. Circulation 79: 304–311

Sobolski J, Kornitzer M, de Backer G et al 1987 Protection against heart disease in the Belgian Physical Fitness study: physical fitness rather than physical activity. American Journal of Epidemiology 125: 601–610

Sports Council 1992 Allied Dunbar National Fitness Survey. Activity and Health Research. Sports Council American College of Sports Medicine 1993 Position stand on physical activity, physical fitness and hypertension. Medicine and Science in Sports and Exercise 25: i–x

Stamler R, Stamler J, Gosch F C 1989 The primary prevention of hypertension by nutritional-hygienic means: final report of randomised clinical trial. Journal of the American Medical Association 262: 1801–1807

Stefanick M L, Wood P D 1994 Physical activity, lipid and lipoprotein metabolism and lipid transport. In: Bouchard C, Shepherd R J, Stephens T (eds) Physical activity, fitness and health: International proceedings and Consensus statement. Human Kinetics, Champaign IL, p 417–431

Stephens T, Jacobs D R, White C C 1985 A descriptive epidemiology of leisure time activity. Public Health Reports 100: 147–158

Superko H R 1991 Exercise training, serum lipids, and lipoprotein particles: is there a change threshold? Medicine and Science in Sports Exercise 23: 677–685

Thompson P D 1996 The cardiovascular complications of vigorous physical activity. Archives of Internal Medicine 156: 2297–2302

Thompson P D 1996 The cardiovascular complications of vigorous physical activity. Archives of Internal Medicine 156: 2297–2302

Thompson P D, Funk E J, Carleton R A, Sturners W Q 1982 Incidence of death during jogging in Rhode Island from 1975 through 1980. Journal of the American Medical Association 2535–2538

Thompson P D, Klocke F J, Levine B D, VanCamp S P 1994 Task force 5. Coronary artery disease. Journal of the American College of Cardiology 24: 845–899

Tofler G H, Mittleman M A, Muller J E 1996 Physical activity and the triggering of myocardial infarction: the case for regular exercise. Heart 75: 323–325

Tofler G H, Stone P H, Maclure M et al 1990 Analysis of possible triggers of acute myocardial infarction. American Journal of Cardiology 66: 22–27

Van Baak M 1998 Exercise and hypertension. British Journal of Sports Medicine 31(1): 17–21

Wilhelmsen L, Svardsudd K, Korsan-Bengtson K, Larrson B, Welin L, Tibblin G 1984 Fibrinogen as a risk factor for stroke and myocardial infarction. New England Journal of Medicine 311: 501–508

25

Strength training in older individuals

Marc T. Galloway

KEY POINTS

1. Strength training is now generally recommended for physical activity and health, for both younger and older individuals.
2. Current evidence suggests that muscle retains its ability to respond to training throughout life.
3. Strength training can effectively restore many of the functional impairments observed in older individuals.
4. Resistance training has a beneficial effect on bone health, making it especially applicable to both pre- and postmenopausal women at risk of osteoporosis.
5. Exercise prescriptions are helpful for older individuals undertaking a resistance training regimen, and the volume of exercise should be individualized to avoid frustration and encourage compliance.

INTRODUCTION

The specific health advantages associated with a regular exercise program have been described in other chapters of this text and will not be elaborated on here. It appears, however, that the adoption of a regular exercise program may be beneficial in avoiding many of the functional declines observed with aging (Schilke 1991). Resistance training has been adopted for a variety of purposes over the last half of this century. In the late 1940s, Delorme introduced aggressive resistance exercises as a method to speed recovery following orthopedic injury (Delorme 1945). He later introduced the concepts of employing a low number of repetitions with a heavy weight to build muscle strength and the use of lighter weights with higher numbers of repetitions to produce gains in muscle endurance (Delorme & Watkins 1948, Gallagher & Delorme 1949). Resistance training has been routinely accepted as an adjunct to enhance sports performance. The benefits of strength training, however, are not restricted to the young or to athletes. Over last 10 years, the American Heart Association, the American Association of Cardiovascular and Pulmonary Rehabilitation, the American College of Sports Medicine (ACSM), and the US Surgeon General have all included strength training in their recommendations for physical activity and health (ACSM 1998a,b)

This chapter reviews the changes that occur within skeletal muscle as a consequence of aging and the potential benefits of strength training in older individuals. In addition, this chapter will seek to provide a stepwise approach to the formulation of an exercise prescription that integrates strength training into a balanced fitness program.

THE EFFECT OF AGING

Age-related muscle weakness is a major contributor to the high rate of injury observed in older individuals and to the functional limitations present in this population. The aging process is characterized by gradual decline in a variety of physiologic parameters that reflect progressive deterioration of biologic function. The loss of muscle bulk with accompanying decline in muscle strength and endurance have historically been perceived as inevitable consequences of aging. While declines in musculoskeletal function are apparent from observation of the general population, review of the performance records from world-class masters athletes suggests the preservation of significant function throughout life (Galloway & Jokl 1996). Indeed, considerable controversy remains with regard to the etiology and reversibility of age-related alterations in the musculoskeletal system.

Age-related changes in muscle

Muscle strength peaks between the second and third decades of life and does not begin to decline until the age of 50 (Hurley 1995). Between the ages about 50 and 70, a 12–15% decrease per decade in concentric muscle strength has been observed (Hurley 1995). In addition, a gender-based difference in the rate, degree, and mode of strength decline has been reported. Concentric

muscle strength in women has been reported both to peak and to begin its decline earlier than in men (Hurley 1995).

Loss of muscle mass is the major contributor to age-related strength loss (Porter et al 1995). Replacement of muscle by fibrous and adipose tissue has been reported (Rice et al 1989). Fat-free body mass has been shown to decrease by 15% between the third and eighth decades of life (Evans 1997). These changes reflect a loss of muscle protein in addition to infiltration of muscle by fatty tissue. Muscle atrophy that accompanies aging is primarily the result of a loss of muscle cells (Lexell et al 1983). There appears to be an equal loss of type I (slow twitch) and type II (fast twitch) muscle fibers with the aging process (Lexell et al 1988).

An alternative mechanism for aging atrophy is a reduction in the size of individual muscle fibers. Examination of whole muscle preparations show that the reduction in the size of type II fibers is greater than that observed in the type I fiber population, resulting in a greater percentage of the muscle being composed of type I fibers (Lexell et al 1983). The functional implications of these findings are a relatively greater reduction in the speed and power-producing properties of the older muscles.

PRINCIPLES OF STRENGTH TRAINING

The physiologic response of muscle to an exercise regimen is proportional to the volume of work performed by the muscle and varies in accordance with the manner in which the muscle is loaded. Endurance training involves prolonged cyclical muscle activity of the large muscle groups. Endurance exercises promote an increase in aerobic capacity, as reflected by increased mitochondrial density and increased myoglobin content, and induce a relative hypertrophy of type I muscle fibers. Only minor increases in whole-muscle cross-sectional area are seen in response to this form of exercise.

Resistance training exercise regimens are designed to overload muscle by utilizing weights in the 6–10 repetition maximum (RM) range. Progressive resistance training results in greater increases in muscle size, strength, and speed of contraction than do endurance programs. As might be expected, type II fibers are affected to a greater extent than are type I fibers with these types of exercises.

The degree to which a muscle can be trained is in part dependent upon the genetic potential of the individual. While this factor comes into consideration in training athletes, it is usually not an issue for older individuals whose strength levels do begin to approach their genetic potential. Significant gains in strength are apparent in response to a 6-month training program involving heavy resistance exercises in middle-aged and older men and women (Hakkinen et al 1988). Gains in strength were greater than would have been predicted by the changes in muscle bulk for the older age groups, suggesting that neural adaptations are an important mechanism for initial strength gains in this population (Hakkinen et al 1998). The loss of spinal motor neurons, and consequently motor units, occurs with increasing age, is one of the mechanisms leading to age-related strength loss, and can be detected as early as age 60 in men (Booth et al 1994). It is not known whether an aggressive resistance training program can alter this process (Booth et al 1994).

RESULTS OF RESISTANCE TRAINING
Muscle strength

Improvement in muscle strength has consistently been observed following the adoption of resistance training exercises by older people (Fiatarone et al 1990, Jette et al 1999, Krebs et al 1998). Studies of power lifters lend insight into the cellular mechanisms underlying resistance exercise-associated strength gains. The cellular response to resistance training includes increases in the cross-sectional area of muscle fibers and increases in the number of fibers expressing MHC IIA subunits (Kadi et al 1999). In addition, there are increases in the number of myonuclei, satellite cells, and fibers expressing early myogenesis following strength training (Kadi et al 1999).

Clinical studies examining strength gains in response to resistance exercise indicate that significant improvement in muscle function is not limited by age (Fiatarone et al 1990). Strength gains of up to 174% have been reported following resistance training in nursing home residents up to 96 years of age (Fiatarone et al 1990). Krebs et al (1998) reported an 18% improvement in lower extremity strength following 6 months of resistance exercises employing elastic tubing in a group of individuals whose mean age was 75. Similar strength gains have been demonstrated by other investigators utilizing low-resistance exercise with elastic tubing in elderly patients (Mikesky et al 1994).

Rehabilitation

Strength training has long been an accepted part of rehabilitation following athletic injury. Muscle weakness is a common complaint of patients with cardiac disease. Resistance training in this setting has been demonstrated to improve peak exercise performance and endurance. Cardiac rehabilitation employing resistance training correlates with improvement in indicators of emotional health as well as with overall quality of life measures (McCartney 1998).

Aggressive resistance exercises appear to hold promise in the treatment of patients with chronic low back pain. Lumbar extension exercises with the pelvis stabilized and employing one set of 8–15 repetitions are performed once a week to improve strength, muscle cross-sectional area, and vertebral bone density in patients with chronic low back pain (Carpenter & Nelson 1999). The positive response to this program was long-lasting and independent of diagnosis (Carpenter & Nelson 1999).

Resistance exercises are an important component in the treatment of osteoarthritis (McCubbin 1990). Muscle weakness as a result of pain and disuse is frequently found in patients with osteoarthritis. Exercise that focuses on the quadriceps muscles aids in alleviating many of the symptoms associated with knee arthrosis. Muscle weakness is also apparent in patients with hip arthritis and is reflected by a positive Trendelenburg sign. Exercises emphasizing strengthening of the hip abductor muscles can produce significant functional improvement of patients with hip arthritis as well as following total hip arthroplasty. Likewise, significant functional gains can be seen in the upper extremities of patients with glenohumeral osteoarthritis and concomitant rotator cuff pathology in response to a rotator cuff strengthening program. Explosive-type resistance training programs are beneficial in enhancing athletic performance. These types of exercise, however, are inappropriate in older individuals because of a higher risk of injury.

Functionality

The potential benefit of resistance training may be greatest for the frail elderly. These individuals suffer from the greatest degree of functional impairment and loss of independence. Exercise has also been shown to enhance postural stability, increase walking velocity, and reduce the potential for falls (Butler et al 1998, Smith & Gilligan 1991). Krebs et al (1988), in a randomized study of the effect of strength training on gait, found significant improvements in gait stability as reflected by peak side-to-side movement velocity and a more stable base of support. Even the relatively minor strength gains following the low-resistance exercise utilized in their study resulted in significant enhancement of gait stability in their subjects. Greater benefit may be realized using a more strenuous exercise regimen. Fiatarone et al (1990) reported a 48% increase in mean tandem gait speed in very old institutionalized individuals in response to an 8-week program of high-intensity resistance exercise.

EXERCISE PRESCRIPTION
Overview

The use of an exercise prescription is helpful for individuals undertaking a new program of resistance training. The exercise prescription, in general, involves the performance of a pre-participation inventory, the establishment of defined exercise goals, and specification of the type and volume of resistance training to be employed. The use of an exercise prescription is especially important for previously inactive individuals. In addition to identifying potential contraindications to exercise, the use of an exercise prescription encourages compliance through the establishment of a set of attainable goals. Moreover, the exercise prescription provides a useful guide for the gradual progression of exercise intensity, thereby reducing the risk of injury.

The pre-participation inventory

The initial step in the formulation of an exercise prescription is the needs assessment or inventory. The needs inventory takes into account the individual's age, health status and current level of fitness. The development of a resistance training program for the elderly must accommodate many specific limitations that are unique to this population (Barry 1986). These may include reduced cardiac reserve and a variety of coexistent cardiovascular conditions, such as hypertension and coronary artery disease. The overall functional status of the individual must also be taken into account before a particular exercise program is specified. Those who have been inactive for long periods may need to begin with a strengthening program which utilizes isometric muscle contractions, and then progress to isotonic exercises, in which resistance is provided by very light weights or elastic tubing. A history of prior musculoskeletal injuries and/or other disabilities must also be considered when designing an appropriate strengthening program for older people.

Establishing attainable goals

The establishment of realistic goals can greatly improve compliance with the prescribed regimen. Fitness goals should reflect the long-term objectives of the individual, in addition to defining a set of checkpoints that subjects can use to monitor their progress. Strict control of the rate of exercise progression in these individuals is essential for avoiding injury. The 10% rule is a useful guide in these individuals. Using this principle, the duration and/or intensity of a specific exercise is increased at no greater rate than 10% per week. The 10% rule provides a useful practical guideline for those individuals involved in non-supervised muscle strengthening activities. In general, older individuals should be directed to a program of generalized flexibility and strengthening before becoming involved in a specific sport.

Exercise volume

The musculoskeletal response to resistance training is dependent on the total volume of the work done by the muscle and the mode of muscle contraction. The number of sets and repetitions performed with the weight, as well as the amount of weight lifted determines the volume of work performed by muscle. Variation of the lifted load and the number of repetitions performed can influence the degree to which hypertrophy or endurance of the muscle is promoted. The most important variable in any resistance training program is the load applied to the muscle. By convention, loads are designated by the number of repetitions that can be performed throughout the full range of motion on the exercised joint. For example, the magnitude of weight that can be lifted only once through the full range of motion, utilizing good form, is designated the one repetition maximum (1 RM).

The greatest gains in muscle strength are produced by resistance exercises performed using a weight that can be lifted for 10 repetitions (10 RM range). Decreasing the amount of weight (to the 12–20 RM range) will promote increases in muscle endurance, but will provide a lesser stimulus to muscle hypertrophy. The intensity of a resistance workout correlates most closely in the development of muscle strength, whereas the total training volume appears most important for development of muscle endurance.

Resistance training protocols utilizing 1–6 RM loads are categorized as high-intensity. These protocols are most appropriate for younger individuals preparing for vigorous sports competition. Moderate-intensity exercises are exemplified by programs that stipulate loads in the 8–12 RM range. This level of strength training is appropriate for most middle-aged and older individuals. Resistance training programs that utilize a weight load in the 12–15 RM range are recommended for cardiac patients as well as elderly and more frail individuals (Feigenbaum & Pollock 1999).

A traditional weight training protocol involves exercises that are performed using three sets of exercise for 3 days a week. Pollock et al (1993) studied the effect of extension exercises on cervical strength and found larger improvements when exercises were performed twice a week as compared with once a week. More recently, the need for multiple sets of an exercise performed on a given day have come into question (Feigenbaum & Pollock 1999). A study examining strength gains in response to high-intensity knee extension exercises found no difference between regimens employing one or three sets of the exercise (Starkey et al 1996). Similarly, a 2 day/week training program has been shown to produce 80% of the strength gains seen in response to a 3 day/week program (Braith et al 1989). In addition, splitting a workout into two daily sessions of shorter duration may be advantageous for the development of muscle power and hypertrophy, as well as neuromuscular adaptations (Hakkinen & Kallinen 1994).

The amount of time required to complete an exercise program has a direct impact on compliance. Since compliance is a major issue with any exercise program, and especially so in middle-aged and older populations, a conditioning program that utilizes one set of repetitions is advantageous (Feigenbaum & Pollock 1999). On the basis of these studies, it would appear that the expected strength gains resulting from a protocol requiring only one set of repetitions would not differ substantially from those employing greater numbers of sets. Protocols requiring fewer numbers of sets may be associated with a reduced risk of overuse injury.

The frequency of exercise training (number of sessions per week) must be stipulated in the exercise prescription. Theoretically, any resistance training regimen must allow sufficient time for muscle recovery between sessions without promoting a detraining effect. Most resistance training programs for athletes build in 48 h of rest between sessions, thereby resulting in a 3 day/week weight-lifting protocol. Feigenbaum & Pollock (1999) noted a significant variation in response to the frequency of training between the major muscle groups, and concluded that a greater frequency of training correlates with increased strength gains.

Gillam (1981) studied the response to training using the bench-press exercise. He quantified differences in strength gains produced by regimens that employed training either 1, 2, 3, 4, or 5 days/week over a 7-week period. Strength gains were greatest in the 5 day/week group (41%). Those training 3 or 4 days/week experienced similar strength gains (32 and 29%, respectively) which were superior to the increases measured in subjects training only 1 or 2 days/week (20 and 24%, respectively) (Gillam 1981). While there appears to be a direct correlation between strength gain in the upper extremity and the frequency of resistance training, these data clearly indicate that a significant strength increase (20%) can result even from a single training session per week.

This finding has important implications when applied to older individuals. In this population, a 20% improvement in upper extremity function can translate into significant functional gains. The greatest gains in strength occur in response to moving from an active lifestyle to one that includes at least the weekly participation in resistance training activities. The frequency of training is of secondary importance for individuals whose primary goals are health-related and in whom time constraints are a significant factor. For individuals wishing optimal strength gain, a training frequency of at least 3 days/week is a more appropriate strategy for the extremities.

Fewer training sessions per week may be required for the postural muscles (Feigenbaum & Pollock 1999). In a review of the effect of training frequency on lumbar extension strength, Graves et al (1990) found no significant strength differences between protocols employing exercises once, twice or three times a week (40, 41 and 37%, respectively). Similar findings are seen in the neck region where a twice weekly training regimen confers similar strength gains to a three times a week protocol (DeMichele et al 1997). Both these training regimens produced results superior to those seen in a once a week training effort. There is some evidence to suggest that strength gains in the lumbar spine can be maintained using a significantly lower volume of work. Lumbar spine extension strength was noted to be maintained for up to 12 weeks by a program in which resistance exercises were performed as infrequently as once every 4 weeks (Tucci et al 1992).

When choosing the most appropriate training frequency, one must consider the specific needs and functional deficits of the patient. A 3 day/week training regimen affords the advantages of optimal strength gains while allowing adequate time for muscle recovery and lessening the risk of overuse injury inherent in more aggressive resistance training programs. A training frequency of twice a week is sufficient for muscles

---

Box 25.1 Resistance training exercises

- Chest press
- Shoulder press
- Triceps extension
- Biceps curl
- Leg extension
- Latissimus pull down
- Lower back expansion
- Abdominal curl/crunch
- Toe raise
- Leg curl

---

of the trunk and spine and only slightly less effective than more frequent training protocols for enhancing strength gains in the extremities. Recommendation of a twice a week training frequency encourages greater compliance and may be more acceptable for many previously inactive older individuals undertaking resistance training. Programs that employ resistance training twice a week can produce between 80 and 90% of the strength gains experienced by untrained individuals undertaking a more frequent lifting regimen (Graves et al 1994).

Resistance training is an important component of any comprehensive fitness program. Current recommendations by the American College of Sports Medicine are that one set of exercises targeting the major muscle groups be performed using a weight that can be lifted 8–12 times. Exercises should be performed 2–3 days/week. A sample of representative exercises is listed in Box 25.1. While additional sets of exercises employing a heavier weight can result in further strength development, the current recommendations provide for optimal strength development with the least amount of time investment. This is important, since resistance training programs lasting more than 60 min carry higher rates of drop-out (ACSM 1998a,b).

Exercise equipment

The type of resistance exercise will in part depend on the starting condition of the participant. Resistance exercise training can involve calisthenics, the use of variable-resistance machines, elastic bands, free weights, or plyometric exercises that involve the use of explosive movements such as jumping to enhance muscle action. For more frail individuals, strengthening should be initiated using exercises that employ isometric muscle contractions. The weight of the

extremity provides the resistance, thereby minimizing the risk of joint injury. As strength and coordination improve, elastic tubing can be introduced, and the joint can be exercised throughout its full range of motion.

Higher levels of conditioning can be achieved utilizing weights. Free weights are ideal for younger subjects as they require greater proprioceptive feedback and dynamic control than are necessary with more constrained variable-resistance machines that utilize weight stacks. Free weights, however, must be used cautiously in older populations. Older individuals who desire to use free weights should be advised to begin with very light weights and always to use a spotter.

Variable-resistance machines with weight stacks have been advocated as ideal for strength training in older individuals (Feigenbaum & Pollock 1999). In addition to lessening the risk of injury, these systems allow more gradual increases in the weight used and afford greater support and protection of the axial skeleton during the weight-lifting exercise (Feigenbaum & Pollock 1999). Variable-resistance machines have the additional advantage of allowing the performance of upper extremity strengthening exercises without requiring a tight grip on the bar. This is important in older populations, where forceful gripping has been shown to increase the risk of exercise-induced hypertension (Feigenbaum & Pollock 1999). Moreover, variable-resistance systems are more efficient, allowing the participant to move through the exercise regimen in less time.

CONCLUSIONS

Progressive resistance exercises hold promise for the treatment of many of the age-associated declines in musculoskeletal function. Increasing age is associated with a decrease in maximal oxygen utilization as well as reductions in fat-free body mass and muscle strength which lead to diminished endurance and impaired physical function. Reductions in gait speed and stability accompany these changes, and result in loss of independence and increased risk of injury. On a cellular level, elderly individuals demonstrate a relative loss of muscle fibers, with a relatively greater loss being present among the type II muscle fiber subtype. The metabolic potential of older muscle, however, remains relatively unaffected and current evidence would suggest that muscle retains its ability to respond to training throughout life.

Strength training can effectively restore many of the functional impairments that are observed in older individuals. Moreover, strength training is important for the maintenance of bone health. Osteoporosis and osteoporosis-related fractures are a major source of morbidity and mortality in the aging population. Progressive resistance exercises stimulate bone formation and peak bone density in young people. In addition, strength training retards age-related bone loss in older people. The effect of resistance training on bone health makes it especially applicable to both pre- and postmenopausal women who are at risk of osteoporosis.

The use of an exercise prescription is especially helpful for older individuals undertaking a resistance training regimen. In the initial assessment, the individual's current level of fitness and concurrent physical limitations are determined. Long-term and short-term goals are outlined at the start of a program to encourage compliance and to assist in avoiding injury. The response of any muscle to a strength training program is dependent on the volume of work performed in addition to the type of exercise (isometric, isotonic, etc.) and mode of muscle contraction (concentric or eccentric). In general, there appears to be an advantage in performing multiple sessions of resistance training per week.

Current recommendations for older individuals wishing to maintain generalized fitness is that one set of an exercise be performed 3 days a week for the major muscle groups utilizing a weight that can be lifted for 10–12 repetitions. Such a protocol appears to confer significant benefits while minimizing the risk of injury. The volume of exercise prescribed must be individualized to avoid frustration and encourage compliance. Gradual

progression of the volume of exercise should be encouraged at the onset of a resistance training program and is essential to avoiding injury.

REFERENCES

American College of Sports Medicine 1998 American College of Sports Medicine Position Stand. Exercise and physical activity for older adults. Medicine and Science in Sports Exercise 30(6): 992–1008

American College of Sports Medicine 1998 American College of Sports Medicine Position Stand. The recommended quantity and quality of exercise for developing and maintaining cardiorespiratory and muscular fitness, and flexibility in healthy adults. Medicine and Science in Sports Exercise 30(6): 975–991

Barry H C 1986 Exercise prescriptions for the elderly. American Family Physician 34(3): 155–162

Booth F W, Weeden S H et al 1994 Effect of aging on human skeletal muscle and motor function. Medicine and Science in Sports Exercise 26(5): 556–560

Braith R W, Graves J E et al 1989 Comparison of 2 vs 3 days/week of variable resistance training during 10- and 18-week programs. International Journal of Sports Medicine 10(6): 450–454

Butler R N, Davis R et al 1998 Physical fitness: benefits of exercise for the older patient. 2. Geriatrics 53(10): 46, 49–52, 61–62

Carpenter D M, Nelson B W 1999 Low back strengthening for the prevention and treatment of low back pain. Medicine and Science in Sports Exercise 31(1): 18–24

Delorme T L 1945 Restoration of muscle power by heavy resistance exercise. Journal of Bone and Joint Surgery 27: 645–667

Delorme T L, Watkins A L 1948 Techniques of progressive resistance exercise. Archives of Physical Medicine 29: 263–273

DeMichele P L, Pollock M L et al 1997 Isometric torso rotation strength: effect of training frequency on its development. Archives of Physical Medicine and Rehabilitation 78(1): 64–69

Evans W 1997 Functional and metabolic consequences of sarcopenia. Journal of Nutrition 127(suppl 5): 998–1003S

Feigenbaum M S, Pollock M L 1999 Prescription of resistance training for health and disease. Medicine and Science in Sports Exercise 31(1): 38–45

Fiatarone M A, Marks E C et al 1990 High-intensity strength training in nonagenarians. Effects on skeletal muscle. Journal of the American Medical Association 263(22): 3029–3034

Gallagher J, Delorme T 1949 The use of the technique of progressive resistance exercise in adolescence. Journal of Bone and Joint Surgery 31-a: 847–858

Galloway M, Jokl P 1996 Age and sports participation: the effect of aging on muscle function and athletic performance. Sports Medicine and Arthroscopy Review 4: 221–234

Gillam G M 1981 Effects of frequency of weight training on muscle strength enhancement. Journal of Sports Medicine 21: 432–436

Graves J E, Pollock M L et al 1994 Exercise, age, and skeletal muscle function. Southern Medical Journal 87(5): S17–22

Graves J E, Pollock M L et al 1990 Effect of training frequency and specificity on isometric lumbar extension strength. Spine 15(6): 504–509

Hakkinen K, Kallinen M 1994 Distribution of strength training volume into one or two daily sessions and neuromuscular adaptations in female athletes. Electromyography in Clinical Neurophysiology 34(2): 117–124

Hakkinen K, Kallinen M et al 1998 Changes in agonist-antagonist EMG, muscle CSA, and force during strength training in middle-aged and older people. Journal of Applied Physiology 84(4): 1341–1349

Hurley B F 1995 Age, gender, and muscular strength. Journal of Gerontology Part A: Biological Sciences, Medical Sciences 50: 41–44

Jette A M, Lachman M et al 1999 Exercise – it's never too late: the strong-for-life program. American Journal of Public Health 89(1): 66–72

Kadi F, Eriksson A et al 1999 Cellular adaptation of the trapezius muscle in strength-trained athletes. Histochemical Cell Biology 111: 189–195

Krebs D E, Jette A M et al 1998 Moderate exercise improves gait stability in disabled elders. Archives of Physical Medicine and Rehabilitation 79(12): 1489–1495

Lexell J, Henriksson-Larsen K et al 1983 Distribution of different fiber types in human skeletal muscles: effects of aging studied in whole muscle cross sections. Muscle and Nerve 6(8): 588–595

Lexell J, Taylor C C et al 1988 What is the cause of the ageing atrophy? Total number, size and proportion of different fiber types studied in whole vastus lateralis muscle from 15- to 83-year-old men. Journal of Neurological Science 84(2–3): 275–294

McCartney N 1998 Role of resistance training in heart disease. Medicine and Science in Sports Exercise 30 (suppl 10): S396–402

McCubbin J A 1990 Resistance exercise training for persons with arthritis. Rheumatic Diseases Clinics of North America 16(4): 931–943

Mikesky A E, Topp R et al 1994 Efficacy of a home-based training program for older adults using elastic tubing. European Journal of Applied Physiology 69(4): 316–320

Pollock M L, Graves J E et al 1993 Frequency and volume of resistance training: effect on cervical extension strength. Archives of Physical and Medical Rehabilitation 74(10): 1080–1086

Porter M M, Vandervoort A A et al 1995 Aging of human muscle: structure, function and adaptability [see comments]. Scandinavian Journal of Medicine & Science in Sports 5(3): 129–142

Rice C L, Cunningham D A et al 1989 Strength in an elderly population. Archieves of Physical Medicine and Rehabilitation 70(5): 391–397

Schilke J M 1991 Slowing the aging process with physical activity. Journal of Gerontology Nursing 17(6): 4–8

Smith E L, Gilligan C 1991 Physical activity effects on bone metabolism. Calcified Tissue International 49(suppl): S50–54

Starkey D B, Pollock M L et al 1996 Effect of resistance training volume on strength and muscle thickness. Medicine and Science in Sports Exercise 28(10): 1311–1320

Tucci J T, Carpenter D M et al 1992 Effect of reduced frequency of training and detraining on lumbar extension strength. Spine 17(12): 1497–1501

* This material is based upon work supported by the US
Department of Agriculture, under agreement No.
58–1950–9–001. Any opinions, findings, conclusion, or
recommendations expressed in this publication are those of
the author(s) and do not necessarily reflect the view of the
US Department of Agriculture.

26

Soft tissue responses to exercise in the elderly*

Maria A. Fiatarone Singh

KEY POINTS

1. Loss of adipose tissue in response to exercise is proportional to the energy deficit induced, and is minimal without concurrent dietary energy restriction.
2. Fat is lost preferentially from central stores with both progressive resistance training and cardiovascular endurance training in the elderly.
3. The most critical exercise-related factor leading to muscle hypertrophy is the relative intensity of the load imposed on the muscle.
4. Lean mass accretion with progressive resistance training in the elderly is attenuated by very advanced age, inadequate protein and calorie intake, and certain chronic diseases.
5. Autocrine and paracrine functions of endogenously produced insulin-like growth factor I in muscle appear to play a central role in the myogenic and anabolic responses to progressive resistance training.
6. The soft tissue response to resistive exercise (increased muscle, decreased fat) offers the best combination of adaptations for many elderly individuals, in particular those with chronic wasting diseases, functional impairment, central obesity and its metabolic complications of glucose and lipid metabolism, degenerative arthritis and mobility disorders, and neurologic deficits.

INTRODUCTION

Exercise has specific effects on soft tissues which are determined by the modality, quantity and intensity of the exercise itself, the underlying nutritional milieu of the individual, particularly in relation to energy balance, and the demographic and clinical characteristics of the older adult. The complexity of such interacting forces increases with age, resulting in a somewhat heterogeneous range of soft tissue responses to habitual exercise in the elderly. In this chapter, the adaptations to exercise which occur in adipose tissue and skeletal muscle will be considered, with a particular emphasis on the structural responses to musculoskeletal loading. Identification of exercise-related variables and other factors which affect this soft tissue response will be provided where such evidence exists. Functional adaptations to progressive resistance training and other forms of exercise are covered elsewhere in this volume and will not be reviewed here. Finally, the clinical implications of this soft tissue adaptation to exercise are discussed in relation to age-related changes in body composition, common geriatric diseases, and nutritional considerations in this population.

EFFECTS OF EXERCISE ON ADIPOSE TISSUE QUANTITY AND DISTRIBUTION

Observational studies of normals and master athletes

Increases in body weight, body fat and central (truncal and visceral as opposed to appendicular and subcutaneous) fat distribution with advancing age typify cross-sectional and longitudinal studies of body composition. Many epidemiological studies suggest a role for physical activity as a modifier of these 'age-related' changes in weight and body composition (Bortz 1982, 1989). In most populations which have been studied, the decline in energy expenditure through physical activity is even greater than the decline in energy intake with age, leading to an energy surfeit which must be stored as fat (Roberts et al 1992, 1994). For example, Meredith et al (1987) showed that the variance in percentage body fat was very closely related to number of hours of training per week in runners aged 20–60, but was not explained by age, suggesting that the usual pattern of increasing fat may not be genetically determined or inevitable, but at least modifiable by lifestyle choices.

In general, even individuals who are not athletes, but who simply classify themselves as more active in daily life, have lower body weight, body mass index (BMI), percentage body fat and less central adiposity than sedentary age-matched peers (Romieu et al 1988, Thune et al 1997). DiPietro et al (1993) found that these associations strengthened with older age groups (at least up to the age of 54) and more intensive activities, although walking was significantly associated with leanness and by far the most prevalent activity reported among the 18 682 participants in the US Behavioral Risk Factor Surveillance System Survey. Of particular importance for the elderly are the observations that the metabolically dangerous visceral adiposity associated with hyperlipidemia, hypertension, insulin resistance and ultimately diabetes and atherosclerosis is inversely related to both habitual activity levels and aerobic fitness categories (Barakat et al 1988, Blair et al 1989, Seidell et al 1991).

Interpretation of such cross-sectional investigations as cited above is obviously limited by the possibilities that differential survival will influence body composition values of older age groups, that obesity itself may preclude physical activity (i.e. obesity causes inactivity rather than the converse), and that genetic factors that influence body weight and composition may also influence activity levels. Longitudinal studies are therefore better suited to address the potential usefulness of exercise as a means of influencing body composition in older adults. In general, these studies show similar trends in that there is an inverse relationship between activity level and adipose tissue accumulation with age, although the associations tend to be far less dramatic than in cross-sectional studies (Tuomilehto et al 1985).

Cross-sectional studies of master athletes have yielded important insights into the effect of exercise on body weight and composition in old age, because exercise habits are more easily quantified than in the general population, and more sophisticated body composition measurements have often been utilized in these subjects. For example, Prately et al (1995) studied master runners and non-obese (body fat <25%) sedentary controls aged 50–70 years, and found no difference in mean BMI, fat-free mass (FFM) or percentage body fat, but found lower central obesity in the athletes. Waist-to-hip ratio, as the index of central obesity, was the only independent predictor of glucose disposal rates in multiple regression analysis, again demonstrating the metabolic importance of the fat distribution patterns exhibited by the master athletes.

Exercise intervention trials to modify body fat stores and distribution in normals and obese older adults

Major reviews and meta-analyses provide little evidence for the ability of exercise to significantly modify body weight or total body fat as an isolated intervention in normal elders (Ballor & Keesey 1991, Epstein & Wing 1980, King et al 1991, Thompson et al 1982), even after 1 year of training. As shown in Box 26.1, the most significant losses of weight and body fat occur in studies of men, in which relatively high doses and durations of exercise are utilized, and the response appears to be most robust in younger populations who are not morbidly obese. However, in an uncontrolled trial, Schwartz et al (1991) studied healthy young and old men after 6 months of intensive aerobic training (5 days/week for 45 min at 85% of heart rate reserve), and found that small but significant decreases in weight (2.5 kg), percentage body fat (2.3%), total body fat mass (2.4 kg) and waist-to-hip ratio (2%) accompanied exercise training only in the old men. Importantly, more than 20% decreases in subcutaneous truncal and visceral abdominal fat deposits were seen by CT scan in the old men. Fat was lost preferentially from storage sites which were initially the largest. This study is significant for demonstrating, for the first time, major changes in regional fat distribution via exercise in the absence of dietary restriction, large losses of weight or total body fat mass. It suggests that aerobic exercise alone may improve the metabolically undesirable central deposition of fat (Bengtsson et al 1993), even without dieting in healthy older men. However, extrapolation of these data to potential benefits in obese older adults is limited by the quasi-experimental design, non-obese subjects studied, lack of women in the trial and the high dose (5 days/week) and intensity (85% of heart rate reserve) of training, which may not be sustainable in clinical populations such as older obese women.

Similar results on central obesity were reported by Kohrt et al (1992) following 9–12 months of intensive endurance training in weight-stable healthy older men and women. It is not clear, however, that exercise of the intensity used in such studies and others with similar findings could be adhered to by individuals with chronic illness or significant obesity at baseline, or even that similar adaptations would take place in such individuals. Studies employing low-to-moderate level aerobic exercise have typically not demonstrated the same ability to decrease fat mass or shift fat distribution as seen in these higher intensity regimens (Franklin et al 1978, Pollock et al 1971).

There are very limited data on the efficacy of exercise as an isolated treatment for reduction of body fat in already obese individuals, and no randomized controlled trials using only aerobic exercise in the treatment of obesity in the elderly. In a study of middle-aged obese women, Despres et al (1991) found that aerobic exercise resulted in reductions in abdominal adipose tissue as well as the ratio of subcutaneous abdominal to thigh fat, indicating preferential losses of central adiposity, just as has been seen in non-obese older adults, as described above (Kohrt et al 1992, Schwartz et al 1991).

In summary, there is no evidence to date from randomized clinical trials in obese elderly subjects that aerobic exercise without dietary restriction can significantly lower body weight, percentage body fat, central adiposity or lipid profiles. Other reasons to advocate such exercise in this group, however, include increases in aerobic fitness (Ruoti et al 1994) and insulin sensitivity (Hersey et al 1994, Katzel et al 1995), which may occur with exercise independently of weight loss in the elderly.

Like aerobic training, progressive resistive exercise in the absence of dietary energy restriction appears to have only a small impact on total body weight or adipose tissue mass in young or old individuals. However, there is evidence of reduction in intra-abdominal fat stores with resistance training in two studies of normal-weight elderly subjects. Treuth et al (1995) reported that 14 women (mean age 67 years) who undertook moderate-intensity progressive resistance training for 16 weeks had significant reductions (10%) in intra-abdominal fat areas as well as decreased subcutaneous fat, with no overall changes in body weight or composition. Treuth et al (1994) also found similar results after strength training in 51 to 71-year old men, who lost 8% of truncal fat. Thus, like aerobic training (Kohrt et al 1992, Schwartz et al 1991), resistance training appears capable of reducing metabolically undesirable central fat deposits in the absence of weight loss or caloric restriction in the normal-weight elderly.

Box 26.1 Factors predictive of greater adipose tissue losses via exercise

- Induction of an overall energy deficit
- Greater dose of exercise (intensity and duration)
- Male gender
- Younger age
- Lower body mass index

Mechanisms of adipose tissue loss with exercise

Although relative body fat certainly appears to have genetic determinants which influence the metabolism and storage of adipose tissue, ultimately fat deposition can only occur if energy expenditure falls below energy intake, resulting in a positive energy balance. Conversely, loss of fat tissue requires a negative energy balance, regardless of whatever alterations in fat and other substrate oxidation may be achieved by modulation of diet composition and physical activity levels (Roberts et al 1996). Energy expenditure and intake may both be influenced by aerobic and resistance training in unique ways, as shown in Table 26.1. It is of note that energy expenditure specific to the type of exercise employed may not be the most important factor in choosing an exercise modality for weight loss. Rather, the regularity and dose of exercise, its effects on other components of energy expenditure as well as concomitant changes in dietary intake are likely to be far more important determinants of efficacy in reducing body fat.

Resistance training studies in the healthy elderly suggest favorable shifts in energy balance even in the absence of weight loss or increases in fat-free mass, which may be mechanistic in the reduction in obesity described above. Campbell et al (1994) reported that total energy requirements for weight maintenance are increased approximately 15% after 12 weeks of resistance training in older men and women, primarily due to increases in resting metabolic rate, as well as the energy requirements of the exercise itself. Treuth et al (1995) also described increased resting energy expenditure as well as fat oxidation after resistance training in postmenopausal women. The increase in resting metabolic rate may be due to both increased muscle mass itself and increased protein turnover (breakdown and synthesis) within existing muscle as it repairs damage or responds to anabolic signals. Over the long term, such adaptations within muscle tissue may significantly affect energy balance and contribute to the maintenance of a healthful body weight while minimizing fat deposition.

There are no trials yet of progressive resistance training as an isolated intervention to induce weight loss in obese older adults, but studies from younger individuals suggest that it is unlikely to induce substantial losses of body fat without dietary alteration. The combination of weight-lifting and hypocaloric dieting has been of increasing interest in recent years, however. There is one randomized controlled trial comparing resistance training with endurance training after hypocaloric dieting in obese older women. After 11 weeks of dieting, Ballor et al (1996) randomly allocated 18 older women to moderate-intensity resistance or aerobic exercise training for an additional 12 weeks. Weight remained stable in the weight-lifters, as the decline in fat mass was more than replaced by a gain in fat-free mass. By contrast, the endurance training group lost both fat and fat-free mass, which combined to produce a significant drop in total body weight.

Changes in energy expenditure specific to the resistive exercise appear to be important in the mediation of these alterations in body fat in Ballor et al's (1996) study. Resistance training increased resting energy expenditure by 5% (79 kcal/day), although not sufficiently to offset the 15% decline which had been induced by the hypocaloric diet, whereas aerobic exercise did not affect metabolic rate. In addition, the thermic effect of a meal, which had also been reduced by dieting, was 8% higher after weight training, and again unchanged by aerobic exercise. Thus, overall, more favorable body composition profiles and energy

Table 26.1 Alterations in energy balance potentially related to adipose tissue reduction with exercise

Effect	Observed with aerobic training in the elderly	Observed with resistance training in the elderly
Excess energy expenditure in exercise session	Yes	Yes
Increased spontaneous physical activity level apart from prescribed exercise	No	Yes
Increased resting metabolic rate	Variable	Yes
Increased fat oxidation	Yes	Yes
Increased thermic effect of feeding	Variable	Yes
Increased energy requirements of larger muscle mass	No	Yes
Increased protein turnover in skeletal muscle	Variable	Yes
Better adherence to hypocaloric diet	Yes	No

balance changes could be attributed to resistance exercise in this study of diet-restricted women, despite the greater weight loss in the aerobic exercise group. In the long-term control of body weight and adipose tissue deposition, these body composition and energy expenditure adaptations seen with resistance training may be extremely important in minimizing the tendency for weight and fat to be regained after dieting has ceased (weight cycling) (van Dale & Saris 1989).

EFFECTS OF EXERCISE ON LEAN BODY MASS AND MUSCLE MASS

Specificity of training in epidemiological and intervention studies

In contrast to the relatively consistent data on body weight, fat, and fat distribution and exercise, consensus on the ability of exercise to prevent age-related losses of lean body mass has not yet been reached. Due to the relative difficulty in accurately estimating muscle mass in population studies, the ability of habitual activity to modify age-related changes in this specific compartment of lean mass is even more controversial. Although it is often assumed that age-related losses of muscle are attenuated in physically active individuals, review of the available data demonstrates little or no effect of exercise on this parameter (Forbes 1992). Most studies suggest that aerobic activities such as walking have, at most, a modest effect on lean mass retention, and rates of loss in longitudinal follow-up have not differed by physical activity level. The higher lean body mass sometimes seen in active adults may be due to a combination of genetic factors, higher socioeconomic status, lower burden of disease and better nutritional state, all factors which are associated with higher levels of physical activity and which may serve to minimize rates of muscle loss with age.

An example of the specificity of the adaptation of lean tissue to various exercise modalities is provided by Klitgaard et al's (1990) cross-sectional observations of elderly runners, swimmers, weight-lifters and untrained young and old men (28 vs. 69 years). The trained men had participated in sports in their youth, and had been actively training in their current sport for 12–17 years prior to study. Whole muscle cross-sectional area as assessed by computed tomography (CT) scanning of the arm and leg, as well as mean fiber cross-sectional area of vastus lateralis and biceps brachii/brachialis muscles in weight-lifters were the

same or higher than in young controls. By contrast, older endurance-trained athletes had no more muscle mass than old sedentary men. For example, muscle area was 20–24% lower in old compared with young sedentary men, whereas the weight-lifters had 18–29% larger muscle areas than their sedentary peers, making them comparable to men 40 years younger than themselves. This specificity of progressive resistance training for the preservation or augmentation of muscle mass in older men is consistent with most epidemiological studies of non-athletes, which show similar rates of decline in lean tissue with age, despite varying levels of endurance-type activities.

Limited longitudinal data are available on lean tissue changes in either master athletes or non-athletic populations in relation to exercise levels. Pollock et al (1987) described increased fat mass and decreased fat-free mass over 10 years in 50 to 82-year-old runners, despite continued endurance training and competition. However, a subset of the men who added weight-lifting to their running during this time were able to maintain their fat-free mass over the decade of observation.

These differential effects of exercise modality on lean body mass are reflected in the distinct adaptations within skeletal muscle observed after training, as outlined in Box 26.2. Aerobic training produces little or no change in mean cross-sectional area of muscle fibers, but rather induces changes in the processes responsible for oxygen extraction and utilization for metabolism, as well as the ability to take up and store glucose more efficiently, allowing greater intensities and quantities of aerobic work to be performed. Resistance training, on the other hand, if it is of sufficient intensity and duration, increases the size of muscle fibers and leads to both damage and regeneration of myofibrils associated with an array of changes in protein turnover and growth factors.

Potential mechanisms of heterogeneous response of muscle to progressive resistance training

There are numerous studies in normal healthy older adults which indicate that high-intensity resistance training is associated with increases in lean body mass or muscle area, usually with minimal alteration of total body weight (Cartee 1994, Charette et al 1991, Lillegard & Terrio 1994, McCartney et al 1995). However, the observed adaptive response of skeletal muscle to resistance training in these studies is quite variable, likely influenced by the intensity and duration of the intervention, subject characteristics and the precision of the

---

Box 26.2 Comparison of skeletal muscle adaptations to progressive resistance training and aerobic training

Progressive resistance training
- Increased type I and II mean fiber cross-sectional area
- Increased amino acid delivery and uptake into muscle
- Increased myofibrillar protein synthesis
- Increased protein breakdown
- Z-band and myofibrillar damage
- Increased IGF-I appearance and activity
- Developmental myosin isoform appearance in mature and small fibers
- Myogenic process involving satellite cell activation, proliferation and differentiation
- Small to moderate increases in oxidative enzyme capacity
- Variable changes in capillary density

Aerobic training
- Increased mitochondrial density
- Increased oxidative enzyme capacity (e.g. citrate synthase, succinate dehydrogenase)
- Increased glycogen storage
- Increased GLUT-4 transporter content
- Increased capillary density; new capillary formation
- Minimal or no increase in mean fiber area
- Shift to higher proportion of type IIa and lower proportion of type IIb fibers

---

measurement technique itself. Typically, the largest relative changes are seen regionally in cross-sectional area of individual muscle fibers on biopsy specimens, or CT scan analyses of muscle area, whereas whole body measures of lean body mass show more modest changes (Nelson et al 1996). Muscle hypertrophy is specific to the trained muscle groups, thus apparently being mediated by local rather than systemic factors. As shown in Table 26.2, muscle fiber cross-sectional area changes on biopsy have varied from decreases of 12% to increases of 62% in various studies, which may be due to training differences and subject characteristics, as well as error due to sampling and precision inherent in the muscle biopsy technique (Cartee 1994, Evans 1996).

Unfortunately, most studies to date have included only healthy individuals (Brown et al 1990, Campbell et al 1994, Charette et al 1991, Frontera et al 1988, Larsson 1982, Lexell et al 1995, Pyka et al 1994), and little clinical information other than age to allow insight into the wide range of muscle tissue responsiveness to weight-lifting regimens. However, as can be seen in Figure 26.1, age is clearly inversely related to the degree of muscle hypertrophy achieved, even when training techniques are quite similar, and all are within the moderate- to high-intensity range (60–90% of the one repetition maximum) which produces optimal increases in maximal force production. Gender does not significantly influence muscle fiber responsiveness in these studies. The FICSIT trial allowed us to look at a wider range of clinical characteristics which might predict lean tissue responsiveness, due to the very advanced age, chronic diseases and nutritional deficiencies present in this nursing

Table 26.2 Changes in muscle fiber cross-sectional area with progressive resistance training in the elderly

Study	n	Gender	Mean age (years)	Health status	Intensity[a]	Duration (weeks)	Type I change with exercise (%)	Type II change with exercise (%)
Larsson (1982)	6	Men	59	Healthy	Moderate	12	37.8*	51.5*
Frontera et al (1988)	12	Men	66	Healthy	High	12	33.5***	27.6***
Brown et al (1990)	14	Men	63	Healthy	High	12	14.0 (BB)[b]	30.2* (BB)
Charette et al (1991)	19	Women	70	Healthy	Moderate	12	7.3	20.1*
Pyka et al (1994)	11	Mixed	69	Healthy	Moderate	30	48.3**	61.7**
Campbell et al (1994)	12	Mixed	65	Healthy	High	12	4.6	2.7
Lexell et al (1995)	20	Mixed	74	Healthy	High	11	13.0* (BB) −4.0	17.0* (BB) −8.0
Pu et al (1997)	17	Women	80	CHF	High	10	9.5	13.6
Fiatarone Singh (1998)	26	Mixed	87	Frail	High	10	4.6	−11.5

[a] Moderate = 60–75% of one repetition maximum as progressive training load; high = 75–90% of one repetition maximum as progressive training load.
[b] BB = results from biopsy of the biceps brachii. All other values represent vastus lateralis biopsies.
*$P <0.05$, **$P <0.01$, ***$P <0.001$, compared with controls or baseline value.

A

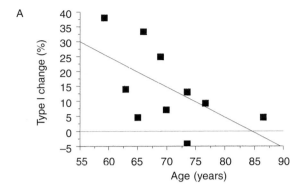

B

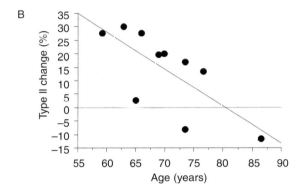

Figure 26.1 Relationship between the hypertrophic response of type I (A) and II (B) fibers to progressive resistance training and the age of the study group. The graphs include all published trials of moderate- to high-intensity progressive resistance training (above 60% of the 1 RM) of 10–15 weeks' duration in which the vastus lateralis or biceps brachii muscle was biopsied. Each symbol represents the mean age of the study group reported. There was an inverse relationship between the relative increase in fiber area and the study group age. For type I fibers, $r = -0.584$, $P = 0.077$; for type II fibers, $r = -0.726$, $P = 0.018$). Intensity of training within this range and gender were unrelated to this hypertrophic response in a multivariate regression model including age. (Data are taken from Brown et al 1990, Charette et al 1991, Campbell et al 1994, Fiatarone et al 1994, Frontera et al 1988, Larsson 1982, Lexell et al 1995, Pyka et al 1994, Pu et al 1997).

home population (Fiatarone et al 1994). In this study, depressive symptoms were associated with lower physical activity levels at baseline ($r = -0.446$, $P < 0.05$), as well as diminished regenerative and functional adaptations to resistance training within skeletal muscle. Increased muscle area was related to higher dietary energy intake before and during the trial, and greater presence of insulin-like growth factor I in skeletal muscle at baseline, and was only significantly

increased in type II fibers in those exercising subjects who consumed a 360 kcal/day supplement in addition to regular meals. In the only other biopsy study to date of chronically diseased individuals (Pu et al 2000), it was found that older women with congestive heart failure, like the frail nursing home residents, had modest, non-significant increases in fiber area after 10 weeks of high-intensity training, despite robust gains in muscle strength, endurance and functional performance.

Taken together, the existing literature suggests that both exercise-related variables and individual characteristics contribute to the wide range of lean tissue responsiveness to resistance training. The factors thus far identified as important in this regard are summarized in Box 26.3. Because hypertrophy requires synthesis of new proteins and structural changes, neural adaptation is the primary cause of immediate changes in strength in response to resistance training, and longer periods of training are associated with greater gains in muscle tissue. Exercise which does not involve high loading forces on the muscle is generally ineffective with regard to gains in both strength and muscle mass. Although it is possible to see changes in whole body lean tissue with progressive resistance training even in the face of hypocaloric dieting in healthy middle-aged and older women (Ballor et al 1988, 1996), in chronically diseased elderly subjects, even eucaloric energy intake appears to inhibit muscle growth, and energy supplementation was necessary to induce significant hypertrophy with weight-lifting exercise (Fiatarone et al 1994). Further research is required to separate out the effects of advanced age, nutritional deficiencies, hormonal status, disease attributes and extreme sedentariness in clinical populations who may

---

Box 26.3 Factors associated with more robust hypertrophic response of skeletal muscle to progressive resistance training in the elderly

Training factors
- Higher intensity of applied load (relative to one repetition maximum)
- Eccentric and concentric loading
- Longer duration of training

Subject characteristics
- Younger age
- Relatively healthy clinical status
- Previously untrained status
- Positive energy balance before and during training
- More IGF-I present in skeletal muscle at baseline

impair their ability to augment lean tissue with this mode of exercise relative to healthy peers.

Mechanisms underlying increased muscle mass after progressive resistance training

Ultimately, the increase in muscle mass in response to resistance training requires synthesis of new proteins as well as contribution of new myonuclei to preserve the nuclear:cytoplasmic ratio of mature, multinucleated muscle fibers. These myonuclei must come from sources extrinsic to mature muscle fibers, whose nuclei are incapable of cell division after embryonic development. Some of the possible factors contributing to training-induced hypertrophy are listed in Box 26.4. Muscle can respond to loading in the absence of anabolic factors such as estrogen and testosterone, and even in the face of marginal protein and energy intake, although all of these factors may augment the training effect. Although hypothalamic integrity in relation to growth hormone secretion is necessary for early growth and development, it does not appear to be critical to the local hypertrophy in response to loading, and exogenous administration has generally not been shown to successfully augment muscle size or strength in the elderly (Taafe et al 1996, Wolfe 1998). Insulin-like growth factor I (IGF-I) is primarily produced in the liver in response to hypothalamic growth hormone secretion, but it can also be synthesized in skeletal muscle itself, apparently in response to local factors. The autocrine (produced in and acting on muscle fibers) and paracrine (produced in muscle and acting on neighboring cells such as satellite cells) functions of IGF-I cover a spectrum of activities necessary for myogenesis and anabolism, as listed in Box 26.5.

Box 26.4 Potential mechanisms of skeletal muscle adaptation to progressive resistance training

- Changes in anabolic hormone (estrogen, androgens) secretion/activity
- Increased hypothalamic growth hormone secretion/activity
- Increased paracrine/autocrine activity of IGF-I
- Regenerative response to mechanical damage and subsequent inflammation
- Increased amino acid delivery to muscle via increased regional blood flow
- Increased dietary energy intake
- Increased dietary protein intake

Box 26.5 Known effects of IGF-I on skeletal muscle

- Increased muscle protein synthesis rate
- Decreased ubiquitin-mediated protein degradation
- Increased uptake of amino acids from circulating pools
- Increased RNA synthesis
- Increased DNA content
- Increased expression of muscle-specific proteins, myogenic regulatory factors
- Activation and proliferation of satellite cells
- Induction of myoblast differentiation, fusion

Although hyperplasia, or new muscle fiber formation, has never been conclusively demonstrated in humans in response to exercise (Taylor & Wilkinson 1986), satellite cell activation has been seen after synergist muscle ablation in conjunction with compensatory hypertrophy in young rats (Salleo et al 1980). Sporadic examples of activated satellite cells, myoblasts and myotubes were identified morphologically by electron microscopy in post-exercise samples in a study of frail nursing home residents (Fiatarone et al 1994), although the extent of their appearance could not be quantified. Therefore, quantitative immunohistochemical staining for embryonic and neonatal myosin was undertaken in these specimens, in order to localize the fibers in which regenerative adaptations were occurring. These developmental myosin isoforms are normally seen only early in fetal development or as a regenerative response to pathologic damage to muscle. We saw developmental myosin staining in both large mature fibers and very small fibers after exercise, suggesting that regeneration could be occurring by way of hypertrophy of mature fibers, as well as activation of the kinds of myogenic precursor cells seen by electron microscopy.

A suggested pathway by which progressive resistance training could lead to augmentation of muscle mass is shown in Figure 26.2. Local mechanical stretching and loading may lead to damage and inflammation of myofibrils, particularly if the eccentric forces are high (Fielding et al 1993). We have seen that increases in muscle damage after resistance training are highly correlated with increases in IGF-I and embryonic myosin staining in muscle, suggesting that damage may initiate a regenerative response mediated by IGF-I. Myogenic processes are required to provide the myonuclei which can either form new fibers or be incorporated into enlarging mature fibers. Anabolic processes are necessary for protein synthesis resulting in new myofibril formation. More work is needed to define the specific exercise factors and individual characteristics which influence these pathways, so that optimal gains in muscle mass are achieved in the elderly.

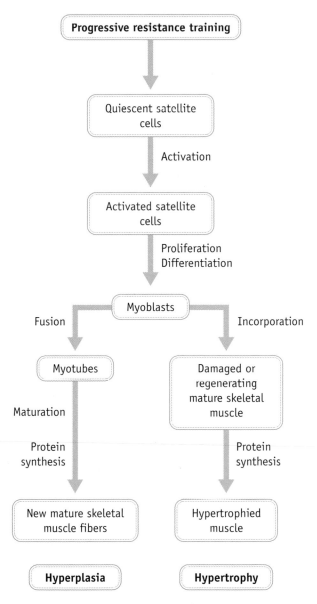

Figure 26.2 Proposed model of muscle growth in response to progressive resistance training. Myogenic and anabolic processes both contribute to loading/stretch/damage-induced adaptations in skeletal muscle. The myogenic process of proliferation and differentiation is necessary for both new and hypertrophied cell formation. Hypertrophy requires anabolic processes to promote protein synthesis as well. Each step in this pathway has been shown to be stimulated by autocrine and paracrine actions of IGF-I.

CONCLUSIONS

Exercise in the elderly has the potential to induce major adaptations within the soft tissue compartments, affecting quantitative tissue stores, regional distribution patterns and qualitative aspects such as rates of fat oxidation in adipocytes, glucose homeostasis, skeletal muscle protein turnover, mitochondrial respiration, oxygen extraction, blood flow regulation and functional capacity (force, power, endurance, mobility). The effects observed are quite specific to the modality and dose of exercise employed, and thus consideration of the functional and clinical benefits of most concern to the individual should underlie the exercise prescription in the elderly. Many of the most common chronic diseases and syndromes in the elderly are related to the amount of fat and lean tissue present, as shown in Box 26.6, emphasizing the central role of body composition in health and function in the aging population.

Loss of total body and central fat mass is best achieved by a combination of decreased energy intake and increased energy expenditure secondary to exercise. Progressive resistance training is particularly valuable in this regard, as it is tolerable in obese, sedentary patients with chronic disease, mobilizes the metabolically dangerous visceral adipose tissue, prevents the loss of lean tissue accompanying hypocaloric dieting, and increases basal energy expenditure, thermic effect of feeding, and energy expenditure in overall physical activity, thus minimizing weight cycling. However, regular aerobic exercise has been shown to have the important ability to enhance compliance with an energy-restricted diet, the critical long-term factor in successful weight maintenance. It is not yet known if resistance training shares this same capacity to enhance behavioral change. Although much of the morbidity related to excess adiposity requires preventive efforts early in life, there is evidence that modification of this risk factor may have

Box 26.6 Clinical syndromes in which modulation of soft tissue mass by exercise may be preventive (P) or therapeutic (T)

Decreased total or visceral adipose tissue mass
Atherosclerosis (P,T)
Breast cancer (P)
Colon cancer (P)
Degenerative arthritis (P,T)
Diabetes mellitus (P,T)
Gout (P,T)
Hyperlipidemia (P,T)
Hypertension (P,T)
Low back pain (P,T)
Low self-esteem (P,T)
Mobility impairment, disability (P,T)
Peripheral vascular disease (P,T)
Sleep apnea (P,T)
Stroke (P)
Vascular impotence (P)
Venous disease (P,T)

Increased muscle mass
Chronic obstructive pulmonary disease (T)
Chronic renal failure (T)
Congestive heart failure (T)
Diabetes mellitus (P,T)
Frailty, functional decline (P,T)
Gait and balance disorders, falls (P,T)
HIV infection (T)
Low back pain (P,T)
Neuromuscular disease (T)
Osteoporosis (P,T)
Parkinson's disease (T)
Protein-calorie malnutrition, marasmus (T)
Rheumatoid arthritis (T)
Stroke (T)

clinical benefits even after disease has already become overt, as in the case of diabetes, sleep apnea, hypertension and degenerative arthritis, for example.

Augmentation of muscle mass or prevention and treatment of age- and disease-related sarcopenia is only reliably achieved with high-intensity progressive resistance training begun in mid- or late life and continued indefinitely. The adaptations at the cellular level which promote muscle accretion include both myogenic and anabolic pathways, predominantly resulting in hypertrophy of existing mature muscle fibers. The process includes enhanced myofibrillar protein synthesis as well as incorporation of new myonuclei resulting from activation of satellite cell pools. IGF-I and other growth factors appear to play a central role in this process, whereas, by contrast, exogenous administration of such hormones has not been shown to replicate the functional gains which accompany endogenous activation via resistance training. Such augmentation of muscle mass and function is important in the clinical management of many common geriatric syndromes, and in particular may relieve the disability associated with sarcopenia in many chronic diseases such as renal failure, emphysema, congestive heart failure and rheumatoid arthritis.

Although the soft tissue response of both fat and muscle appears to be attenuated with advanced age, much of this may be attributable to concurrent disease in this cohort (which lessens the actual intensity of exercise prescribed or achieved) or to coexistent nutritional deficiencies of either protein or energy. Nonetheless, the soft tissues retain a remarkable degree of plasticity in response to exercise through the last decades of life. More research is needed in clinical populations to optimize training regimens and co-therapies (nutritional, pharmacological, hormonal) so as to achieve maximal soft tissue responses to exercise. In addition, long-term monitoring of clinical and functional outcomes of such adaptation will further establish the critical role of exercise in the medical management and quality of life of the elderly.

REFERENCES

Ballor D, Keesey R 1991 A meta-analysis of the factors affecting exercise-induced changes in body mass, fat mass, and fat-free mass in males and females. International Journal of Obesity 15: 717–726
Ballor D L, Harvey-Berino J R, Ades P A, Cryan J, Calles-Escandon J 1996 Contrasting effects of resistance and aerobic training on body composition and metabolism after diet-induced weight loss. Metabolism: Clinical and Experimental 45(2): 179–183
Ballor D L, Katch V L, Becque M D, Marks C R 1988 Resistance weight training during caloric restriction

enhances lean body weight maintenance. American Journal of Clinical Nutrition 47: 19–25

Barakat H, Burton D, Carpenter J 1988 Body fat distribution, plasma lipoproteins and the risk of coronary heart disease of male subjects. International Journal of Obesity 12: 473–480

Bengtsson C, Bjorkelund C, Lapidus L, Lissner L 1993 Associations of serum lipid concentrations and obesity with mortality in women: 20 year follow-up of participants in prospective population study in Gothenburg, Sweden. British Journal of Medicine 307: 1385–1388

Blair S, Kannel W, Kohl H 1989 Surrogate measures of physical activity and physical fitness: evidence for sedentary traits of resting tachycardia, obesity, and low vital capacity. American Journal of Epidemiology 129: 1145–1156

Bortz W M 1982 Disuse and aging. Journal of the American Medical Association 248: 1203–1208

Bortz W M 1989 Redefining human aging. Journal of the American Geriatric Society 37(11): 1092–1096

Brown A, McCartney N, Sale D 1990 Positive adaptations to weight-lifting training in the elderly. Journal of Applied Physiology 69(5): 1725–1733

Campbell W W, Crim M C, Young V R, Evans W J 1994 Increased energy requirements and changes in body composition with resistance training in older adults. American Journal of Clinical Nutrition 60(2): 167–175

Cartee G D 1994 Aging skeletal muscle: response to exercise. Exercise & Sport Sciences Reviews 22: 91–120

Charette S, McEvoy L, Pyka G et al 1991 Muscle hypertrophy response to resistance training in older women. Journal of Applied Physiology 70(5): 1912–1916

Despres J-P, Pouliot M, Moorjani S 1991 Loss of abdominal fat and metabolic response to exercise training in obese women. American Journal of Physiology 24: E159–167

DiPietro L, Williamson D F, Caspersen C J, Eaker E 1993 The descriptive epidemiology of selected physical activities and body weight among adults trying to lose weight: the Behavioral Risk Factor Surveillance System survey 1989. International Journal of Obesity and Related Metabolic Disorders 17(2): 69–76

Epstein L, Wing R 1980 Aerobic exercise and weight. Addictive Behaviors 5: 371–388

Evans W J 1996 Reversing sarcopenia: how weight training can build strength and vitality. Geriatrics 51(5): 46–47, 51–53; quiz 54

Fiatarone M A, O'Neill E F, Ryan N D et al 1994 Exercise training and nutritional supplementation for physical frailty in very elderly people. New England Journal of Medicine 330: 1769–1775

Fiatarone Singh M A 1998 Body composition and weight control in older adults. In: Lamb D R, Murray R (eds) Perspectives in exercise science and sports medicine, vol 11. Exercise, nutrition and control of body weight. Cooper, Carmel, IN, p 243–293

Fielding R A, Manfredi T J, Ding W, Fiatarone M A, Evans W J, Cannon J G 1993 Acute phase response in exercise. III. Intramuscular mediators of inflammatory injury. American Journal of Physiology 265: R166–172

Forbes G 1992 Exercise and lean weight: the influence of body weight. Nutrition Reviews 50: 157–161

Franklin B A, Besseghini I, Golden L H 1978 Low intensity physical conditioning: effects on patients with coronary heart disease. Archives of Physical Medicine and Rehabilitation 59(6): 276–280

Frontera W R, Meredith C N, O'Reilly K P, Knuttgen H G, Evans W J 1988 Strength conditioning in older men: skeletal muscle hypertrophy and improved function. Journal of Applied Physiology 64: 1038–1044

Hersey W C R, Graves J E, Pollock M L et al 1994 Endurance exercise training improves body composition and plasma insulin responses in 70- to 79-year-old men and women. Metabolism: Clinical and Experimental 43(7): 847–854

Katzel L I, Bleecker E R, Colman E G, Rogus E M, Sorkin J D, Goldberg A P 1995 Effects of weight loss vs aerobic exercise training on risk factors for coronary disease in healthy, obese, middle-aged and older men. A randomized controlled trial [see comments]. Journal of the American Medical Association 274(24): 1915–1921

King A, Haskell W, Taylor C, Kraemer H, DeBusk R 1991 Group- vs home-based exercise training in healthy older men and women: a community-based clinical trial. Journal of the American Medical Association 266: 1535–1542

Klitgaard H, Mantoni M, Schiaffino S et al 1990 Function, morphology and protein expression of ageing skeletal muscle: a cross-sectional study of elderly men with different training backgrounds. Acta Physiologica Scandinavica 140: 41–54

Kohrt W M, Obert K A, Holloszy J O 1992 Exercise training improves fat distribution patterns in 60- to 70-year-old men and women. Journal of Gerontology 47(4): M99–105

Larsson L 1982 Physical training effects on muscle morphology in sedentary males at different ages. Medicine and Science in Sports and Exercise 14: 203–206

Lexell J, Downham D, Larsson Y, Bruhn E, Morsing B 1995 Heavy-resistance training in older Scandinavian men and women: short- and long-term effects on arm and leg muscles. Scandinavian Journal of Medicine and Science in Sports 5: 329–341

Lillegard W A, Terrio J D 1994 Appropriate strength training. Medical Clinics of North America 78(2): 457–477

McCartney N, Hicks A, Martin J, Webber C 1995 Long-term resistance training in the elderly: effects on dynamic strength, exercise capacity, muscle, and bone. Journal of Gerontology 50A(2): B97–B104

Meredith C N, Zackin M J, Frontera W R, Evans W J 1987 Body composition and aerobic capacity in young and middle-aged endurance-trained men. Medicine and Science in Sports and Exercise 19: 557–563

Nelson M, Fiatarone M, Layne J et al 1996 Analysis of body-composition techniques and models for detecting change in soft tissue with strength training. American Journal of Clinical Nutrition 63: 678–686

Pollock M, Miller H, Janeway R, Linnerud A, Robertson B, Valentino R 1971 Effects of walking on body composition and cardiovascular function of middle-aged men. Journal of Applied Physiology 30: 126–130

Pollock M L, Foster C, Knapp D, Rod J L, Schmidt D H 1987 Effect of age and training on aerobic capacity and body composition of master athletes. Journal of Applied Physiology 62(2): 725–731

Pratley R, Hagberg J, Rogus E, Goldberg A 1995 Enhanced insulin sensitivity and lower waist-to-hip ratio in master athletes. American Journal of Physiology 268: E484–490

Pu C, Johnson M, Forman D, Piazza L, Fiatarone M 1997 High-intensity progressive resistance training in older women with chronic heart failure. Medicine and Science in Sports and Exercise 29: S148

Pu C T, Johnson M T, Forman D E, Hansdorff J M, Roubenoff R, Fielding R A, Fiatarone Singh M A 2000 The effects of high-intensity strength training on skeletal muscle and exercise performance in older women with heart failure: a randomized control trial. Journal of Applied Physiology, in press

Pyka G, Taaffe D R, Marcus R 1994 Effect of a sustained program of resistance training on the acute growth hormone response to resistance exercise in older adults. Hormone and Metabolic Research 26(7): 330–333

Roberts S, Young V, Fuss P et al 1992 What are the dietary energy needs of elderly adults? International Journal of Obesity 16: 969–976

Roberts S B, Fuss P, Dallal G E et al 1996 Effects of age on energy expenditure and substrate oxidation during experimental overfeeding in healthy men. Journal of Gerontology. Series A, Biological Sciences & Medical Sciences 51(2): B148–157

Roberts S B, Fuss P, Heyman M B et al 1994 Control of food intake in older men. Journal of the American Medical Association 272(20): 1601–1606

Romieu I, Willett W C, Stampfer M J et al 1988 Energy intake and other determinants of relative weight. American Journal of Clinical Nutrition 47(3): 406–412

Ruoti R G, Troup J T, Berger R A 1994 The effects of nonswimming water exercises on older adults. Journal of Orthopaedic and Sports Physical Therapy 19(3): 140–145

Salleo A, Anastasi G, LaSpada G, Falzea G, Denaro M 1980 New muscle fiber production during compensatory hypertrophy. Medicine and Science in Sports and Exercise 12(4): 268–273

Schwartz R S, Shuman W P, Larson V et al 1991 The effect of intensive endurance exercise training on body fat distribution in young and older men. Metabolism: Clinical and Experimental 40(5): 545–551

Seidell J C, Cigolini M, Deslypere J P, Charzewska J, Ellsinger B M, Cruz A 1991 Body fat distribution in relation to physical activity and smoking habits in 38-year-old European men. The European Fat Distribution Study. American Journal of Epidemiology 133(3): 257–265

Taafe D, Jin I, Hoffman A, Marcus R 1996 Lack of effect of recombinant human growth hormone (GH) on muscle morphology and GH-insulin-like-growth factor expression in resistance-trained elderly men. Journal of Clinical Endocrinology and Metabolism 81: 421–425

Taylor N, Wilkinson J 1986 Exercise-induced skeletal muscle growth: Hypertrophy or hyperplasia? Sports Medicine 3: 190–200

Thompson J, Jarvic G, Lahey R 1982 Exercise and obesity: etiology, physiology and intervention. Psychological Bulletin 91: 55–79

Thune I, Brenn T, Lund E, Gaard M 1997 Physical activity and the risk of breast cancer. New England Journal of Medicine 336: 1296–1300

Treuth M, Hunter G, Szabo T, Weinsier R, Goran M, Berland L 1995 Reduction in intra-abdominal adipose tissue after strength training in older women. Journal of Applied Physiology 78(4): 1425–1431

Treuth M, Hunter G, Weinsier R, Kell S 1995 Energy expenditure and substrate utilization in older women after strength training: 24-h calorimeter results. Journal of Applied Physiology 78(6): 2140–2146

Treuth M, Ryan A, Pratley R et al 1994 Effects of strength training on total and regional body composition in older men. Journal of Applied Physiology 77: 614–620

Tuomilehto J, Jalkanen L, Salonen J T, Nissinen A 1985 Factors associated with changes in body weight during a five-year follow-up of a population with high blood pressure. Scandinavian Journal of Social Medicine 13(4): 173–180

van Dale D, Saris W 1989 Repetitive weight loss and weight regain: effects on weight reduction, resting metabolic rate, and lipolytic activity before and after exercise and/or diet treatment. American Journal of Clinical Nutrition 49(3): 409–416

Wolfe J 1998 Growth hormone: a physiological fountain of youth? Journal of Anti-Aging Medicine 1(1): 9–25

27

Management of musculoskeletal overuse injuries in aging, including master athletes

Yuji Nabeshima   Masahiro Kurosaka
Shinichi Yoshiya   Kosaku Mizuno

KEY POINTS

1. There is a higher incidence of sports-related injuries among older athletes, in part due to the reduced flexibility and range of motion of their joints.
2. There is some evidence that exercise reduces the deterioration of the aging musculoskeletal system.
3. Pre-existing orthopedic problems, e.g. osteoarthritis, meniscal tear and hallux valgus, are strongly related to overuse injuries, especially in aging athletes.
4. Treatment principles of overuse injuries in aging athletes are basically the same as those in young athletes.

INTRODUCTION

Overuse injuries are among the major sports-related musculoskeletal injuries encountered in sports medicine. They are a common problem in younger athletes participating at a high level of competition, and as such there is much information in the literature on injuries in these athletes. However, there is less information available on overuse injuries in aging athletes. In order to understand the features and specific aspects of this problem, in this chapter we present a review of previous studies, our own clinical experience, and summarize the current knowledge.

BASIC SCIENCE

The musculoskeletal system is an integrated unit, which consists of the myofascial compartment, tendons, osteotendinous junctions, and bones. Overuse injuries can be seen in all four components. Compartmental syndrome, tendinopathy (including insertional tendinopathy), and stress fracture are common clinical features.

The myofascial compartment consists of a group of muscles, a major artery, and a nerve bounded by bone and relatively inelastic fascia (Teitz 1989). Increased pressure within a closed compartment damages the muscles and nerves and diminishes tissue perfusion, which may lead to an ischemic injury (Caplan et al 1987). Common causes of increased compartment pressures include bleeding into a compartment, edema following partial or temporary ischemia, and crushing injuries (Caplan et al 1987).

The role of the musculotendinous junction, a common site of muscle injuries, is to transmit the force produced in the muscle to the tendon. The myotendinous junction is composed of the interdigitations between the sarcolemma of each muscular fiber and tendon collagen fibrils, which are separated from the basal membrane of the sarcolemma (Selvanetti et al 1997). The structure and function of the tendon have been widely investigated (Gelberman et al 1987). The primary function of the tendon is to effectively transmit muscle tension to the bone. Tendons are composed of dense, regularly arranged collagen fibrils. Most of the tendon consists of type I collagen, with a small amount of type III collagen. The outer surface of the tendon is enveloped in a sheath of fine connective tissue (epitenon), whose inner surface is continuous with the endotenon, a thin membrane of loose connective tissue binding collagen fibers in fascicles and also carrying blood vessels, lymphatics, and nerves (Selvanetti et al 1997). In some tendons, the epitenon is surrounded by a loose areolar tissue (paratenon), allowing free movements of the tendon against surrounding tissues. The peritenon is composed of both the epitenon and the paratenon. In those areas where the movement of tendons causes too much friction, the paratenon is developed as a double-layered synovial sheath (tenosynovium) (Selvanetti et al 1997).

There are two types of tendon insertions into the bone. In direct insertions, tendon fibers can be divided into superficial and deep fibers. The main fibers in direct insertion sites are deep fibers which meet the bone at a right angle. The deep fibers inserted into the bone have four distinct zones (Cooper & Misol 1970, Woo et al 1987): the tendon tissue, the fibrocartilage, the mineralized fibrocartilage, and the bone. Another form of insertion is called indirect insertion. The superficial fibers predominate at indirect insertion sites. Thus insertion of the fibers into the bone is mainly through fibers blending with the periosteum (Benjamin et al 1986, Woo et al 1987).

Bone serves as a storehouse for calcium and, early in life, as a producer of blood cells. The bone functions predominantly to transmit loads in association with muscles and gravity. Bone is composed predominantly of mineralized organic matrix on a collagen framework. A longitudinal orientation of collagen fibers increases the tensile strength of bone, and a transverse orientation increases its compressive strength. The collagen, mostly type I, accounts for about 90% of the organic matrix of the bone, with 10% composed of proteoglycans and other proteins (Teitz 1989). Biomechanical data show that bones are able to elongate approximately 0.75% of their original length before permanent deformation occurs. While the collagenous component is primarily responsible for resisting tensile stresses, the mineral component is responsible for resisting compression (Teitz 1989).

EFFECTS OF AGING ON THE MUSCULOSKELETAL SYSTEM

Noyes & Grood (1976) reported the effects of aging on human cadaveric anterior cruciate ligaments. They discovered much less stiffness and maximum force in the older donor group, as well as a smaller amount of energy absorbed. Woo et al (1991) aligned the ligament axis with the load cell axis more accurately and found a significant reduction in the material properties of human cadaveric anterior cruciate ligament–bone units between the ages of 20 and 80 years. Aging collagen has increased stability to thermal denaturing and reduced solubility (Viidik 1979). In addition to alteration of the collagen the connective tissue undergoes a generalized decrease in water content (Menard & Stanish 1989). Stabilization of collagen with maturity enhances tissue strength, while a loss of water and elastin reduces tissue plasticity (Morein et al 1978).

Another important threat to the aging musculoskeletal system is osteoporosis, especially in women. Osteoporotic bone alteration could represent a serious threat to aging athletes, particularly if they begin their sporting program at or above 50 years of age. For those individuals who remain active throughout their lives, osteoporosis is of less concern, since physical activity partially counteracts the process of demineralization (Menard & Stanish 1989). Regardless of age, bone responds to muscular traction and gravitational loading by increasing in thickness, strength, calcium concentration, nitrogen levels, hydroxyproline, and DNA (Booth et al 1975, Sinett 1986, Twomey & Taylor 1985).

In contrast, many authors have demonstrated a smaller effect of aging on skeletal muscle. The number of muscle fibers and motor units does not decrease with age, and the percentage of muscle fiber types remains the same (Aniansson et al 1980, Essen-Eustausson & Bovees 1986, Green 1986). The relatively few age-related changes in the skeletal muscle that have been reported are as follows:

- A decrease in mitochondrial volume occurs with no change in number (Green 1986).
- Grouping of fiber types occurs.
- Lipofuscin granules develop for unknown reasons.
- A decline in fiber area develops, particularly after age 60–70 years (Aniansson et al 1980, Essen-Eustausson & Borees 1986).
- The total collagen content in whole muscles appears to increase continuously with age (Alnaqeeb et al 1984).
- Muscle strength decreases beyond the age of 50 such that, at age 65, individuals maintain between 75 and 80% of their peak strength (Åstrand 1986).
- Ultrastructural investigation has shown that age-related changes in type I fibers are Z-band streaming and formation of nemalin-like structures, while type II fibers undergo fragmentation, loss of Z-materials and increased lipofuscin (Sato et al 1986).

Reduced flexibility and range of motion of joints are among the deleterious effects of aging, contributing to the higher incidence of sports-related injuries in older athletes. Brown (1993) found that orthopedic and physical factors such as obesity, history of previous joint injury and osteoarthritis, foot deformity, limited range of dorsiflexion of the ankle, and hip flexor tightness were factors strongly related to the development of joint pain in controlled exercise in the elderly.

Does exercise alter or reduce this deterioration of the aging musculoskeletal system? Vailas et al (1985) demonstrated that the concentration of tendon glycosaminoglycans in 28-month-old rats with free access to voluntary running wheels in cages was equivalent to the level found in 9-month-old sedentary rats, suggesting that voluntary exercise slowed the decline in galactosamine-containing glycosaminoglycans with aging. Viidik (1979) has developed several models demonstrating that training will enhance the failure strength of tendons and ligaments.

CLINICAL FEATURES OF OVERUSE INJURIES IN AGING

Overuse injuries are defined as musculoskeletal damage as a consequence of repetitive and cumulative microtrauma imposed on the tissues. Overuse injury can occur even if the tissue is stressed under the level of yielding strength when forces exceed the basal adaptive capacity of the structures. Also, if repetitive stress is applied frequently and there is not sufficient time for the tissue to go through intrinsic repair, some forms of overuse injuries will develop (Selvanetti et al 1997). Overuse injuries can result from poor training technique, malalignment, poor equipment, and an unfavorable environment (Teitz 1989). Moreover, pre-existing orthopedic problems such as osteoarthritis, meniscal tear, hallux valgus, and flattening of the plantar arch etc. are strongly related to overuse injuries, especially in aging athletes (Brown 1993).

Overuse injuries found clinically in the extremities are tendinitis, stress fractures, and compartment syndromes. They usually occur in sports activity, especially in endurance sports and sports demanding skill and power (Selvanetti et al 1997).

The most common clinical conditions are insertional tendinopathies such as epicondylitis, Achilles tendinopathy, and jumper's knee (Fig. 27.1). Hip adductor syndrome is recognized as chronic tendinopathy not only at the insertion site but also near the myotendinous junction of the muscle involved, mostly the adductor longus muscle (Jarvinen et al 1997). Another type of overuse injury related to the tendon is iliotibial band friction syndrome. It is an overuse injury caused by excessive rubbing of the band over the lateral femoral epicondyle during sports activities with repetitive knee flexion and extension (Franco et al 1997). On the other hand, hamstring syndrome with pain around the ischial tuberosity is a different category of tendon-related overuse injuries. It is caused by the tight piriformis muscle and tendon which compress and irritate the main trunk of the sciatic nerve (Orava 1997).

Overuse injuries seen in tendon or tendon–bone insertion are usually called tendinitis, and recently tendinopathy has been suggested as a better descriptive term. These disorders can be classified according to their anatomical site and histopathological pattern. Inflammation of the paratenon is classified as paratenonitis. Symptomatic overload of the tendon with vascular disruption and inflammatory repair response is defined as tendinitis, while intratendinous degeneration due to atrophy is called tendinosis (Fig. 27.2) (Selvanetti et al 1997).

Diagnosis of tendon-related overuse injuries is not very difficult in typical cases. History of overuse and

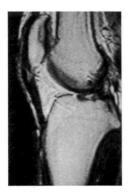

Figure 27.1 Insertional tendinopathy in a soccer player. Sagittal T_2-weighted image shows relatively high signal at the proximal end of the patella tendon.

repeated painful episodes during activities are necessary for diagnosis. The clinical findings of tendon overuse injuries include tenderness, pain on motion under resistance, and pain on tendon stretching. Although most tendon injuries can be evaluated fully by medical history and clinical assessment, some types of tendon overuse injuries may require additional imaging for localization and characterization.

Stress fractures nowadays are generally associated with athletic activities, although they were commonly seen in soldiers in the past. In fact, some types were known as 'march fractures'. Stress fractures are defined as partial or complete fractures depending upon the extent of the fracture line (Fig. 27.3). Stress on the bone may be imposed by impact, muscle pull, or muscle fatigue. The most common site of involvement is the tibia, but almost all of the lower extremity bones as well as some of the upper extremity bones may be injured as a result of overuse. Clinical diagnosis of stress fractures is relatively easy if physicians take a precise history and physical findings, although bone tumors may be part of the differential diagnosis in some cases. Pain increases with activity and distinct tenderness can be detected in the involved bone. Radiographs usually show a fracture line through the bone surrounded by a sclerotic shadow without displacement. New periosteal callus may or may not be seen. Bone scans and magnetic resonance imaging (MRI) are very useful in the case of negative radiographs (Fig. 27.4).

Wiley et al (1987) described the clinical pictures of exertional compartmental syndrome as the presence of crampy muscle pain precipitated by a fixed workload. Other terms that have been used are Volkmann's ischemia, traumatic tension in muscles, impending

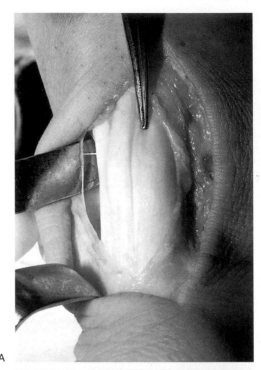

A

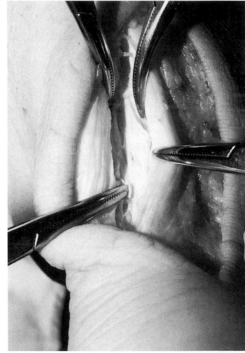

B

Figure 27.2 A: Peritendinitis with tendinosis of the Achilles tendon in a rugby football player. B: Note the thickened paratenon and degenerated nodular portion in the midsubstance of the tendon.

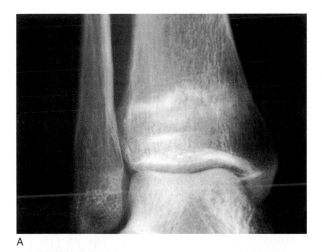

A

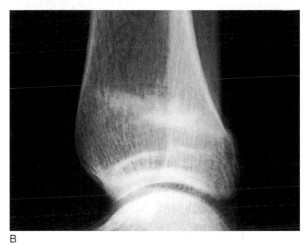

B

Figure 27.3 A,B: Stress fracture of the tibia in a marathon runner.

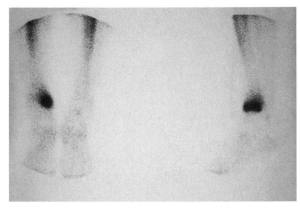

Figure 27.4 Stress fracture of the tibia in a volleyball player. The bone scan shows focally increased activity at the medial malleolus.

ischemic contracture, anterior tibial syndrome, and calf hypertension. The appearance of pain, sensory symptoms, or muscle weakness requires a thorough examination to rule out a compartmental syndrome. Also, the passive muscle stretch test will cause pain if the muscle is ischemic. Tissue pressure should be measured in questionable cases. Patients with chronic compartmental syndrome usually have high resting pressures and consistently require prolonged periods of time for compartmental pressures to return to pre-exercise levels. In order to confirm diagnosis of chronic compartmental syndrome, compartmental pressures can be measured before and immediately after exercise and after a recovery period of 10–20 min. Teitz (1989) reported that resting pressures of 108 athletes with

leg pain ranged from 18 to 28 mmHg, with a mean of 22 mmHg, whereas the resting mean pressure of asymptomatic controls was 8 mmHg. After exercise, mean compartmental pressure in the symptomatic patients was 80 mmHg with a range from 48 to 135 mmHg. On the other hand, the mean pressure was 26 mmHg in the control population. In the controls, it took approximately 1 min to return to resting pressure. In the symptomatic patients, return to resting pressures averaged 40 min.

What are the differences between overuse injuries in the aging population and those in young athletes? Aging athletes are often the victims of two types of injury: those that they incurred in their youth, and those that result from their current training regime (Menard & Stanish 1989). Usually they have degenerative tissue problems in the musculoskeletal system which have resulted from chronic overuse or trauma experienced over years of athletic stress. They may have lower limb malalignment such as varus or valgus knee and calcaneus varus/valgus. Joint space narrowing with varus/valgus knee with previous meniscal surgery is a typical example. Brown (1993) examined the occurrence of injury or painful episodes that limit participation in two groups, in the age range 60–72 years, who participated in either low-intensity mobility exercise or moderate-intensity aerobic training. Participants in the moderate-intensity training group exhibited various complaints, such as knee and foot pain, plantar fasciitis, compartmental syndrome, muscle strain (hamstrings or hip adductors), and stress fractures. Participants with pre-existing orthopedic abnormalities had a higher incidence of painful episodes than those without previous orthopedic problems. Brown concluded that obesity, history of previous joint injury and osteoarthritis, foot deformity, limited range of ankle dorsiflexion, and hip flexor tightness seemed to have a close relationship to the development of painful episodes, including overuse injuries.

In summary, degenerative problems and previous orthopedic lesions, as well as age-associated loss of flexibility, are the factors which are believed to be associated with overuse injuries in aging populations, including master athletes.

MANAGEMENT OF OVERUSE INJURIES

The principles of treatment of overuse injuries in aging athletes are basically the same as in young athletes. Conservative treatment involving rest, ice and heat, taping, non-steroidal anti-inflammatory drugs (NSAIDs), stretching, muscle strengthening, and bracing is usually recommended (Brown 1993). Icing is useful in the first few days after the injury to decrease swelling and pain, while heat may be used later in the healing process to promote remodeling of the scar tissue (Teitz 1989). Administration of NSAIDs generally inhibits the synthesis of the prostaglandins and lowers the increased vascular permeability. However, over-suppression of the inflammatory response by drugs may also influence a reparative reaction, and thus decreased tissue regeneration may occur. If significant inflammation persists, these drugs are usually useful in reducing it, and fibroblasts can synthesize new collagen (Teitz 1989). Muscle strengthening, taping and bracing may be helpful to prevent further damage to the injured tendons and ligaments.

In addition to these therapeutic modalities, it is important to consider those factors thought to be significant in preventing further damage to overuse injuries (Teitz 1989). Consideration of intensity and duration of activity level is essential, and activity level should be determined according to the ability and physical status of each individual. Exercise technique is also an important factor. Reasonable and effective motion of each performance puts less stress on the musculoskeletal system and reduces the risk of overuse injuries. For example, dancers who always use the rectus femoris to raise their legs to the front will develop rectus femoris tendinopathy. If they use the iliopsoas muscle, which is a much stronger hip flexor, they can achieve this performance more effectively with less risk of tendinopathy. Players should choose equipment, e.g. tennis rackets and shoes, which reduce the shock transferred from the ball or ground. The environment may also contribute to overuse injuries. Running on hard ground such as asphalt, exercising on sloping ground, and activities in very cold or hot environments must be conducted carefully.

Some injuries, such as stress fracture in the femoral neck, hamstring syndrome or severe persistent tendinopathy, may require surgical treatment.

Consideration should be given to the management of overuse injuries in aging athletes (Menard & Stanish 1989). First, considering the relative lack of adaptability of such athletes, the factors which are related to overuse injuries, such as intensity and technique of exercise, equipment and environment, should be carefully controlled and individualized. Secondly, often elderly athletes exhibit some degree of degeneration in their musculoskeletal and cardiovascular systems. Relatively lower stress will cause overuse injuries, and degenerative conditions could influence the process of healing. Consequently, it will take older athletes a longer time to return to sports activities than is the case with younger athletes. Older athletes may discontinue participation in athletic activities after a long period of treatment. Therefore, it is important to educate them about the characteristics of the injuries and the physical background, and about the need to continue with relatively mild exercise, such as swimming and cycling, during the treatment period. Finally, consideration of psychological stability is important for athletes, since they can often become very despondent about their injuries. Sports medicine doctors are advised not to state definitively that athletes will need to stop their activities in order to facilitate treatment.

CONCLUSIONS

The overall picture of overuse injuries in aging populations has been described. A proper approach to the management of overuse injuries in elderly athletes requires a sound knowledge of anatomy, morphology and physiology, and a thorough understanding of clinical pathology. It should be realized that aging athletes have some degree of degeneration in the musculoskeletal system and that they may also have some previous orthopedic abnormalities. Therefore, comprehensive treatment is required in the management of overuse injuries in this population, including modification of training style and equipment, improvement of the environment, appropriate drugs and physical therapy, taping and bracing, and a suitable psychological approach.

REFERENCES

Alnaqeeb M A, Alzrid N S, Eoldspink E 1984 Connective tissue changes and physical properties of developing and aging skeletal muscle. Journal of Anatomy 139: 677–689

Aniansson A, Erimby B, Nygaard E 1980 Muscle fiber composition and fiber area in various age groups. Muscle and Nerve 2: 271–272

Åstrand P O 1986 Exercise physiology of the mature athlete. In: Sutton J R, Brock R M (eds) Sports medicine for the mature athlete. Benchmark Press, Indianapolis, p 3

Benjamin M, Evans E J, Copp L 1986 The histology of tendon attachments to bone in man. Journal of Anatomy 149: 89–100

Booth F W, Gould E W 1975 Effects of training of endurance exercise on bone dimensions, collagen and calcium in the aged male rat. Exercise and Sport Sciences Reviews 3: 83–112

Brown M 1993 Physical and orthopaedic limitations to exercise in the elderly. In: Buckwalter J A, Goldberg V A, Woo S L Y (eds) Musculoskeletal soft-tissue aging: Impact of mobility. American Academy of Orthopaedic Surgeons, Rosemont, ch 16, p 209–216

Caplan A, Carlson B, Faulkner J, Fischman D, Garrett W Jr 1987 Skeletal muscle. In: Woo S L Y, Buckwalter J A (eds) Injury and repair of the musculoskeletal soft tissue. American Academy of Orthopaedic Surgeons, Park Ridge, IL, ch 6, p 209

Cooper R R, Misol S 1970 Tendon and ligament insertion: a light and electron microscopic study. Journal of Bone and Joint Surgery 52A: 1–21

Essen-Eustausson B, Borees O 1986 Histochemical and metabolic characteristics of human skeletal muscle in relation to age. Acta Physiologica Scandinavica 126: 107–114

Franco V, Cerullo G, Gianni E, Puddu G 1997 Iliotibial band friction syndrome. Operative Techniques in Sports Medicine 5(3): 153–156

Gelberman R, Goldberg V, An K N, Banes A 1987 Tendon. In: Woo S L Y, Buckwalter J A (eds) Injury and repair of the musculoskeletal soft tissue. American Academy of Orthopaedic Surgeons, Park Ridge, IL, ch 1, p 5

Green H J 1986 Characteristics of aging human skeletal muscles. In: Sutton J R, Brock R M (eds) Sports medicine for the mature athlete. Benchmark Press, Indianapolis, p 17

Jarvinen M, Orava S, Kujula U M 1997 Groin pain (adductor syndrome). Operative Techniques in Sports Medicine 5(3): 133–137

Menard D, Stanish W D 1989 The aging athletes. American Journal of Sports Medicine 17: 187–196

Morein G, Goldefter L, Kobyliansky E 1978 Changes in the mechanical properties of rat tail tendons during post natal osteogenesis. Anatomy and Embryology 154: 121–124

Noyes F R, Grood E S 1976 The strength of the anterior cruciate ligament in human and rhesus monkeys: age-related and species-related changes. Journal of Bone and Joint Surgery 58A: 1074–1082

Orava S 1997 Hamstring syndrome. Operative Techniques in Sports Medicine 5(3): 143–149

Sato T, Akatsuka H, Kito Y 1986 Age changes of myofibrils of human minor pectoral muscle, mechanics of aging and development. Mechanisms of Ageing and Development 34: 297–304

Sclvanetti, Cipolla M, Puddu G 1997 Overuse tendon injuries: basic science and classification. Operative Techniques in Sports Medicine 5(3): 110–117

Sinett P 1986 Aging and disease. Australian Family Physician 15(2): 123–127

Teitz C C 1989 Overuse injuries. In: Teitz C C (ed) Scientific foundation of sports medicine. B C Decker, Toronto, ch 13, p 299

Twomey L, Taylor J 1985 Age changes in lumbar intervertebral discs. Acta Orthopaedica Scandinavica 56: 496–499

Vailas A C, Pedrini V A, Pedrini-Mille A, Holloszy J O 1985 Patellar tendon matrix changes associated with aging and voluntary exercise. Journal of Applied Physiology 58: 1572–1576

Viidik A 1979 Connective tissues – possible implications of the temporal changes for the aging process. Mechanisms of Ageing and Development 9: 267–285

Wiley J P, Clement D B, Doyle D L, Tauton J E 1987 A primary care perspective of chronic compartment syndrome of the leg. The Physician and Sportsmedicine 15: 111–120

Woo S L Y, Hollis J M, Adams D J 1991 Tensile properties of the human femur-anterior cruciate ligament-tibia complex: The effects of specimen age and orientation. American Journal of Sports Medicine 19: 217–225

Woo S L Y, Maynard J A, Butler D L et al 1987 Ligament, tendon, and joint capsule insertions to bone. In: Woo S L Y, Buckwalter J A (eds) Injury and repair of the musculoskeletal soft tissue. American Academy of Orthopaedic Surgeons, Park Ridge, IL, ch 4, p 133

28

Balance in the older person: effects of age and disease

Graham K. Kerr
Charles J. Worringham

KEY POINTS

1. The increased occurrence of falls in the elderly are a major cause of injury and disability.
2. Age-related physiological changes to the sensory and musculoskeletal systems affect balance and gait.
3. Changes in vision, such as age-related maculopathy, increase postural instability.
4. The deterioration in proprioception that occurs with normal ageing and as a consequence of diabetic peripheral neuropathy affects balance and gait.
5. Age-related impairments of the vestibular system increase postural instability.
6. Impaired muscle function is associated with instability during balance, gait and other tasks.

INTRODUCTION

The maintenance of balance while standing and walking relies on intact visual, proprioceptive, vestibular and motor systems. However, the interactions between these systems may be altered in people with sensory and/or motor impairment, which can result from a range of different injuries and diseases, as well as normal age-related changes. Many conditions can disturb normal balance, including both disorders affecting brain structures such as the cerebellum and those whose effect is more peripheral, particularly in the three key sensory systems, vision, proprioception and the vestibular system. In the following sections of this chapter, we review some of the important features of the more common disorders that affect balance.

INCIDENCE OF FALLS AND HEALTH CARE IMPLICATIONS

The increased occurrence of falls with advancing age is a significant cause of mortality, morbidity and disability, affecting not only the individuals concerned, but the health care system and the broader community. It is estimated, for example, that by the age of 85, approximately half of all injury-related deaths arise from falls, with between one-third and a quarter of all people over 65 reporting a fall in the previous year (Blake et al 1988). Although many of these events may cause only minor injuries, others result in serious disabling injuries, including fractures of the hip and head injuries. The indirect effects of falls include the costs of health care, estimated to exceed $10 000 for each person hospitalized as a result of a fall in the USA. Data from a recent Australian study of community-dwelling adults over the age of 70 showed that, in a 12-month period, 49% of the subjects fell, and 23% fell more than once; 9% suffered fractures and 10% strains or other moderate injuries as a result of the fall. Many of these events occurred during activities such as walking, often under altered sensory or environmental conditions (Hill et al 1999). Predisposition to falling also contributes to reduced quality of life and placement of people in institutional care (Lord 1996).

AGE-RELATED CHANGES THAT AFFECT FALLS AND BALANCE

There is widespread agreement that falls result from multiple factors – both environmental (e.g. trip and slip hazards) and biological (age-related changes in strength, coordination and sensory systems, such as vision, contributing to falls) (Lord 1996, Stelmach & Worringham 1985). Decreased joint range of motion and muscle strength, as well as alterations in anthropometric variables (decreased height, increased kyphosis), are all age-related effects on the musculoskeletal system that affect postural stability during quiet stance and gait. Age-related changes to the sensory and motor systems also contribute to increased postural instability and predisposition to falls.

Standing postural sway is greater in the elderly, and muscle onsets in reaction to a perturbation are slower, although the same pattern of muscle response organization is maintained (Woollacott 1993). Lateral instability is increased in older adults and is a predictor of falling. To compensate for disturbances to their postural balance, older adults take more lateral steps than young adults to maintain balance (Woollacott & Tang 1997).

There are pronounced changes in gait due to ageing that ensure that upright stance is not compromised. Older people adopt a more rigid posture, take shorter steps and strides and have lower cadence. These adaptive strategies minimize the ground reaction forces when the foot strikes the ground during each step, which can cause instability if not controlled for (Woollacott & Tang 1997). The more rigid posture adopted allows stabilization of the upper body, the head and the direction of gaze. However, there is greater acceleration of the head in older adults during walking, potentially leading to a difference in the visual motion and vestibular cues to regulate upright posture during walking.

Older people take longer to implement an avoidance strategy when walking (Patla 1993), and use a more conservative strategy when stepping over obstacles, such as slower crossing speeds, shorter heel-to-obstacle distance after crossing, and a shorter crossing-step length. Foot clearance when stepping over obstacles remains similar to that of young adults, although it is not clear whether this is due to slower speed during motion. Attention demand during walking is also greater in older people than in young adults (Teasdale et al 1993).

VISION AND BALANCE

During quiet stance, the visual cues provided by small movements of the body with respect to the external visual environment may be used to ensure stable postural control. When visual cues are degraded by ocular disease such as retinitis pigmentosa, age-related maculopathy (ARM) and diabetic retinopathy, postural instability is increased. People with visual impairment are more likely to have falls. They are also more dependent on visual information to judge the orientation of their body to the environment, particularly when there is conflict between sensory cues (Lord 1996).

The age-related changes in the visual system, including decreased visual acuity and contrast sensitivity, are predictors of falls. Of the two, contrast sensitivity is a more important predictor. Decreased contrast sensitivity, particularly at low and intermediate spatial frequencies, may impair perception of edges such as steps and curbs, thereby contributing to an increased risk of falling (Lord 1996).

Visual control of walking is altered with ageing, particularly when a change of movement is required. Impaired visual function decreases mobility and common obstacles such as curbs and stairs result in slower movements and larger foot clearances when visual acuity is degraded. Decreased contrast sensitivity also has a strong relationship to decreased mobility performance and postural stability in subjects with poor vision (Elliott et al 1995).

Age-related maculopathy

Age-related maculopathy (ARM) is the leading cause of severe and irreversible visual impairment in the older population (Hampton & Nelsen 1992) and is predicted to become more prevalent in our society. It affects 1.2–1.8% of the general population, rising to 18.5% over the age of 85, with a marked preponderance of women affected. The impact of ARM on visual function is significant, resulting in loss of visual acuity, contrast sensitivity, colour vision problems, adaptation difficulties and central visual field defects. This loss of sensitivity of central visual field function probably has a significant impact on postural stability of patients with ARM, as central vision plays a key role in postural stability (Paulus et al 1984). Thus, the efficacy of visual input in postural stability is significantly reduced in people with ARM (Elliott et al 1995, Turano et al 1996). The magnitude of postural stabilization is strongly related to increased motion displacement thresholds and binocular scotomas within the central 5° of the visual field (Turano et al 1996). People with ARM also have significantly poorer mobility performance under low illumination levels. In addition, they complain of problems in mobility, including difficulties with street crossings and seeing traffic lights (Lovie-Kitchin & Bowman 1985).

As an adaptation to the disease process, people with ARM rely more on proprioceptive information during the maintenance of quiet stance (Elliott et al 1995, Turano et al 1996). However, in conditions where other sensory systems are unreliable for postural control, there is an increased risk of falling because normal visual cues are either degraded or unavailable (Lord 1996).

The ability to integrate different sources of sensory information is therefore crucial if people are to adapt to alterations in their sensory and motor systems due to injury or disease. This ability is especially important in the control of balance. However, elderly adults have difficulties in adapting to alterations in sensory information and show decreased postural stability when visual and proprioceptive information is changed (Hay et al 1996). This has implications for the assessment of postural changes that occur as a result of age-related visual deterioration. People with ARM may have markedly different abilities for compensating to altered visual information than do younger people with other visual deficits.

Although upright posture can be maintained without vision, when there are deficits in the proprioceptive and vestibular systems, there is an increased reliance on vision for maintaining postural stability. This is evident in diabetic peripheral neuropathy, where deficits in proprioception around the ankle joint cause impairment in balance when vision is occluded. Indeed, this population has an increased incidence of falls arising from alterations in postural control (Cavanagh et al 1993). Similarly, visual impairment will induce a compensatory bias in postural control towards the use of other senses. Thus, in situations in which increased reliance would normally be placed on visual mechanisms, such as when standing or walking on a slippery or uneven surface, people with visual impairment are more prone to falling (Lord 1996).

PROPRIOCEPTION AND BALANCE

During standing and walking, proprioceptive information from sensory receptors in muscles, tendons, joints and skin informs the central nervous system (CNS) of the orientation of the body and of its position and velocity. Proprioceptive information not only contributes to an internal representation of the vertical orientation of the body (Gurfinkel et al 1995), but is also used to establish our sense of body shape, size and orientation. It is therefore essential for continuous, integrative control of voluntary human movement and enables us to interact appropriately with our environment (Gandevia & Burke 1992).

Sensory receptors in the legs and feet are able to sense changing muscle lengths and the different pressures applied. This information is used to control the centre of mass of the body to ensure that it lies within the body's base of support. These inputs from the lower limbs are used by the CNS to coordinate and control sequential rotations of body and limb segments, particularly during locomotion, and for balance control.

Several aspects of proprioceptive information are affected as a consequence of normal ageing. Cutaneous vibratory sensation and joint sensation deteriorate with age. This loss of sensation is not only a common finding with increasing age, affecting some

50% of the elderly without neurological disease (Horak 1992), but is also associated with the risk of falling because of the central role played by proprioceptive inputs in balance. The degradation of proprioceptive information means that even the most routine of daily tasks, including standing and walking, require visual feedback and intense concentration. Uncoordinated gait often results, and postural stability is compromised (Cavanagh et al 1993, Inglis et al 1994). Thus, although movement is still possible when proprioception is absent or degraded, its control is significantly affected.

Diabetes and diabetic peripheral neuropathy

In 1990, it was estimated that 3.8% of the Australian population were diagnosed with diabetes mellitus and that 900 000 Australians would acquire the disease by the year 2000 (International Diabetes Institute 2000). The alteration of the metabolism of carbohydrates, fats and proteins produced by diabetes mellitus is largely due to inadequate control of blood glucose levels by insulin. This hyperglycaemic state can cause significant vascular complications, leading to eye disease and reduced vision (retinopathy), kidney disease (nephropathy) and complications affecting the peripheral nervous system (diabetic neuropathy).

Diabetic peripheral neuropathy is a complication of diabetes mellitus which results from damage to the peripheral nerves, and affects some 60% of diabetic patients. Several types of diabetic peripheral neuropathy have been identified, the most common of which is distal symmetric polyneuropathy; this predominantly affects the sensory system, but also affects the motor and autonomic systems to varying degrees. The symptoms of distal symmetric polyneuropathy include sensations of burning, tingling, numbness, paraesthesiae and loss of sensation. These deficits typically appear first in the toes and lower half of the lower limbs, then in the fingertips, and steadily progress proximally (Thomas & Tomlinson 1993). The progression of distal symmetric polyneuropathy is consistent with a 'dying back' process of neuronal degeneration, whereby the distal portions of the longest nerves are affected first. These symptoms may be slight initially and go unnoticed for several years because nerve damage usually occurs over a long period of time.

Peripheral neuropathy is the single most significant factor in the development of ulceration and lower extremity amputation. The combined effects of sensory, motor and autonomic disturbances to the lower limb result in increased plantar pressures, reduced skin viability, foot deformities and loss of protective sensation. When these factors are combined with peripheral vascular disease, the foot is subject to an increased risk of injury and a reduced ability to heal, prolonging infection and increasing the risk of gangrene.

The ability to sense movement of the ankle is impaired in people with diabetic peripheral neuropathy. The threshold for detection of movement onset has been found to be significantly increased for dorsi- and plantarflexion movements of the ankle joint (Simoneau et al 1995), which are extremely important for the control of posture. Alterations in gait pattern have been observed in people with diabetic peripheral neuropathy. Patients with peripheral neuropathy have a perception of decreased safety in challenging sensory environments (e.g. in the dark), an increased risk of injury during gait, and an increased incidence of falls (Cavanagh et al 1993).

Depending on the severity, people with diabetic peripheral neuropathy are more unstable, as indicated by increased sway during quiet stance (Cavanagh et al 1993). They exhibit a hip strategy of postural control and delayed onset and scaling of their muscular responses to postural perturbations (Inglis et al 1994). Most of these effects are probably due to impaired somatosensory feedback and the consequent decrease of reflexes and decreased muscle strength. This indicates that, in diabetic peripheral neuropathy, the way in which posture and balance are organized and controlled by the CNS may be altered. As proprioceptive information is used by the CNS to maintain and update an internal reference for upright posture, postural alterations can be expected.

THE VESTIBULAR SYSTEM AND BALANCE

The vestibular system is also involved in the control of normal stance (Allum & Pfaltz 1985). However, the vestibular system probably contributes less to overall postural stability than do the proprioceptive and visual systems, because thresholds for perception of sway during standing are much higher for vestibular senses (Fitzpatrick & McCloskey 1994).

Nevertheless, the vestibular system exerts a major influence over the control of balance, so that impairments in its function may lead to symptoms that include postural instability, and, in some instances, directly to falls. The vestibular system shows degeneration with age and is susceptible to various disorders, of which three are most prominent: vestibular neuritis, Ménière's disease and benign paroxysmal positional vertigo (Baloh & Honrubia 1990, Büttner 1999).

Vestibular neuritis

Mainly a disorder affecting people in the middle years of life, between the third and sixth decades, vestibular neuritis not infrequently follows a viral infection of the upper respiratory tract, but may also be the consequence of a vascular disorder. Its onset is acute, with patients experiencing a bout of vertigo, often quite serious, for a period that may extend from some hours to several days. The vertigo is experienced even when the patient remains motionless. Unlike some other conditions affecting the vestibular system, there are no effects on hearing. The cause of these symptoms, and its effect on balance, reviewed below, is a decreased firing rate in fibres leading from the vestibular receptors. The condition usually affects just one side. This disorder is a peripheral one, but its symptoms may be mimicked by some CNS conditions. For example, multiple sclerosis, when producing plaques in parts of the brain stem, can lead to similar deficits.

Balance in patients with vestibular neuritis is frequently affected. Not only will they locate the visual vertical inaccurately and misjudge the 'subjective straight ahead', but they may also show postural imbalance and be susceptible to falls towards the affected side.

Vestibular neuritis tends to resolve gradually even without treatment, over a period of a few days up to about 6 weeks. This improvement is likely to be the result of vestibular compensation – an adaptive process whereby the abnormal input from the periphery no longer produces the same effect centrally. However, many people continue to experience some level of symptoms, and these residual effects may include poor balance. In particular, manoeuvres that include rapid head motions may spark instability and a possible fall. 'Vestibular exercises' may be valuable in promoting compensation, as are whole body movements that can promote the restoration of a person's balance control.

Ménière's disease

One of the more common afflictions of the vestibular system, Ménière's disease can strike a person at any age, but is more typically seen in people in their 30s and 40s. Again, vertigo is the primary symptom, but unlike vestibular neuritis, it tends to be in recurrent episodes lasting a few minutes or a few hours. In addition, it is often accompanied by other symptoms, including tinnitus which is frequently subjectively loud, fluctuating loss of hearing, and sometimes by a sensation of 'fullness' of the ear. The disease results from endolymphatic hydrops. Because of excessive production and/or inadequate reabsorption of endolymph, membranes retaining the endolymph rupture, leading to mixing of endolymph and perilymph. The former has a substantially higher potassium concentration, which may activate the sensory structures of the vestibular system, giving rise to signals of movement and position that do not reflect the person's actual posture.

Ménière's disease, in contrast to vestibular neuritis, may often afflict a person bilaterally. The acute phase, with recurrent attacks whose frequency and duration are most variable, gives way to an often prolonged chronic phase with reduced symptoms. Balance is often impaired markedly in the acute phase, but relatively subtle balance impairments are normal for the chronic phase. Thus, a person may appear to have essentially normal postural control, but may be especially reliant on proprioceptive and visual cues. Where these are removed, either in clinical testing or in conditions of poor illumination, visual deficits and/or neuropathy (see previous sections), the patient may have noticeably impaired balance.

A minority of Ménière's disease sufferers may have a more serious postural complication, whereby they experience sudden and unpredictable falls, often with no attempt to prevent the fall or protect themselves. These 'drop' attacks, or 'Turmakin otolithic crises' are thought to represent a special form of Ménière's disease in which the otolith system, as opposed to the semicircular canals, is involved. Not surprisingly, they frequently result in injury.

Benign paroxysmal positioning/positional vertigo (BPPV)

A third condition that can lead to poor balance control and which results from a disturbance of normal vestibular function is benign paroxysmal positional vertigo. Short-duration vertigo spells (up to slightly more than half a minute) are induced when the person repositions the head, typically from an upright position to one with the affected side downwards, relative to gravity. The underlying process is described as benign, since it has a relatively straightforward physical cause. It involves clots of material, presumed to be derived from otoconia, forming a plug which exerts forces on the cupula when the critical position is adopted. This gives rise to misleading sensory signals. The canal most frequently affected is the posterior semicircular canal. Because of its orientation, the sitting to lying movement induces forces that shift the plug towards the cupula, thus producing an attack. Predisposing factors include viral infections and other flu-like symptoms, noted by many patients in the period preceding the first attack, but head trauma has also been reported as an underlying cause. Furthermore, a number of patients report having had a previous bout of vestibular neuritis. However, many cases are labelled as idiopathic. BPPV is increasingly seen with advancing age, with one estimate that nearly a third of all adults will have had at least one episode by the time they reach the age of 70.

Combined with the vertiginous symptoms, postural imbalance is often experienced. Since attacks in this particular condition are specifically triggered by head movements, special risks are present in conditions when a person with BPPV is liable to make such movements. A construction worker, for example, standing on a ladder but quickly looking up to check for obstacles or a fellow worker, might trigger an attack that leads to a fall from height.

BPPV tends to resolve over a variable period (weeks to months), but in some individuals it never fully subsides and may still leave a deficit in balance control. A notable feature of treatment is the often spectacular success of various 'liberatory' manoeuvres. These will not be reviewed here, but a common feature is that the patient undergoes a set of movements designed to impel the plug away from the cupula and towards the ampulla, with the goal of having it settle in the utricle, where its presence is quite benign. Nevertheless, despite the absence of clinical symptoms, postural control deficits can still be observed. Dynamic posturography showed impaired balance in patients 3 days and again at 1 month following the Semont liberatory manoeuvre, for example (Di Girolamo et al 1998).

MOTOR OUTPUT

Thus far, a variety of impairments in sensory systems have been outlined, together with their effects on balance control. Of course, even if one assumes that an individual had the ideally functioning visual, proprioceptive and vestibular systems, balance may still be affected because of impairments in the selection and programming of balance-related muscle actions, or because of peripheral motor dysfunction.

A variety of well-known neurological diseases can produce deteriorations in balance primarily because of motor output as opposed to sensory dysfunction. These include not only idiopathic Parkinson's disease and cerebellar disease, involving the two principal subcortical motor loops, but less common pathology such as progressive supranuclear palsy, a form of parkinsonism in which one hallmark is a propensity to fall backwards. In addition to their typical manifestation in hemiplegia, ischaemic or haemorrhagic strokes may also affect balance specifically, especially if occurring near the midline of the cerebellum or in other sites participating in balance control.

To maintain balance, or to engage a postural reflex in the event of an impending fall, the CNS must not only be able to generate an appropriate set of muscle commands, but also send them rapidly to the participating muscles. Obviously, demyelinating disease may decrease this rate, but age alone is associated with marked loss of nerve conduction velocity. In turn, the musculature must be capable of generating sufficient force to execute the required motions or torques to counteract imbalance – a frequent problem for the elderly. The role of muscle strength as a determining factor in the maintenance of balance depends on several issues. As a general rule, the more impaired are the non-muscle components of balance (e.g. poor proprioceptive acuity), the more dependence will be placed on the ability to generate high muscle forces. This is because the forces required to retain balance increase as the centre of mass approaches the edge of the base of support, or has greater velocity, or both. Both situations occur with increased frequency when sensory losses are evident. Empirically, several authors have found associations between decreased muscle strength and instability or actual falls. For example, Scarborough et al (1999) reported in a group of older adults that greater quadriceps strength was positively associated with dynamic stability during both gait and rising from a chair. Indeed, lower extremity strength limits the lowest level of chair from which older people can rise successfully. Furthermore, aspects of muscle function other than maximum isometric strength may be particularly important, e.g. the rate of force development, which is also correlated with instability in older adults (Izquierdo et al 1999). Decline in muscle strength with age, especially in females, has also been taken to explain why, in obstacle avoidance and balance recovery tasks, older people and females perform worse than younger subjects and males in those tasks with large force requirements (Schultz et al 1997).

CONCLUSIONS

1. Impaired balance and consequent falls represent a substantial and growing societal burden, especially in the older section of the population.
2. Vision has a major role in balance control, especially in compensating when other senses are lost or degraded. Age-related maculopathy is one common visual disorder of the elderly which has demonstrable effects on balance.
3. Of all the sensory inputs, proprioception is the most crucial for normal balance control. Not only does proprioceptive function deteriorate with normal ageing, but it is also impaired by various diseases, notably diabetic peripheral neuropathy.
4. A range of vestibular dysfunctions can impair balance as well as giving rise to vertigo and other symptoms. Of the three most common disorders, benign paroxysmal positional vertigo is not only the most prevalent, but also has the strongest association with advancing age.
5. Central processes and the organization of balance-related motor commands can be disrupted by neurological disease of the CNS, notably those affecting the basal ganglia and cerebellum.
6. Decreased muscle strength has minimal effects on some balance tasks, but can impose significant limitations on others. The rate of force production, rather than simple maximal isometric strength, is an important factor. Impaired muscle function is associated with instability during gait and with impairments in tasks such as rising from a chair.

REFERENCES

Allum J, Pfaltz C 1985 Visual and vestibular contributions to pitch sway stabilization in the ankle muscles of normals and patients with bilateral vestibular deficits. Experimental Brain Research 58: 82–94

Baloh R, Honrubia V (eds) 1990 Clinical neurophysiology of the vestibular system. FA Davis, Philadelphia

Blake A J, Morgan K, Bendall M J et al 1988 Falls by elderly people at home: prevalence and associated factors. Age Ageing 17: 365–372

Büttner U (ed) 1999 Vestibular dysfunction and its therapy. Karger, Basel

Cavanagh P, Simoneau G, Ulbrecht J 1993 Ulceration, unsteadiness, and uncertainty: the biomechanical consequences of diabetes mellitus. Journal of Biomechanics 26(suppl 1): 23–40

Di Girolamo S, Paludetti G, Briglia G, Cosenza A, Santarelli R, Di Nardo W 1998 Postural control in benign paroxysmal positional vertigo before and after recovery. Acta Oto-Laryngologica 118: 289–293

Elliott D B, Patla A E, Flanagan J G, Spaulding S, Rietdyk S, Strong G, Brown S 1995 The Waterloo vision and mobility study: postural control strategies in subjects with ARM. Ophthalmology and Physiological Optics 15: 553–559

Fitzpatrick R, McCloskey I 1994 Proprioceptive, visual and vestibular thresholds for the perception of sway during standing in humans. Journal of Physiology 478: 173–186

Gandevia S C, Burke D 1992 Does the nervous system depend on kinesthetic input to control natural limb movements? Behavioural and Brain Sciences 15: 615–633

Gurfinkel V S, Ivanenko Y P, Levick Y S, Babakova I A 1995 Kinesthetic reference for human orthograde posture. Neuroscience 68: 229–243

Hampton G R, Nelsen P T 1992 Age-related macular degeneration. Principles and practice. Raven Press, New York

Hay L, Bard C, Fleury M, Teasdale N 1996 Availability of visual and proprioceptive afferent messages and postural control in elderly adults. Experimental Brain Research 108: 129–139

Hill K, Schwarz J, Carroll S 1999 Falls among healthy, community-dwelling, older women: a prospective study of frequency, circumstances, consequences and prediction accuracy. Australian & New Zealand Journal of Public Health 23: 41–48

Horak F 1992 Effects of neurological disorders on postural movement strategies in the elderly. In: Vellas B, Toupet M, Rubenstein L, Albarede J L, Christen Y (eds) Falls, balance and gait disorders in the elderly. Elsevier, Paris, p 137–151

Inglis J T, Horak F B, Schupert C L, Jones-Rycewicz C 1994 The importance of somatosensory information in triggering and scaling automatic postural responses in humans. Experimental Brain Research 101: 159–164

International Diabetes Institute 2000 Online. Available: http://www.idi.org.au

Izquierdo M, Aguado X, Gonzalez R, Lopez J L, Hakkinen K 1999 Maximal explosive force production capacity and balance performance in men of different ages. European Journal of Applied Physiology & Occupational Physiology 79: 260–267

Lord S R 1996 Instability and falls in elderly people. In Lafont C, Baroni A, Allard M et al (eds) Facts and research in Gerontology (Falls, gait and balance disorders in the elderly). Springer, New York, pp 125–139

Lovie-Kitchin J, Bowman K 1985 Senile macular degeneration. Butterworth, Woburn, MA

Patla A E 1993 Age-related changes in visually guided locomotion over different terrains: major issues. In

Stelmach G, Homberg V (eds) Sensorimotor impairment in the elderly. Kluwer Academic, Amsterdam, p 231–252

Paulus W M, Straube A, Brandt T 1984 Visual stabilization of posture: physiological stimulus characteristics and clinical aspects. Brain 107: 1143–1163

Scarborough D M, Krebs D E, Harris B A 1999 Quadriceps muscle strength and dynamic stability in elderly persons. Gait and Posture 10: 10–20

Schultz A B, Ashton-Miller J A, Alexander N B 1997 What leads to age and gender differences in balance maintenance and recovery? Muscle and Nerve 5: S60–64

Simoneau, G G, Ulbrecht J S, Derr J A, Cavanagh P R 1995 Role of somatosensory input in the control of human posture. Gait & Posture 3: 115–122

Stelmach G, Worringham C 1985 Sensorimotor deficits related to postural stability: implications for falling in the elderly. Clinics in Geriatric Medicine 1: 679–694

Teasdale N, Lajoie Y, Bard C, Fleury M, Courtemanche R 1993 Cognitive processes involved for maintaining postural stability while standing and walking. In Stelmach G, Homberg V (eds) Sensorimotor impairment in the elderly. Kluwer Academic, Amsterdam, p 157–168

Thomas P K, Tomlinson D R 1993 Neuropathies predominantly affecting sensory or motor function. In: Asbury A K, Thimas P K (eds) Peripheral nerve disorders 2. Butterworth-Heinemann, Oxford, p 59–94

Turano K A, Dagnelie G, Herdman S J 1996 Visual stabilization of posture in persons with central visual field loss. Investigative Ophthalmology & Visual Science 37: 1483–1491

Woollacott M 1993 Age-related changes in posture and movement. Journal of Gerontology 48: 56–60

Woollacott M, Tang P 1997 Balance control during walking in the older adult: research and its implications. Physical Therapy 77: 647–661

29

Exercise in inflammatory arthritis and osteoarthritis

David Perry

KEY POINTS

1. Traditional teaching has recommended rest as treatment for synovitis.
2. Research confirms that active exercise can increase inflammatory changes in acute synovitis.
3. Immobility is associated with adverse effects on cartilage.
4. Aerobic conditioning exercise programmes benefit patients with inflammatory synovitis and osteoarthritis.
5. Symptoms and signs (e.g. joint score) may decrease in patients with low-grade chronic synovitis after aerobic exercises.
6. The long-term effects of exercise on synovitis and cartilage need further research.

INTRODUCTION

Although there is increasing evidence of benefit, active exercise in patients with inflammatory synovitis remains a contentious issue. When analysing the current evidence, it is important to differentiate between the systemic effects of exercise and the local supportive effect of specific loading exercise or stretching programmes applied across an articulation. It is also essential to assess the patient's current status carefully in terms of active inflammatory synovitis. Furthermore, any associated systemic complications, particularly pleuropericardial or vasculitic, must be fully evaluated first.

The reason why exercise in patients with inflammatory synovitis remains such a dilemma for rheumatologists in particular is that, traditionally, they have promoted rest and local joint immobilization as one of the mainstays of the early management of active synovitis. This does not, however, preclude the prescription of active exercise in less inflammatory phases. This chapter will therefore analyse the current evidence for the value of exercise in arthritis and attempt to distinguish between exercise levels which are beneficial and those which may be detrimental to the health of joints. It will deal initially with the potential systemic effects of exercise on the joint in animals and humans, and then review the evidence for any benefit from the local effects of loading or stretching exercise to improve joint function in inflammatory disease and osteoarthritis. Furthermore, although rest has been shown to have some relatively short-lived benefits in synovitis, prolonged immobilization is clearly deleterious to the health of bone and articular cartilage, and is the basis of the immobilization model of osteoarthritis in animals. Therefore, as a starting point, it is necessary to review briefly the rationale for rest in the active phase of synovitis and any evidence that exercise *per se* may aggravate synovitis.

EFFECTS OF REST ON SYNOVITIS

In-patient bed rest with or without individual joint immobilization has largely been abandoned by rheumatologists, partly through improvements in pharmacological agents and partly due to the imperatives of cost and reducing bed numbers. Studies such as Mills et al (1971) and Lee et al (1974) showed modest improvement in joint symptoms with rapid equilibration to the level of a non-rest group after discharge. Furthermore, other admission factors such as diet, medication or physiotherapy may have modified the disease process, despite attempts to control for these. Similarly, joint immobilization studies show only short-term benefits. Gault & Spyker (1969), in a study of 3 weeks immobilization with unilateral splintage, reported that improvements in finger joint movement and grip were no longer demonstrable compared with the unsplinted side by 1 week after remobilization. Splintage remains a useful short-term measure for particularly troublesome joints, and night splintage can be used to prevent deformity. Long-term immobilization leads to predictable degenerative articular cartilage changes which form the basis of the standard experimental model of osteoarthritis in rabbits (Fu et al 1998, Langenskiold et al 1979).

LOCAL EFFECTS OF EXERCISE ON ACTIVE SYNOVITIS

Several animal studies lend support to the view that exercise may aggravate synovitis when started inappropriately in an active phase. Fam et al (1990) reported that knee joints of rabbits with acute calcium pyrophosphate-induced synovitis, when exercised by normal cage activity or passive range movement (ROM) exercises, developed higher synovial fluid white cell (WBC) counts than immobilized knees. There was also more synovial oedema, vasodilatation and synovial lining disruption in the active groups.

In more chronic synovitis, after repeated injection of calcium pyrophosphate, synovial fluid WBC counts were comparable in exercised and non-exercised animals, but the immobilized knees exhibited less synovial cell hyperplasia, villous hypertrophy, cellular infiltration and fibrosis and, in contrast, more adverse cartilage effects. This is in keeping with the practical view that there needs to be a balance between 'too little and too much' exercise even in patients with chronic synovitis.

Furthermore, Merritt & Hunder (1983) showed that, in acute urate-induced synovitis in rabbits, isometric exercises (without joint motion) did not increase inflammatory features, but passive ROM exercises were associated with increased intra-articular temperature and synovial fluid WBC counts. Although this might suggest that joint motion, not exercise *per se*, is responsible for deleterious effects on the inflamed joint, Blake et al (1989) reported that isometric quadriceps exercise in rheumatoid patients with knee synovitis resulted in a significant rise in intra-articular pressure. The authors postulated the potential risk from these pressure changes of hypoxic-reperfusion injury. They further suggested that this might explain apparent improvement of synovitis through exercise by the mechanism of hypoxic-reperfusion autosynovectomy.

SYSTEMIC EFFECTS OF EXERCISE AND POTENTIAL EFFECTS ON THE SYNOVIUM

While several research studies show that local exercise effects may in some situations aggravate synovitis, what can be concluded from the potential systemic effects of exercise on the synovium? It is first necessary to review some of the data in relation to stress and inflammatory synovitis. Acute exercise induces many physiological changes, including changes in levels of the stress hormones and in the number and distribution of peripheral white blood cells. Catecholamines produced through exercise are probably responsible for the immediate leucocytosis and redistribution of lymphocyte subsets, whereas cortisol is likely to be the cause of the delayed neutrophilia, lymphopenia, monocytopenia and oesinopenia which occur some hours after the finish of even a short period of fairly intensive exercise. The well known anti-inflammatory properties of cortisol may have important effects on the synovium after exercise, and β-endorphins, which are produced with generally similar kinetics to cortisol after exercise, may modify local musculoskeletal pain and centrally affect mood.

Interrelationships between the immune system, neuropeptides and associated endocrine processes were more clearly defined in the 1980s, with corticotrophin-releasing hormone (CRH) highlighted as the central focus of the psychoneuroimmunological endocrine axis (Sternberg et al 1989). Many diverse chemicals can increase CRH release in the paraventricular nucleus of the hypothalamus (Box 29.1). This results in activation of the sympathetic nervous system and the hypothalamic–pituitary axis. The immediate result of the stress response is a rise in blood sugar, heart rate and blood pressure with higher levels of arousal. Other effects of the stress response are summarized in Box 29.2, and may exert action on the inflammatory process, particularly changes in glucocorticoids and natural killer cells.

Box 29.1 Factors which can increase corticotrophin-releasing hormone release

- Interleukin-1
- Interleukin-6
- TNF (tumour necrosis factor)
- Eicosanoids
- Platelet activity factor
- Acetylcholine
- Serotonin

Box 29.2 Effects of the stress response

- Increased mesolimbic dopamine
- Melantoin
- Natural killer cells
- Somatostatin
- Glucocorticoids
- Decreased growth hormone
- Somatomedin C

Box 29.3 β-endorphin effects

- Increased interleukin-2
  — autologous mixed lymphocyte reaction (MLR)
- Decreased T rosette formation
  — lymphocyte proliferation
  — inhibitory effects of PGE_2

The stress response is at first beneficial, but is eventually turned off by corticotrophin, β-endorphin and glucocorticoids. Chronic elevation of the CRH response, which can be seen after pathologically intensive exercise, causes anorexia, weight loss and immune suppression. On the other hand, chronically reduced CRH secretion may be associated with chronic fatigue syndrome. An interesting experimental model is the Lewis rat, characterized by a streptococcal cell wall-induced inflammatory (rheumatoid-like) synovitis associated with a hypofunctional CRH neuron. This poor function leads to hypoadrenalism which increases susceptibility to inflammatory arthritis.

B-endorphin, which turns off CRH, can affect many pathways and is proinflammatory (Box 29.3). Eventually, in animals, endogenous secretion or exogenous administration of cortisol inhibits effector T cells, B lymphocytes and macrophage activation, with decreased cytokine production. However, these mechanisms have not been verified in humans, so that any clinical significance remains speculative. Nevertheless, on current evidence it would appear inadvisable to allow a patient with recent synovitis, even if inactive at the time, to undertake very intensive exercise likely to cause fatigue as this might cause a relapse of synovitis, quite apart from any local deleterious effects due to repetitive loading of any abnormal joints.

POTENTIAL BENEFITS OF AEROBIC CONDITIONING EXERCISE IN PATIENTS WITH RHEUMATOID ARTHRITIS (RA)

Aerobic conditioning exercise has been shown, in many studies in rheumatoid arthritis, to produce beneficial effects, not only improving aerobic capacity, but also functional ability. Harkcom et al (1985) investigated 20 women with RA and compared three groups at different exercise intensities on a cycle ergometer for 12 weeks. Exercise intensity was maintained at 70% of maximum heart rate at 50 rpm for 15, 25 or 35 min, performed as five bouts separated by 1-min rest periods. Aerobic capacity increased in all the exercise groups, and, importantly, the count of tender joints (joint score) decreased from 32.9 to 19.9. The latter finding raises the possibility of systemic effect, which could have been cortisol-driven, but unfortunately this was not evaluated. This, however, lends support to the view that moderate chronic rheumatoid synovitis (as evidenced by the mean joint score of 32.9) is not a contraindication to active conditioning exercise programmes. It should be noted as a caveat that in this study there was a mild increase in pain levels after exercise, despite the fall in joint count.

Combined exercise regimes in RA

Ekblom et al (1975) failed to show changes in joint counts in 23 RA patients treated as in-patients for 6 weeks with muscle strengthening and mobility exercises for 5 days/week. This group performed additional strength work and cycle ergometry compared with 11 controls, who only performed the basic programme. Both groups showed an increase in muscle strength, but only the first group showed improvement in physical performance and aerobic capacity. Review of the patients at 6 months revealed that only six out of 23 continued to exercise at high levels (at least four times per week), although no relapse of disease was recorded. This may, however, only reflect selection of a group with a better prognosis in a study with quite small numbers.

Nordemar et al (1976, 1981) also published several studies in RA patients following moderate and intensive cycle ergometry which showed improved muscle function without increasing joint symptoms. They also reported significantly greater increases in type 2 than in type 1 muscle fibre size compared with pre-exercise atrophic changes. Furthermore, in a longer-term review, they reported that there was no change in oxygen consumption or heart rate compared with a control group, but there was improved ability in activities of daily living (ADL) and less progressive radiological changes. However, this relatively small study of 23 patients may again reflect patient selection rather than an effect of exercise on erosive disease. Larger studies are clearly needed to evaluate this interesting finding further.

Lyngberg et al (1988), in a study involving 20 RA patients, also showed reduction of swollen joints by about 40%, including the knees and ankles, despite repetitive action through cycle ergometry, in addition to a programme of dynamic strength and stretch work. A control group who were instructed in the latter programme only, which they were to perform at home, failed to follow the programme probably because of its complexity as well as the lack of supervision. This raises important issues of choice of suitable programmes for individual patients and their likely compliance.

Van Deusen & Harlowe (1987) reported combining T'ai-Chi Ch'uan, frequently prescribed in China for RA according to Kirsteins et al (1991), ROM stretch and relaxation techniques. They reported that, 4 months after completion of an 8-week programme, there was still recordable benefit in upper limb mobility. Perlman et al (1990) also described post-test improvements in 53 RA patients following a regime of 2 h twice weekly aerobic dance exercises combined with stretching and strengthening for 16 weeks. Improvements were seen in joint swelling, pain, health status rating and psychological assessment.

In summary, there is now sufficient evidence from many studies to confirm the safety of aerobic conditioning exercises for RA patients, if commenced during periods of moderate- or low-grade inflammatory activity. There are also clear benefits from combining such programmes with strengthening and stretching regimes. Longer-term studies are necessary, however, to evaluate the possibility of modification of disease progression raised by Nordemar's (1981) paper. Only studies with very large numbers of patients are likely to clarify such a possibility because of the complexity of the disease process and therapeutic intervention, as well as selection bias.

EXERCISE IN ANKYLOSING SPONDYLITIS (AS)

Rheumatologists have for years stressed the need for patients with ankylosing spondylitis to perform a regular exercise programme to try to retain some spinal mobility and avoid deterioration in posture. However, there is surprisingly little published work to evaluate the important components of spinal stiffness and pain, maximal in the early morning and late evening, probably mirroring the circadian rhythm of cortisol. Improvement in symptoms generally follows everyday activity, with thoracic mobility reaching its maximum at midday. A recent postal questionnaire response from 90 out of 125 AS patients contacted (Tench et al 1998) suggested that either they fail to appreciate the importance of regular exercise or the chronicity of their disease leads to non-compliance. Only 34% confirmed that they were following a daily programme, and 22% responded that they had performed no exercises in the preceding month. There are studies showing that regular exercise improves symptoms, mobility and function in the short term, but little is known or established about potential long-term effects on disease progression and outcome.

O'Driscoll et al (1978) showed significant improvement in neck movement, especially lateral flexion, in 25 AS patients following 3 weeks of intensive in-patient physiotherapy, compared with nine inactive controls. In Kraag's (1990) study, 26 AS patients, when compared with 27 non-exercised AS controls, showed significant improvement in function and finger floor distance (?hamstring stretch rather than increased spinal flexibility), but not in Schober's test, after 4 months of home physiotherapy. A rather anecdotal report from Rasmussen & Hansen (1989), in a study of 47 AS patients, stated that 18 of the group, who were undergoing 90-min weekly training sessions and who had suffered from the disease for 5 years, showed no disease progression. Without a control group, this is likely to reflect patient selection and natural history rather than any treatment effect, but clearly a long-term controlled study is needed to investigate this interesting report.

Most studies have assessed traditional spinal exercise programmes in patients with AS. However, Carbon et al (1996) showed, in 11 AS patients without hip disease or active knee joint involvement, that a brief period (30 min) of cycle ergometry exercise at around 70% $\dot{V}O_{2\,max}$ leads to a short-term improvement in spinal flexibility. This study concluded that lower limb exercises can elicit short-term benefits by a systematically mediated mechanism and the authors are currently investigating the role of cortisol or other factors in this effect.

THE ROLE OF EXERCISE IN ESTABLISHED OSTEOARTHRITIS (OA)

Although the beneficial role of exercise in the management of patients with inflammatory joint disease is becoming more widely accepted because of increasing research evidence, there is considerably less evidence for benefit in osteoarthritis. Furthermore, the mechanical impact loading effects of exercise on degenerative cartilage merits careful analysis. Pain from OA load-bearing joints, when persistent, will inhibit muscle function. Reduced joint mobility may be the result of this or the cause of further muscle dysfunction. The logic, therefore, of aiming to restore muscle strength and stretch is clear, but there is little evidence that this will then protect against further cartilage damage. Few exercise programmes have been subjected to carefully controlled studies. Rehabilitation programmes in patients with anterior cruciate ligament (ACL)-deficient knees have produced conflicting data in terms of protection against the development of degenerative change in the long-term ACL-deficient knee of unoperated patients.

In a well-controlled study of ultrasound and exercise in 69 patients with knee osteoarthritis, Falconer et al (1992) showed increased ROM and walking speed after 4 weeks of stretching exercises followed by ROM and isometric strengthening exercises. There was no difference between patients treated with or without ultrasound, but also no non-exercise controls.

Although traditionally there is a general reluctance to advise load-bearing exercises in established OA, studies of low-impact aerobic conditioning exercises have not shown adverse effects on joint symptoms. However, it could still be possible that symptoms of increasing articular damage are being masked by other systemic effects. Beals et al (1985), studying patients with RA and OA, failed to show increased joint symptoms after a vigorous session of cycle ergometry in 18 patients with OA. Kovar et al (1992) showed a reduction in knee pain and an improvement in 6-min walking distance and AIMS physical activity assessment in a randomized controlled study of 8 weeks of fitness walking in 107 patients with OA of the knee. Minor et al (1988, 1989) also showed an improvement in the aerobic capacity of OA and RA patients, confirming that both groups were deconditioned.

CONCLUSIONS

The role of exercise in both inflammatory arthritis and osteoarthritis is being increasingly evaluated. Our current state of knowledge still points to reduced activity and controlled muscle strengthening, stretching and ROM exercises as the correct management of patients in an active inflammatory phase. However, there is now considerable evidence that carefully selected patients with less active synovitis not only benefit through improved aerobic capacity and resultant well-being, but also may experience improved joint symptoms and function. It is too early to draw conclusions about possible long-term modification of the disease process and it will be difficult to examine this interesting possibility without very carefully controlled studies.

Improvements in aerobic capacity and well-being generally appear more impressive in RA patients than in OA or AS subjects and probably reflect the poorer physical status of RA patients due to their systemic as well as articular disease.

REFERENCES

Agudelo C A, Schumacher H R, Phelps P 1972 Effect of exercise on urate crystal-induced inflammation in canine joints. Arthritis and Rheumatism 15: 609–616

Baslund B, Lyngberg K, Anderson V 1993 Effect of 8 weeks bicycle training on the immune system of patients with rheumatoid arthritis. Journal of Applied Physiology 75(4): 1691–1695

Beals C A, Lampman R M, Banwell B F et al 1985 Measurement of exercise tolerance in patients with rheumatoid arthritis and osteoarthritis. Journal of Rheumatology 12: 458–461

Blake D R, Merry P, Unsworth J et al 1989 Hypoxic-reperfusion injury in the inflamed human joint. Lancet 1: 289–293

Carbon R J, Macey M G, McCarthy D A, Pereira F P, Perry J D, Wade A J 1996 The effect of 30 minutes cycle ergometry on ankylosing spondylitis. British Journal of Rheumatology 35: 167–177

Ekblom B, Lovgren O, Alderin M 1975 Effect of short term physical training on patients with rheumatoid arthritis. A six month follow-up study. Scandinavian Journal of Rheumatology 4: 87–91

Falconer J, Fam A G, Schumacher H R J R, Clayburne G 1990 Effect of joint motion on experimental calcium pyrophosphate dihydrate crystal induced arthritis. Journal of Rheumatology 17: 644–655

Falconer J, Hayes K W, Chang R W 1992 Effect of ultrasound on mobility in osteoarthritis of the knee. A randomised clinical trial. Arthritis Care and Research 5: 29–35

Fam A G, Schumacher H R Jr, Clayburne G et al 1990 Effect of joint motion on experimental calcium pyrophosphate dihydrate crystal induced arthritis. Journal of Rheumatology 17: 644–655

Fu L L K, Maffulli N, Yip K M H, Chan K M 1988 Articular cartilage lesions of the knee following immobilisation or destabilisation for 6 or 12 weeks in rabbits. Clinical Rheumatology 17: 227–233

Gault S J, Spyker J M 1969 Beneficial effect of immobilisation on joints in study using sequential analysis. Arthritis and Rheumatism 12: 34–44

Harkcom T M, Lampman R M, Banwell B F, Castor C W 1985 Therapeutic value of graded aerobic exercise training in rheumatoid arthritis. Arthritis and Rheumatism 28: 32–39

Kirsteins A E, Dietz F, Hwang S M 1991 Evaluating the safety and potential use of a weight bearing exercise, Tai Chu Chuan for rheumatoid arthritis patients. American Journal of Physical Medicine and Rehabilitation 70: 136–141

Kovar P A, Allegrante J P, MacKenzie C R 1992 Supervised fitness walking in patients with osteoarthritis of the knee: a randomised controlled trial. Annals of Internal Medicine 116: 529–534

Kraag G, Stokes B, Groh J et al 1990 The effects of comprehensive home physiotherapy and supervision on patients with ankylosing spondylitis – a randomized controlled trial. Journal of Rheumatology 17: 228–233

Lee P, Kennedy A C, Anderson J, Buchanan W W 1974 Benefit of hospitalisation in rheumatoid arthritis. Quarterly Journal of Medicine 43: 205–214

Langenskoild A, Michelsson J E, Videman T 1979 Osteoarthritis of the knee in rabbits produced by immobilisation: attempts to achieve a reproducible model for studies on pathogenesis and therapy. Acta Orthopaedica Scandinavica 50: 1–14

Lyngberg K, Danneskoild-Samsoe B, Halskov O 1988 The effect of physical training on patients with rheumatoid arthritis: changes in disease activity, muscle strength and aerobic capacity. A clinically controlled minimised cross-over study. Clinical and Experimental Rheumatology 6: 253–260

McCarthy D, Dale M M 1988 The leucocytosis of exercises: a review and model. Sports Medicine 6: 333–336

Merritt J L, Hunder G G 1983 Passive range of motion, not isometric exercises, amplifies acute urate synovitis. Archives of Physical Medicine and Rehabilitation 64: 130–131

Mills J A, Pinals R S, Ropes M W, Short C L, Sutcliffe J 1971 Value of bed rest in patients with rheumatoid arthritis. New England Journal of Medicine 284: 453–458

Minor M A, Hewett J E, Webel R R et al 1988 Exercise tolerance and disease related measures in patients with rheumatoid arthritis and osteoarthritis. Journal of Rheumatology 15: 905–911

Minor M A, Hewett J E, Webel R R et al 1989 Efficacy of physical conditioning exercise in patients with rheumatoid arthritis and osteoarthritis. Arthritis and Rheumatism 32: 1396–1405

Nordemar R, Enblom B, Zachrisson L, Lundqvist W 1981 Physical training in rheumatoid arthritis: a controlled long term study I. Scandinavian Journal of Rheumatology 10: 17–23

Nordemar R, Edström L, Ekblom B 1976 Changes in muscle fibre size and physical performance in patients with rheumatoid arthritis after short-term physical training. Scandinavian Journal of Rheumatology 5: 233–238

Nordemar R 1981 Physical training in rheumatoid arthritis: a controlled long term study II. Functional capacity and general attitudes. Scandinavian Journal of Rheumatology 10: 25–30

O'Driscoll S J, Jayson M I V, Baddeley H 1978 Neck movements in ankylosing spondylitis and their responses to physiotherapy. Annals of the Rheumatic Diseases 37: 64–66

Perlman S G, Connell K J, Clark A 1990 Dance based aerobic exercise for rheumatoid arthritis. Arthritis Care and Research 3: 29–35

Rasmussen J O, Hansen T M 1989 Physical training for patients with ankylosing spondylitis. Arthritis Care and Research 2: 25–27

Sternberg E M, Hill J M, Chrowsos G P et al 1989 Inflammatory mediator-induced hypothalamic-pituitary-adrenal axis activation is defective in streptococcal cell wall arthritis-susceptible Lewis rats. Proceedings of the National Academy of Sciences, USA 86: 2374–2378

Tench C M, Jawad A S M, Perry J D 1998 A study to assess the use of alternative therapies in a population of outpatients with ankylosing spondylitis and their compliance with conventional therapy. British Journal of Rheumatology Abstracts Supplement 2

Van Deusen J, Harlowe D 1987 The efficacy of the ROM dance programe for adults with rheumatoid arthritis. American Journal of Occupational Medicine 41: 90–95

Wallace D J 1987 The role of stress and trauma in rheumatoid arthritis and systemic lupus erythematosus. Seminars in Arthritis and Rheumatism 16: 153–157

30

Management of osteoarthritis of the knee in middle-aged physically active patients

Henry Ching Lun Ho
Kai Ming Chan   Christer Rolf

KEY POINTS

1. Osteoarthritis is not simply a condition caused by the mechanical wear and tear of ageing, nor is it caused by inflammation.
2. Epidemiological studies demonstrate a striking increase in the prevalence of osteoarthritis with advancing age.
3. No definite cure for osteoarthritis is known.
4. Successful treatment of osteoarthritis cannot be achieved without addressing the joint as a whole.
5. The treatment of osteoarthritis of the knee in middle-aged active patients requires an accurate assessment of the disease severity, gauged by subjective pain perception and functional deficit.

INTRODUCTION

The management of osteoarthritis in the middle-aged physically active patient is a controversial issue. Some may be master athletes, while others wish to participate in various recreational activities as a way of maintaining good health. Being former elite athletes, some of these patients may also have sustained a previous cruciate ligament tear resulting in functional instability. Despite treatment, the latter group is at a greater risk of developing osteoarthritis.

Osteoarthritis involves not only the articular cartilage, but also all the surrounding passive stabilizers, i.e. soft tissues such as the joint capsule and synovial lining. Successful treatment cannot be achieved without addressing the joint as a whole. Most available treatment measures are purely symptomatic, and no definite cure is known.

The prevalence of osteoarthrosis in any population is difficult to determine accurately because of difficulties in establishing a well defined diagnosis, and also because of the recurrence of symptoms over a period of time. Epidemiological studies based on symptoms, clinical examination and radiographic evaluation demonstrate a striking increase in its prevalence with advancing age (Lawrence et al 1989). The percentage of people with mild, moderate or severe radiographic changes in at least one joint increases progressively from 5% of people younger than 25 to more than 80% of people older than 75 (Praemer et al 1992). Despite this strong association between age and osteoarthrosis, the relationships between joint use, ageing and joint degeneration are far from clear. Furthermore, the changes seen in the articular cartilage from older people differ from those seen in young individuals with osteoarthrosis, and normal lifelong use has not been shown to cause osteoarthrosis *per se*. Therefore, osteoarthrosis is not simply a condition caused by the mechanical wear and tear of ageing, nor is it caused by inflammation. Rather, there is a regressive sequence of cellular and matrix alterations resulting in the loss of structure and function of the articular cartilage accompanied by cartilage repair and bone-remodelling reactions (Buckwalter & Martin 1995). Because of this process, the degeneration of the articular cartilage is not uniformly progressive, and the rate of degeneration varies between individuals and between joints. Occasionally, degeneration occurs rapidly, but most of the time it occurs over many years and may stabilize or even decrease.

The effect of joint use on degeneration has been well investigated. Moderate and probably even strenuous regular activity does not cause or accelerate the development of osteoarthrosis in normal joints with normal articular cartilage, alignment, proprioception, innervation and stability. In fact, activities which induce cyclical loading stimulate matrix synthesis, whereas prolonged static loading or the absence of loading and motion causes degradation of the matrix and eventual joint degeneration (Buckwalter & Lane 1996). Despite this importance of regular activity for the maintenance of joint health, studies of individuals in different occupations, such as farmers, construction site workers, metal workers, miners and pneumatic drill operators, have suggested that certain activities are associated with acceleration of the degenerative process. These include repetitive, intense joint loading (Buckwalter & Lane 1996, Buckwalter et al 1995), such as repetitive lifting, an awkward work posture, vibration, continuously repeated movements and a working speed that is determined by a machine.

Sports which involve high-impact or torsional loading with pivoting, such as soccer and basketball, may also accelerate joint degeneration, in addition to there being a higher risk of ligamentous injuries. Different types of sport have different intensity, rate and frequency of impact and torsional loading, of which amongst the highest are competitive football, baseball, squash, rugby, water skiing, downhill skiing and karate. These involve great amounts of pivoting of the knee and are likely to cause ligament injures and subsequent articular degeneration. On the other hand, recreational swimming, stationary cycling, rowing, skiing, golf, walking, water aerobics, jogging and ballroom dancing involve lower impact and torsional loading, and are unlikely to cause injury and degeneration (Buckwalter & Lane 1997). Those individuals with joint conditions such as joint incongruity, abnormal joint mechanics, as with ligamentous insufficiency, and malalignment problems are more likely to suffer osteoarthrosis when exposed to high-impact and torsional joint loading (Buckwalter & Lane 1996).

Athletes who have previously sustained meniscal injuries and have undergone partial meniscectomy are at increased risk of osteoarthritis. Up to 89% of these patients develop arthritic changes, and between 2 and 50% suffer some restriction in sport. In addition, between 2 and 25% stop sport altogether (Rangger et al 1997). Patients over the age of 30 with chondral damage have the worst functional outcome after this procedure.

MANAGEMENT

Many attempts have been made to treat this condition. So far, no one has ever managed to reverse the pathological process and return the knee joint to its former healthy state. Secondary OA, caused by trauma, infection and haemophilia, is only found in a minority of cases and the majority of patients belong to the so-called idiopathic group. Therefore, the available traditional methods of treatment have been primarily aimed at controlling the symptoms and functional deficit.

The patient's age, functional disability and pain, and level of expectation of the treatment have to be considered. For example, a professional middle-aged athlete may wish to continue in sport at a more intense level than an office executive who takes part in the odd weekend game of golf or tennis. Clearly, the requirements of these two groups at the extreme ends of the spectrum must be considered. Consequently, a thorough history and clinical examination are essential. Osteoarthritis causes recurrent pain and stiffness, particularly after prolonged periods of rest such as sleep, loss of joint function and effusion. All these components require accurate assessment and documentation for one to be able to assess the subsequent treatment efficacy. Pain is very subjective and is subject to temporal variation. A study by Scott & Huskisson (1979) showed that the recorded level of pain based on the visual analogue scale is different depending on whether patients have access or not to their previous pain scores. Moreover, misleading assessments are particularly likely after prolonged treatment, as the patients' memory of their initial state fades. The functional impairment inflicted on the patient is perhaps easier to quantify and qualify. Lequesne (1997) devised the algofunctional indices for the hip and the knee joints, and found it useful as a means of assessing the severity of functional deficit and evaluating and comparing the efficacy of different treatment modalities.

After a thorough assessment of the patient's symptoms and disabilities, the treatment strategies can be broadly divided into the following categories:

Patient education and psychological support. This is particularly important for athletes who view the onset of the osteoarthritis as the end of their active lifestyle. It is all too easy to slip into an inactive state which has the detrimental effect of weight gain and hence increased load across the knee joint and further progression of the condition. Another important aim of this mode of treatment is to improve patient compliance.

Non-operative management. This includes the modification of contributing factors such as weight-bearing sports and high-impact loading sports which increase the load on the joint. Rather than giving up sport altogether, the emphasis of management should be on modification of sports activity. Sports such as swimming, golf, stationary cycling and rowing, which involve low-impact loading, should be encouraged, as these improve muscle strength, joint motion and patient mobility. Measures which reduce the intensity of impact loading include wearing special impact-absorbing shoes, playing on special impact-relieving surfaces, and maintaining good muscle strength and tone. In addition, participation in a variety of sports can minimize a repeated pattern of excessive joint motion and loading.

Physiotherapy. This improves the strength of muscle acting across the joint and reduces joint stiffness. This form of therapy is especially important in unstable joints such as those seen in anterior cruciate ligament injuries. Muscle strengthening exercises such as quadriceps training can reduce disability and pain and may even eliminate the need for drug treatment.

Pharmacological management. This traditionally involves the use of non-steroidal anti-inflammatory drugs (NSAIDs). These drugs have important side-effects, classically gastrointestinal disturbances such as peptic ulceration, gastritis and oesophagitis, and can also lead to renal impairment. They must be used with caution, and should not be prescribed until a full history of the patient's health and analgesic requirements has been obtained. Their use should be avoided if the simpler treatment modalities mentioned above can provide equal or, in some cases, better relief of pain and disability. A recent overview showed that paracetamol is attracting growing interest as a less toxic alternative to NSAIDs. While the differences in efficacy between NSAIDs is only marginal, the toxic side-effects vary tremendously. More recent research is aimed at reducing these side-effects while maintaining drug efficacy. The addition to NSAIDs of cytoprotective drugs such as misoprostil is established, but makes them more costly. One theoretically feasible way of overcoming the unwanted side-effects is by administering the NSAID as a topical gel. However, studies have shown conflicting results. Indeed, when released in high concentrations through the skin, these drugs do become detectable in the blood. Opioids such as dextropropoxyphene may be used with paracetamol in patients intolerant to NSAIDs.

An important measure is to prevent further cartilage damage *per se*. The synovial fluid normally plays this role, and the introduction of its main component, hyaluronic acid, into the joint by intra-articular injection has been well studied (Lussier et al 1996). Hyaluronic acid is also an important component of the articular cartilage matrix and promotes the aggregation of proteoglycans. By supplementing the viscoelastic properties of the synovial fluid, it can protect the cartilage by increasing its shock-absorbing capacity. The biological half-life of hyaluronic acid is about 15–20 h. Moreover, the introduction of exogenous hyaluronic acid is also thought to stimulate endogenous hyaluronic acid production, and to restore the protective layer over the hyaline cartilage. The drug is usually given as a course of three weekly injections and a second course may also be given after several months. Studies have shown that a 77% improvement in pain and an 87% improvement in activity level after a single course can be achieved. The duration of benefit is about 8 months. It has a good safety record with only a low complication rate involving local skin reactions such as pain, swelling and redness at the injection site which may be related to the injection technique.

Surgical treatment. This includes arthroscopy, osteotomy and total knee arthroplasty, all of which will be discussed in greater detail below.

ARTHROSCOPIC MANAGEMENT

Arthroscopy is a minimally invasive alternative to the traditional surgical treatments such as osteotomy and joint replacement. The three main criteria to satisfy for the use of arthroscopy in the management of osteo-arthritis are as follows:

- Failure of conservative treatment. The patient should have at least tried a minimum of 6 months of a rigorous programme of anti-inflammatory medication, physiotherapy, exercise, and reduction or modification of activities.
- Significant impairment of activities of daily living and athletic performance.
- Reluctance to undergo major joint reconstructive surgery.

It is vitally important that the patient fully understands that an arthroscopy, in this context, is purely a time-buying procedure that can provide good palliation of pain, and at the same time defers more major surgical procedures to a later date. In a large follow-up study by Ogilvie-Harris & Fitsialos (1991), 68% of the patients had at least 2 or more years of relief of pain after arthroscopic debridement and lavage; 53% were still relatively symptom-free after 4 years. Less favourable results were found in patients with bicondylar disease and valgus malalignment. Arthroscopic surgery is more likely to fail if one or more of the following factors are involved (Chan et al 1994).

- varus malalignment of more than 20°, or valgus malalignment of more than 30°
- significant joint instability, particularly combined with severe radiological features
- significant obesity
- unrealistically high expectations.

Thus, patient selection is crucial for the success of this operation. This procedure can be performed under either general or local anaesthesia with or without tourniquet. The arthroscope allows the direct visual-

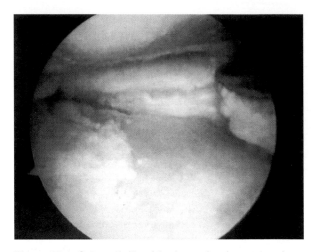

Figure 30.1 Osteoarthritis of the knee showing exposed bone and loose articular cartilage flap.

ization of the joint to help us detect areas of cartilage wear and defects, meniscus tears and ligament injuries (Fig. 30.1). It is essential to map out such pathologies clearly and to plan treatment accordingly. The role of repair of meniscal tears in this age group is debatable, and most meniscal tears will be partially excised if the meniscal fragment is causing impingement on the articular surfaces during normal joint motion. The meniscus involved is trimmed to restore a stable rim with continuous longitudinal fibres. Furthermore, areas of inflammatory synovitis within the knee may be excised. Fragmented articular cartilaginous debris can be removed with minute shears or jaws. All such procedures can provide pain relief with removal of sources of locking, such as loose chondral fragments (Chan et al 1994). Another way in which arthroscopy may relieve pain is by the washing-out effect of inflammatory mediators such as cytokines and other as yet unidentified chemicals which are thought to contribute to both pain and progressive cartilage damage (Smith et al 1997).

For many years clinicians have investigated ways of restoring the damaged articular cartilage to its former state, but have made little progress until the last two decades. Implantation of artificial matrices, growth factors, perichondrium, periosteum (Buckwalter & Lohmander 1994), and transplanted chondrocytes (Brittberg et al 1994) and mesenchymal cells (Shapiro et al 1993) can stimulate the formation of cartilaginous tissue in osteochondral and chondral defects. In addition, certain operative techniques to stimulate cartilage regrowth have been studied, including drilling and burring the subchondral bone to cause bleeding in the hope of producing a fibrin clot containing the relevant growth factors and stem cells to the defective surface (Menche et al 1996) (Figs 30.2 and 30.3). However, comparative studies are often limited by differences in patient selection and operative techniques. So far, there are no large-scale prospective randomized controlled clinical trials to fully define the role of these methods in the management of osteoarthritis. In addition, the response of the joint to these treatments is currently variable and unpredictable. Studies have shown the formation of a fibrocartilaginous articular surface that varies in composition from dense fibrous tissue with little or no type II collagen to hyaline cartilage-like tissue with predominantly type II colla-

gen. Moreover, some authors have shown an increase in joint space thickness, but failed to demonstrate any correlation with relief of symptoms (Bert & Maschka 1989). This may indicate limitations in patient selection in terms of age, disease severity and distribution, and differences in individual pain perception. Another factor contributing to the failure of these treatment of modalities may be that the fibrocartilage lacks the structure, composition, mechanical properties and durability of natural hyaline cartilage. Further studies are required to establish the role of these methods.

Another method of managing the problem of articular cartilage loss which is gaining particular interest together with the advent of newer and more sophisticated arthroscopic instruments is the technique of mosaic-plasty osteochondral grafting (Fig. 30.4). This involves the harvesting of a small osteochondral graft either from a non-weight-bearing donor area of the same knee joint (autograft), such as the patella, femoral condyle or proximal part of the fibula (Outerbridge et al 1995), or from other sources (e.g. human allograft) and its implantation in a mosaic-like

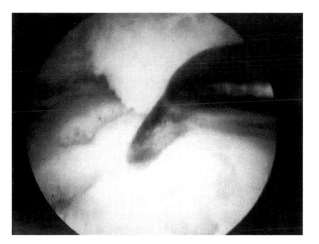

Figure 30.2 Microfracture: the exposed bone is penetrated.

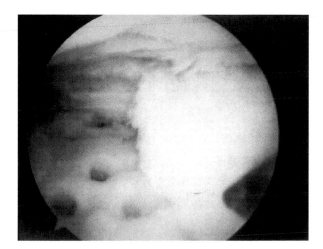

Figure 30.3 Microfracture: fibrocartilage is expected to fill the raw eburnated surface.

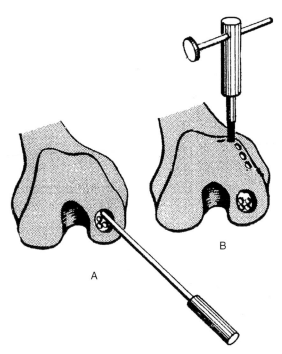

Figure 30.4 Arthroscopic autogenous osteochondral mosaic-plasty. A: The area defective of articular cartilage is prepared. B: A non-weight-bearing area of the joint is chosen from which osteochondral grafts are taken to fill the defective region.

fashion into areas of focal cartilage defect of the weight-bearing surface. A recent study by Hangody et al (1997) yielded encouraging results at 5-year follow-up. Better results in terms of return to normal activity, competitive sports and work and relief of pain were obtained when compared with a similar group treated with abrasion arthroplasty. In addition, there was preservation of structural integrity and composition with evidence of good bonding of the hyaline osteocartilaginous graft to the neighbouring hyaline cartilage at the new site. However, it is only effective in knee joints with localized areas of cartilage loss, and has no place in joints with more generalized osteoarthritis.

OSTEOTOMY

Osteotomy is the next operative option and should only be considered if the above-mentioned simpler and more conservative treatment measures fail to control the patient's symptoms and maintain a satisfactory level of activity. The surgical technique should take into consideration the future possible need for total knee replacement in terms of preserving adequate bone stock and obtaining good lower limb biomechanics. Osteotomy is most appropriate for unicompartmental osteoarthritis of the knee without joint contracture, with an arc of motion of at least 100°, a low adductor moment, metaphyseal bowing, intact ligaments, no severe osseous defects or intra-articular osteophytes and the ability to tolerate immobilization in a cast if this is the planned method of fixation (Grelsamer 1995). Osteotomy can allow a patient to return to a high level of physical activity. According to one study by Nagel et al (1996), many patients can return to activities such as running and jumping, i.e. the type of sport which could lead to damage to the components of a total knee arthroplasty. Eighty-two per cent of the patients in their study were satisfied with their functional outcome, and would have the operation again given the same situation.

The rationale for osteotomy is based on the theory that excess varus or valgus deformity leads to excessively high forces, causing progressive damage to the articular cartilage and osteoarthritis in predominantly one compartment of the knee joint. The patient selected for osteotomy must have sufficient clinical evidence of unicompartmental disease and satisfy the aforementioned criteria based on the information obtained from the history, clinical, radiological and arthroscopic examinations. Having obtained standing long-leg radiographs of the lower limbs to include the hip, knee and ankle joints, the mechanical and anatomical axes of the lower limbs are measured, and a careful preoperative plan is made. The exact site, degree of varus or valgus correction and the method of fixation vary from patient to patient as well as from surgeon to surgeon. When osteoarthritis is mainly confined to the medial joint compartment, the usual site of the osteotomy is at the level of the proximal tibia either below or above the level of the tibial tuberosity. The decision on which of these levels to choose can have important effects on the rate of bony union, the tension of the collateral ligaments and the height of the patella relative to the knee joint in some groups of patients. The overall effect of the osteotomy is to create a valgus knee and various authors suggest different degrees of overcorrection of the varus deformity, as this has been widely considered to affect the long-term success of the operation. In general terms, tibial osteotomy can take the form of a lateral closing wedge, a medial opening wedge or a dome (barrel-vault) osteotomy. The last of these three does not affect leg length or ligamentous tension, which some have considered important in the outcome of the operation.

There are several options for fixing the tibia once the osteotomy has been made, including staples alone or cast alone, or a combination of these. External fixation is also used by some. Immobilization in a cast or relying on staples alone requires a strong osseous hinge. Immobilization in a cast can be uncomfortable especially in hot climates, and can cause stiffness and loss of motion at the knee joint. External fixation requires meticulous care of the pin sites. The results of long-term follow-up after tibial osteotomy appear in some cases to be related to the postoperative alignment of the lower limb, and a slight overcorrection of the varus deformity is recommended to a degree which is yet to be defined universally. Also, better results are found if the procedure is done for earlier stages of osteoarthritis in lighter and younger patients. When osteoarthritis is predominantly found in the lateral knee compartment in a valgus knee, the osteotomy is usually performed at the level of the distal femur, especially if the deformity is more significant. The fixation involves a plate placed either medially or laterally.

While osteotomy may be a useful procedure for relieving pain and improving knee function in younger patients, one must bear in mind the technical difficulties which may arise when the time comes to carrying out a total knee arthroplasty later on in their lives. Examples include wound problems such as healing and infection, difficulty with ligament balancing, problems with aligning the knee prosthesis, entrapment of the common peroneal nerve in scar tissue, and the presence of metalwork such as staples which may require removal through a separate incision. Osteotomy is otherwise a good interim surgical measure in the younger patients.

OSTEOARTHRITIS IN THE UNSTABLE KNEE

While the above treatments are applicable to middle-aged active patients with only degenerative knees, one must not forget to mention those who also suffer from instability, due, for example, to anterior cruciate ligament tear from a previous sporting injury. As one would expect, knee instability from previous cruciate ligament tear with progressive medial compartment degenerative arthritis, as in a varus knee, is a common scenario in the athletic world. It can be envisaged that this complex combined problem is likely to increase with the ever-mounting enthusiasm to participate in sport as part of one's leisure activity.

The role of high tibial osteotomy alone or in combination with an anterior cruciate ligament reconstruction, either simultaneously or as a delayed procedure, has attracted much interest and controversy. To tackle this challenging problem, the surgeon has to distinguish the symptoms of pain from those of instability and, at the same time, be able to evaluate the relative contribution of each to the patient's disability. A retrospective study by Lattermann & Jakob (1996) used a symptom-orientated approach. Such patients were divided into three main categories depending on their symptomatology and clinical assessment:

- patients aged 38–48 years who complained of pain as their main symptom, especially during light activity, and occasionally of instability
- patients aged 25–40 with significant instability symptoms and who additionally complained of pain during light activity
- patients under 20 to 35 years of age who had severe instability and pain with moderate activity, and who performed sport at a competitive level.

These three groups received, respectively, high tibial osteotomy alone, high tibial osteotomy and later anterior cruciate ligament reconstruction if instability persisted, and a combined high tibial osteotomy with anterior cruciate ligament reconstruction. The group receiving high tibial osteotomy alone had effective pain relief from the operation, and an additional stabilizing effect was experienced by some. This latter effect has been explained by some to be due to an alteration

in knee kinematics and the formation of osteophytes. For the other two groups who received anterior cruciate ligament reconstruction as well, there was little difference in terms of overall pain relief, knee stability and function, whether this latter procedure was done simultaneously or as a staged procedure. These patients have usually suffered severe damage to their knees, and a return to previous high levels of intense physical activity may not be possible. The combined approach may, however, provide adequate symptom relief as well as knee stability during active daily activity. The concerns about the combined approach include the increased operating time, a greater amount of surgery which, in theory, may hinder early reconstruction of the anterior cruciate ligament graft, graft rupture, graft misplacement, peroneal nerve palsy, deep vein thrombosis, and under- or overcorrection of varus alignment. Nonetheless, high rates of patient satisfaction have been achieved by some authors (Latterman & Jakob 1996).

While this combined approach is attractive when treating a knee with simultaneous knee pain and instability, the selection of patients for this procedure is very important. These patients should understand that they have suffered significant damage to their knees, and some preoperative counselling regarding activity modification and postoperative expectations ought to be an integral part of the management process. Only those who have significant instability either at the time of high tibial osteotomy or as a persistent symptom should be considered for additional stabilization surgery. Those who have predominantly pain with less instability may be managed with high tibial osteotomy alone.

On the other hand, Shelbourne & Stube (1997) evaluated a series of patients who had chronic instability with evidence of knee degenerative osteoarthritis who were treated with only an autogenous patellar tendon–bone anterior cruciate ligament reconstruction. They reported an overall improvement in subjective parameters such as pain, stability and activity level. The degree of improvement was greater in those with medial compartmental rather than lateral compartmental osteoarthritis, and those with bicompartmental disease did less well.

Anterior cruciate ligament reconstruction in the middle-aged

The role of anterior cruciate ligament reconstruction in middle-aged patients has been thoroughly investigated, and several studies report results comparable to those performed in younger age groups (Heier et al 1997). Plancher et al (1998) recorded excellent results at follow-up to 55 months. The mean age of their patients was 45 years. All patients were satisfied with their operation, with a return to cycling activities at a mean of 4 months, a return to jogging at 9 months, skiing at 10 months, and tennis at 12 months. None of the patients had instability symptoms. The authors found that the patients who had operative treatment had better results in terms of achieving greater knee stability and pain relief than those who had non-operative treatment with or without knee brace. Arthrofibrosis was not found to be a problem in the operated group. The rate of dissatisfaction was noted to increase with the duration of follow-up amongst those patients who received non-operative treatment. The rate of re-injury was also lower in the operated patients. Overall, they concluded that, in selected mature athletes, operative intervention together with strict adherence to the regimented rehabilitation programme can offer a good chance of return to pre-injury levels of sports activity and a lower incidence of re-injury.

TOTAL KNEE REPLACEMENT

The last of the surgical options for managing osteoarthritis of the knee is total knee replacement. This procedure has not been widely practised in active young or middle-aged patients because of the main concern regarding the possibility of aseptic loosening due to wear debris generated during their active lives. Because of the potential for numerous revision operations in the course of a lifetime, total knee replacement has generally been reserved for patients over the age of 60. However, a recent study by Diduch et al (1997), investigating 103 primary total knee replacements for osteoarthritis in young active patients with a mean age of 51 years (ranging from 22 to 55), revealed promising long-term results in terms of the survival of the prosthesis and high levels of sporting activity achieved postoperatively. Most of their patients were able to change from sedentary, desk-type work with limited walking on even ground to an occupation that involved light labour such as nursing or truck driving and some recreational activities such as cycling, cross-country skiing or swimming after the operation. One-quarter of their patients were able to take part in strenuous farm or construction work and competitive cycling or cross-country skiing, or were able to participate in tennis or downhill skiing. Regular walking for 2 miles was the most common activity and cycling was the second most common. Other activities included golf, treadmill exercise, aerobics, tennis and using a stair-climbing machine. Apart from the high level of activity achieved, their study, which is the longest follow-up of total knee replacements for patients in this relatively young age group, revealed an overall survival rate of the implant of 94% at 18 years. Long-term studies of this type are currently lacking, and further work has to be done to support such promising results. Until then, one must proceed along this mode of treatment with caution, and for most patients, a more conservative approach is more appropriate.

CONCLUSIONS

In essence, it can be seen that the treatment of osteoarthritis of the knee in middle-aged active patients is complex and requires an accurate assessment of the disease severity gauged by subjective pain perception and functional deficit. The management options can be summarized as in Table 30.1.

Table 30.1 Management options for osteoarthritis of the knee in middle-aged active patients

Severity	Treatment
Mild	Physiotherapy, analgesia, modification of exacerbating factors, viscosupplementation
Moderate pain and disability	Viscosupplementation, arthroscopy, cartilage resurfacing (abrasion and burr arthroplasty), mosaic-plasty, ?chondrocyte transplantation, ?perichondral grafts
Moderate pain and disability with disease mainly confined to one compartment	Osteotomy
Moderate with instability	Osteotomy alone, osteotomy + anterior cruciate ligament reconstruction, anterior cruciate ligament reconstruction alone
Severe pain and disability	Total knee replacement

It can be seen that the main areas of advance and research should concentrate on restoring the articular cartilage damage to as near 'normal' as possible, but many uncertainties lie ahead, especially the long-term outcome of such procedures. Every consideration should be made to preserve bone stock and delay total knee arthroplasty as late as possible, since knowledge of its long-term results in this relatively young age group is currently lacking. The other area of contention is the unstable knee with osteoarthritis. Patients with such a complex problem usually have sustained significant injury to the knee and may have adjusted their activities to a lower level of intensity. The treatment goal in these cases has to be clearly defined.

REFERENCES

Bert J M, Maschka K 1989 The arthroscopic treatment of unicompartmental gonoarthrosis. Arthroscopy 5: 25–32

Brittberg M, Lindahl A, Nilsson A, Ohlsson C, Isaksson O, Peterson L 1994 Treatment of deep cartilage defects in the knee with autologous chondrocyte transplantation. New England Journal of Medicine 331: 889–895

Buckwalter J A, Lane N E 1996 Aging, sports and osteoarthritis. Sports Medicine and Arthroscopy Review 4: 276–287

Buckwalter J A, Lane N E 1997 Current Concepts: Athletics and osteoarthritis. American Journal of Sports Medicine 25(6): 873–881

Buckwalter J A, Lohmander S 1994 Current concepts review. Operative treatment of osteoarthrosis. Current practice and future development. Journal of Bone and Joint Surgery 76A: 1405–1418

Buckwalter J A, Martin J A 1995 Degenerative joint disease. Clinical Symposia, Summit, New Jersey, Ciba-Geigy

Buckwalter J A, Lane N E, Gordon S L 1995 Exercise as a cause of osteoarthritis. In: Kuettner K E, Goldberg V M (eds) Osteoarthritic disorders. The American Academy of Orthopaedic Surgeons, Rosemount, IL, p 405–417

Chan K M, Chien P, Tseng G H C 1994 Arthroscopic surgery of degenerative arthritis of the knee – a 'miniaturized house cleaning' procedure. Journal of the Hong Kong Medical Association 46(3): 182–186

Diduch D R, Insall J N, Scott W N et al 1997 Total knee replacement in young, active patients. Long-term follow-up and functional outcome. Journal of Bone and Joint Surgery (Am) 79(4): 575–582

Grelsamer R P 1995 Current concepts review. Unicompartmental osteoarthritis of the knee. Journal of Bone and Joint Surgery (Am) 77A(2): 278–292

Hangody L, Kish G, Karpati Z et al 1997 Arthroscopic autogenous osteochondral mosaicplasty for the treatment of femoral condylar articular defects. A preliminary report. Knee Surgery, Sports Traumatology, Arthroscopy 5(4): 262–267

Heier K A, Mack D R, Moseley J B et al 1997 An analysis of anterior cruciate ligament reconstruction in the middle-aged patients. American Journal of Sports Medicine 25(4): 527–532

Latterman C, Jakob R P 1996 High tibial osteotomy alone or combined with ligamentous reconstruction in anterior cruciate ligament-deficient knees. Knee Surgery, Sports Traumatology, Arthroscopy 4(1): 32–38

Lawrence R, Hochberg M, Kelsey J L et al 1989 Estimates of the prevalence of selected arthritic and musculoskeletal diseases in the United States. Journal of Rheumatology 16: 427–441

Lequesne M G 1997 The algofunctional indices for hip and knee osteoarthritis. Journal of Rheumatology 24(4): 779–781

Lussier A, Cividino A A, McFarlane C A et al 1996 Viscosupplementation with Hylan for the treatment of osteoarthritis: findings from clinical practice in Canada. Journal of Rheumatology 23(9): 1579–1585

Menche D S, Frenkel S R, Blair B et al 1996 A comparison of abrasion burr arthroplasty and subchondral drilling in the treatment of full-thickness cartilage lesions in the rabbit. Arthroscopy 12(3): 280–286

Nagel A, Insall J N, Scuderi G R et al 1996 Proximal tibial osteotomy. A subjective outcome study. Journal of Bone and Joint Surgery (Am) 78(9): 1353–1358

Ogilvie-Harris D J, Fitsialos D P 1991 Arthroscopic management of the degenerative knee. Arthroscopy 7(2): 151–157

Outerbridge H K, Outerbridge A R, Outerbridge R E 1995 The use of a lateral patella autologous graft for the repair of a large osteochondral defect in the knee. Journal of Bone and Joint Surgery 77A: 65–72

Plancher K D, Steadman J R, Briggs K K et al 1998 Reconstruction of the anterior cruciate ligament in patients who are at least forty years old. A long-term follow-up and outcome study. Journal of Bone and Joint Surgery (Am) 80(2): 184–197

Praemer A, Furner S, Rice D P 1992 Musculoskeletal conditions in the United States. The American Academy of Orthopaedic Surgeons, Park Ridge, IL

Rangger C, Kathrein A, Klestil T, Glotzer W 1997 Partial meniscectomy and osteoarthritis. Implications for treatment for athletes. Sports Medicine 23(1): 61–68

Scott J, Huskisson E C 1979 Accuracy of subjective measurements made with or without previous scores: an important source of error in serial measurement of subjective states. Annals of the Rheumatic Diseases 38: 558–559

Shapiro F, Koide S, Glimcher M 1993 Cell origin and differentiation in the repair of full thickness defects of articular cartilage. Journal of Bone and Joint Surgery 75A: 532–553

Shelbourne K D, Stube K C 1997 Anterior cruciate ligament (ACL)-deficient knee with degenerative arthrosis: treatment with an isolated autogenous patella tendon ACL reconstruction. Knee Surgery, Sports Traumatology, Arthroscopy 5(3): 150–156

Smith M D, Triantafillou S, Parker A 1997 Synovial membrane inflammation and cytokine production in patients with early osteoarthritis. Journal of Rheumatology 24(2): 365–371

31

Sport after total joint arthroplasty

William J. Mallon
Thomas Parker Vail

KEY POINTS

1. The single most frequent indication for joint replacement is relief of pain, but restoration of function is becoming increasingly important as younger and healthier patients consider the operation.
2. Individual patients considering a prosthetic implant must be given a realistic expectation of future function and performance.
3. Important parameters to consider when deciding on joint replacement with a view to return to sporting activity are the joint in question, the implant design, and the sport in which the patient wants to participate.
4. Routine follow-up is essential to recognizing and treating some of the complications that will arise from increased use of an implant.

INTRODUCTION

During the past 20 years, the number of total joint replacement procedures performed through the world has increased steadily (Praemer et al 1992). Frequently, patients who are considering joint replacement wish to return to recreational sports. Less common but more highly publicized is the goal of participation in competitive or professional sports, notably the return of Bo Jackson to professional baseball after his hip replacement. Although the single most frequent indication for replacing a joint is the relief of pain, the restoration of function has become increasingly important as younger and generally healthier patients consider joint replacement.

Although physical activity is generally associated with good health, there is evidence that some occupations and sports activities are associated with increased rates of osteoarthritis (Felson 1988, Klunder et al 1980, Marti et al 1989, Vingård et al 1991, 1993). A realistic expectation for function and performance of a prosthetic implant is important for a patient trying to weigh the pros and cons of joint replacement surgery. Specific decisions must be individualized for each patient, but a general understanding of the demands of a particular sport and its relevance to the joint being replaced is also important. The relevant issues surrounding the decision to replace a joint and the patient's postoperative athletic performance depend on which joint is being replaced, the implant design, and the particular sporting activity in which the patient wishes to participate.

ANATOMIC LOCATION
Hip and knee replacement

Hips and knees are the most frequently replaced joint with the best-analyzed outcomes (Charnley 1979, Joshi et al 1993, Wroblewski 1986). Results have varied with the type of prosthesis used as well as the surgical approach. In a recent review of the outcome of 330 Charnley total hip arthroplasties with cement after a minimum of 20-year follow-up, 32 (10%) of the 322 hips that had been followed up had been revised secondary to loosening because of infection, aseptic loosening, or dislocation (Schulte et al 1993). Twenty-two of the 98 acetabular components in the 98 patients who survived a minimum of 20 years were loose, compared with only seven of the femoral components. These results reflect the experience of a single surgeon performing cemented total hip arthroplasty using the Charnley prosthesis during a time when the cement was finger-packed without a cement plug or cement pressurization. Improved cement technique and use of a porous, cementless acetabular socket show early promise, with a lower rate of acetabular and femoral loosening at 5 years of follow-up (Harris 1994). The experience with early cementless femoral components (Callaghan 1993, Capello et al 1994, Heekin et al 1993, Woolson & Maloney 1992) has not been as favorable as with the cemented components, with the exception of more extensively coated designs (Engh et al 1994). Newer designs of cementless femoral components in total hip arthroplasty that include circumferential

coating, better fit, distal polishing, and decreased bending stiffness hold future promise. The 7-year results of a hydroxyapatite-coated femoral component compare favorably with the best cemented series, with some favorable bone remodeling noted radiographically (Manley 1995). Some authors have reported a lower rate of postoperative limp and earlier return to activity when a posterior approach to the hip is used rather than the anterolateral (Callaghan 1993).

Total knee arthroplasty has improved with changes in component design during the last decade. Problems with metal-backed patellar components have been resolved by returning to all-polyethylene patellar components and a few designs with improved metal-backed polyethylene. Outstanding results with success rates >95% at 10 years have been reported with cruciate sparing (Ewald & Christie 1987), cruciate sacrificing (Insall 1993, Ranawat et al 1989), and mobile bearing implants (Buechel & Pappas 1989). The use of metal-backed, cemented tibial components has reduced the incidence of radiolucent lines when compared with the all-polyethylene tibial components within the first 5 years. Fixation with cement is the standard for both tibia and femur. Although some authors have reported success using cementless fixation in knee arthroplasty, others have had failures (Engh et al 1994, Hungerford et al 1989). The fixation in cementless knees is less reliable, although fibrous fixation has been shown to perform well clinically over many years. The subvastus approach to the knee has been reported to decrease recovery time after total knee replacement. However, the final outcome using this approach has not differed from a standard midline approach.

Shoulder replacement

Total shoulder replacement and humeral hemiarthroplasty have been uniformly successful clinically. Hemiarthroplasty has traditionally been reserved for fractures and more active patients. Integrity of the rotator cuff plays a major role in the outcomes of the arthroplasty, with rotator cuff-deficient shoulders having less successful outcomes. Cementless humeral components and cemented glenoid components have been the standard. Loosening and radiographic lucencies of and about the glenoid have been the major concern, although radiographic lucencies have not always correlated well with clinical loosening. Although most shoulder replant surgeons will allow certain patients to return to sports, notably golf (Collis 1974, Lemos & Healy 1997, Mallon 1992), no scientific studies have yet been published concerning return to sports after total shoulder replacement.

Elbow replacement

The standard today is a constrained arthroplasty such as the Coonrad–Morrey design. Although these implants have fared well clinically, significant limitations are imposed on patients that are not consistent with most sporting activities (Collis 1974, Mallon 1992).

Ankle replacement

Total ankle replacement is still considered experimental at this point. Newer cementless designs may have promise, but in general this procedure is reserved for the sedentary patient, in particular the patient with rheumatoid arthritis. Failures in all patients have been uniformly high. Return to weight-bearing sports after a total ankle replacement is not thought to be advisable (Mallon 1992).

IMPLANT DESIGN

For all current designs of joint replacements with a bearing surface, the limiting factor in the longevity of the implant is wear of the polyethylene liner. It has been well established that polyethylene wear particles can lead to lysis of bone with subsequent loss of structural integrity of bone and loosening of the implant (Chew & Lev 1992, Harris 1994). Design features that can minimize wear include a highly polished metal surface, enhanced polyethylene quality, sterilization of polyethylene in a non-oxidizing environment, ion-implanted metal surfaces, and the avoidance of concentrated loading on the polyethylene surface.

Favorably, polyethylene loading can be achieved in total hip arthroplasty by choosing a minimum polyethylene thickness of 6 mm (Brand et al 1994), and using a 26 or 28 mm femoral head rather than a 32 mm femoral head (Crowninshield et al 1980). The prosthesis should provide exact restoration of the femoral offset to ensure proper tension and moment arm for the abductor muscles. The choice of materials is somewhat controversial, with polished chrome–cobalt metal articulating with ultrahigh-molecular-weight polyethylene being most common. Ceramic femoral heads can provide a decreased surface roughness, but some designs have been prone to fracture (Ranawat et al 1989) and third-party wear. For younger, active patients, the use of constrained implants and elevated

lip liners should be discouraged because of the decreased safe zone for dislocation, and the potential for increased wear secondary to liner impingement. Avoiding screw holes and other conduits for debris is advantageous.

Design features in total knee arthroplasty can also affect joint loading and polyethylene wear (Livermore et al 1990). For active individuals, limited prosthetic constraint is desirable while achieving some polyethylene–metal conformity. Hinged designs that do not allow roll-back or torsional movement are associated with a high rate of loosening (Andriacchi et al 1986). A curved polyethylene design that achieves a broad metal–polyethylene contact area throughout the range of motion will limit high polyethylene stresses in flexion. A minimum polyethylene thickness of 8 mm at the tibiofemoral articulation is desirable (Brand et al 1994). Patellofemoral conformity and contact area in flexion are also very important for active individuals with >110° of flexion. Finally, the issue of whether to save or sacrifice the cruciate is debated and unresolved. However, it is clear that if the cruciate is saved, the joint must not be elevated, and the ligaments must be properly balanced to achieve the desired postoperative range of motion (Andriacchi et al 1986). Increased flexion causes increased patellofemoral stresses, which may be increased further by aggressive sports, a condition that may lead to more patellofemoral problems. Rotation of the total knee arthroplasty may cause incongruity of the otherwise congruous articulation. This increases peak stresses in the polyethylene and may lead to premature wear.

TYPES OF SPORT

Although the outcome of total joint replacement has been extensively studied, participation in sports after joint replacement has not. Historically, sports have been discouraged. Charnley (1979) discouraged his patients from anything more strenuous than walking. The basic question to be answered is whether participation in sports will decrease implant longevity by increasing the rate of wear, the rate of loosening, or the rate of complications. If one looks at the question from a purely mechanical point of view, it is apparent that the bearing surface wear rate is directly related to the cycles of use. Increased cycles of use for a given period will lead to increased wear of the bearing surface. Increased impact loading has a negative impact on wear rates. Does this simplistic mechanical fact mean that outcomes for joint replacement in patients participating in sport will be unacceptably diminished?

Definitive answers to this question do not exist in the orthopaedic literature, but some limited information on sports participation after joint arthroplasty can be studied to give some idea of the possible trends.

Published information on sports participation after joint arthroplasty is both retrospective and limited in scope, and much of it is anecdotal (Andriacchi et al 1982, Dubs et al 1983, Kilgus et al 1991, Mallon 1992, Mallon & Callaghan 1992, 1993, McGrory et al 1995, MacNicol et al 1980, Minns et al 1993, Ritter & Meding 1987, Stiehl & deAndrade 1995, Visuri & Honkanen 1980, White 1992). The most recent articles detail recommendations of staff surgeons, fellows, and residents at the Mayo Clinic (McGrory et al 1995), and recommendations for activity after joint replacement (Lemos & Healy 1997, Stiehl & deAndrade 1995, Vail et al 1996). Our own recommendations (see Tables 31.1 and 31.2) are consistent with these studies and, to some extent, based upon them.

The type of sport and the extent of participation will have great bearing on the extent to which a joint implant might be adversely affected. In general, sports can be roughly divided into high-, intermediate-, and low-impact for this discussion (Table 31.1) (McGrory et al 1995). The factors taken into consideration when categorizing a particular activity and its suitability for participation after joint replacement include the degree of repetition, the magnitude of joint loading, and the potential for violence. Repetitive loading can lead to fatigue failure of the prosthetic parts or the

Table 31.1 Sports participation for patients with joint replacements based upon level of impact loading (based on Vail et al 1996)

Level of impact	Examples	Recommendations
Low	Stationary cycling Calisthenics Golf Stationary skiing Swimming Walking Ballroom dancing Water aerobics	● Can improve general health ● Desirable for most patients, but may increase rate of wear ● Orthotics and activity modifications can reduce impact loads ● Concentration on conditioning and flexibility rather than strengthening
Potentially low	Bowling Fencing Rowing Isokinetic weight-lifting Sailing Speed walking Cross-country skiing Table tennis Jazz dancing and ballet Bicycling	● Desirable for most patients, but may increase rate of wear ● Requires preactivity evaluation, monitoring and development of guidelines by surgeon ● Balance and proprioception must be intact ● Orthotics and activity modifications can reduce impact loads ● Emphasize high number of repetitions with minimal resistance
Intermediate	Free weight-lifting Hiking Horseback riding Ice skating Rock climbing Low-impact aerobics Tennis In-line skating Downhill skiing	● Appropriate only for selected patients ● Require preactivity evaluation, monitoring and development of guidelines for participation by surgeon ● Excellent physical condition is necessary ● Orthotics, impact-absorbing shoes and activity modification are frequently necessary
High	Baseball/softball Basketball/volleyball Football Handball/racketball Jogging/running Lacrosse Soccer Water skiing Karate	● Should be avoided ● Significant probability of injury and need for revision

Table 31.2 Sports participation for patients with joint replacements based upon anatomic location of arthroplasty (based on Vail et al 1996)

Sport	Acceptable	Possible	Not recommended
Ballet dancing	Shoulder	Hip, knee	
Ballroom dancing	Hip, knee, shoulder		
Baseball/softball			Hip, knee, shoulder
Basketball			Hip, knee, shoulder
Bicycling	Hip, knee, shoulder		
Bowling	Hip, knee	Shoulder	
Calisthenics		Hip, knee, shoulder	
Cross-country skiing	Hip, knee, shoulder		
Downhill skiing	Shoulder	Hip, knee	
Fencing		Hip, knee	Shoulder
Football			Hip, knee, shoulder
Golf	Hip, knee, shoulder		
Handball/racketball		Shoulder	Hip, knee
Hiking	Shoulder	Hip, knee	
Horseback riding	Hip, knee, shoulder		
Ice skating	Hip, knee, shoulder		
In-line skating	Hip, knee, shoulder		
Jazz dancing	Shoulder	Hip, knee	
Jogging/running	Shoulder	Hip, knee	
Karate			Hip, knee, shoulder
Lacrosse			Hip, knee, shoulder
Low-impact aerobics	Hip, knee, shoulder		
Rock climbing		Hip, knee, shoulder	
Rowing	Hip, knee	Shoulder	
Sailing	Hip, knee, shoulder		
Soccer		Shoulder	Hip, knee
Speed walking	Hip, knee, shoulder		
Stationary cycling	Hip, knee, shoulder		
Stationary skiing	Hip, knee, shoulder		
Swimming	Hip, knee	Shoulder	
Table tennis		Hip, knee, shoulder	
Tennis		Hip, knee, shoulder	
Volleyball			Hip, knee, shoulder
Walking	Hip, knee, shoulder		
Water aerobics	Hip, knee, shoulder		
Water skiing		Hip, knee	Shoulder

disruption of the implant–bone interface. Violent loading has the potential for causing catastrophic complications such as fracture and dislocation.

Golf has been the best-studied activity after joint replacement, although the reports by Mallon (1992) and Mallon & Callaghan (1992, 1993) were retrospective and only documented that return to play was a possibility. In general, these results showed that most golfers experienced some discomfort after playing golf with either a hip or knee replacement. Hip replacements performed slightly better than knee replacements in terms of less pain. In golfers with knee replacements, those with a left knee replacement (for right-handed golfers) had more difficulty (Mallon 1992, Mallon & Callaghan 1992, 1993).

More recently, Mullick et al (1997) studied the effects of hip replacement on tennis players. They studied 58 tennis players who had undergone 75 hip replacements and concluded that all of their patients were satisfied with the result and their increased ability to participate in tennis after the operation.

Classification of sports by the degree of impact loading during participation may give some clues to the acceptability of a sport after joint arthroplasty. We have classified sports into low-, potentially low-, intermediate-, and high-impact loading, and summarized the recommendations in Table 31.1.

Accidents do occur and are more common in the group of high-impact sports. Unfortunately, fractures about components and dislocations with associated ligament injury are far more difficult to deal with than simple mechanical failure of most implants. Many overactive patients may simply need a polyethylene liner exchange which, although a major operation, will involve less pain and recovery time than a major revision. Others may require fixation of a periprosthetic fracture or revision to substitute for an injured ligament. Physicians will almost universally recommend that patients restrict their activities following complications of joint arthroplasty related to sports activity.

For total hip and knee replacement, recovery times may vary, but, in general, patients may be capable of returning to low- and intermediate-impact sports as early as 4–6 months postoperatively. Adherence to the precautions for the specific joint and the routine exercises are critical to rehabilitation. If the patient has not participated in the sport before or for some extended time, cautious return to the activity is recommended. A few general guidelines can be given:

- Pain should not accompany the activity for the ensuing 24 h, and, if it does, discussion with the surgeon should occur before further resumption of sports.
- Sport modifications to minimize joint loading should be encouraged.
- Frequent rest periods on resuming the sport should be taken.
- Return to prior levels of sporting activity should be done gradually.

Critical to the patient's understanding is the knowledge that recovery times vary dramatically from one patient to another.

CONCLUSIONS

In interested patients, intelligent participation in recreational sports should be a routine part of the preoperative discussion for those considering total joint replacement. For total hip, knee, and shoulder replacement patients, it may be one of the major concerns, and most patients with shoulder replacements may return to some limited sporting activities.

Aerobic activity should be encouraged in all joint replacement patients. Nevertheless, a thorough and thoughtful discussion of the risks of accelerated wear, aseptic loosening, and even castastrophic failure must be included. Advanced design features may be appropriate for the more aggressive athlete, but they must be applied only after highlighting the potential complications of the design. Routine follow-up is critical to recognizing and treating some of the complications that will arise with the increased use of the implant.

For each patient with arthritis, the functional limitations are different. Physicians must help the aging athlete make the appropriate choices regarding joint replacement surgery, knowing that they may be approaching or exceeding the limit of the design of the implants available, but realizing that the choice to participate in sports after arthroplasty is an individual one. The psychological and overall health benefits of sports participation may lead many joint arthroplasty recipients to choose to continue actively engaging in their favorite sports.

REFERENCES

Andriacchi T P, Galante J O, Fermier R W 1982 The influence of total knee-replacement design on walking and stair climbing. Journal of Bone and Joint Surgery (Br) 64: 1328–1335

Andriacchi T P, Stanwyck T S, Galante J O 1986 Knee biomechanics and total knee replacement. Journal of Arthroplasty 1: 211–219

Brand R A, Pedersen D R, Davy D T, Kotzar G M, Heiple K G, Goldberg V M 1994 Comparison of hip force calculations and measurements in the same patient. Journal of Arthroplasty 9: 45–51

Buechel F F, Pappas M J 1989 New Jersey low contact stress knee replacement system: ten-year evaluation of meniscal bearings. Orthopedic Clinics of North America 20: 147–177

Callaghan J J 1993 The clinical results and basic science of total hip arthroplasty with porous-coated prostheses. Journal of Bone and Joint Surgery (Am) 75: 299–310

Capello W N, Sallay P I, Feinberg J R 1994 Omniflex modular femoral component: two- to five-year results. Clinical Orthopedics and Related Research 298: 54–59

Chandler H P, Reineck F T, Wixson R L, McCarthy J C 1981 Total hip replacements in patients younger than thirty years old. Journal of Bone and Joint Surgery (Am) 63: 1426–1434

Charnley J 1979 Low-friction arthroplasty of the hip: theory and practice. Springer-Verlag, Berlin

Chew F S, Lev M H 1992 Polyethylene osteolysis. American Journal of Roentgenology 159: 1254

Collis D K 1974 Degenerative diseases and golf. In: The neck, shoulder and upper extremities in sports (and special golf panel). Postgraduate Course of the American Academy of Orthopaedic Surgeons, Eugene, OR, July

Crowninshield R D, Brand R A, Johnston R C et al 1980 The effect of femoral stem cross-sectional geometry on cement stresses in total hip reconstruction. Clinical Orthopedics and Related Research 146: 71–77

Dubs L, Gschwend N, Munzinger U 1983 Sport after total hip arthroplasty. Archives of Orthopaedic and Trauma Surgery 101: 161–169

Engh C A, Hooten J P Jr, Zettl-Schaffer K F, Ghaffarpour M, McGovern T F, Macalino G E, Zicat B A 1994 Porous-coated total hip replacement. Clinical Orthopedics and Related Research 298: 89–96

Ewald F, Christie M I 1987 Results of cemented total knee replacement in young patients. Orthopaedic Transactions 11: 442

Felson D T 1988 Epidemiology of hip and knee osteoarthritis. Epidemiologic Reviews 10: 1–28

Harris W H 1994 Osteolysis and particle disease in hip replacement: a review. Acta Orthopaedica Scandinavica 65: 113–123

Heekin R D, Callaghan J J, Hopkinson W J, Savory C G, Xenos J S 1993 The porous-coated anatomic total hip prosthesis, inserted without cement: results after five to seven years in a prospective study. Journal of Bone and Joint Surgery (Am) 75: 77–91

Hungerford D S, Krackow K A, Kenna R V 1989 Cementless total knee replacement in patients 50 years old and under. Orthopedic Clinics of North America 29: 131–145

Insall J N 1993 Total knee replacement. In: Insall J N (ed) Surgery of the knee. Churchill Livingstone, New York, p 677–718

Joshi A B, Porter M L, Trail I A, Hung L P et al 1993 Long-term results of Charnley low-friction arthroplasty in young patients. Journal of Bone and Joint Surgery (Br) 75: 616–623

Kilgus D J, Dorey F J, Finerman G A M, Amstutz H C 1991 Patient activity, sports participation, and impact loading on the durability of cemented total hip replacements. Clinical Orthopedics and Related Research 269: 25–31

Klunder K J, Rud B, Hansen J 1980 Osteoarthritis of the hip and knee joint in retired football players. Acta Orthopaedica Scandinavica 51: 925–927

Lemos M J, Healy W L 1997 Activity after replacement of the hip, knee, or shoulder. Orthopedics (special edn) Summer/Fall 7–9

Livermore J, Ilstrup D, Morrey B 1990 Effect of femoral head size on wear of the polyethylene acetabular component. Journal of Bone and Joint Surgery (Br) 72: 518–528

McGrory B J, Stuart M J, Sim F H 1995 Participation in sports after hip and knee arthroplasty: review of the literature and survey of surgeon preferences. Mayo Clinic Proceedings 70: 342–348

MacNicol M F, McHardy R, Chalmers J 1980 Exercise testing before and after hip arthroplasty. Journal of Bone and Joint Surgery (Br) 62: 326–331

Mallon W J 1992 Total joint replacement and golf. In: McCarroll J R, Stover C S, Mallon W J (eds) Feeling up to par: medicine from tee to green. F A Davis, Philadelphia

Mallon W J, Callaghan J J 1992 Total hip replacement in active golfers. Journal of Arthroplasty 7(suppl): 339–346

Mallon W J, Callaghan J J 1993 Total knee participation in active golfers. Journal of Arthroplasty 8: 299–306

Manley M (ed) 1995 Seven-year results on HA femoral components of total hip replacements. Osteonics Corp., Allendale, NJ

Marti B, Knobloch, Tschopp A, Jucker A, Howald H 1989 Is excessive running predictive of degenerative hip disease? Controlled study of former elite athletes. British Medical Journal 299: 91–93

Minns R J, Crawford R J, Porter M L, Hardinge K 1993 Muscle strength following total hip arthroplasty: a comparison of trochanteric osteotomy and the direct lateral approach. Journal of Arthroplasty 8: 625–627

Mullick T, Mont M A, Silberstein C, Hungerford D S 1997 Epidemiological characterization of tennis players who have undergone a total hip arthroplasty. Orthopaedic Transactions 20: 876

Praemer A, Furner S, Rice D P 1992 Musculoskeletal conditions in the United States. American Academy of Orthopaedic Surgeons, Park Ridge, IL, p 127–141

Ranawat C S, Padgett D E, Ohashi Y 1989 Total knee arthroplasty for patients younger than 55 years. Clinical Orthopedics and Related Research 248: 27–33

Ritter M A, Meding J B 1987 Total hip arthroplasty: can the patient play sports again? Orthopaedics 10: 1447–1452

Schulte K R, Callaghan J J, Kelley S S, Johnston R C 1993 The outcome of Charnley total hip arthroplasty with cement after a minimum twenty-year follow-up: the results of one surgeon. Journal of Bone and Joint Surgery (Am) 75: 961–975 [Comment: Journal of Bone and Joint Surgery (Am) 1993; 75: 959–960; erratum: Journal of Bone and Joint Surgery (Am) 1993; 75: 1418]

Stiehl J B, deAndrade J R 1995 Activities after replacement of the hip and knee. Orthopedics (special edn) 1: 32–33

Vail T P, Mallon W J, Liebelt R A 1996 Athletic activities after joint arthroplasty. Sports Medicine and Arthroscopy Reviews 4: 298–305

Vingård E, Alfredsson L, Goldie I, Hogstedt C 1993 Sports and osteoarthrosis of the hip: an epidemiologic study. American Journal of Sports Medicine 21: 195–200

Vingård E, Alfredsson L, Goldie I, Hogstedt C 1991 Occupation and osteoarthrosis of the hip and knee: a register-based cohort study. International Journal of Epidemiology 20: 1025–1031

Visuri T, Honkanen R 1980 Total hip replacement: its influence on spontaneous recreation exercise habits. Archives of Physical Medicine and Rehabilitation 61: 325–328

White J 1992 No more bump and grind. The Physician in Sportsmedicine 20: 223–228

Woolson S T, Maloney W J 1992 Cementless total hip arthroplasty using a porous-coated prosthesis for bone ingrowth fixation: $3\frac{1}{2}$-year follow-up. Journal of Arthroplasty 7: 318–328

Wroblewski B M 1986 Fifteen- to twenty-one year results of the Charnley low-friction arthroplasty. Clinical Orthopedics and Related Research 211: 30–35

32

Health benefits of Tai Chi Chuan in older individuals

*Guo Ping Li   Ling Qin
Kai Ming Chan*

KEY POINTS

1. Tai Chi Chuan is a safe exercise for the elderly, and is effective in the maintenance of neuromuscular coordination, muscle strength, flexibility, and cardiorespiratory and immunoendocrine function.
2. Tai Chi Chuan has the potential to retard bone loss and, thereby, prevent osteoporosis and related fracture.
3. Tai Chi Chuan can improve psychological well-being in the elderly and enhance social independence.
4. It has significant advantages over other forms of physical activity, in that it is cheap, safe, can be practiced without special facilities, and is not affected by the weather.

INTRODUCTION

Due to the increased standard of health care and advanced technological development in most modern societies, there has been a gradual expansion of the section of the population over 60 years old. This group of physically active individuals may have more time for leisure pursuits as a result of retirement. In some countries, these citizens have the privilege to engage in recreational physical activities that best suit them.

Tai Chi Chuan (TCC) dates back hundreds of years in historical Chinese culture. For centuries, TCC has been a popular form of martial arts in Oriental culture. In the West, it has become popular to incorporate TCC as an exercise and therapeutic option. A large number of experimental investigations, epidemiological studies and clinical trials in both the Chinese and Western literature offer strong evidence of the health benefits to the elderly through regular practice of TCC. Research to determine the significance of TCC in prevention or deceleration of bone loss and related fracture is underway. All these findings will add a new dimension to the prevention and management of chronic diseases in the elderly through participation in their favorite exercise, TCC.

In this chapter, we will analyze the medical and scientific aspects of Tai Chi Chuan with specific reference to its effect on the physical and psychological well-being of the older individual engaged in this regular form of physical activities.

TAI CHI CHUAN AND ITS DEVELOPMENT

Tai Chi Chuan (TCC), also called Tai Chi Quan, Taijiquan, or Tai Chi, was developed by Chen Yuting of China in the mid-16th century (late Ming to early Qing dynasty of China), and matured into a jewel of the Chinese cultural heritage (Chen 1985).

Tai Chi meaning 'supreme ultimate', and *Chuan* meaning 'fist') was first perceived as a form of shadow boxing. It was subsequently transformed into a martial art. A unique attribute of TCC is its gentle movements designed to dissipate force through the body while changing pose. Movement can be vigorous or gentle, with a slow and rhythmic harmony.

Over the centuries, a number of TCC schools evolved and various TCC styles developed. The Yang, Chen, Sun and Wu styles are four of the most popular. The classic Yang TCC consists of 108 poses. It takes about half an hour to complete the set. In a meeting of TCC masters convened by the Chinese National Athletic Committee in 1956, a combined TCC form integrating the essence of each TCC school was defined. A simplified 48- and 24-pose TCC was later developed for the promotion of TCC across different population strata (Wang et al 1995, Xu 1994). Whether it is the classical or a simplified style, there are three essential features:

- a naturally extended and relaxed body yet with an awareness of proper trunk alignment, accompanied by deep breathing in reaching the target posture
- a tranquil but alert mind, with the body commanded by the subconscious mind (body–mind harmony)
- well-coordinated sequences of both isometric and isotonic segmental movements in all body movements (Figs 32.1–32.4).

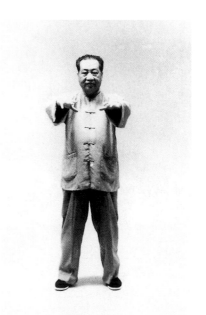

Figure 32.1 Commencing position of Tai Chi Chuan (performed by Mr Shuren Wei, fifth generation of Yang-style Tai Chi Chuan) – standing with feet apart, raise arms forward and upward, bend knees and push palms down.

It is believed that TCC movements seek to balance the so-called 'Qi' (vital energy) in the body's meridians. While performing TCC, deep breathing and concentration are essential to strengthen this vital energy and attain a body–mind harmony. TCC has long been practiced by elderly Chinese people to maintain fitness and health, reduce illness, rehabilitate and prolong life (Li & Ji 1995, Lin 1993, Xu 1994, Zhang 1994).

Alongside the popularity of TCC in China, it is also growing in popularity in both the Far East and Western countries. Chinese immigrants and governmental and civil cultural exchange programs have contributed to this increase in popularity. TCC is a low-cost and effective health promotion intervention. In the West, it can be a promising treatment modality to cope with the escalating health care expenditure on chronic illness and disability of the elderly brought about by the aging population. Interest in the health benefits of TCC has accelerated remarkably, and has led to a growing amount of research in this area.

HEALTH BENEFITS FOR THE ELDERLY

The health benefits of TCC have been extolled throughout the Chinese literature. However, not until

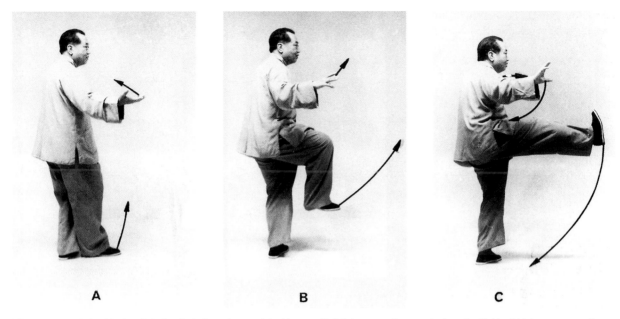

Figure 32.2 Kick with the right heel. A: Step forward, hold arms. B: Lift knee and separate hands. C: Heel kick, arms apart.

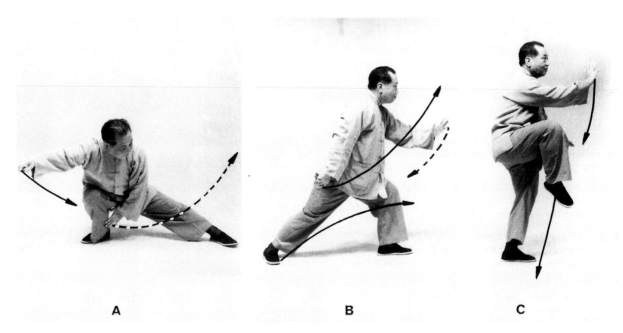

Figure 32.3 Snake creeps down, left side. A: Crouch stance, threading palm. B: Bow stance, standing up. C: Lift knee and upturn palm.

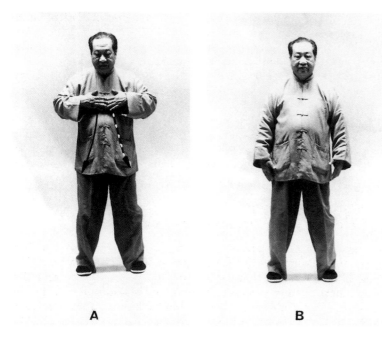

A **B**

Figure 32.4 Closing form of Tai Chi Chuan. A: Holding arms and extending them forward. B: Pushing arms downward and resting them by the sides of the hips.

recent decades has attention been focused on examining the scientific evidence of these claims. Table 32.1 summarizes several early cross-sectional and longitudinal studies in China conducted by the People's Sports and Exercise Publication (1976, 1983) and the An Wei Science and Technology Publication (1983), respectively. These findings suggest that TCC is beneficial to health, especially for the elderly and people with chronic disease. In addition, elderly people who practice TCC regularly showed improvement in selected physiological and pathological variables.

Similar studies have been initiated in the West. In 1990, the American National Institute on Aging started the FICSIT (Frailty and Injuries: Cooperative Studies on Intervention Techniques) trials, which explored the contribution of TCC to the physiological, behavioral and environmental aspects related to frailty or falls in elderly individuals (Province et al 1995). In comparing the performance of elderly subjects practicing TCC with baseline rates of those undertaking other forms of exercise, favorable cardiovascular, respiratory, hormonal and psychological responses were noted, with the improvements maintained over years.

Table 32.1 Changes in selected measures after TCC practice in the over-60s

Condition	TCC	Controls
Occurrence of spondylitis (%)	23.8	47.2
Occurrence of osteoarthritis (%)	14.3	79.4
Occurrence of degeneration/deconditioning (%)	25.8	47.2
Ability to touch the floor with the hands (%)	85.7	20.6
Average resting systolic blood pressure (mmHg)	134	154
Recovery of blood pressure after a 30-s, 20 repeated sit–stand exercise (%), within 3 min	90.2	22.4
Air exchange (L/min)	79	64.3
Incidence of developing atherosclerosis (%)	37.5	46.4
Sit–stand 20 times in 30 s (%)	No abnormal heart beats	35 abnormal heart beats
Behavioral test outcomes indicative of anxiety, anger, sadness, depression and loneliness (%)	92.3 improved	71.6 worse
High-density lipoprotein (mg)	Reduced by 14.5	No change

Psychosocial well-being

Physical activity helps to relieve symptoms of anxiety and depression and hence improve psychological well-being. TCC does more than other forms of physical activity as it emphasizes the importance of 'body–mind harmony'. Moreover, while practicing TCC, it is necessary to concentrate the body's vital energy (*Qi*) at the 'Dan Tian' (an acupoint) to reach a slow but deep and rhythmic breathing. This helps to regulate sympathetic and parasympathetic nervous systems during the excitation–inhibition transition (Li & Ji 1995).

Brown et al (1995) evaluated 69 healthy women (54.8 ± 8.3 years) after randomly assigning them into the control group (C), moderate-intensity walking group (MW), low-intensity walking group (LW), low-intensity walking plus relaxation response group (LWR), and TCC-type program (TCC). Women in the TCC group experienced significant reduction in mood disturbance (tension, depression, anger, confusion, and total mood disturbance) and an improvement in general mood (Table 31.2). The results indicate that TCC may have great therapeutic potential for persons with clinical symptoms of mental disorder, such as depression, anxiety, and chronic fatigue.

Apart from the beneficial effects on general psychosocial well-being, Wolf et al (1996) reported that regular practice of TCC could reduce the risk of multiple falls in the elderly by 47.5%, due to a reduced fear of falling response and intrusiveness response after TCC intervention (Table 32.3).

Jin (1992) also reported a significant increasing heart rate, noradrenaline exertion in urine and decreasing salivary cortisol concentration in a group of 33 TCC practitioners aged 66–77, as compared with 33 aged-matched controls. These data suggest that regular practice of TCC helps to relieve tension, depression, fatigue and anxiety, which implies an improved psychological well-being.

Cardiorespiratory system

Premature aging of the cardiovascular system is a major factor in the aging process. It is characterized by attenuation and loss of elastic fibers in the vessel walls, atherosclerotic plaques, calcareous deposit in the media, and narrowing of the lumens. These structural changes lead to a decrease in the velocity of blood flow and oxygen concentration in the circulating blood, and hamper the heart function.

Several studies suggest that TCC has positive effects on the maintenance of cardiorespiratory function in the elderly (Chen et al 1995, Lai et al 1995, Lan et al

Table 32.2 Psychological variables in pre- and post-test scores from 69 women (age 54.8 ± 8.3 years). (After Brown et al 1995)

| Variables | Test | Groups | | | | | Multiple comparisons |
		MW	LW	LWR	TCC	C	
POMS	Pre-test	122.4 ± 8.2	103.0 ± 4.8	110.4 ± 5.2	133.9 ± 15.4	128.8 ± 12.7	TCC > LW,
Total	Post-test	100.0 ± 5.4	101.8 ± 5.6	102.9 ± 6.2	90.4 ± 4.6	116.7 ± 10.6	LWR, C
POMS	Pre-test	7.8 ± 2.1	4.7 ± 1.3	5.0 ± 1.1	12.4 ± 4.1	9.6 ± 2.4	TCC > LW,
Anger	Post-test	3.3 ± 1.4	3.7 ± 0.9	2.9 ± 1.2	2.4 ± 1.1	7.9 ± 2.1	LWR, C
POMS	Pre-test	8.7 ± 1.5	6.0 ± 0.9	6.5 ± 1.3	10.1 ± 3.8	9.0 ± 2.3	TCC > LW,
Tension	Post-test	4.3 ± 0.8	5.7 ± 1.3	6.2 ± 1.7	1.4 ± 0.4	6.9 ± 1.7	LWR
POMS	Pre-test	5.8 ± 1.1	3.7 ± 0.6	6.1 ± 1.0	7.4 ± 2.5	7.5 ± 1.8	TCC > LWR
Confusion	Post-test	4.0 ± 0.7	3.7 ± 0.7	4.9 ± 1.0	2.0 ± 0.4	4.7 ± 1.4	
POMS	Pre-test	8.4 ± 2.5	4.7 ± 1.2	4.4 ± 1.2	11.6 ± 2.9	11.7 ± 3.7	TCC > LW
Depression	Post-test	3.3 + 1.1	4.5 ± 1.2	5.3 ± 1.7	2.9 ± 1.3	9.1 ± 3.2	
LSES mood	Pre-test	18.3 ± 0.8	20.1 ± 0.6	18.9 ± 0.5	17.9 ± 0.9	17.7 ± 0.7	TCC > C
	Post-test	18.8 ± 0.9	19.9 ± 0.6	19.4 ± 0.5	19.6 ± 0.5	18.2 ± 0.9	
Body	Pre-test	103.7 ± 5.7	86.4 ± 4.3	95.6 ± 3.9	105.3 ± 4.2	91.3 ± 6.4	MW > C
cachexis	Post-test	88.8 ± 7.6	79.9 ± 4.8	90.5 ± 3.9	94.7 ± 4.9	98.1 ± 7.0	

C, control group; LSES, life satisfaction in the elderly scale; LW, low intensity walking group; LWR, low-intensity walking plus relaxation response group; MW, moderate-intensity walking group; POMS, profile of mood states; TCC, TCC-type program.

Table 32.3 Time differences for psychosocial well-being outcome variables. (After Wolf et al 1996)

	Pre-TCC	15 weeks TCC	4 months post-TCC
	TCC (n = 60)		
Not at all afraid (%)	43	53	47
Somewhat afraid (%)	33	39	37
Fairly afraid (%)	13	2	8
Very afraid (%)	10	7	8

1996, Li et al 1994). Lan et al (1996) investigated the cardiorespiratory function, flexibility and body composition of 66 TCC practitioners aged 70 ± 4 years, each with around 12 years of training. The subjects exercised 4.3 times/week, 50 min per session, with an intensity equivalent to 70% of their maximum heart rate. During peak exercise the TCC group, which included both men and women, showed a significant 19% increase in $\dot{V}O_2$, O_2 pulse and work rate as compared with the sedentary control group (Table 32.4). Li et al (1994) also conducted a study in 20 women aged 58–65 in which the subjects were recruited to practice TCC for a month. Echocardiography results before and after the training period were compared. They showed that the thickness of the left ventricle, contraction amplitude, and blood supply of ventricle walls improved. Heart rate and blood pressure were lowered, whereas stroke volume and ejection fraction increased. Similar findings were observed in another study by Chen et al (1995), in which blood rheological tests were evaluated in TCC practitioners with a training history of over 5 years. Cardiac output had increased significantly by increased stroke volume, while heart rates had decreased. TCC movements demand endurance. They enhance the catalysis and breakdown of the trypsin lipase system on the endothelial layers of capillaries into triglyceride.

Plasminogen activator inhibitor (PAI) levels in blood plasma are significantly lower than those in the control and coronary heart disease groups.

Aging reduces the elasticity of lung tissue with atrophy of the pulmonary alveoli, resulting in up to a 50% decrease in oxygen exchange in elderly people, when compared with young adults. In an ordinary breath, only one-seventh of total gas capacity in the alveoli is exchanged, yet by taking a deep breath, the volume of gas exchanged jumps to one-third. Since TCC emphasizes slow, deep and rhythmic breathing, the thoracic cavity is expanded and the elasticity of lung tissues is increased, thus contributing to improved alveolar ventilation, increased alveolar-to-arterial gas exchange and reduced respiratory frequency.

Immunoendocrine system

Function of both the immune and endocrine systems also declines with aging. Available data suggest that TCC exercise might have positive effects on the endocrine system. From a cross-sectional study of 51 TCC teachers with a mean age of 69, it is evident that long-term TCC exercise can maintain euthyroid status, with secretion of thyroid hormone at a level of 0.93 ± 0.2 ng/mL, significantly higher than that of age- and sex-matched controls. Testosterone concentration is also maintained at 680 ng/cL, a level comparable to that of healthy adults (Zhang 1994). In addition, TCC enhances the functions of the pituitary gland, ensuring that the metabolism of the whole body is favorably regulated.

TCC exercise exposes the body to mild and appropriate levels of stress, which present favorable stimuli to hematopoietic organs, such as bone marrow, spleen and the lymph nodes (Xia et al 1991). Stress triggers secretion of erythropoietin and leukocyte-stimulating factor, and speeds up the formation and maturation of

Table 32.4 Cardiorespiratory variables of TCC and control groups. (After Lan et al 1996, with permission)

	Men		Women	
	TCC (n = 22)	Control (n = 18)	TCC (n = 19)	Control (n = 17)
$\dot{V}O_{2\ peak}$ (L/kg per min)	26.9 ± 4.7	$21.8 \pm 3.1^*$	20.1 ± 2.9	$16.5 \pm 2.0^*$
Peak O_2 pulse (mL/beat)	10.3 ± 2.4	$8.7 \pm 1.5^*$	7.0 ± 1.4	$5.6 \pm 0.7^*$
Peak work rate (W)	140 ± 30	$118 \pm 27^*$	96 ± 17	$78 \pm 17^*$
Ventilatory threshold of $\dot{V}O_2$ (mL/kg per min)	15.6 ± 3.3	$12.3 \pm 1.8^*$	12.6 ± 3.0	$10.9 \pm 1.8^*$
Ventilatory threshold (work rate, W)	70 ± 24	$52 \pm 12^*$	45 ± 16	$35 \pm 15^*$

Data are means $\pm$ SD.
$^*P <0.05$, comparing the group differences between TCC and control groups.

erythrocyte and hemoglobin. This leads to positive physiological adaptation in the blood system, and enhances immune function. Zhang (1990) studied immunoglobulin (IgG, IgA, IgM and IgE) levels in 30 elderly TCC practitioners and found a significant increase in IgG and IgM levels in men, and in IgM levels in women.

Neuromuscular coordination – balance

Observable alterations in posture, movement patterns and gait with advancing age are characterized by varying degrees of slowed movement, reduced range of motion, reduced muscle strength, increased flexed posture, reduced arm swing, and decreased unilateral weight shifts and stance times (Wolf et al 1996). One major consequence of these alterations is reduced balance capacity. This has repeatedly been proved to be an intrinsic risk factor of falls in the elderly (King et al 1994).

Falls and related injuries are the leading global medical problems of the elderly. In the USA alone, approximately 30% of persons over 65 years of age fall at least once every year, with multiple events in about half of them. About 10–15% of falls caused serious injuries, such as hip and distal radius fractures or soft tissue injuries. Substantial morbidity and mortality associated with falls in the elderly contribute to high medical costs. Fall survivors exhibit greater functional decline than non-fallers in their daily living, and physical and social activities (Blake et al 1988). Physical activity is one of the prescriptions to prevent falls in the elderly.

TCC demands well-coordinated and balanced movements in moving forward and backward. A number of studies confirm that regular TCC exercise improves or maintains one's balance, posture stability and flexibility. This translates in a decreased incidence of falls (Wolf et al 1996, Wolfson et al 1996). TCC also improves the function of the central nervous system in coordinating proprioceptive sense and balance organs (Fan 1994). Wolf et al (1996) compared TCC with an exercise control group and computerized balance training to evaluate the effects of TCC intervention over a period of 15 weeks with a 4-month follow-up. Falls were monitored continuously throughout the study in 200 subjects (162 women and 38 men) with a mean age of 76.2 years. TCC exercise delayed the onset of first or multiple falls in older individuals, with a substantial reduction of 47.5% in the rate of fall occurrence. This reduction was associated with a concomitant significant improvement in fear of falling after TCC training. The findings are of significance, as one of the more pervasive objectives of many geriatric therapeutic interventions is to improve or maintain balance in order to promote functional independence and eliminate or reduce fall-related events.

Another 2- to 4-year follow-up study from a planned meta-analysis of the FICSIT trial in the USA (Province et al 1995) also showed strong evidence that exercise programs could decrease the incidence of falls. In their cooperative studies, 100–1323 subjects aged 60–75 years in seven different regions were randomly assigned to various formal exercises or control programs. Results indicated that there was more reduction of falls if the exercise, such as TCC, included some activities for improving balance. Based on this scientific evidence, the American College of Sports Medicine recently published a position paper (ACSM 1998) stating that:

The optimal program for older women would include activities that improve strength, flexibility and coordination which may indirectly but effectively decrease the incidence of osteoporotic fractures by lessening the likelihood of falling.

Prevention of osteoporosis and fracture

A major intrinsic risk factor of fracture is osteoporosis. It primarily affects older persons and especially postmenopausal women (Dambacher et al 1998, Riggs & Melton 1986). Current estimates suggest that 1 in 4 postmenopausal women will suffer from an osteoporotic fracture. Osteoporotic fractures are the fifth most common finding in an elderly patient's medical history. The lifetime risk of fractures is 40% for women and 13% for men from their 50th birthday (Lau et al 1996). Without appropriate preventive measures, hip fractures may increase by 60% in the following 30 years. Early prevention, however, may reduce more than half of these fractures (Riggs & Melton 1986).

Available evidence indicates only that strength, power, and impact loading exercises can increase or maintain bone mineral density (BMD) and that reduction in bone mass occurs in women with decreased activity or inactivity (Dalsky et al 1988, Bassey 1995). As grip strength correlates significantly with BMD in elderly women (Lau et al 1993), and regular TCC exercise maintains and improves muscular strength (Guo & Hong 1995), TCC as a low-weight-bearing physical activity may be effective in decelerating bone loss and preventing osteoporosis. It also plays a role in counteracting the negative effects of estrogen deficiency in BMD in postmenopausal women.

The only documented study on the potential beneficial effects of regular TCC exercise on the skeleton dates back to 1983 (An Wei Science and Technology Publication 1983). Radiographic evaluation of 31 elderly subjects who practiced TCC for over 10 years showed that the shape of their spine remained structurally 'normal' and the percentage of deformation of vertebral bodies among the TCC subjects was 36.6%. This is much lower than in the control group (63.8%). In addition, the mobility of the spine was greater in the TCC group than in the control group.

With the recent development in non-invasive BMD measurement techniques, the BMD at various anatomic sites or even whole body BMD and its changes can be accurately and precisely monitored. The authors' research group has started a randomized controlled trial to investigate the effects of low weight-bearing TCC on balance, muscle strength and BMD in community-dwelling postmenopausal women in Hong Kong (Fig. 32.5). Results will be compared with women participating in brisk walking and a control program. Subjects with habitual exercise of more than 5 years are also evaluated. Our preliminary findings reveal that postmenopausal women with habitual exercise show significantly higher bone mass than those without regular physical activity. One-year participation in TCC or brisk walking retards loss in volumetric BMD in both the distal radius and distal tibia, when measured with peripheral quantitative computed tomography (pQCT), however not in areal BMD in the spine and proximal femur measured by Dual-Energy X-ray absorptometry (DXA) (Chan et al 2000, Qin et al 2000). Non-invasive technology is not available at present to monitor the potential benefits of TCC on the improvement or maintenance of bone structure quality with 1-year exercise intervention. Long-term follow-up studies are needed to reveal the potential beneficial effects of exercise intervention on BMD of the subjects.

TAI CHI CHUAN AS A THERAPEUTIC REGIME

Scientific evidence shows that, if appropriately prescribed and conducted, TCC exercise not only produces substantial health benefits in the elderly, but is also an alternative form of therapeutic regime for common health problems in older people.

The US Centers for Disease Control and Prevention and the American College of Sports Medicine (ACSM) recently recommended that activity for improving the cardiorespiratory system should use large muscle groups, be maintained for a prolonged period, and be rhythmic and aerobic in nature. This recommendation coincides with the practice of TCC, which features gentle and rhythmic movements. Moreover, the intensity of TCC is well within the recommended levels (Wolf et al 1997):

- intensity should correspond to 60–90% of maximal heart rate
- duration should be 20–60 min of aerobic activity
- frequency should be 3–5 days/week.

TCC is a unique form of low-impact, low-velocity physical activity that involves no jumping. Lower limb joints, particularly the knee and ankles, are often sites of degenerative joint disease in the elderly, and TCC

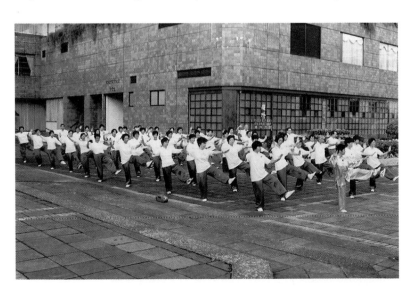

Figure 32.5 A group of postmenopausal women in Hong Kong practicing Tai Chi Chuan (TCC) in a randomized study on potential effects of TCC in prevention of osteoporosis and fall-related fracture.

appears to be a good and safe exercise. No adverse effects are reported on the active range of motion or weight-bearing joint integrity in patients with rheumatoid arthritis or myocardial infarction, or in osteoporotic patients (Henderson et al 1998).

Fear of falling is a dominant factor that prevents the elderly from participating in physical activity. Those who are motivated to start an exercise program often withdraw shortly after. In the Atlanta FICSIT study (Wolf et al 1996), subjects over 70 years old were randomly divided into three groups: TCC, individualized balance training (BT), and exercise control education (ED). After 15 weeks, both the TCC and BT groups showed increased confidence in balance and movement, but only TCC subjects reported positive changes in lifestyle. Many of the subjects in the TCC group incorporated TCC exercise into their daily routine, and approximately half of the subjects continued additional TCC classes voluntarily. We had a similar experience in our study on postmenopausal women. The drop-out rate in the TCC group was lower, with fewer complaints of back or joint pain, as compared with the group performing brisk walking.

Many forms of physical activity are suitable for the elderly, such as brisk walking, jogging, swimming, playing tennis or other ball games, cycling, dancing and low-impact aerobics such as TCC. This last activity, however, has definite advantages over the other forms of exercise. It is cheap, safe, convenient to practice, requires no special equipment or space, and is not affected by weather conditions. It can be practiced individually or in a group. TCC is also a vehicle for social interaction through which the elderly can seek assistance and support from other elderly individuals facing similar health problems. TCC may also enhance independence by decreasing the need for assistance in the activities of daily life (Guo & Hong 1995, Li & Ji 1995).

Despite the common consensus of TCC as a comparatively safe form of physical activity for the elderly, special precautions must be taken:

- Practice TCC step by step. For the elderly, especially those with chronic diseases, monitoring of their cardiovascular, respiratory, nerve and motor systems is recommended. It is advisable to consult a doctor or sports medicine specialist for a prescription on TCC styles and workload before commencing a TCC program. It is also important to consult a physician if experiencing pain or severe exhaustion after a workout.
- Self-supervision and self-perception. If there are symptoms of chest pain, chest distress or shortness of breath, stop exercise immediately. The appropriate workload can be determined by measuring the pulse

rate recovery, i.e. the pulse rate returns to the resting level 5 min after the TCC session.

- The body movements with individually adequate velocity should be emphasized, with a balanced mind concentration and strength distribution. Correct respiration pattern is an integral part of an effective workout.
- Most TCC movements are executed with the knees bent and/or standing on one leg. People suffering from arthritis may experience pain during workout. Knees should only be flexed to a tolerable degree. In case of increased pain, the workload or style of movements should be reduced or readjusted.

CONCLUSIONS

Tai Chi Chuan is more than just a safe and popular exercise for the elderly. It is effective in the maintenance of neuromuscular coordination, muscle strength, flexibility, and cardiorespiratory and immunoendocrine function. It has great potential to retard bone loss and thus prevent osteoporosis and related fracture. It also plays a crucial role in the improvement of the psychological well-being of the elderly and the enhancement of their social independence.

The intensity of TCC exercise fulfills the guidelines on exercise prescription by the Chinese National Athletic Committee, Chinese Sports Editorial Board, and the American College of Sports Medicine. In addition, TCC has significant advantages over other forms of physical activity, being cheap, safe, convenient to practice without special equipment or space, and unaffected by weather conditions.

The world population is aging. The number of people aged over 65 will rise from 390 to 800 million by 2025, with a life expectancy of 73 years (Lau 1997). Morbidity accompanying aging places a great burden on health care systems worldwide. TCC excels as a promising treatment modality for chronic illness and disability in the elderly. Further study is warranted to delineate its effect in the treatment of chronic diseases such as coronary artery disease, hypertension, gastrointestinal dysfunction, arthritis, and established osteoporosis.

REFERENCES

American College of Sports Medicine 1998 Position stand: exercise and physical activity for older adults. Medicine and Science in Sports and Exercise 30(6): 992–1008

An Wei Science and Technology Publication 1983 Health care and exercise of old age. An Wei Science and Technology Publication, China

Blake A J, Morgan J, Bendall M J 1988 Falls by elderly persons at home: prevalence and associated factors. Age and Ageing 17: 365–372

Brown D R, Wang Y, Ward A et al 1995 Chronic psychological effects of exercise and exercise plus cognitive strategies. Medicine and Science in Sports and Exercise 27(5): 765–775

Chan K M, Au S K, Choy W Y et al 2000 Beneficial effect of one-year Tai Chi in retardation of bone loss in postmenopausal women. Journal of Bone and Mineral Research 15 (suppl 1): S439

Chen M L, Yuan G L, Wei J W, Zhao H B, Xu L M 1995 Effects of Taijiquan and 18-form Qigong training on serum t-PA, PAI activities in aged people. Journal of the Shanghai Physical Education Institute 19(3): 66–68

Chen X W 1985 Chen's Taijiquan. Beijing, People's Sports and Exercise Publication Chinese Sports Editorial Board. Simplified 'Taijiquan'. Beijing China Informational Book Trading Corporation, China

Dalsky G P, Stocke K S, Ehsani A A, Slatopolsky E, Lee W C, Birge S J Jr 1988 Weight-bearing exercise training and lumbar bone mineral content in postmenopausal women. Annals of Internal Medicine 108: 824–828

Dambacher M A, Neff M, Kissling R, Qin L 1998 Highly precise peripheral quantitative computed tomography, bone density, loss of bone density and structures: consequences for prophylaxis and treatment. Drugs and Aging 12(1): 15–24

Fan G L 1994 Mental training through Taijiquan. Journal of Zhejiang Sports Science 16(5): 28–29

Guo J R, Hong Y L 1995 Improvement of motor ability through Taijiquan exercise in aged individuals. Journal of the Tianjin Physical Education Institute 11(14): 14–17

Henderson N K, White C P, Eisman J A 1998 The roles of exercise and fall risk reduction in the prevention of osteoporosis. Endocrinology and Metabolism Clinics of North America 27(2): 369–387

Jin P 1992 Efficacy of Tai Chi, brisk walking, meditation, and reading in reducing mental and emotional stress. Journal of Psychosomatic Research 36(4): 361–370

King M B, Judge J O, Wolfson L 1994 Functional base of support decreases with age. Gerentology 49(6): 258–263

Lai J S, Lan C, Wong M K, Teng S H 1995 Two-year trends in cardiorespiratory function among older Tai Chi Chuan practitioners and sedentary subjects. Journal of the American Geriatrics Society 43(11): 1222–1227

Lan C, Lai J S, Wong M K, Yu M L 1996 Cardiorespiratory function, flexibility, and body composition among geriatric Tai Chi Chuan practitioners. Archives of Physical and Medical Rehabilitation 77(6): 612–616

Lau E M C 1997 Osteoporosis in Asia – crossing the frontiers. World Scientific, Singapore

Lau E, Woo J, Leung P C 1993 Low bone mineral density, grip strength and skin-fold thickness are important risk factors for hip fracture in Hong Kong Chinese. Osteoporosis International 3(2): 66–69

Lau E, Chan H, Woo J 1996 Normal ranges for and the prevalence of vertebral fracture in Hong Kong Chinese. Journal of Bone and Mineral Research 11(9): 1364

Leaders 1995 Exercise in primary prevention of osteoporosis in women. Annals of the Rheumatic Diseases 54: 861–862

Li H Q, Ji S X 1995 Health promotion and therapeutic effects, and the mechanism of Taiji practice. Journal of the Shanghai Physical Education Institute 19(13): 95–98

Li S Y, Wang W J, Liu B 1994 Changes in cardiac function before and after practicing Yang's Taijiquan in aged female individuals. Journal of Shandong Sports Science 10(23): 11–12

Lin S T 1993 Aging process of population and Taijiquan practice. China Sports History 2: 11–13

People's Exercise and Sports Publication, Sports and Exercise Building Group 1976 Knowledge of sports and exercise physiology. People's Exercise and Sports Publication, Canton, China

People's Sports and Exercise Publication, Aging in Medical Science Research Group 1983 Behavior of Tai Chi and non-Tai Chi participants. People's Sports and Exercise Publication, Canton, China

Province M A, Hadley E, Hornbrook M C et al 1995 The effects of exercise on falls in elderly patients. Journal of the American Medical Association 273(17): 1341–1347

Qin L, Au S K, Choy W Y, Leung P C, Neff M, Dambacher M A, Lau E, Chan K M 2000 Regular Tai Chi exercise retards bone loss and decline of bone structure and bone strength index in postmenopausal women. Journal of Bone and Mineral Research 15(suppl 1): S437

Riggs B L, Melton L J 1986 Involution osteoporosis. New England Journal of Medicine 314: 1676–1686

Wang Y Q, Wei S R, Qi Y 1995 Yang's Taijiquan. Beijing, People's Sports and Exercise Publication, China

Wolf S L, Barnbart H X, Kutner N G, McNeely E, Coogler C, Xu T S and the Atlanta FICSIT Group 1996 Reducing frailty and falls in older person: an investigation of Tai Chi and computerized training. Journal of the American Geriatrics Society 44: 489–497

Wolf S L, Coogler C E, Xu T 1997 Exploring the basis for Tai Chi Chuan as a therapeutic exercise approach. Archives of Physical and Medical Rehabilitation 78(8): 886–892

Wolfson L, Whipple R, Derby C et al 1996 Balance and strength training in older adults: intervention gains and Tai Chi maintenance. Journal of the American Geriatrics Society 44: 498–506

Xia Y J, Zhang Y, Tan Z B 1991 Investigation on the effect of Taijiquan practice on the health condition of middle age intellectuals. Chinese Journal of Sports Medicine 10(3): 174–175

Xu C 1994 Wellness of Taijiquan (II). Journal of Zhonghua Wushu 6: 4–6

Zhang G D 1990 Effect of 48-form Taijiquan and Yiqi Yangfei Qigong on the serum immunoalbumin content. Journal of the Beijing Physical Education Institute 4: 12–14

Zhang Q Q 1994 Taijiquan – the best measures of preserving health and anti-aging process. Journal of Zhonghua Wushu 6: 23–24

33

Alpine skiing in the elderly

Arnold Koller

KEY POINTS

1. About 90% of all sudden cardiac deaths among downhill skiers occur in males over the age of 34. A steep increase in sudden cardiac death risk is observable in male skiers above the age of 50. In addition, older skiers are at increased risk for skiing injuries.
2. No increased sudden cardiac death risk is found for persons practising alpine sports regularly. Compared with cross-country skiing and jogging, the frequency of sudden cardiac death frequency in alpine skiing is markedly lower.
3. For non-extreme skiing activities, the external and internal forces are within reasonable limits, and one should expect positive effects from these activities as long as they are executed within reasonable limits.
4. Alpine skiing is characterized by substantial demands on both the aerobic and anaerobic metabolism. Despite the apparently high energy demand, a unique feature of alpine skiing is the reliance on high force production, especially during sustained slow eccentric muscle contraction.
5. Ageing is reportedly associated with coronary heart disease, hypertension, diabetes and a variety of musculoskeletal problems.
6. It is necessary to have reasonably frequent comprehensive expert medical evaluation. Moreover, individually adjusted pre-practice training prior to skiing is recommended for elderly skiers.

INTRODUCTION

Skiing is a popular winter sport in alpine regions all over the world. People can ski from the age of 3 to age 70 and beyond. Skiing is fun, and there are many elements which go into making it fun. Certainly, part of it is the thrill of pitting one's wits and physical ability against nature, but for others the attraction is the excitement of the speed that can be attained while skiing. Most people are in some way attracted to speed (Leach 1994).

Virtually the only major drawbacks to skiing are the injuries which skiers may suffer. Although recreational skiing has become safer due to the use of better equipment, particularly safety binding, recent epidemiological data have shown that older adults (>45 years) are at increased risk from skiing injuries. Moreover, other studies suggest that mortality increases with age. A steep increase in risk is observable in male skiers above the age of 50 (Table 33.1) (Burtscher et al 1997). Alpine skiing is a thrilling event, but that thrill comes with a relatively high risk of injury, particularly in elderly subjects. Moreover, such vigorous exercise may actually increase the risk of a heart attack in sedentary men at high risk of heart disease (Barinaga 1997). What factors contribute to this increase in risk observable in elderly skiers? While skiers have come to accept this inherent risk, I believe that there are ways to reduce it.

DEFINING THE ELDERLY

Who are the elderly? Defined in terms of chronological age, the elderly usually include individuals aged 65 years and older. In contrast, the World Health Organization has adopted the following classification system: middle age, 45–59; elderly, 60–74; old, 75–90; very old, over 90. Whatever classification is adopted, the elderly constitute a group characterized by con-siderable variation in physiological, mental and functional capacity. Furthermore, dissimilarities among subgroups are often so pronounced that it can be misleading to consider the elderly as a single group. These dissimilarities include genetic make-up, lifestyle, place of residence and living arrangement (Alter 1996).

EXTERNAL LOADING

The external forces reported in the literature are not excessive in alpine skiing when compared with other sporting activities, but ski-specific force applications (e.g. excessive mogul skiing) may create high internal local stresses (Nigg et al 1997). The internal forces, however, are the forces which are of importance when deciding whether a specific skiing activity is 'safe' and can be recommended to a specific person (Nigg et al 1997).

LOADING OF THE HIP JOINT DURING SKIING ACTIVITIES

In a recent study, loading of the hip joint was quantified during various alpine and cross-country skiing activities, and was compared with heel-toe running (Nigg et al 1997). Cross-country skiing was reported to have slightly smaller hip joint loading than heel-toe running. Hip joint loading in alpine skiing was reported to be lower than heel-toe running for skiing long turns on flat slopes, and slightly higher than heel-toe running for skiing short turns on flat slopes and long turns on steep slopes. However, the loading of the hip joint was substantially higher than for heel-toe running for skiing short turns on steep slopes and for skiing small moguls (Nigg et al 1997). Interestingly, impact forces at the hip joint were only observed during heel-toe running, not during the various alpine and cross-country skiing activities. Therefore, the external and internal forces are within reasonable limits for non-excessive skiing activities (Nigg et al 1997). However, as with most other sports activities, the loading of the locomotor systems increases substantially when extreme situations are encountered. These may occur due to the selection of the activity (e.g. excessive mogul skiing) or due to the loss of control during skiing activity (e.g. a fall). In such situations, forces may be excessive and cause an injury. Biomechanical or epidemiological studies, however, provide only information about controlled situations.

Table 33.1 Annual death risk among Austrian downhill skiers of different age groups

Age (years)	Number of deaths from 1986 to 1995 per annual number of skiers	Annual death rate per 100 000 downhill skiers
1–15	27/572 900	0.5
16–29	49/1 043 600	0.5
30–44	31/736 600	0.4
45–59	35/283 800	1.2
>59	43/8600	5.0

Oesterreichischer Alpenverein, 1997.

Potential risks associated with skiing in the elderly

In this context, three conditions prevalent in the geriatric population require special consideration. First, ligaments, tendons and muscles in the elderly are less elastic and pliable. Generally, this change is due to decreased water content (i.e. dehydration), increased crystalline orientation, calcification and replacement of elastic fibres with collagenous fibres (Alter 1996). Consequently, these less elastic tissues are potentially subject to an injury such as sprains or strains (Alter 1996). If an elderly person has been bedridden or immobilized, or is in an advanced state of deconditioning, osteoporosis may be present. Other conditions that require special precaution are degenerative and inflammatory arthritis, i.e. osteoarthritis and rheumatoid arthritis.

ASPECTS OF MUSCLE PROPERTIES AND USE IN ALPINE SKIING

Energy demand in skiing

Alpine skiing is characterized by substantial demands on both aerobic and anaerobic metabolism (Tesch 1995).

Maximal aerobic power in alpine skiers

Oxygen consumption may be substantial in skiing, and the energy requirement has been calculated to approximate 120% of the maximal oxygen uptake (Tesch 1995). It appears that, in both absolute and relative terms, advanced skiers are able to utilize a higher fraction of their maximal aerobic power than less advanced skiers. Moreover, it appears that skiing *per se* does not promote adaptations of the magnitude typically shown in endurance athletes (Tesch 1995). However, it must be remembered that skiing has a positive side: it can be conducive to good health. Skiing is an excellent sport for conditioning, as it is largely aerobic (Leach 1994), and aerobic activity is necessary to ward off heart disease (Barinaga 1997). Skiing requires one to be in good shape, and doctors frequently advise their patients to 'get into shape to ski rather than ski to get in shape', thus fighting the systematic off-snow aerobic conditioning.

Potential risks associated with skiing in the elderly. Maximal aerobic capacity, as assessed by maximal oxygen uptake, declines with age in both men and women (Fig. 33.1) (Tanaka et al 1997). The decrease

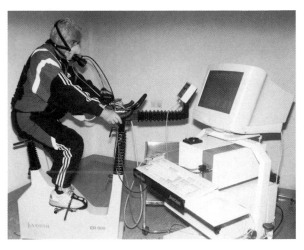

Figure 33.1 Maximal oxygen consumption testing in a 68-year-old alpine skier. Oxygen consumption may be substantial in skiing. Maximal aerobic capacity declines with age, but there is evidence to suggest that regularly performed endurance exercise may attenuate the loss of aerobic capacity with advancing age.

reduces physical work and results in older individuals working closer to maximum effort when performing a given submaximal task by reducing their functional reserve capacity (Tanaka et al 1997). In addition, maximal aerobic capacity has recently been shown to be an independent risk factor for all-cause and cardiovascular disease mortality (Tanaka et al 1997). There is some evidence to suggest that, in men, regular endurance exercise may attenuate the loss of maximal aerobic capacity with advancing age (Tanaka et al 1997). In contrast, the results of recent longitudinal studies in endurance-trained compared with sedentary men suggest as great or greater rates of decline in maximal aerobic capacity as those previously reported in sedentary men (Tanaka et al 1997). The corresponding data in women provide evidence that the absolute, but not the relative, rate of decline in maximal aerobic capacity with age may be greater in highly physically active women compared with sedentary healthy peers. Although endurance-trained women appear to have a greater decline in maximal oxygen uptake with age, their absolute levels are substantially higher than those of their sedentary peers throughout the adult age range studied. Moreover, only a few endurance-trained women had maximal oxygen uptake values lower than 32.5 mL/kg per min, the level below which age-adjusted mortality starts to increase in women.

Therefore, from the standpoint of preventive gerontology, the endurance-trained elderly skiers possess higher levels of physiological functional capacity and, based on recent epidemiological data, lower risk of mortality (sudden cardiac death) than do sedentary skiers (Burtscher et 1997).

Anaerobic metabolism in alpine skiing

The anaerobic component is substantial in alpine skiing (Tesch 1995). This is illustrated by the pronounced lactate accumulation noticed after intense recreational skiing. During intense recreational skiing, the demands on the glycolytic system are high and cause lactic acid levels to rise from resting values of approximately 1 mmol/kg to over 25 mmol/kg of muscle (Leach 1994). Such high lactic acid content in the muscle fibres inhibits further glycogen breakdown and may also interfere with the muscle contractile process. Extended reliance on glycolysis (e.g. for over 2 min) for energy will result in fatigue and eventual exhaustion, as the internal environment of the muscle fibres becomes acidic. Fatigued muscles are able to absorb less energy before reaching the degree of stretch that causes injury (muscle strain). The relevance of this system to human performance and physical fitness throughout the age spectrum is underscored in a recent review paper (Cahill et al 1997), and contrasted with the aerobic energy system.

Potential risks associated with skiing in the elderly. Until recently, it has been assumed that there is an obligatory loss of strength with age (Cahill et al 1997). It is now known that this loss can be modified by anaerobic training. There is also ample evidence that the anaerobic energy system is highly trainable in the elderly (Cahill et al 1997). According to Rogers & Evans (1993):

loss of strength and the decline in the muscle's metabolic capacity can no longer be considered as an inevitable consequence of the aging process.

Glycogen use in alpine skiing

Glycogen utilization may be substantial during the course of a day in leisure skiing. Glycogen content before and after a day of skiing, respectively, averaged 89 and 43 mmol/kg wet weight (Nygaard et al 1978, Tesch 1995). Several studies have demonstrated a decrease in resting muscle glycogen content during the course of a few days of intense skiing (Nygaard et al 1978, Tesch 1995). Low glycogen levels may have detrimental effects on performance while skiing. Thus, individuals who exhaust their glycogen levels through previous vigorous exercise show marked impairment in sustaining high force output during repeated knee extensions (Berg et al 1995). Hence, glycogen depletion of a similar magnitude would most likely also hamper ski performance.

Fibre type composition in alpine skiers

Elite skiers do not show a distinct fibre type profile (Tesch 1995). The lack of a fibre type profile in elite skiers corroborates the findings of no selective glycogen depletion, and the high demands on both aerobic and anaerobic energy utilization and endurance as well as the performance of slow, and preferentially eccentric, muscle actions (involving forced lengthening of active muscle) in alpine skiing (Tesch 1995). Nygaard et al (1995) reported that, among a group of beginners, the FTb (fast-twitch subtype b) fibres showed a higher degree of depletion than did the slow-twitch fibres. The FTb fibres did not show any noticeable depletion in the experienced skiers. In addition to the slow-twitch fibres, however, the group of excellent skiers had some 80% of the FTa (fast-twitch subtype a) fibres partially depleted after skiing.

Potential risks associated with skiing in the elderly. There is a progressive, age-related decrease in muscular strength, in the size of fast-twitch muscle fibres, and in the proportion of fast-twitch muscle fibres (Fig. 33.2) (Cahill et al 1997). The reported reasons for strength loss include a decrease in the total number of muscle fibres, whole muscle atrophy, muscle fibre atrophy, impaired excitation–contraction coupling, denervation of fast-twitch fibres, and decreased ability or complete inability to activate high-threshold (fast-twitch) motor units. Both muscle mass and strength decline with age. This decline is associated with an increased risk of falls, hip fractures and adverse physiological changes, such as glucose intolerance and loss of bone mineral density (Lindle et al 1997). Consequently, these changes may predispose elderly individuals to osteoporosis, atherosclerosis and diabetes, as well as to functional limitations in activities such as alpine skiing (Lindle et al 1997). It appears, however, that older subjects respond similarly to younger subjects to resistance training, specifically with remarkable degrees of improvement in strength (Cahill et al 1997). Anaerobic training by the elderly induces the biological adaptation of hypertrophy of fast-twitch muscle fibres (Cahill et al 1997).

Muscular strength in alpine skiers

Despite the apparently high energy demand, a unique feature of alpine skiing is the reliance on high force

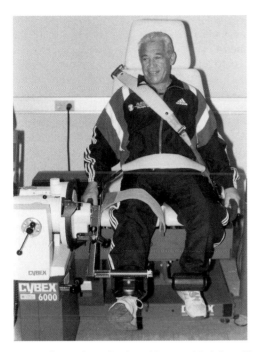

Figure 33.2 Strength testing in a 68-year-old alpine skier on an isokinetic dynamometer. Comparing alpine skiing with other sporting activities, the demand for high force and power from the muscles is very high. There is a progressive, age-related decrease in muscular strength, but resistance training by the elderly may attenuate this decrease.

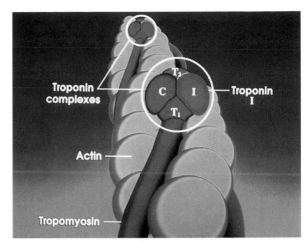

Figure 33.3 Schematic of a part of the thin filament showing the actin helix, tropomyosin coiled coil, and troponin complex. Eccentric exercise, such as alpine skiing, causes a rapid dissociation and/or degradation with rapid removal of skeletal troponin I.

production, especially during maintained slow eccentric muscle action (Berg et al 1995, Leach 1994, Tesch 1995). The observed slow average joint angular movements in skiing also contradicts the common portrayal of alpine skiing as an explosive sport (Berg et al 1995). Considering the superior force output during eccentric compared with concentric muscle actions may be warranted or even required to meet the force demand of a turn. The knee- and hip-extensor muscles of the inside leg use a stretch shortening cycle during the turn. In contrast, the knee- and hip-extensor muscles of the outside leg are loaded predominantly eccentrically after the pole is touched. The metabolic cost at any given power output is substantially lower during eccentric exercise than during concentric exercise (Tesch 1995). Moreover, muscle fatigue is less during eccentric exercise than during concentric exercise. In this context, despite the observation of reliance on eccentric muscle action, the oxygen demand may tax or even exceed maximal aerobic power during giant-slalom skiing (Tesch 1995).

In addition, recent results provide evidence that the high muscle force associated with eccentric contraction or length change occurring during eccentric contraction causes a rapid dissociation and/or degradation with rapid removal of skeletal troponin I (Fig. 33.3) (Sorichter et al 1997). These findings support the concept that eccentric exercise initiates a series of events that result in rapid disruption of the cytoskeletal network and contractile apparatus, which could be the mechanism for deterioration of the contractile response and loss in force generation (Koller et al 1997, Sorichter et al 1997). This prolonged loss in contractile force can result in lowered performance during skiing and may cause inability to recover from injury-producing falls (Koller et al 1997).

Exercise increases the rate of glucose uptake into the contracting skeletal muscles (for review, see Hayashi et al 1997). This effect of exercise is similar to the action of insulin on glucose uptake, and the mechanism through which both stimuli increase skeletal muscle uptake involves the translocation of GLUT-4 glucose transporters to the plasma membrane and transverse tubules. Most studies suggest that exercise and insulin recruit distinct GLUT-4-containing vehicles and/or mobilize different pools of GLUT-4 proteins originating from unique intracellular locations. The ability of exercise to utilize insulin-independent mechanisms to increase glucose uptake in skeletal muscle has important clinical implications, especially for patients with diseases associated with peripheral insulin resistance, such as non-insulin-dependent diabetes mellitus (Hayashi et al 1997). The muscle glucose transporter

(GLUT-4) content, however, is particularly affected by unaccustomed eccentric exercise, and it has been suggested that decreased GLUT-4 content may be an important factor for the delayed glycogen resynthesis pattern after this type of muscle activity (Kristiansen et al 1997).

Finally, the first objective of a recent study was to find out whether basal and/or active muscle energy metabolism is altered in isolated mouse extensor digitorum longus muscle injured by eccentric contractions (Warren et al 1996). Measurements of basal oxygen consumption and isometric tetanus oxygen recovery costs were made along with estimates of the anaerobic contribution from measurements of lactate and pyruvate release. On finding a decreased contraction economy in the injured muscle, the second objective of this study was to determine whether the decreased economy could be attributed to (1) an increased ATP hydrolysis relative to force production; and/or (2) an increased substrate consumption relative to ATP resynthesis. In conclusion, this study showed that contraction economy is decreased but basal energy metabolism is not elevated in muscles during the 2 h after injury initiation. The decreased economy was attributed to two factors. First, in skinned fibres isolated from the injured muscles, the ratio of maximal actomyosin adenosinetriphosphatase activity to force was up by 37%, suggesting uncoupling of ATP hydrolysis from force production. Second, increased reliance on anaerobic metabolism along with the fluorescent microscopic study of mitochondrial membrane potential and histochemical study of ATP synthase suggested an uncoupling of oxidative phoshorylation in injured muscles.

Potential risks associated with skiing in the elderly. The results of a recent study indicate that concentric strength levels begin to decline in the fourth rather than in the fifth decade, as previously reported (Lindle et al 1997). Contrary to previous reports, and most relevant to skiing, there is no preservation of eccentric compared with concentric strength in men or women (Lindle et al 1997). Nevertheless, the decline in eccentric strength with age appears to start later in women than in men and later than concentric strength did in both sexes (Lindle et al 1997).

Although it is attractive to attribute the increased incidence of skiing injuries, typically occurring in the afternoon, or after a few days on vacation (Tesch 1995), to the decline in muscle strength, glycogen depletion (Nygaard et al 1978), impaired muscle glycogen resynthesis (Kristiansen et al 1997), decreased contraction economy (Warren et al 1997), or disruption of

the cytoskeletal network and contractile apparatus (Koller et al 1997), there are no data to support this hypothesis.

Taken together, recent studies lead to a model of muscle injury following eccentric exercise such as alpine skiing (Koller et al 1997) that is sensitive to muscle fibre deformation and may involve rather selective proteolysis of structural proteins (Sorichter et al 1997). The dissolution of these proteins then leads to the ultrastructural abnormalities that have been widely reported in animals and humans. Interestingly, the magnitude of injury induced by stretches of maximally activated muscle fibres of mice and rats increases in old age (Brooks & Faulkner 1996). The increased susceptibility of muscles in old animals to contraction-induced injury resides at least in part within the myofibrils (Brooks & Faulkner 1996).

Impaired exercise-stimulated glucose transport is present when severe insulin resistance of muscle glucose transport and decreased muscle GLUT-4 mRNA and protein levels are caused by unaccustomed eccentric exercise (Hayashi et al 1997). Because it is now known that exercise-stimulated glucose transport is impaired after severe eccentric exercise (Kristiansen et al 1997), future studies should help us to elucidate the effects of alpine skiing on glucose transport in the insulin-resistant state.

Muscle activity

A recent study demonstrated the activity patterns of 12 muscles during three styles of skiing that represent a broad spectrum of current techniques (Hintermeister et al 1997). The primary result from this comparison of skiing styles is the general trend for increasing muscle activity from wedge to parallel and giant slalom turns. Co-contraction of muscles surrounding the knee and hip joints was evident in all styles of skiing. It should be noted that these data are for accomplished skiers. Muscular activity for beginners would most probably be different. Karlsson et al (1978) noted that the patterns of muscle activity from a competitive skier had more distinct bursts of activity and relaxation, whereas those from a recreational skier were active for longer periods of time. It may be that beginners skiing in a wedge would demonstrate greater muscular activity than is registered in more advanced skiers. Also, in contrast to weight-bearing and jumping exercises, it appears from EMG data that, during giant-slalom skiing, muscle strain is repeatedly maintained for several seconds at remarkably high levels (Berg et al 1995).

BALANCE AND PROPRIOCEPTION CHANGES

Balance is an important component in skiing. The most important objective in alpine technique is the regulation of dynamic equilibrium (Mester 1997). Sensory impairments involving visual, auditory, vestibular and proprioceptive modalities may affect balance (Alter 1996). With progressive degeneration of the proprioceptors due to ageing, knowledge of one's position in space can be severely impaired. This ability is further compromised by a reduction in peripheral vestibular excitability. Eventually, these changes in postural stability are manifested as an increase in body sway. With increasing age, the visual contribution to equilibrium becomes the predominant method for assessing body position. Eventually, it too can become compromised. Consequently, the risk of falling increases as the loss of balance becomes increasingly severe.

PHYSIOLOGICAL DEMAND ON THE CARDIOVASCULAR SYSTEM

The Multiple Risk Factors Intervention Trial (MRFIT) study suggested that vigorous exercise may actually increase the risk of a heart attack in sedentary men who have a high risk of heart disease (Barinaga 1997). Alpine skiing increases blood pressure, while also raising heart rate, indicating a high cardiovascular stress during skiing (Table 33.2). Those men, however, who did some form of sustained exercise had significantly lower death rates (sudden cardiac death) than those who did not (Burtscher et al 1997).

Table 33.2 Cardiac troponin T concentrations[a] in 12 male downhill skiers (mean age 67 ± 2.1 years) during the course of a day's leisure skiing

Number of skiers	Troponin T concentrations (ng/mL)
11	<0.05
1	Between 0.05 and 0.1

[a] Cardiac troponin T is a regulatory contractile protein that is only released into the blood following damage to the myocardial cells. Recently, it has been demonstrated that capillary blood can be used as sample material for the measurement of cardiac troponin T with a rapid and easy-to-operate compact benchtop instrument (Cardiac reader, Boehringer Mannheim, Mannheim, Germany) and immunoassays in strip format (Koller & Klingenschmid 1998). This facilitates the biochemical detection of myocardial injury in individuals participating in vigorous exercise, such as alpine skiing.

Altitude must be discussed as an additional risk factor alongside physical exertion, in particular for elderly people (Leach 1994). Breathing and respiration will be affected by lowered partial pressure of oxygen in atmospheric air, such as at high altitude, and can be of concern to those skiers who are predisposed to acute mountain sickness and related pathologies (Leach 1994).

CONCLUSIONS

1. Ageing can be defined as the age-related deterioration of physiological functions necessary for the survival and fertility of an organism. Common age-related diseases linked to these functions include coronary heart disease, hypertension, diabetes and a variety of musculoskeletal problems. Therefore, these seniors have a reduced margin of safety. Skiing in the elderly can be potentially hazardous. Thus, it is necessary to have reasonably frequent comprehensive expert medical evaluation.
2. The deterioration of physiological functions and common age-related diseases linked to these functions, however, can no longer be considered as an inevitable consequence of the ageing process. Thus, exertion tests and an individually adjusted preparatory form of training prior to practising skiing must be recommended for elderly skiers. The goals of this preparation period are to re-establish and improve upon the skier's aerobic power, anaerobic endurance or strength endurance, strength and flexibility. It is critical that balance and proprioception (awareness of body position) exercises are also incorporated into an elderly skier's training programme.
3. Proprioceptive fitness is a much neglected factor by skiers. Here quality and quantity meet. The quality of the 'communication' between our sensors and the peripheral and central nervous systems is an important 'fitness'

feature, which requires quality preparation and maintenance. Every episode of muscle soreness, every microtrauma and every macrotrauma affect negatively the quality of that link, which may be the difference between taking a minor fall and leaving the slopes on a stretcher. Based on recent research, elderly skiers should emphasize balance, coordination drills and agility exercises in their training programmes all year round, to try to reduce the rate of season-ending injuries.

4. One of the most important elements in a programme aimed at injury reduction in the elderly is the development and maintenance of a strong and balanced musculoskeletal system. Congenital features, micro- and macrotrauma can be sources of muscle imbalance. Muscle imbalance can be defined as a muscle which is tight-weak or stretch-weak. A muscle may have 'trigger points', which can arise gradually from repetitive microtrauma, or from macrotrauma. Once in place, these trigger points provide the environment for alteration of posture, movement pattern, deconditioning and pain, thus leading to an increased susceptibility to injury. This is why a correction programme based on a thorough analysis of the movement pattern should stretch tight muscles and strengthen weak ones.

5. In addition to both environmental and personal (e.g. skiing ability) factors, equipment factors may also influence the risk of injury. For example, a softer ski requires lower levels of muscle activity than a stiffer ski, which is what most experts and racers use.

6. Warm-up and cool-down can be critical to a skier's preparation. A recent article (Nicholas 1997) presents some of the more recent information on this topic, and a basic guideline for practical applications.

REFERENCES

Alter M J 1996 Science of flexibility, 2nd edn. Human Kinetics, Leeds

Barinaga M 1997 How much gain for cardiac gain? Science 276: 1324–1327

Berg H E, Eiken O, Tesch P A 1995 Involvement of eccentric muscle actions in giant slalom racing. Medicine and Science in Sports and Exercise 27(12): 1666–1670

Brooks S V, Faulkner J A 1996 The magnitude of the initial injury induced by stretches of maximally activated muscle fibres of mice and rats increases in old age. Journal of Physiology 492(2): 573–580

Burtscher M, Nachbauer W, Kornexl E, Mittleman M A 1997 Fitness, cardiovascular stress, and SCD-risk in downhill skiing. In: Müller E, Schwameder H, Kornexl E, Raschner C (eds) Science and skiing. E & FN Spon, London, ch 4, p 504–512

Cahill B R, Misner J E, Boileau R A 1997 The clinical importance of the anaerobic energy system and its assessment in human performance. The American Journal of Sports Medicine 25(6): 863–872

Hayashi T, Wojtaszewski J F P, Goodyear L J 1997 Exercise regulation of glucose transport in skeletal muscle. American Journal of Physiology 273 (Endocrinology and Metabolism 36): E1039–1051

Hintermeister R A, O'Connor D D, Lange G W, Dillman C J, Steadman J R 1997 Muscle activity in wedge, parallel, and giant slalom skiing. Medicine and Science in Sports and Exercise 29(4): 548–553

Karlsson J, Eriksson A, Forsberg A, Kallberg L, Tesch P 1978 The physiology of alpine skiing. United States Ski Coaches Association, Park City

Koller A, Kliengenschmid K 1998 Cardiac troponin T and myoglobin in capillary whole blood samples. Scandinavian Journal of Medicine and Science in Sports 8: 344–345

Koller A, Gebert W, Sorichter S et al 1997 Troponin I – a new marker of muscle damage in Alpine skiing. In: Müller E, Schwameder H, Kornexl E, Raschner C (eds) Science and skiing. E & FN Spon, London, ch 4, p 528–539

Kristiansen S, Jones J, Handberg A, Dohm G L, Richter E 1997 Eccentric contractions decrease glucose transporter transcription rate, mRNA, and protein in skeletal muscle. American Journal of Physiology (Cellular Physiology 41): C1734–1738

Leach R E 1994 Alpine skiing, 1st edn. Blackwell Scientific, Oxford

Lindle R S, Metter E J, Lynch N A, Fleg J L, Fozard J L, Tobin J, Roy T A, Hurley B F 1997 Age and gender comparisons of muscle strength in 654 women and men aged 20–93 yr. Journal of Applied Physiology 83(5): 1581–1587

Mester J 1997 Movement regulation in Alpine skiing. In: Müller E, Schwameder H, Kornexl E, Raschner C (eds) Science and skiing. E & FN Spon, London, ch 3, p 333–348

Nicholas D 1997 The warm-up and cool-down can be critical to your preparation. Ski Racing 30(3): 27

Nigg B M, van den Bogert A J, Read L, Reinschmidt C 1997 Load on the locomotor system during skiing. A biomechanical perspective. In: Müller E, Schwameder H, Kornexl E, Raschner C (eds) Science and skiing. E & FN Spon, London, ch 1, p 3–27

Nygaard E, Eriksson E, Nilsson P 1978 Glycogen depletion pattern in leg muscle during recreational downhill skiing. In: Figueras J M (ed) Skiing safety II, International series on sport sciences 5. University Park Press, Baltimore, p 273–278

Rogers M A, Evans W J 1993 Changes in skeletal muscle with aging: effects of exercise training. Exercise and Sport Sciences Reviews 21: 65–102

Sorichter S, Mair J, Koller A et al 1997 Skeletal troponin I as a marker of exercise-induced muscle damage. Journal of Applied Physiology 83(4): 1076–1082

Tanaka H, Desouza C A, Jones P P, Stevenson E T, Davy K P, Seals D R 1997 Greater rate of decline in maximal aerobic capacity with age in physically active vs. sedentary healthy women. Journal of Applied Physiology 83(6): 1947–1953

Tesch P A 1995 Aspects on muscle properties and use in competitive Alpine skiing. Medicine and Science in Sports and Exercise 27(3): 310–314

Warren III G J, Williams J H, Ward C W, Matoba H, Ingalls C P, Hermann K M, Armstrong R B 1996 Decreased contraction economy in mouse EDL muscle injured by eccentric contractions. Journal of Applied Physiology 81(6): 2555–2564

34

Racket sports for older individuals

Scott A. Lynch
Per A. F. H. Renström

KEY POINTS

1. Sports activities have positive effects on both physical and mental well-being.
2. Aging is associated with a decreased ability to withstand and avoid excessive stress.
3. Cardiac events are the major risk factor for older athletes.
4. Racket sport players with a history of heart disease should undergo Holter-EKG, exercise stress test and check-up prior to returning to play.
5. Musculoskeletal problems are usually related to those tissues that tend to break down during the aging process.
6. Doubles play provides lower rates of exertion than singles play and may result in lower cardiac risk and fewer musculoskeletal problems.

INTRODUCTION

Racket sports have become more popular among older individuals. This is due to the increased awareness by the general public of the beneficial effects of exercise. In addition, as the population continues to live longer and has more leisure time during the retirement years, athletic activities and the benefits and problems associated with athletics will become more evident.

BENEFITS OF EXERCISE

Physical activity has been associated with several health benefits. It has been shown to help keep the serum lipid profile within low cardiovascular risk levels. The relationship between lipids and artherosclerosis has been well documented, as has been the relationship between atherosclerosis and heart disease. Therefore, if the lipid profile can be controlled, presumably the rate of heart disease can be reduced. Diet and some drugs play an important role in controlling serum lipids. But physical activity has also been shown to improve the lipid profile by raising the level of HDLs (high-density lipoproteins) and lowering the level of LDLs (low-density lipoproteins). In addition, regular endurance training enhances insulin sensitivity and improves glucose utilization. Although the exact level of activity required to provide benefits to the lipid profile and to reduce cardiovascular risk has not been determined, it is likely that physical activity and cardiovascular risk has a 'dose–response' effect. The best effects are shown when comparing sedentary with highly active populations.

In addition to the benefits of altering the lipid profile, physical exercise also provides benefits in other ways. Both the respiratory and cardiovascular systems can adapt to higher loads with repeated regular training. Exercise increases maximal cardiac output, muscle blood flow, oxygen extraction from the lungs, and maximal oxygen uptake. Maximal oxygen uptake, however, does have a normal tendency to decrease with advancing age. This is primarily due to the decreased cardiac output that occurs with the aging process. However, it is well established that individuals who exercise regularly have higher maximal oxygen uptake and a lower rate of decline due to aging than their sedentary counterparts. In a 10-year follow-up study comparing former athletes with non-athletes, there was a continued and widening gap between the two groups in relation to motor skills and maximal oxygen uptake (Slezynski 1991). This indicates that physical activity can provide continued benefit for remarkably long periods of time.

The psychological benefits of exercise have been appreciated for a long time. Many athletes describe a euphoric effect of exercise and a general sense of well-being. Some even describe a type of 'jogger's addiction'. The exact cause of this is unknown, but there is some evidence that exercise causes central nervous system modulation and regulation of endorphins.

Age-related changes occur in all tissues of the body. Skeletal muscle loses some of its elasticity, ligaments and tendons undergo a reduction in strength and stiffness, and articular cartilage undergoes changes in its matrix and structural content. All of these are likely responsible for the perceived reduction in the body's ability to withstand and recover from injuries as it ages. However, as pointed out above, all is not lost, as many of these age-related changes can be diminished by the effects of regular exercise. Controlled loading, stress and motion have been shown to be beneficial for normal and healing structures. This has been well documented for injured ligaments, tendons, and bone.

RACKET SPORTS

The beneficial effects of athletics have been shown in the previous section. How then does this relate to racket sports in particular? There is very little on this subject in the literature. The majority of the work is related to cardiac risks and has been performed on tennis players, as this is by far the most popular of the racket sports. Most of the work can be extended from tennis to other sports, but some care must be exercised since the level of competitiveness and exertion can vary greatly not only between specific sports, but also within sports. Players are not all equally aggressive, nor do they play at the same level. Play that may be very strenuous for some may not provide much of a challenge for others. The important aspect is to determine the safe and beneficial range for each individual. The first thing to realize is that tennis can contribute to death. One study from Germany documented 115 deaths as a result of playing tennis (Parzeller & Rasche 1994). The great majority of these were due to cardiovascular events and nearly all the players were over the age of 40. Roughly half of the cardiac deaths occurred during training and the other half during competition. A few deaths were also reported in badminton, table tennis, and squash, with the average age of these deaths being slightly lower than that of the tennis players. The authors felt that this was due both to the more vigorous nature of the sport and to the relative popularity of tennis in the older age group as opposed to the younger participants of the other sports.

If we wish to avoid these problems, an accurate assessment of the risk of tennis playing must be made. The athlete and physician can then determine at what level of play participation can safely be accomplished, particularly in relation to cardiac risk factors. Seventeen tennis players with cardiovascular heart disease were examined in a study in Germany (Wendt & Schmidt 1994). Holter monitor, exercise stress tests and a variety of different cardiovascular and blood tests were performed during different types of play. Of those patients with no arrhythmias either during Holter monitoring or exercise, none developed arrhythmias during tennis. Of those patients with arrhythmias, some developed more and some fewer during play. Certainly the risk of sudden death in the first group is increased. Of the different types of play examined, competitive tennis caused higher anaerobic thresholds than practice. Reducing the number of balls in the competitive tennis from four to one provided some anaerobic relief. Overall, doubles play had the lowest anaerobic threshold and would be the most suitable play for athletes with cardiovascular disease. The tennis players also experienced reductions in potassium level, magnesium, and hematocrit, which were felt to be related to fluid replacement by water.

Changes in heart rate and blood biochemistry have also been observed in older squash players (Lynch et al 1992). Both in practice and in sequential match play during tournaments, dramatic increases in heart rate and catecholamine levels were seen. In addition, potassium levels decreased. The authors postulated that this combination could lead to sudden cardiac arrhythmias and potential death.

Playing tennis does, however, have many benefits. It is an effective and fun way to maintain cardiovascular exercise and provide the benefits as previously described. Tennis is also a means of maintaining weight-bearing activities to resist bone loss and to provide coordination training to maintain balance and function. Tennis has been shown to provide benefits in muscular strength and fatigue resistance (Laforest et al 1990). The increased strength may provide better impact resistance for joints and their surrounding tissues. By maintaining function, the risk of falling can be reduced. By reducing the number of falls, the rate of osteoporotic hip fractures can possibly be reduced as well. This would have a major impact not only the lifestyle and life expectancy of the individual, but also on the direct and indirect costs to society.

Studies examining the ability of older individuals to participate in moderate-intensity activities reveal that painful episodes occur more frequently in the older population. In studies incorporating low-level jogging into programs for individuals over the age of 60, about 60% will report at least one painful episode over a 1-year period. The knee is by far the most common area of injury. Most of the painful episodes, however, respond quickly to conservative measures such as rest, anti-inflammatory drugs, stretching, and activity modification. Factors that may predispose to painful episodes are obesity, osteoarthritis, weakness, and joint deformity. Overuse injuries are more prominent in the older population. Exercise-induced overuse injuries accounted for 70% of the older athlete injuries in one prospective analysis, as compared with 41% of younger athlete injuries. The most common areas of injury were the knee, shoulder, Achilles tendon, and

posterior tibialis tendon. Athletes with other medical conditions, such as diabetes or hypertension, may have further degeneration of their tissues, and may have fewer reserves available to combat injury. For racket sports, there is no reason to refute the basic premise of the above work. However, because of the nature of the quick starts and stops, and the repetitive overhead motion, particularly of the serve, foot and ankle as well as shoulder problems may be more common. To combat this, it may be prudent to advise some older athletes to change to doubles play. This can reduce the amount of repetitiveness, limit the number of quick starts and stops, and reduce the cardiovascular risk, while still providing an effective and enjoyable form of exercise.

From a musculoskeletal standpoint, the majority of injuries in the older athlete are due to overuse problems. This is primarily due to the breakdown and degeneration of tissue that occurs with the aging process. Early osteoarthritis and chondral or degenerative meniscal injuries are not uncommon in this age group, and these problems can sometimes affect player participation. In addition, we see higher rates of injury to the posterior tibialis tendon and Achilles tendon.

Degenerative meniscus tears

The menisci transmit between 50 and 100% of the load across the knee. Forces across the knee can range from two to four times body weight. Therefore, it is not surprising that injuries to the menisci are common in middle-aged and elderly players.

Meniscus tears can occur from an acute twisting event, but they can, and often do, occur without specific trauma. In older tennis players, meniscal injuries usually occur by degeneration as a result of the aging process.

For acute tears, sudden pain will occur following a twisting event. Degenerative tears will have a more gradual onset of symptoms, but an acute tear can occur to an already weakened degenerative meniscus. If a tear is present, some minor swelling and aching may occur. For large tears, locking of the knee may occur, but locking is unusual in the older athletes.

Patients with symptomatic meniscal tears will usually have tenderness over the joint line and discomfort with extremes of range of motion. The diagnosis is usually apparent from the combination of the patient history and physical examination. In difficult or unusual cases, an MRI can verify the diagnosis with excellent accuracy. Arthroscopy can be used both to verify and to treat the lesion.

Many meniscus tears have no or few symptoms. An initial treatment of physical therapy to strengthen the quadriceps and hamstrings and control the swelling may give the injury a chance to become asymptomatic. This is usually done for about 4–6 weeks. If the athlete does not respond to therapy, the tear can be removed by arthroscopic surgery.

The rehabilitation time and return to tennis after an excision of a partial tear depend on the location and extent of the meniscus injury. If the tear is small, return to pre-injury level will be approximately 2–4 weeks postsurgery. A return to tennis after 1–3 months is most common.

Degenerative joint disease and chondral lesions

Damage to the intra-articular surface is common among older athletes. These chondral lesions are commonly located on the undersurface of the patella, and on the medial femoral condyle. Damage and/or removal of a meniscus cartilage can predispose the knee to chondral lesions.

Players with chondral injuries may complain of start-up pain following a prolonged period of sitting, and may have intermittent swelling and pain.

Major degenerative joint disease is verified on conventional weight-bearing radiographs. Localized minor chondral lesions are best diagnosed by arthroscopy. MRI can sometimes show chondral lesions, but the accuracy to date is not very good. However, new MRI techniques are emerging that look more promising.

Treatment of chondral injuries is very difficult. Small full-thickness cartilage lesions can be treated with drilling or picking of the area. This is an attempt to increase blood flow to induce a healing response. For lesions that do not respond to this, some new techniques have been investigated, including periosteal transplant, periosteal transplant with cultured chondrocytes, and osteochondral transplant. The results of these techniques are difficult to predict, but it does appear that in the short term many patients are improved. For all of the techniques, however, it is unknown how well the repaired tissue will hold up under vigorous stress, such as racket sports.

For athletes with generalized degenerative joint disease, the above surgeries are not useful. Education and activity modification are the keys in this case. Switching to doubles play may be able to prolong the athlete's tennis career. Muscle strengthening exercises may transfer some of the load away from the chondral surfaces. For chronic cases, arthroscopic debridement may be tried, but the long-term results of this are generally not good. In the long term, when the problem begins to affect activities of daily living and/or sleep, total joint replacement is indicated. This will not return an athlete to vigorous sport, because the mechanical joint cannot withstand the stress. However, some light doubles play may be possible if the player is careful to avoid twisting and jumping.

Chondral injuries represent a difficult problem. Treatment options in present-day medicine are not very good and offer unpredictable results. Those with chondral lesions who continue to play run the risk of accelerating the degenerative changes. How rapidly these changes will progress is unpredictable. An individual decision must be made by assessing symptoms, possible risks, and psychological and cardiovascular benefit of continuing to play.

Posterior tibial tendon rupture

Posterior tibialis tendon problems usually occur in middle-aged females, and complete rupture prior to this time is unusual. This is not a common injury in tennis players, but it may occur in the over 45 age group. Treatment of complete rupture is difficult with an uncertain outcome, so it is important to recognize the symptoms prior to rupture.

Tendon ruptures are frequently not recognized despite a well described presentation and relatively consistent physical findings. The common presenting history is that of a preceding posterior tibial tendon tenosynovitis. This is then followed by a minor ankle injury. Often the patient will not seek treatment immediately because of the relatively minor amount of pain. On physical examination, patients will have mild tenderness along the posterior tibial tendon. In the standing position, they may display the characteristic flat-foot deformity. When viewed from behind, patients will appear to have 'too many toes' due to the collapsed arch and valgus heel alignment. They will have difficulty standing on their toes.

Once rupture occurs, treatment is difficult. Surgical treatment will usually not restore normal foot alignment, particularly in chronic cases, but it generally does improve function. Surgical repair or reconstruction of the tendon is only indicated with flexible foot deformities that can be passively corrected. If there is a rigid flat-foot deformity, and conservative treatment with shoe wear changes and orthotics has been unsuccessful, surgical fusion of the hindfoot joints can be helpful.

Once rupture occurs, return to tennis playing, even with good treatment, will be difficult. This is why it is important to recognize and treat the symptoms aggressively before rupture occurs.

Complete Achilles tendon ruptures

Achilles tendon ruptures are relatively common in tennis and the incidence seems to be rising because of an increasing number of older athletes. The tendon is particularly vulnerable during eccentric gastrocnemius-soleus loading with the knee in extension. The tendon is more vulnerable during middle age as the normal tendon tissue starts to degenerate. This process begins at about the age of 30–35 years. The region between 2 and 6 cm above the calcaneal insertion is the most common area of rupture because of its relatively poor blood supply.

Most ruptures occur without previous symptoms. The rupture is usually accompanied by an audible 'pop'. There is some immediate pain, but it is usually not too severe. A defect will occur in the tendon between 2 and 6 cm above the insertion. If significant swelling occurs, the defect may not be palpable. Patients will be unable to stand on their toes, but many will still be able to generate some active plantarflexion, although it will be weakened. Thompson's squeeze test will confirm the diagnosis. This test is performed by squeezing the calf muscle and examining the foot for the expected plantarflexion response. It is best performed with the patient kneeling on a chair, or lying on the stomach. The absence of plantarflexion confirms an Achilles tendon rupture.

Achilles tendon ruptures can be treated by cast or by surgical repair. Conservative treatment with a cast may be successful if treatment is initiated within 48 h. However, casting has a higher risk of re-rupture, and has more prolonged muscle weakness. Re-rupture rates for non-operatively treated patients have been about 18%.

More recently, several studies have advocated a non-operative functional rehabilitation program that emphasizes relatively early motion (Thermann et al 1995). The typical protocol consists of a walking cast for 3–6 weeks, followed by a progressive rehabilitation program with decreasing heel lifts. Early results of this technique have shown outcomes in non-athletes that are similar to surgical treatment in terms of strength and return to function, and this technique has a lower complication rate. However, caution should be used until better prospectively randomized trials are available.

As compared with the standard non-operative treatment, patients with surgical repair have significantly lower rates of re-rupture, higher rates of resuming sports activities at the same level, lesser degrees of calf atrophy and fewer complaints 1 year after injury (Cetti et al 1993). There is, however, a higher complication rate with surgery, including delayed healing, skin slough, and infection (Lo et al 1997).

Following a complete Achilles tendon rupture treated by surgical repair, return to full tennis playing is usually possible at about 4–6 months. Return after non-operative treatment varies considerably, with return to full tennis activity sometimes possible after 8–12 months.

Chronic Achilles tendinopathy

Tendinosis is most likely due to a failure of the tissue to adapt to the physical load of recurrent microtrauma. Degenerative changes precede spontaneous rupture of tendons in most players (Kannus & Jozsa 1990).

Tendon degeneration is probably exacerbated by malalignment syndromes such as excessive pronation. The inside of the Achilles tendon is placed under increased tension when the foot is placed in hyperpronation. Achilles overuse injury with tendon swelling can also be caused by a non-healing partial tear.

Typical presenting complaints with chronic Achilles tendinopathy are a gradual onset of pain and stiffness in the Achilles tendon. If the patient can recall a more sudden onset, the chronic problems are often caused by a non-healed partial tear. The pain typically increases with activity and is somewhat relieved by rest. A tender nodule will usually develop along the tendon, and pain will be increased with passive dorsiflexion and toe standing or walking. MRI can reveal the extent and size of the injury.

Treatment of Achilles tendinosis should be directed at treating the cause of the injury. Orthotics to correct malalignments are often helpful, and shoes with a good heel support and a heel wedge may prevent excessive pronation. Correction of training errors and a properly organized exercise prescription are the key components in a successful program. Tendon strength is a direct function of its microstructure. The microstructure responds favorably to tension and motion. It is therefore important to stimulate protective motion as early as possible. Eccentric training provides the maximum achievement of load (Fyfe & Stanish 1992). Stretching is used extensively in the treatment of overuse injuries. Function and activity level in chronic tendon injuries are mostly dictated by the athlete's pain.

The indication for surgical treatment of chronic Achilles tendinopathy is persistent pain and loss of athletic performance, with symptoms typically lasting longer than 6 months. The goal of surgery is to remove any degenerative tissue and to relieve external pressure on the tendon. This induces vascular ingrowth and creates new and better organized scar tissue. Following surgery on the Achilles tendon, about 70–80% of athletes make a successful comeback. Return to sports such as tennis and running is usually delayed for 4–8 months after surgery. Twenty per cent, however, need repeat surgery, and about 3–5% are forced to abandon their sports careers because of these injuries (Kvist 1991).

CONCLUSIONS

1. Sports activities help to control lipid profiles, enhance insulin production, improve cardiovascular function, and regulate endorphin release.
2. Skeletal muscle, ligaments, and tendons all undergo age-related matrix changes that make them more vulnerable to injury.
3. Cardiovascular events are the most common cause of death during tennis playing.
4. Athletes with a history of cardiovascular heart disease should have a complete work-up prior to return to racket sports. Evaluation should include Holter monitor and a stress test. These tests can assist in return to play recommendations.
5. The majority of musculoskeletal injuries are due to overuse problems, with the most common areas of injury being the knee, shoulder, and Achilles tendon.
6. Doubles play provides the lowest level of anaerobic threshold. Presumably, this results in fewer adverse cardiac events and fewer overuse injuries.

REFERENCES

Cetti R, Chirstensen S, Ejsted R, Jensen N M, Jorgensen V 1993 Operative versus nonoperative of Achilles tendon rupture. American Journal of Sports Medicine 21: 791–804

Fyfe I, Stanish W 1992 The use of eccentric training and stretching in the treatment and prevention of tendon injuries. Clinical Journal of Sports Medicine 11: 601–624

Kannus P, Jozsa L 1990 Histopathological changes preceding spontaneous rupture of a tendon. Journal of Bone and Joint Surgery 73A: 1507–1525

Kvist M 1991 Achilles tendon injuries in athletes. Sports Medicine 18: 173–201

Laforest S, St Pierre D M, Cyr J, Gayton D 1990 Effects of age and regular exercise on muscle strength and endurance. European Journal of Applied Physiology and Occupational Physiology 60(2): 104–111

Lo I, Kirkley A, Nouweiler B, Kumbhare D A 1997 Operative versus nonoperative treatment of acute Achilles tendon ruptures: a quantitative review. Clinical Journal of Sports Medicine 7(3): 207–211

Lynch T, Kinirons M T, O'Callaghan D, Ismail S, Brady H R, Horgan J H 1992 Metabolic changes during serial squash matches in older men. Canadian Journal of Sports Sciences 17(2): 110–113

Parzeller M, Rasche C 1994 Death in sports: comparison between tennis, table-tennis, badminton, and squash. In: Krahl H, Pieper H-G, Kibler W B, Renström P A (eds) Proceedings – Tennis: Sports Medicine and Science, Essen, Germany, May 19–21, p 246–251

Slezynski J 1991 Former athletes physical fitness. Journal of Sports Medicine and Physical Fitness 31(2): 218–221

Thermann H, Zwipp H, Tscherne H 1995 Functional treatment concept of acute rupture of the Achilles tendon. Unfallchirurg 98(1): 21–32

Wendt T, Schmidt T 1994 Are tennis players still allowed to play tennis without cardiac risk following a myocardial infarction or a coronary revascularization (PTCA, CABG)? In: Krahl H, Pieper H-G, Kibler W B, Renström P A (eds) Proceedings – Tennis: Sports Medicine and Science, Essen, Germany, May 19–21, p 240–245

35

The scientific rationale for the conservative management of soft tissue dysfunction in athletes

Glenn Hunter

KEY POINTS

1. Time pressures in the sporting arena often lead to appropriate treatments being applied at inappropriate times, retarding rather than facilitating the healing process.
2. Complete restoration to optimal values of all factors that contribute to normal function is essential to avoid further dysfunction.
3. Conservative management has, for a very long time, been selected on the basis of belief and convention rather than controlled, objective and reproducible evidence.
4. Modern evidence-based approaches, while bringing scientific refinement to conservative management, are somewhat hindered by the large number of variables associated with the treatment of humans, and the paucity of histological data on pathological mechanisms.
5. At present, many assumptions have to be made in the application of conservative management approaches, and it is important that these are recognized as such.

INTRODUCTION

The goal of rehabilitation is to return patients to their desired level of activity in the shortest and safest possible time. In sport and exercise medicine, time is usually of the essence and this has led to a search for ways to accelerate the healing process. However, there is little evidence to date to indicate that this can be achieved. Indeed, succumbing to the time pressures of the sporting arena is likely to lead to instances where appropriate treatments are applied at inappropriate times, satisfying the coach and the psychological thirst of the athlete, but retarding rather than facilitating the recovery process.

In addition to the time demands, the rehabilitation process is further complicated by the knowledge that the athlete, once recovered, will usually place stresses of considerable magnitude and frequency on the site of dysfunction. There is, therefore, little room for error in the rehabilitation process, and complete restoration to optimal values of all the factors that contribute to normal function is essential to avoid further dysfunction.

The majority of the soft tissue injuries occurring in sport are managed conservatively, and for centuries the application of conservative treatments has been based on art rather than science. Many treatment approaches were selected on the basis of belief and convention rather than controlled, objective and re-producible evidence. The current climate of evidence-based medicine has generated a healthy atmosphere of scientific challenge, and conservative treatment approaches are being subjected to critical analysis to establish their scientific credibility.

Despite the scientific refinement that evidence-based medicine will have on the clinical reasoning process relating to conservative treatment, the process is unlikely to develop into a 'hard' science because of the large number of variables associated with the treatment of human subjects and the lack of valid, sensitive and reliable measurement tools currently available to quantify these variables. This difficulty is manifest in the clinical reasoning process where the clinician attempts to quantify vague constructs such as emotional and psychological state, biomechanical response of the tissue to load, and identification of the exact pathology to formulate a diagnosis. The process is further hindered by the fact that ethical and surgical limitations combined with a comparative lack of research evidence into common soft tissue dysfunctions occurring in sport, have resulted in sparse histological data to aid the study of exact pathological mechanisms.

Although conservative treatments have received considerable focus in the research literature, the combination of unspecified diagnoses and the large number of confounding variables often make the inclusion of manipulation and control into a research design difficult, and yet their absence results in reduced confidence in any results generated. Currently, therefore, many assumptions have to be made in the application of conservative treatment approaches. These assumptions are a necessary and 'healthy' part of the clinical reasoning process as long as they are acknowledged as assumptions and that they filter into a process of diligent inquiry aimed at testing and eventually developing theories.

This chapter will review and explore some of the assumptions used in the clinical reasoning process typically involved in the application of conservative treatment, and, where possible, highlight some of the scientific problems encountered in this process.

PRINCIPLES OF CONSERVATIVE MANAGEMENT OF SOFT TISSUE DYSFUNCTION

Conservative management consists of the use of non-operative methods to treat dysfunction. Once the pathology has been deemed suitable for a conservative approach, a multitude of treatment philosophies are available. These approaches can be linked together by common stages in the rehabilitation process. Each of these stages presents scientific challenges in terms of generating reliable evidence, and they can be listed as follows:

- Establishing the aetiology of injury
- Establishing a hypothesis regarding the site and classification of tissue pathology
- Establishing outcome measurers to evaluate the effectiveness of any treatment intervention
- Analysis of treatment options with regards to the pathology and stage of the healing process
- Discussion with the patient of clinical findings and goal-setting.

Each of the above will be considered in turn.

ESTABLISHING THE AETIOLOGY OF INJURY

To aid the diagnostic process and to prevent the dysfunction from recurring, it is important to identify the aetiological factors which may have produced the dysfunction. Analysis of these factors involves the consideration of intrinsic, extrinsic and task-related factors (Fig. 35.1).

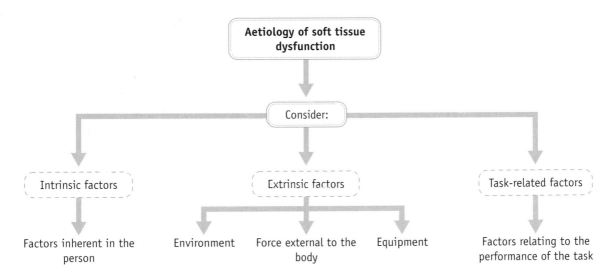

Figure 35.1 Factors to consider in determining the possible aetiology of soft tissue dysfunction (see Caine et al 1996 for a deeper review of this area).

In many instances, it is idealistic to think that the exact cause of the dysfunction can be established, due to the likely multifactorial nature of the aetiology. It is therefore worth remembering that many statements of causative relationships are extremely conjectural, and care should be taken when assessing the validity of such relationships (Meeuwisse 1994, Watson 1997). Recognition of this fact does create a difficult clinical tension between the need for evidence-based decisions and the current lack of evidence on which to base these decisions. Until more convincing evidence becomes available, the temporary solution lies in the acceptance that assumptions have to be made, that the process is one of trial, error and evaluation, but that the process should be based on the current evidence in this field.

Many aetiological theories which relate in particular to the insidious onset of soft tissue dysfunction are based on tests that relate physical measurement to the incidence of injury. For example, measurements of flexibility, muscle imbalance and excessive pronation have all been linked by association to soft tissue dysfunction. In reviewing studies of this type, it should be remembered that correlation does not always imply causation, and that many of these tests have poor repeatability, validity and sensitivity. The lack of well-conducted prospective studies is also evident.

Currently, most approaches to identifying the aetiology of injury relate to the analysis of the rela-tionship between stress and strain, whereby the activity of the athlete imposes a stress on the body which, in turn, induces a strain in the body tissues. Dysfunction indicates an inability of the body tissue to cope with this strain, and therefore attempts are made in treatment to reduce the strain by decreasing the magnitude or volume of the applied stress. An example of the logic used in this line of reasoning is that 'anti-pronation' orthotics are claimed to affect the range, time or rate of pronation. If this claim is valid, this would decrease the strain in a tissue that is overloaded by excessive pronation, e.g. the tibialis posterior. This line of logic is used to validate many treatments, but whether any treatments actually produce an effect over and above that of natural healing, and if so, whether this effect is due to the proposed mechanism of action, has yet to be established in many cases.

The aetiological assumptions that have to be made in the clinical decision process are tested with regard to the effect of the intervention in reducing the rate of injury recurrence or the patient's symptoms. Because other factors that may influence the patient's symptoms cannot be controlled, it is difficult to say that any change was solely due to the correction of one specific aetiological factor. Future research into this multivariate area by the use of multicentre prospective studies should reduce the amount of trial and error made in this clinical process.

ESTABLISHING A HYPOTHESIS REGARDING THE SITE AND CLASSIFICATION OF TISSUE PATHOLOGY

Clinically, manual tests are often used to apply tension to the tissues under the area of the patient's symptoms or to the tissue(s) that could refer to the area of the patient's symptoms. These tests are used to assess the range, quality and limiting factors of the movement, and a hypothesis is formulated with regard to the tissue responsible for the symptoms. The sensitivity of many of these tests is influenced by the experience of the examiner.

Understanding of the site of the pathology is important, as assumptions regarding the anatomy and biomechanics of the tissue influence the rehabilitation protocol used.

The pathology is also a significant factor in influencing the choice of conservative treatment, as many modalities are applied on the basis of their claimed effects on the pathology. However, although imaging techniques are rapidly increasing the understanding of certain pathologies, the classification and histology of many soft tissue lesions remains speculative and the correlation between imaging and actual clinical pictures is uncertain or poor.

With regard to chronic soft tissue dysfunction, evidence is accumulating to suggest that there is a group of patients in whom psychosocial factors appear to be responsible for the prolonged nature of their symptoms. The approach in these patients lies in addressing the altered psychosocial factors rather than adopting a treatment modality that models their pain as being of mechanical origin and applies 'treatments' that are physical in nature. Research into this area is opening new avenues in the process of clinical reasoning (Burton et al 1995, Waddell et al 1993).

ESTABLISHING OUTCOME MEASURES TO EVALUATE THE EFFECTIVENESS OF ANY TREATMENT INTERVENTION

Establishing suitable subjective and physical markers prior to the application of a treatment is a way of attempting to assess the effect of the intervention. Because of the individual nature of most treatment modalities, this process takes the simplified form of a single case study whereby a baseline measurement is taken, an intervention is applied, and the baseline measurement reassessed. Any change in the baseline measurement is assumed to be due to the applied treatment. Of course, this type of research design does not preclude the possibility of some other factor (or factors) producing the change. Nevertheless, the use of either subjective and/or physical outcome markers forms an important, although fallible, component of the clinical reasoning process (Leibenson & Yeomans 1997).

More research is required to establish the validity, reliability and sensitivity of many outcome measures to produce more confidence in the data generated.

ANALYSIS OF TREATMENT OPTIONS WITH REGARD TO THE PATHOLOGY AND STAGE OF THE HEALING PROCESS

Once a hypothesis has been generated regarding the site of tissue dysfunction, a rehabilitation programme is developed by focusing on primary and secondary considerations (Fig. 35.2).

The challenge in rehabilitation lies in being able to influence the primary and secondary considerations without one aggravating the other. Both are important in the rehabilitation process, but work on the secondary factors must not be at the expense of aggravating the pathology.

Primary consideration

The primary consideration is the area and pathology assumed responsible for the patient's symptoms. The clinician chooses a treatment modality on the basis of therapeutic intention, i.e. a treatment that produces a physiological effect that is most likely to have a beneficial influence on the pathology. Our lack of understanding of exact pathological mechanisms, as evidenced by the current debate surrounding the degenerative versus inflammatory models of tendon pathology, combined with the lack of scientific investigation into many of the proposed biological mechanisms of action, highlights the current speculative nature of treatment choice.

Conservative treatments which address the primary site of dysfunction have been mostly electrothermal, with ice, heat, ultrasound and laser being some of the more common modalities in use. With many of these modalities, their proposed mechanism of action has yet to show its clinical effectiveness.

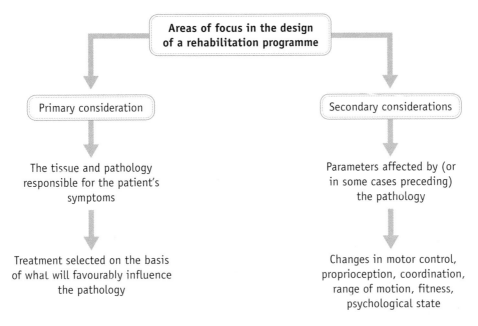

Figure 35.2 Areas for consideration in the design of a rehabilitation programme.

A more recent approach has been the application of early controlled mechanical load to the healing tissue, which is thought to produce benefits in terms of increased collagen and matrix effects which result in a 'better quality' of healing in the tissue (Culav et al 1999). While encouraging, this approach currently draws the majority of evidence from animal studies.

The stages of the healing process, although variable, can be a useful guide to the clinical reasoning process in terms of influencing the time of application of these treatment procedures.

The healing process of soft tissues

Soft tissue pathology usually results in inflammatory or degenerative processes in the tissue. Due to methodological difficulties, more is understood about inflammatory than degenerative processes.

Inflammatory healing process

From the time of injury, the tensile strength of the affected tissue decreases, and an inflammatory cascade ensues with the ultimate aim of increasing the tensile strength of the tissue. During the healing process, the improvement in tensile strength passes through three

stages: the lag, regeneration and remodelling phases (Fig. 35.3).

These stages are of variable time length, being influenced by many factors. Each of the stages facilitates

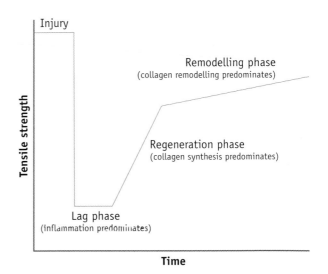

Figure 35.3 Hypothetical model of the relationship between tensile strength and time during the healing process.

the others, and although they are not as clearly delineated as in Figure 35.3, they can be used as a guide to the clinical reasoning process.

The lag phase. During this time period, the tensile strength of the tissue does not improve and therefore it is vulnerable to further injury. The wound is stabilized by a weak fibrin bond, which, if disrupted, will exacerbate the inflammatory response.

This time period typically lasts 3–5 days, and is driven by an inflammatory reaction that is necessary and important for preparing the wound for the regeneration phase (Barlow & Willoughby 1992). Clinically, attempts are made to reduce the inflammatory reaction by the use of rest, ice, compression and elevation (RICE) or by the use of non-steroidal anti-inflammatory drugs (NSAIDs). It is likely that these modalities reduce the secondary effects of the inflammation rather than the initial inflammatory reaction. These modalities may help to reduce pain levels and reduce the amount of fibrin at the site of tissue damage which relates to the amount of scar tissue formation. However, the scientific evidence for the value of these methods in reducing the inflammatory process is currently controversial, with the majority of the positive evidence indicating short- but not long-term benefits of application (Leadbetter 1995).

In some cases, attempts are made to accelerate the inflammatory process, with the aim of promoting earlier macrophage activity and hence an earlier commencement of the regeneration phase. Electrotherapy modalities such as ultrasound and laser are used with this intention, although the in vitro evidence has yet to be supported by the purported in vivo evidence of effectiveness (Nyanzi et al 1999).

The general consensus appears to be that the lag phase is a period of control, where the inflammatory process is controlled by the use of rest, ice compression and elevation. This is a time when the patient's symptoms are predominantly due to chemical mediators. Therefore, this time period is not compatible with a treatment approach that produces mechanical input, e.g. frictions.

The application of ice receives much clinical discussion regarding methods of application and length of time of application. For many years, ice has been applied using a vasodilatation/vasoconstriction model based on the Lewis hunting reaction. Using this model, the ice has to be removed before vasodilatation occurs. The problems are that this time period is extremely variable and that the original work performed by Lewis on the finger may not be valid in other areas of the body. Ice may be more effective if its

application were based around the principle of preventing secondary hypoxia. In this model, it is assumed that further cellular damage may occur following injury due to the hypoxic environment of the tissue. The ice is applied for 20–30 min with the assumption that the metabolism of the cells will be decreased, enabling them to cope in the hypoxic environment (Knight 1995).

Taping is also useful during the lag phase, so that some movement is allowed, but movements that will tension the site of tissue damage are prevented.

Due to the pressures of time, the injured area is typically rested for 24–48 h post-injury and then active attempts are made to restore movement. The author believes that the lag phase is critical to the successful healing of the damage tissue and that any intervention which produces tension at the specific site of tissue damage will only retard the healing process and may promote chronic pain due to central sensitization from increased nociceptor bombardment. This opinion is based on histological studies of the healing process and has not been subjected to scientific testing.

Regeneration phase. The appearance of the fibroblast signals the 'start' of this phase. During this phase, tensile strength increases rapidly due to the rate of collagen synthesis. The tensile strength of the tissue is influenced by the amount and orientation of collagen cross-links that occur, and this is influenced by the application of careful tension to the site of dysfunction (Gomez et al 1991). On this basis, the use of active or passive movement with the aim of progressively tensioning the site of dysfunction appears to be a valid approach during this phase. It is important to realize that these tensile forces, applied either by a therapist or by the patient, are difficult to quantify in terms of magnitude, rate, frequency and duration, and generally are guided by the reproduction of mild discomfort but not pain. Again, a clinical versus scientific contrast develops between the evidence that loading appears to be important but that clinically this principle is difficult to apply in a quantifiable manner.

In principle, once any hypermobility/laxity has been eliminated, tensile forces should be applied with regard to the functional demands placed on the tissue. For example, the anterior talofibular ligament of the ankle joint would be subjected to progressive tension through plantarflexion and inversion (Hunter 1998).

If the current evidence is valid, correctly applied tension to healing tissue may promote a greater increase in tensile strength, which will reduce the time of the remodelling phase that follows.

Remodelling phase. In this phase, collagen synthesis is matched by collagen degradation, so that the tensile strength develops at a slower rate than during the regeneration phase, and the scar also tends to become stiffer. Random collagen formation may result in a scar that is stiff, but lacking in mechanical properties in relation to the demands of functional loading. Tensioning the wound during this period may help to produce a more extensible scar and influence the remodelling process.

Many of the treatment modalities used in the early stages of the healing process are also used in the remodelling phase. This may not be appropriate, as much of the evidence cited to support the use of these modalities is derived from studies applied during the inflammatory phase of healing, where the biological processes are different from those during the later stages. More studies are required into the effects of modalities during the later stages of the healing process.

The above review of the healing process and its influence on clinical reasoning is based on an inflammatory model with a bias towards the importance of mechanical loading in influencing the process itself. Evidence is accumulating to suggest that a degenerative model may be more relevant in certain tissues, such as tendons (Kannus 1997). Little is currently understood about degeneration of soft tissues, but the application of mechanical load during this process may be a stimulus that induces the inflammation that is required to promote healing. With regard to tendons, there is some interesting evidence to suggest that eccentric loading, in particular, may provide an important stimulus for promoting a healing response, although the exact mechanism of action and specific protocols to be used have yet to be established (Alfredson et al 1998).

Secondary considerations

Secondary considerations are the variables affected by the primary site of tissue damage. For example, following injury to the lateral ligament complex of the ankle joint, the secondary factors that will be affected are alterations in strength, power, endurance and co-ordination of the muscle–tendon unit activity, decreased range of movement, altered proprioception, decreased coordination, decreased skill, altered psychological state and decreased cardiopulmonary performance. These factors form the kinetic environment in which the tissue will function once restored to optimal functional ability.

The current emphasis in rehabilitation has been to move away from the focus on muscle strength to one of developing muscle control, with the muscular recruitment pattern considered important in promoting joint stability. This has led to the development of the muscle imbalance approach, which addresses the active, passive and neurodynamic systems of the body in the correction of dysfunction. This approach is heavily dependent on patient compliance, but interesting protocols have been developed with regard to the treatment of low back pain using spinal stabilization (Norris 1995). More work is required to establish what 'normal' movement is and to assess the clinical effectiveness of this particular approach.

DISCUSSION WITH THE PATIENT OF CLINICAL FINDINGS AND GOAL-SETTING

Involvement of the patient in the formulation of a rehabilitation process is legally mandatory regarding informed consent, but is also essential from the point of view of patient motivation and commitment to the programme.

The majority of rehabilitation programmes are highly dependent on patient compliance, and involvement of patients in the decision process forms an important part of giving the patients a feeling of responsibility for their own treatment. An understanding of the psychological reaction of patients to injury and the process of implementing change is an essential part of the therapist's clinical reasoning skills (Taylor & Taylor 1997).

Research in this area tends to be more qualitative in design, and, coupled with the more quantitative methods of the hard sciences, these methods are sometimes portrayed as less credible in producing evidence relating to cause and effect. It should be remembered that, rather than being two separate approaches to research, qualitative and quantitative approaches are part of the same spectrum and mutually support each other. In areas where the feelings of the subject form the area of study, and where the degree of control and manipulation required for a randomized clinical trial is restricted, qualitative approaches generate many useful hypotheses which can facilitate the process of clinical reasoning.

CONCLUSIONS

Due to the difficulties in implementing appropriate research designs, the conservative treatment process is often difficult to conduct on the basis of scientific logic alone. Experience and, to some extent, 'art' will always form an integral part of the clinical reasoning process. Intuition and speculation based on knowledge and experience are used to generate hypotheses about future treatment approaches, and scientific logic should not stifle this clinical 'creativity' but be used as a guide to keep the creativity in the direction of scientific 'fact' and not fiction.

The development of multicentre studies, valid, reliable and sensitive outcome measures, refined diagnostic techniques, and a culture which seeks to test the many hypotheses that are generated during the process of clinical reasoning will help to redress a balance towards science informing practice rather than art and convention.

REFERENCES

Alfredson H, Pielila T, Jonsson P, Lorentzon R 1998 Heavy load eccentric calf muscle training for the treatment of chronic Achilles tendinosis. American Journal of Sports Medicine 26(3): 360–366

Barlow Y, Willoughby J 1992 Pathophysiology of soft tissue repair. British Medical Bulletin 48(3): 698–711

Burton A K, Tillotson K M, Main C J, Hollis S 1995 Psycho-social predictors of outcome in acute and sub-chronic low back pain trouble. Spine 20: 722–728

Caine D J, Caine C G, Linder K J 1996 Epidemiology of sports injuries. Human Kinetics, Champaign, IL

Culav E M, Clark C H, Merrilees M J 1999 Connective tissues: matrix composition and its relevance to physical therapy. Physical Therapy 79: 308–316

Gomez M A, Woo S L-Y, Amiel D, Harwood F 1991 The effects of increased tension on healing medial collateral ligaments. American Journal of Sports Medicine, 19: 347–354

Hunter G 1998 Specific soft tissue mobilization in the management of soft tissue dysfunction. Manual Therapy 3(1): 2–11

Kannus P 1997 Tendon pathology: basic science and clinical applications. Sports, Exercise and Injury 3: 62–75

Knight K 1995 Cryotherapy in sports medicine. Human Kinetics, Champaign, IL

Leadbetter W B 1995 Anti-inflammatory therapy in sports injury – the role of non-steroidal drugs and corticosteroid injection. Clinics in Sports Medicine 14(2): 453

Leibenson C, Yeomans S 1997 Outcome assessment in musculo-skeletal medicine. Manual Therapy 2(2): 67–74

Meeuwisse W H 1994 Assessing causation in sports injury: a multifactorial model. Clinical Journal of Sports Medicine 4: 166–170

Norris C M 1995 Spinal stabilization – muscle imbalance and the low back. Physiotherapy 81(3): 127–138

Nyanzi C S, Langridge J, Heyworth J R C, Mani R 1999 Randomized controlled study of ultrasound therapy in the management of acute lateral ligament sprains of the ankle joint. Clinical Rehabilitation 13: 16–22

Taylor J, Taylor S 1997 Psychological approaches to sports injury rehabilitation. Aspen, Gaithersberg, p 35–55

Waddell G, Newton M, Henderson, Somerville I, Main D 1993 A fear avoidance beliefs questionnaire and the role of fear avoidance in chronic low back pain and disability. Pain 52: 157–168

Watson A W S 1997 Sports injuries: incidence, causes, prevention. Physical Therapy Review 2: 135–151

Physical activity in disability

SECTION CONTENTS

36

Rehabilitation after cardiac ischaemic event

Toshihito Katsumura

KEY POINTS

1. The principal aim of cardiac rehabilitation is to improve quality of life through preventing a recurrence of myocardial infarction.
2. Modification of coronary risk factors through nutrition instruction and smoking cessation is also essential in cardiac rehabilitation.
3. Cardiac rehabilitation includes patient education about coronary heart disease and coronary risk factors.
4. The risk stratification for a subsequent cardiac event provides signposts for patient management throughout the rehabilitation process.
5. Exercise testing is essential to assess the patient's functional capacity and to evaluate the efficacy of the patient's current medical regimen.
6. Exercise prescription that is based on type, intensity, duration and frequency of exercise is essential for the safety and efficacy of exercise therapy.

INTRODUCTION

In the early 1900s, patients were generally confined to bed rest for 2 months after an acute myocardial infarction, because it was believed that physical activity would result in the development of ventricular aneurysm, heart failure, cardiac rupture and sudden death (Froelicher 1988). Clinicians gradually became aware that early mobilization was not harmful and could help to avoid some of the complications of bed rest, such as pulmonary embolism and deconditioning

(Groden et al 1967). Moreover, aggressive treatment of myocardial infarction during the acute phase resulted not only in shortening of hospital stay but also in changing the concept of cardiac rehabilitation.

The main aim of cardiac rehabilitation was initially to increase exercise performance. However, the focus has changed to preventing recurrence of myocardial infarction, thus improving quality of life and prognosis by reducing coronary risk factors. For this purpose, cardiac rehabilitation includes not only exercise therapy but also psychological consultation and patient education about coronary heart disease and coronary risk factors.

PHYSIOLOGICAL EFFECTS OF EXERCISE IN CARDIAC REHABILITATION

The goal of coronary heart disease therapy is to improve the patient's quality of life and the prognosis of the condition. Exercise has proven effective in achieving this goal.

Cardiovascular physiological effects

One of the major beneficial effects of exercise-based cardiac rehabilitation in patients with ischaemic heart disease is a significant improvement in cardiocirculatory performance and physical work capacity. Both cardiac and peripheral adaptations can contribute to the improvements.

Central changes

Cardiac function. Maximal cardiac output is the product of maximal heart rate and maximal stroke volume. The increase in maximal cardiac output after exercise training in patients with ischaemic heart disease is due to an increase in both stroke volume and maximal heart rate. In normal subjects, maximal heart rate is usually not affected by exercise training. Although animal studies have shown increased myocardial contractility and resistance to hypoxia with exercise training, human data have not consistently shown improved myocardial performance. However, some studies (Redwood et al 1972) have revealed an increase in the left ventricular ejection fraction in patients with ischaemic heart disease after exercise training.

~imal oxygen uptake. Following exercise train-
~ts with ischaemic heart disease show an
maximal oxygen uptake ($\dot{V}O_{2\,max}$), a reflec-
tion of the increased capacity of the cardiovascular system to deliver oxygen and of the muscles to utilize that oxygen. The magnitude of the change is less evident in patients with ischaemic heart disease than in apparently healthy individuals, but the small increases in $\dot{V}O_{2\,max}$ produced by exercise training in these patients often result in significantly improved endurance and quality of life.

Myocardial oxygen uptake. With the effects on $\dot{V}O_{2\,max}$, exercise training results in a reduction in heart rate, systolic blood pressure, level of myocardial oxygen uptake at a given constant submaximal workload and total body oxygen consumption, since the relative workload and resultant heart rate–blood pressure product in an individual patient are both reduced at the same absolute workload after physical training. Therefore, exercise tolerance is generally improved in patients with ischaemic heart disease, at least in part, because exercise training results in a lower level of myocardial oxygen uptake at the same absolute workload that produced ischaemia before exercise training. The benefits of these adjustments can be demonstrated by the greater level of work that can be achieved before angina or ST depression occurs on ECG (Fletcher et al 1994).

Development of coronary collaterals. It is not clear whether exercise training can improve cardiac vascularity and perfusion in humans. Present knowledge does not support the concept that exercise training promotes collateral arterial development in patients with ischaemic heart disease. Improvement of ischaemia most likely occurs by reducing myocardial oxygen uptake rather than by increasing oxygen supply.

Autonomic nervous system changes. Blood and urinary catecholamine levels are lower at rest and during submaximal exercise after physical training, presumably as a result of reduced sympathetic nervous system activity. Parasympathetic tone may also be increased and, with sympathetic adjustments, may account for the slower heart rate and lower arterial blood pressure seen after physical training.

Peripheral changes

Myocardial damage after a cardiac ischaemic event can significantly limit maximal stroke volume during exercise, depending on the extent of infarction and on the degree of residual ischaemia. Therefore, in patients with limited left ventricular function, exercise training appears to reverse the effects of reconditioning primarily through peripheral adaptations.

Improvements in physical work capacity after exercise training may be due to several factors, including greater availability of oxygen to the exercising muscles, greater use of aerobic processes, and/or greater anaerobic capacity. Changes in the skeletal muscles tend to improve oxygen accessibility from the circulation because of the higher myoglobin concentration and greater capillary density, both of which enhance oxygen transport. Skeletal muscle mitochondria also increase, in both size and number, with exercise training, allowing the muscle to rely on the more efficient oxidative metabolism. A greater concentration of oxidative enzymes allows muscles to obtain a larger share of their energy from aerobic rather than anaerobic sources. In so doing, the amount of high-energy phosphates generated from each mole of substrate metabolized is much greater, resulting in increased efficiency of substrate use. Therefore, lactate accumulation is also decreased, and the anaerobic threshold is increased.

Role of exercise in coronary risk factor modification

Physical inactivity is a major modifiable coronary risk factor, along with cigarette smoking, hypertension and hyperlipidaemia. Other risk factors include age, gender, obesity, diabetes mellitus and family history. Of these, hypertension, hyperlipidaemia, obesity and diabetes mellitus may be favourably affected by appropriate physical training.

The effects of endurance exercise on the physiological precursors of atherosclerosis have been evaluated in many studies and extensively reviewed (Hagberg 1990).

Regular dynamic exercise in men is associated with a marked increase in high-density lipoprotein (HDL) cholesterol level, significantly profound when accompanied by weight reduction. In addition, both fasting and postprandial total cholesterol, low-density lipoprotein (LDL) cholesterol, and triglyceride levels tend to be reduced after exercise training in men (Tanz & Weltman 1985). In contrast, endurance training is less likely to increase HDL cholesterol levels in women. For example, in the absence of other interventions, exercise training does not cause HDL cholesterol levels to increase appreciably in older women (Taylor & Ward 1993). Furthermore, high levels of exercise have been required before an appreciable increase in HDL cholesterol levels occurs in younger women (Taylor & Ward 1993).

Moderate-intensity regular physical exercise can play a significant role in achieving proper body weight in overweight subjects when combined with appropriate reduction in caloric intake. Weight loss in men, whether by diet or by exercise, usually results in a reduction in elevated plasma levels of triglycerides, LDL, very low-density lipoprotein (VLDL) and total cholesterol, and an increase in HDL cholesterol levels (Leon 1988). In contrast, exercise during weight reduction may help to prevent the reduction of HDL cholesterol, normally associated with weight reduction by dietary modification alone in women (Taylor & Ward 1993).

Weight loss results in a reduction in high blood pressure and ameliorates associated abnormalities in glucose–insulin dynamics in overweight subjects (Leon 1988). Regular endurance exercise in hypertensive subjects resulted in the reduction by approximately 10 mmHg of both systolic and diastolic blood pressures in many studies (Hagberg 1990), although it is usually not adequate as the sole form of therapy to control blood pressure in these subjects. The most likely mechanism for the decrease in resting blood pressure observed in response to regular exercise is a reduction in body fat and/or attenuated sympathetic nervous system activity (Hagberg 1990).

Exercise training, when associated with a reduction in body weight and fat stores, appears to be associated with an accelerated rate of glucose utilization and increased insulin sensitivity (Leon 1988) in diabetic and non-diabetic subjects. These effects have been shown to persist for as long as 7 days after the cessation of exercise training. Although exercise training results in reduced blood pressure and insulin requirements and increased insulin sensitivity in hypertensive and diabetic subjects, exercise training alone is not sufficient as the sole measure for blood pressure and glycaemic control. Therefore, regular endurance exercise in conjunction with optimal pharmacological therapy can be expected to enhance effectiveness.

Thus, regular endurance exercise can result in significant improvements in a number of cardiovascular risk factors. Exercise training, therefore, serves as a rational component of a more comprehensive cardiac rehabilitation programme that also promotes behavioural changes through patient education to modify cardiovascular risk factors in patients with atherosclerosis. Most cardiovascular rehabilitation programmes now include exercise training and formal programmes in nutritional counselling and smoking cessation as part of a comprehensive programme of non-pharmacological treatment of cardiovascular risks, combined with pharmacological therapy as prescribed by the patient's personal physician.

REHABILITATION PROGRAMME

In the USA, because of the high cost of medical care, the goal of aggressive treatment of myocardial infarction during the acute phase was merely to shorten the length of hospital inpatient stay. Consequently, patients were discharged immediately after acquiring a level of physical activity considered suitable for daily living.

However, under this system the patient could not return to social activity with the physical fitness level acquired at the time of hospital discharge. Therefore, the concept of cardiac rehabilitation which incorporates a phase 1 in-hospital rehabilitation and a phase 2 post-discharge rehabilitation was established. Rehabilitation has subsequently become part of the outpatient environment and is conducted through multiple models.

In 1991, the Japanese Circulation Society published guidelines for exercise therapy for patients with heart disease. According to these, the rehabilitation programme is divided into three phases: the acute phase (from the onset of acute myocardial infarction to hospital discharge for 3–4 weeks), the convalescent phase (from hospital discharge to the return to society for 2 months), and the maintenance phase (for the duration of the patient's life after returning to the community).

Acute phase

In Japan, the Ministry of Health and Welfare first published a manual for acute phase cardiac rehabilitation in 1983 (Fig. 36.1). Since then, the manual has been modified at various institutions. A rehabilitation programme for patients with acute myocardial infarction was developed at the Tokyo Medical University Hachioji Medical Center (Table 36.1). Rehabilitation during stages 1–4 is carried out in the coronary care

unit for 2–4 days, and thereafter in the cardiovascular ward. After each rehabilitation stage, subjective symptoms, blood pressure and electrocardiogram are checked. If the result meets one or more of the following criteria, either the rehabilitation stage will be repeated or further investigations will be considered:

- a rise of at least 30 mmHg or a decline of at least 20 mmHg in systolic blood pressure over resting levels (except in the case of orthostatic hypotension)
- an increase in heart rate greater than 120 beats/min
- a depression of at least 1 mm or an elevation of at least 2 mm in the ST segment, significant arrhythmias, or a bundle branch block
- subjective symptoms such as chest pain, palpitations, shortness of breath, general fatigue, dizziness or fainting.

Preparation for discharge from the hospital

Three factors virtually determine the prognosis of any patient after myocardial infarction: the amount of residual myocardium at risk, the extent of left ventricular dysfunction, and the arrhythmic potential of the cardiac substrate. Predischarge risk stratification is performed to identify patients at risk of death or reinfarction and those at risk who need only conventional therapy to achieve a good prognosis (Krone 1992).

Before hospital discharge or shortly thereafter, patients with recent acute myocardial infarction should undergo standard exercise testing (submaximal at

Table 36.1 AMI rehabilitation programme for uncomplicated patients and successful cases of PTCA or PTCR. (From Tokyo Medical University Hachioji Medical Center 1998, with permission)

Stage	Activity	Measurements	Notes
1	Bed up 30° (15 min)	ECG, BP	In bed
2	Bed up 90° (15 min)	ECG, BP	
3	Sitting without help (30 min)	ECG, BP	
4	Standing (5 min)	ECG, BP	In room, portable toilet
5	Walking (50 m – slow)	ECG, BP	In ward
6	Walking (200 m/4 min)	ECG, BP	
7	Walking (400 m/8 min)		
8	Walking (400 m/6 min) or shower test	ECG, BP	Walking test, shower
9	Walking (800 m/12 min) or light physical exercise		
10	Walking (400 m/5 min)	ECG, BP	Within hospital
11	Physical test (walking up 1–2 flights of stairs at any pace)	ECG, BP	
12	Bath test	ECG, BP	Bath
13	Physical test (walking up 2–4 flights of stairs at any pace)	ECG, BP	
14	Exercise tests		
15	Loading test (5 min)	ECG, BP	
16	Walking outside of hospital (30 min)	ECG, BP	
17	Rehabilitation centre		

ECG = electrocardiogram; BP = blood pressure

Days	1st week (1–7)	2nd week (8–14)	3rd week (15–21)	4th week (22–28)
Places for rehabilitation	CCU	CCU or post CCU	General rehabilitation ward	General rehabilitation ward
Level of physical activity	Immobilization → Bed rest →	Within room	Within ward	Within ward
Intensity (METs)	1 MET →	1–2 METs	2–3 METs	3–5 METs
Main exercise	Assisted upright position[a]	Unassisted upright position[a]; Standing, walking around bed[a]; Walking in room[a]	Walking within hallway 50 m[a], 200 m[a] (times/day 1 2 3 / 1 2 3)	Walking within hallway 500 m[a] (or using stairs, depending on condition) (times/day 1 2 3); Evaluation of exercise capacity upon discharge[b]
Excretion	In bed	In bed or bedside toilet; Bedside toilet or toilet in room	Toilet in ward	Toilet in ward
Hygiene	Partial sponge bath (assisted) →	Full sponge bath (assisted); Dental hygiene, face washing, shaving	Assisted shampoo	Full bath (depending on condition)
Diet	Fast; Liquid diet; Rice porridge (light) (assisted); Rice porridge (medium) (unassisted); Rice porridge (full)	Normal diet	Normal diet	Normal diet
Recreation	Prohibited → Radio (music) →	Newspapers, magazines, TV	Conversation in lobby	Conversation in lobby

1 MET (metabolic equivalent) = resting oxygen uptake ≈ 3.5 mL/kg per min.

[a] Tolerance test.

[b] Master two-step test (single), treadmill, ergometer etc.

Figure 36.1 Cardiac rehabilitation manual. (From Toshima 1983, with permission)

4–7 days or symptom-limited at 10–14 days). The purpose of testing is to:

- assess the patient's functional capacity and ability to perform tasks at home and at work
- evaluate the efficacy of the patient's current medications regimen.
- stratify risk for a subsequent cardiac event.

At the Tokyo Medical University Hachioji Medical Center, patients with recent acute myocardial infarction undergo symptom-limited exercise testing on average 14 days after the acute episode (Table 36.2).

The results of risk stratification (Box 36.1) provide signposts for patient management throughout the rehabilitation process (Pashkow 1993). For example, a patient with poor ventricular function (ejection fraction <30%), abnormal signal-averaged ECG or low exercise capacity should preferably receive cardiac monitoring and exercise supervision in a hospital- or facility-based programme. The patient is not a candidate, at least ini-

tially, for community-based group or unsupervised home rehabilitation. In contrast, a patient with an uncomplicated complete surgical revascularization can undergo symptom-limited exercise testing after having recovered from surgery, and can begin progressive activity at home and continue to exercise in a home- or community-based programme. This patient may need some supervised training to ensure the appropriate understanding of the exercise prescription and for coronary risk factor education and modification.

Convalescent phase

Cardiac rehabilitation is important especially during convalescence. Its purposes during this phase are to improve the impaired physical ability resulting from the decrease in cardiac function and prolonged bed rest after myocardial infarction, and to remove any anxiety over exercise or daily life. Rehabilitation during the convalescent phase is divided into two types: supervised and unsupervised. The choice of a given programme depends on the results of the risk stratification assessment (Japanese Circulation Society 1991).

Supervised rehabilitation programme (hospital- or facility-based)

A rehabilitation programme supervised by doctors, nurses and exercise professionals is usually considered for patients who have suffered a myocardial infarction, and is conducted on an outpatient basis. In a supervised rehabilitation setting, it is possible to increase understanding and information exchange and to promote a personal relationship among the patients.

Box 36.1 Characteristics of low-, intermediate- and high-risk patients. (From Pashkow 1993, with permission)

Low-risk patients
- After uncomplicated coronary revascularization
- ≥7.5 METs 3 weeks after an ischaemic event
- No ischaemia, left ventricular dysfunction or significant arrhythmia

Intermediate-risk patients
- ≤7.5 METs 3 weeks after an ischaemic event
- Angina or 1- to 2-mm ST-segment depression with exercise
- Perfusion or wall motion abnormalities with stress
- History of congestive heart failure
- More than mild but less than severe left ventricular dysfunction
- Late potentials present on signal-averaged electrocardiogram
- Non-sustained ventricular arrhythmia
- Inability to self-monitor exercise or comply with exercise prescription

High-risk patients
- Severe left ventricular dysfunction
- ≤4.5 METs 3 weeks after cardiac event
- Exercise-induced hypotension (≥15 mmHg)
- Exercise-induced ischaemia >2-mm ST-segment depression
- Ischaemia induced at low levels of exercise
- Persistence of ischaemia after exercise
- Sustained ventricular arrhythmia, spontaneous or induced

METs, metabolic equivalents.

Table 36.2 Rating of perceived exertion (RPE). (From Borg 1982, with permission of Human Kinetics)

6	No exertion at all
7	
8	Extremely light
9	Very light
10	
11	Light
12	
13	Somewhat hard
14	
15	Hard (heavy)
16	
17	Very hard
18	
19	Extremely hard
20	Maximal exertion

Moreover, patients and their families will be able to acquire knowledge relevant to the disease and coronary risk factors, as well as gaining motivation to continue exercising.

Unsupervised rehabilitation programme

An unsupervised rehabilitation programme is implemented when facilities for rehabilitation are not available. Most important in an unsupervised programme is that the patients perform the programme safely. Patients with exercise-induced myocardial ischaemia, severe left ventricular dysfunction or serious arrhythmias should be selected with caution. In this programme, exercise intensity should be set relatively low to prevent exercise-related accidents and to avoid compliance problems. Accordingly, patients must be thoroughly instructed on the programme, and should demonstrate a thorough understanding of their exercise limits prior to beginning. Further, the programme also aims to instil the patient with the motivation to exercise.

Maintenance phase

Patients with acute myocardial infarction should continue exercise after returning to social life. The purpose of exercise during this phase is to maintain the physical activity level acquired during convalescence, to prevent the recurrence of myocardial infarction, and to improve the prognosis by improving and avoiding coronary risk factors. Patients must be strongly motivated to continue to exercise, and it is hoped that those around patients will recognize their efforts and support them.

Exercise prescription through exercise testing

Exercise prescription of a different type, intensity, duration and frequency of exercise is essential for the safety and efficacy of exercise therapy. The basic exercise prescription is light- to moderate-intensity aerobic (dynamic) exercise lasting for 20–60 min more than three times a week. The type of exercise should be mainly aerobic, such as walking, jogging, cycling and swimming, using large muscle groups of the lower extremities. However, many occupational and recreational activities require the use of upper body strength as well. Therefore, complementary weight-training programmes are also appropriate for selected low-risk patients (Franclin et al 1991, Stewart 1992). Relative intensity, which can be ascertained by exercise testing, is the most important factor for safety and effi-

cacy. Exercise intensity is determined by factors such as $\dot{V}O_2$, heart rate, or rating of perceived exertion. However, exercise prescription should be modified to suit the individual patient's condition. The following are examples of how exercise prescriptions are developed in two different conditions: the absence and presence of ischaemia or arrhythmias (Fletcher et al 1995).

Prescription in the absence of myocardial ischaemia or significant arrhythmias. Exercise intensity should be 50–80% of $\dot{V}O_{2\,max}$, as determined through exercise testing:

- The target heart rate should be 50–75% of heart rate reserve [(maximum heart rate – resting heart rate) $\times$ 0.5–0.7 + resting heart rate]. The heart rate can be used for the prescription of many types of dynamic lower limb exercises.
- Activities can be prescribed as the target work intensity that achieves the training heart rate after 5–10 min at that workload (steady state). It may be expressed as watts on an ergometer, speed on a treadmill, or in METs.
- Heart rate monitoring using one of the commercially available heart rate monitors is safe, especially for low- to moderate-intensity exercise.
- If an individual intends to walk on a level surface, activity can be prescribed as the step rate assessed on a treadmill to generate the desired heart rate. The usual procedure is to determine the step rate on a treadmill, and then to prescribe the appropriate rate. Step rate can be easily measured, as it requires less skill than counting heart rate. If this approach is used, individuals should be cautioned about avoiding hills. Walking in shopping malls or gyms allows subjects to avoid inclement weather. Exercise should be monitored for the first few sessions while the individual begins regular physical activity, to make sure that the instructions are understood and that the activity is well tolerated.
- Individuals can also judge the intensity of exercise as the rating of perceived exertion, which can be equated to desirable heart rate during laboratory exercise and to their activities. The original scale is a 15-grade category scale ranging from 6 to 20 with a verbal description at every odd number (Table 36.2).
- Activities can progress as increasingly higher tolerance is achieved. The appropriate initial intensity of training is 50–60% of $\dot{V}O_{2\,max}$ or a rating of perceived exertion of 12–13 on a scale of 6–20. After safe activity levels have been established, duration is increased in 5-min increments each week. Later, intensities can be increased as heart rate response to exercise decreases with conditioning.

Exercise prescription in the presence of ischaemia or arrhythmias. An exercise test is essential for this type of prescription. Arrhythmias or ischaemia episodes that require such precautions can vary, but usually include ventricular ectopic beats in sequence, a symptomatic or haemodynamically unstable arrhythmia, chest discomfort believed to be angina, ST depression of 2 mm or more, or a fall in systolic blood pressure of 20 mmHg or more from baseline.

The exercise test is performed in the usual fashion, but the conditioning work intensity is derived from the heart rate associated with the abnormality. If the exercise test continues to high effort levels, the heart rate at 50–60% of maximum can be used if it falls at least 10 beats/min below the abnormal level. Otherwise, the recommended training heart rate is 10 beats/min less than that associated with the abnormality.

Exercise prescription for patients with coronary risk factors. Exercise prescription for these patients is basically the same as that for patients with uncomplicated myocardial infarction. However, exercise prescriptions should be modified according to the risk factors.

For patients with uncomplicated mild to moderate hypertension (systolic blood pressure 140–179 mmHg, diastolic blood pressure 90–109 mmHg; Guidelines Subcommittee of the WHO 1999), exercise intensity should be at a level at which systolic blood pressure does not exceed 200 mmHg during exercise.

For patients with hyperlipidaemia or with mild to moderate uncomplicated non-insulin-dependent diabetes mellitus, the duration should be somewhat longer, and the frequency should be greater to increase energy expenditure.

For obese patients, it is essential to increase energy expenditure. Low-intensity exercise is recommended to increase the consumption of fatty acids during exercise and to prevent musculoskeletal injuries such as low back pain or knee joint pain caused by being overweight.

Management of coronary risk factors

Reduction of coronary risk factors through nutrition instruction and smoking cessation is also essential in cardiac rehabilitation. Rehabilitation programmes stressing non-pharmacological interventions have been shown to achieve significant reductions in total cholesterol levels and LDL, with increases in HDL levels. Exercise, weight management, dietary modification, stress management and smoking cessation have all been shown to improve blood lipid levels. Exercise and moderate consumption of alcohol can also be effective in raising HDL levels (Gaziano et al 1993, Paunio et al 1994).

Smoking induces coronary spasm, reduces the anti-ischaemic effects of beta-blockers, and doubles mortality after myocardial infarction (Barry et al 1989, Dealfield et al 1984, Winniford et al 1987). Smoking cessation reduces the rates of reinfarction and death within 1 year of quitting, although one-third to one-half of patients with acute myocardial infarction relapse within 6–12 months (Burling et al 1984).

CONCLUSIONS

The principal aim of cardiac rehabilitation was initially to increase exercise performance. However, the focus has changed to preventing a recurrence of myocardial infarction, thus improving the quality of life and the prognosis by eliminating coronary risk factors associated with the disease. For this purpose, cardiac rehabilitation includes not only exercise therapy but also psychological consultation and patient education about coronary heart disease and coronary risk factors.

According to the guidelines of the Japanese Circulation Society (1991), the cardiac rehabilitation programmes should be divided into three phases: the acute phase (in hospital), the convalescent phase and the maintenance phase (after discharge). Before discharge from the hospital or shortly thereafter, patients with recent acute myocardial infarction should undergo standard exercise testing. The purpose of testing is to assess the patients' functional capacity and ability to perform tasks at home and at work, to evaluate the efficacy of the patient's current medical regimen, and to stratify risk for a subsequent cardiac event. The results of risk stratification provide signposts for patient management throughout the rehabilitation process.

Exercise prescription is essential for the safety of exercise therapy. The patient may need some supervised training to ensure appropriate understanding of the exercise prescription and for coronary risk factor education and modification.

REFERENCES

Barry J, Mead K, Nabel E G et al 1989 Effects of smoking on the activity of ischemic heart disease. Journal of the American Medical Association 261: 398–402

Borg G 1998 Borg's perceived exertion and pain scales. Human Kinetics, Champaign, IL

Burling T A, Singleton E G, Bigelow G E, Baile W F, Gottlieb S H 1984 Smoking following myocardial infarction: a critical review of the literature. Health and Psychology 3: 83–96

Dealfield J, Wright C, Krikler S, Ribeiro P, Fox K 1984 Cigarette smoking and the treatment of angina with propranolol, atenolol, and nifedipine. New England Journal of Medicine 310: 951–954

Fletcher B J, Dunbar S B, Felner J M, Jesnsen B E, Almon L, Cotsonis G, Fletcher G F 1994 Exercise testing and training in physical disabled men with clinical evidence of coronary artery disease. American Journal of Cardiology 73: 170–174

Fletcher G F, Balady G, Frolicher V F, Hartley L H, Haskell W L, Pollock M L 1995 Exercise standards: a statement for healthcare professionals from the American Heart Association. Circulation 91(2): 580–615

Franclin B A, Bonzheim K, Gordon S, Timmis G 1991 Resistance training in cardiac rehabilitation. Journal of Cardiopulmonary Rehabilitation 11: 99

Froelicher V 1988 Cardiac rehabilitation. In: Parmley W, Chatterjee K (eds) Cardiology. J B Lippincott, Philadelphia

Gaziano J M, Buring J E, Breslow J L et al 1993 Moderate alcohol intake, increased levels of high-density lipoprotein and its subfractions, and decreased risk of myocardial infarction. New England Journal of Medicine 329: 1829–1834

Groden B, Allison A, Show G 1967 Management of myocardial infarction: the effect of early mobilisation. Scottish Medical Journal 12: 435–439

Guidelines Subcommittee of the World Health Organization – International Society of Hypertension Mild Hypertension Liaison Committee 1999 World Health Organization – International Society of Hypertension Guidelines for the Management of Hypertension. Journal of Hypertension 17: 151–183

Hagberg J M 1990 Exercise, fitness and hypertension. In: Bouchard C, Shephard R J, Stephens T, Sutton J R, McPherson B D (eds) Exercise, fitness and health: a consensus of current knowledge. Human Kinetics, Champaign, IL, p 445–466

Japanese Circulation Society 1991 Clinical standard of exercise therapy. Japanese Circulation Journal 55(suppl III): 386–397

Krone R J 1992 The role of risk stratification in the early management of a myocardial infarction. Annals of Internal Medicine 116: 223–237

Leon A S 1988 Physiological interaction between diet and exercise in the etiology and prevention of ischemic heart disease. Annals of Clinical Research 20: 114–120

Pashkow F J 1993 Issues in contemporary cardiac rehabilitation: a historical perspective. Journal of the American College of Cardiology 21(3): 822–834

Paunio M, Heinonen O P, Virtamo J et al 1994 HDL cholesterol and mortality in Finnish men with special reference to alcohol intake. Circulation 90: 2909–2918

Redwood D R, Rosing D R, Epstein S E 1972 Circulatory and symptomatic effects of physical training in patients with coronary-artery disease and angina pectoris. New England Journal of Medicine 286: 959–965

Stewart K J 1992 Weight training in coronary artery disease and hypertension. Progress in Cardiovascular Diseases 35: 159

Tanz Z V, Weltman A 1985 Differential effects of exercise on serum lipid metabolism and lipoprotein levels seen with changes in body weight: a meta-analysis. Journal of the American Medical Association 254: 919–924

Taylor P A, Ward A 1993 Women, high-density lipoprotein cholesterol, and exercise. Archives of Internal Medicine 153: 1178–1184

Toshima H 1983 Study on the development of cardiac rehabilitation system. 1982 Report of achievement of study on cardiovascular disease of the Ministry of Health and Welfare of Japan, 158

Winniford M D, Jansen D E, Reynolds G A, Apprill P, Black W H, Hillis L D 1987 Cigarette smoking-induced coronary vasoconstriction in atherosclerotic coronary artery disease and prevention by calcium antagonists and nitroglycerin. American Journal of Cardiology 59: 203–207

37

Exercise in low back pain patients

David D. FitzGerald

KEY POINTS

1. Selection for exercise therapy in low back pain patients can be divided into clinical subgroups.
2. Definition of subgroups allows appropriate exercise parameters to be set.
3. Injudicious exercise may be, at best, useless, and at worst detrimental to effective rehabilitation.
4. To understand function and subsequent dysfunction, it is necessary to understand how components interact, rather than treating the constituent parts in isolation.
5. 'Relative flexibility', which considers the contribution of individual elements to general movement patterns, forms the basis of an approach to rehabilitation – the movement dysfunction model.

INTRODUCTION

The selection and prescription of appropriate exercise has many parallels with pharmacological interventions. It must be specific, regulated and adapted according to the clinical presentation. At best, injudicious use of exercise may be useless; at worst, it may be provocative and detrimental to effective rehabilitation. This chapter is largely directed towards functional rehabilitation in accordance with one of the primary tenets of exercise prescription – that of specificity. When employing a functional model of rehabilitation, diagnosis is often secondary to the search for a pathological process, contributing factors and regional interactions. Understanding of function and subsequent dysfunction must be based on a knowledge of how components interact, rather than on the isolated analysis of the constituent parts which has been the dominant focus in recent decades.

Sarhmann (1987) provided a clinical framework based on 'movement dysfunction' which applies in a very practical way to rehabilitation strategies. A core element of this construct is the concept of 'relative flexibility' – a hypothesis regarding the contribution of individual elements to general movement patterns. For example, analysing the proportion of thoracic, lumbar and pelvic motion in forward flexion can yield information regarding deficient movement patterns causing increased tissue stress and subsequent pathology. This analysis can be readily tested clinically by evaluating the symptom response with alterations in movement strategies. Whilst it is accepted that our knowledge of this functional interaction is still in its infancy, there is a growing body of data to substantiate the clinical application of this approach (Janda 1978, 1983, Jull & Janda 1987, Kendall et al 1993, Lewit 1999, Richardson et al 1999).

There is likely to be a significant difference between exercise prescription derived from structural/diagnostic-based protocols and those derived from a movement dysfunction model. Given that the aim of rehabilitation is to restore function, what follows is a clinical framework from which rational exercise prescription can be selected and incorporated into rehabilitation programmes specific to clinical presentations. The focus of this chapter is biased towards the practising clinician and, as such, some areas of discussion have yet to be validated through acceptable research methodology, which will hopefully be forthcoming.

GENERAL CONSIDERATIONS FOR PATIENT SELECTION

There are a number of factors which must be considered prior to the utilization of exercise in the management of low back pain patients.

Objective of exercise prescription

Absolute rest should be minimal except in acute low back pain presentations or those likely to require invasive intervention (Deyo et al 1986, Waddell 1998). It is also acknowledged that physical treatment of some form promotes early return to function and reduces the likelihood of chronic disability (Shekelle et al 1992).

There is a growing body of evidence to support the role of both manipulation and exercise therapy in the treatment of musculoskeletal dysfunction (Koes et al 1992a,b). The implications of these findings dictate that restoration of range of motion, restoration of active muscular control and increasing functional capacity are the primary objectives of rehabilitation. The specific protocols to achieve these objectives are detailed later. At the other end of the pathological spectrum – presentations of irreversible pathology, failed surgical intervention, or chronic pain syndromes – prescription of exercise is aimed at optimizing function within the pathological limits, prevention of progressive deterioration, maintaining/improving cardiovascular function and promoting activation of pain inhibitory systems (Harding 1998, Wright 1995). The clinical objective is to improve general functional capacity rather than specific biomechanical issues.

Source of symptoms

The specificity in determining a local source of pain in the lumbar spine is confounded by the shared innervation of multiple structures. This implies that the presenting pain pattern may originate from a number of potential structures (more commonly, multiple sources simultaneously) which cannot be selectively isolated with provocation tests. Most clinical diagnoses rarely implicate most of the anatomical structures capable of producing pain. Discogenic, facet joint and nerve root pathology form the typical triad of diagnostic labels with the majority of low back pain, some 70%, lacking a specific diagnosis other than 'low back pain' (Loeser 1977). From a rehabilitation perspective, the clinical picture correlates better with the changes in function rather than the alleged structural pathology (Lewit 1999). Clearly diagnosed pathology (disc herniation, spondylolisthesis, scoliosis, etc.) can be secondary to changes in function producing a pathological chain of tissue insult. With this as a basis, diagnostic tools such as radiological evaluation form a useful adjunct to comprehensive physical examination but not a substitute for it. It is now well accepted that the poor correlation between symptomatology and radiographic appearance (Arnoldi et al 1975, Dieppe 1989, Witt et al 1984) does not indicate the routine use of X-rays in low back pain (Waddell 1998).

Pathological process

In the acute presentation, the primary objective is the reduction of pain and the promotion of pain-free motion. This will usually require integrated pharmacological, physical and electrotherapeutic treatment. Exercise at this time would typically aim to improve flexibility, using small-range, low-intensity, pain-free movements of the target structures. Other variables such as exercise volume and intensity are dictated by clinical issues relating to the level of tissue irritability (Zusman 1998), treatment response and the anatomical structure involved. This is particularly relevant in peripheral neuropathic pain where neural tissue mobilization should not involve sustained holding (Butler 1991), in contrast to joint and muscle which are more tolerant.

A prerequisite level of pain-free motion is desirable prior to undertaking strength and mobility exercises as part of the management regime and can be difficult to judge for the inexperienced clinician. Recognition should also be given to presentations where central pain states are evident in the symptom characteristics (hyperpathia, secondary hyperalgesia and spontaneous pain). These findings dramatically alter the response properties and cannot be ignored when prescribing exercise. Exercise responses in fibromyalgia (which form a subgroup of the low back pain population) implicate considerably reduced exercise tolerance (Lund et al 1993) and require longer recovery between bouts of exertion. Similar responses are reported in pain management regimes (Shorland 1998).

Another clinical subgroup may be classified as 'acute on chronic' presentations with mixed patterns of pathology. Typically, pain results from an acute inflammatory response at a site of previous pathology, indicating reduced mechanical tolerance with subsequent tissue failure. Frequently, the patient may have some suspicion of dysfunction indicated by increased stiffness, fatiguability or subtle uncoordination, and such findings are often indicators of imminent failure. Conversely, examination of an apparently 'acute onset' injury often reveals evidence of previous subclinical trauma such as tissue thickening, adaptive shortening or restricted joint range. The significant difference between this patient group and the 'acute onset' mechanism is that there may be residual soft tissue changes and functional disturbance from previous episodes, which may perpetuate the problem and slow recovery rates. In the evaluation and treatment of symptoms related to chronic low back pain, it is important to consider the aetiology. It may be related to extrinsic factors, such as poor ergonomics, extreme work environments or excessive spinal load. In this event, adaptations or modifications may allow continued activity. With insidious-onset histories, optimization of intrinsic factors is the primary goal of rehabilitation. Typically this will involve combinations of flexibility, postural stability, strength, coordination and functional re-education.

In the chronic presentation there is less indication for specific modalities (with the exception of transcutaneous electrical nerve stimulation, TENS) or non-steroidal anti-inflammatories, and exercise prescription should involve strength, mobility and coordination exercises simultaneously. Much of this patient group display fear/avoidance behaviour, poor locus of control and are generally deconditioned. The goals of rehabilitation are to address these factors in a multi-disciplinary environment with emphasis on behavioural modification to physical stress.

Prognosis

In general, there is poor correlation between the extent of pathology and the functional impairment. Outcome measures from pain management centres and work hardening programmes indicate a lack of specificity in predicting the likely responders to rehabilitation programmes (Cohen & Cambell 1996) with conflicting reports regarding outcomes (Waddell 1998). In the acute presentation, there is increasing evidence that biopsychosocial factors are more accurate than physical parameters (Watson 2000) in predicting treatment response. However, there are a number of clinical indicators which should be considered when making a prognosis.

Indicators of positive outcomes

- Progressive improvement of pain-free range in accordance with known tissue-healing time
- Progressive reduction of clinical findings in conjunction with symptomatic improvement
- Reduced/lack of fear-avoidance behaviour
- Increasing functional capacity
- Lack of aberrant neuroplasticity.

Indicators of negative outcomes

- Neural tissue irritability
- Spontaneous pain
- Non-mechanical symptom behaviour
- Diffuse, variable, symptom distribution
- Poor association with clinical findings and symptomatology
- Fear-avoidance behaviour.

Mechanical dysfunction

To establish a hypothesis of mechanical pain as the mechanism of symptom generation, typical clinical features are identifiable:

- There should be identifiable aggravating and easing factors.
- Symptoms should correlate with the provoking activity.
- Duration and intensity of symptoms should be proportional to the intensity of provocation.
- Clinical findings should correlate with the region of symptoms.

These indicators are often compounded by the patient's belief systems, psychosocial and general physical state. It is critical that rehabilitation strategies are specific to the components of symptomatology whether dominantly physical or dominantly anxiety/fear-related. Having fulfilled these criteria, the diagnostic task is to determine the pathogenetic chain of dysfunction and assess the correlation with clinical presentations (Lewit 1994). The interdependence of this chain may be anatomically distant from the site of symptoms.

Contraindications

The treating clinician must always be aware of medical conditions which may necessitate caution with exercise prescription or prohibit its application. Absolute contraindications include acute major trauma, acute pain provoked by movement, terminal malignancy, severe cardiac instability or severe respiratory distress. There are many conditions which require caution and continuous monitoring of patient response, but which do not preclude appropriately graded exercise.

SCIENTIFIC PRINCIPLES OF EXERCISE PRESCRIPTION

The components of exercise therapy applicable to low back pain rehabilitation include the following:

- aerobic exercise
- muscle strength/endurance
- flexibility exercise
- coordination/functional training.

Multiple systems, including the cardiovascular, neurological, respiratory, endocrine and musculoskeletal systems, are challenged during therapeutic exercise and undergo specific physiological responses. The musculoskeletal system which is our primary focus. Aerobic exercise is a discipline in its own right and excellent reviews regarding the physiological effects are available (Åstrand 1987, Wolf et al 1993), although detailed consideration is beyond the scope of this discussion. In general terms, aerobic exercise prescription should delineate frequency, intensity, duration, type of activity, initial fitness level and progression targets. There is a growing body of evidence to substantiate the use of aerobic exercise as part of pain management programmes (Gatchel & Turk 1996) and syndromes such as fibromyalgia (Vaeroy & Mersky 1993). The precise mechanisms involved remain speculative but may relate to endogenous opioid stimulation enhancing pain modulation, in conjunction with the typical physiological responses to exercise (Wright 1995, Zusman 1998).

MUSCLE STRENGTH AND LOW BACK PAIN

The significance of muscle dysfunction in the pathogenesis of low back pain is a source of considerable debate (Macintosh et al 1993b, Mirka & Marras 1993, Nouwen 1987, Potvin 1991), although chronic low back pain sufferers demonstrate back and abdominal muscle weakness (Beimborn & Morrissey 1988) and reduced endurance. Some debate relates to the incidence of primary muscle pain as a source of symptoms (Sherman & Arena 1993) and some to the secondary effects of muscle dysfunction on associated structures (Bergmark 1989, Cresswell 1993, Hides et al 1996a,b, Hodges & Richardson 1996, Jull & Janda 1987, Jull et al 1994). In practical terms, these are not mutually exclusive perspectives and probably represent different patient subgroups (Panjabi 1992a,b). Methodological differences aside, the specificity of data collected regarding trunk muscle strength in relation to low back pain is inconclusive. Gross measures of force output from trunk muscles, typically using isokinetic dynamometry, timed sit-ups (Hall et al 1992) or sustained holds, quantify performance rather than specific muscle strength and coordination (Waddell 1998). These measures of performance bear little relationship to pain, disability or work capacity (Newton & Waddell 1993). Moreover, they do not yield information regarding the distribution of stresses within the spinal column and hence a specific target for rehabilitation. This situation has led to a substantial research effort to elucidate the mechanisms of muscular control in the lumbar spine and to optimize rehabilitation strategies. Significant evidence has now accumulated

(Allison et al 1997, Jull & Richardson 1994, O'Sullivan 2000, 1997, O'Sullivan et al 1998, Richardson et al 1999) which implicates a highly specific muscular control system in the lumbopelvic region.

Although all trunk muscles contribute to lumbopelvic control, the obliques, transversus abdominis and multifidus have key roles (Gracovetsky et al 1985, Kendall et al 1983, Richardson et al 1990, 1999, Tesh et al 1987). The obliques and transversus abdominis muscles appear to be particularly vulnerable to disuse and loss of supporting function (Caix et al 1984, Nouwen et al 1987). The gluteus maximus, gluteus medius and iliopsoas muscles also commonly show signs of dysfunction relative to their synergist partners (Janda 1978, Janda & Smith 1980, Sahrmann 1987). Vleeming et al (1997) have also demonstrated important synergies between the oblique abdominals, gluteus maximus, hamstrings and thoracolumbar fascia in stabilization of the pelvic girdle. This contemporary information must be incorporated into therapeutic exercise regimes.

Using this approach, it is imperative to ensure that the relevant muscles are targeted, loaded at the appropriate intensity, and observation made for muscle substitution as task difficulty increases.

To examine and rehabilitate the 'core stabilizing' muscles of the lumbar region, specific test positions and protocols have been established. Two basic assessments in four-point kneeling have been described. Firstly, instruction is given to flex/extend the lumbar spine within the available range whilst maintaining the thoracic spine in neutral (Fig. 37.1). This can be considered a basic proprioceptive test for the lumbar spine and examines the ability to dissociate movement in lumbar segments relative to the rest of the spine. It attempts to examine the coordination between the erector spinae with direct lumbar attachments (multifidus, lumbar longissimus and iliocostalis) and the abdominals. Inability or poor control is indicative of proprioceptive deficiency, loss of active spinal segmental control or generalized coordination deficits of the trunk and pelvic region.

Secondly (Fig. 37.2), to activate the core stabilizers (transversus abdominis and multifidus) simultaneously, instruction is given to position the lumbar spine in neutral lordosis, draw in the abdomen and prevent any change in spinal contour. The lateral abdominal wall can be palpated to assess contraction strength. Facilitation can be used, such as instruction to 'suck in', pull the navel towards the spine, squeeze the pelvic floor or count aloud whilst maintaining the contraction. Vigilant observation for muscle substitution

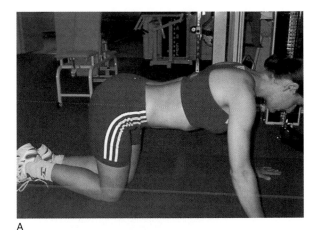

A

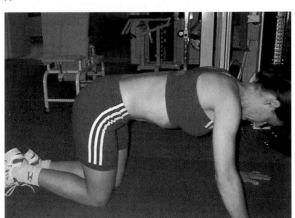

B

Figure 37.1 Basic proprioceptive test for the lumbar spine in four-point kneeling. A: Flexion. B: Extension.

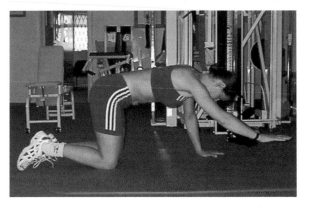

Figure 37.2 Activation of core stabilizers (transversus abdominis and multifidus). The lumbar spine is positioned in neutral lordosis, and then the abdomen is drawn in while preventing any change in spinal contour.

or altered synergies, indicated by arching the back (upper abdominal dominant activation), holding the breath (gross muscle recruitment) or rib cage narrowing (external oblique dominance), should be made.

There is evidence to suggest a link between the ability to perform transversus abdominis contractions and a reduction of symptoms in low back pain (Hodges & Richardson 1996) and spondylolisthesis (O'Sullivan 2000, O'Sullivan & Twomey 1998, O'Sullivan et al 1997). Similar findings have been reported for the lumbar multifidus (Hides et al 1996a,b, Richardson et al 1999). Baseline stability outlined above is a prerequisite to sustaining higher load associated with functional movements or complex motor skills.

BIOMECHANICAL ASPECTS OF FUNCTIONAL REHABILITATION

Having outlined the rationale for functional rehabilitation, it is evident that there are numerous potential causes of movement dysfunction, the precise make-up of which can only be determined by systematic examination. Deficiencies in movement can be broadly classified as either mechanical restrictive dysfunctions or motor control dysfunctions:

• *Mechanical restrictive disorders* refer to any increased tissue tension which distorts movement. This could be articular, ligamentous, fascial or muscular, and requires specific differentiation in order to select appropriate treatments.
• *Motor control dysfunctions* relate to deficiencies in neuromuscular regulation and local muscle incompetence. Specific muscle function testing provides information regarding the mechanical capacity of the muscles under test. Analysis of functional movement evaluates muscle interactions in terms of activation, coordination and force generation. The principles of exercise progression would be from cognitive to associative (O'Sullivan 2000) with final progression to autonomous movement patterns (Shumway-Cook & Wollacott 1995).

These categorizations follow a format from isolated activation of target muscle groups to specific dysfunctional (painful) movement patterns, through to automatic execution of efficient movement patterns in activities of daily living.

To be effective, it requires examination to evaluate functional motion qualitatively, and manual skills to assess the biomechanics of segmental motion. The objective is to evaluate tissue adaptation in regions of increased functional load in advance of gross patho-logical changes appearing through failure. The following exercise protocols are derived from this clinical framework.

FUNCTIONAL EXERCISE PROTOCOLS

Flexion

Biomechanical factors

This terminology has been specifically used as opposed to 'lumbar flexion', which does not occur in isolation during functional movement. The relative flexibility between spine and pelvis has been referred to as lumbopelvic rhythm and some important facts should be considered for rehabilitation purposes. The total range of lumbar sagittal plane rotation is approximately 45° with an average range of 9–14° per segment (Bogduk & Twomey 1991). Allowing for lumbar lordosis implies a range of lumbar flexion between 30° and 35° from an upright starting position. The pelvis must rotate about the femoral heads under control of eccentric hip extensor activity, producing in the region of 60–80° of hip flexion in a ratio of 2:1 hip/spinal motion (Raschke & Chaffin 1996). Attainment of the upright position from flexion is initiated by hip extensors posteriorly rotating the pelvis through range to the upright position. The paraspinal muscles become active approximately midway through this movement at the so-called 'critical point' (Bogduk 1994). Patients with habitual anterior pelvic tilt frequently achieve the upright position by early lumbar hyperextension rather than proportional spinal/pelvic motion. This may produce the characteristic 'catch' sometimes associated with spinal instability (Gertzbein et al 1984, 1985, Pearcy et al 1984) and can often be improved by altering the movement sequence. Synergic proximal trunk stabilization through co-activation of paraspinals and abdominal wall is also a prerequisite (Cresswell 1993, Cresswell & Thorstensson 1989, 1994, Cresswell et al 1992).

Movement dysfunctions

Increases in relative spinal flexion which may be either regional (i.e. thoracic or lumbar) or specific segmental hyperflexion. Whilst it is not possible to define which structures are specifically vulnerable, there are good data on the relative contribution of components resisting flexion (Adams & Dolan 1997). Rehabilitation should focus on optimization of biomechanics in conjunction with desensitizing painful tissue.

Increases in relative pelvic flexion (sagittal rotation) with diminished spinal contribution. This movement pattern is often associated with lumbosacral and sacroiliac symptoms in presentations of hypermobility syndrome, multisegmental spinal stiffness or post-surgical histories. The rationale of treatment is to increase the proportional contribution of spinal motion (regain local mobility) and reduce the contribution of the pelvic component (muscular stabilization).

Protocols for restrictive dysfunction in flexion

Limitation of saggital plane pelvic rotation is evident on straight leg raise (SLR) testing in supine or observation of reduced anterior pelvic motion in standing flexion (typically 60–70° of hip flexion). Full-range lumbar flexion appears as a flattening of the lumbar lordosis in the lower segments and visible flexion in the upper segments. Clinically this is sometimes difficult to assess from observation, and flexion in side-lying or crouched kneeling is useful. The primary objective of exercise prescription is to localize the effect to the target area. For example, repeated forward bending as an exercise will encourage motion in the most flexible regions and could reinforce an existing movement dysfunction.

Useful specific exercises are as follows:

- straight leg raise through doorway (Fig. 37.3)
- leg extension with back against wall
- crouch kneeling
- knee to chest
- arch and hollow in four-point
- flexion over roll
- flexion in sitting
- flexion in sitting (legs extended)
- knee extension in sitting (active lengthening) (Fig. 37.4)
- legs over head in supine.

Protocols for motor control deficits in flexion

The muscular control of spinal flexion has attracted considerable attention from bioengineers, ergonomists, basic scientists and clinicians. Significant recent advances have been made regarding specific patterns of muscle activation to enhance postural stability (Hodges & Richardson 1996, Jull et al 1993, Jull & Richardson 1994, Richardson et al 1999). From a biomechanical perspective, forward bending requires controlled spinal and pelvic motion in a coordinated manner. Spinal flexion is produced by eccentric para-

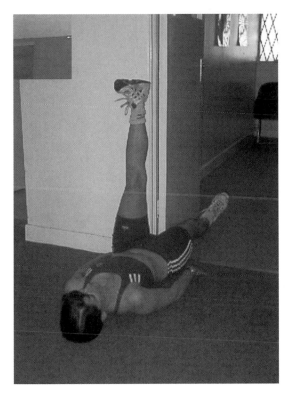

Figure 37.3 Straight leg raise through doorway.

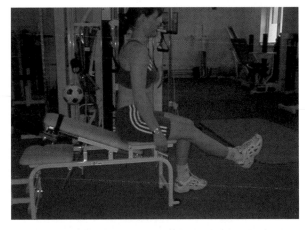

Figure 37.4 Knee extension in sitting (active lengthening)

spinal muscle activity in conjunction with deep abdominal muscle (transversus abdominis) coactivation (Jull & Janda 1987, Jull & Richardson 1994, Richardson et al 1999). Spinal segment control is achieved primarily through multifidus and the lumbar components of longissimus and iliocostalis (Hides et al

1996a,b, Richardson et al 1999). Pelvic rotation is controlled by eccentric hip extensor activity in both hamstrings and gluteus maximus. Gluteus maximus, the primary hip extensor, frequently displays inhibition (Janda 1978, 1983) and represents a sizeable loss to torque generation when its function is compromised. Therefore rehabilitation should address pelvic as well as spinal control.

Useful specific exercises are outlined below:

- core stabilization in four-point (previously described)
- four-point alternate arm lifts
- four-point alternate leg lifts
- four-point kneeling > crouch kneeling (neutral spine)
- forward bend with neutral spine in sitting
- forward bend with neutral spine in standing
- hip extension prone
- bridging (Fig. 37.5)
- forward bending in kneeling (Fig. 37.6)
- forward bending in sitting
- forward bending in standing.

Extension

Biomechanics

This terminology is used to encompass all elements contributing to the movement, including thoracic and lumbar spine, sacroiliac joints and posterior pelvic rotation about the femoral heads. Efficient mechanics dictate a pattern of progressive spinal extension throughout the thoracolumbar region with posterior pelvic rotation and anterior translation (Lee 1999). To achieve this, there must be an adequate range of extension available in the spinal, sacroiliac and hip joints.

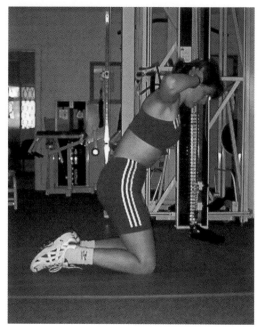

Figure 37.6 Forward bending in kneeling.

The muscular control of this movement requires eccentric work of the rectus and oblique abdominals in conjunction with specific segmental control by multifidus and lumbar longissimus/iliocostalis (Macintosh & Bogduk 1987, Macintosh et al 1993b). The tendency for posterior translation of the spine and anterior translation of the pelvis is opposed by the anterolateral abdominal wall where muscle fibre orientation is horizontal in a sagittal plane and mechanically suited to resisting these forces (Cresswell & Thorstensson 1994).

The significance of lumbar lordosis in low back pain remains debatable (Twomey & Taylor 1994), but extension will obviously increase the existing lordosis. In biomechanical terms, focal stresses localized to individual motion segments are more detrimental than stresses distributed over multiple segments, and rehabilitation should aim to encourage this optimal pattern.

Movement dysfunctions

Segmental hyperextension. This can be observed when assessing the pattern of extension in standing. It is usually associated with sharp, localized midline pain. This is often mistakenly classified as an 'increased lordosis', although the increased movement

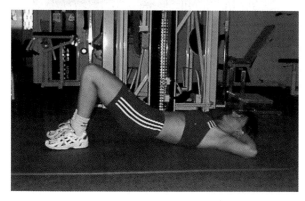

Figure 37.5 Bridging.

is actually localized to a segmental level, rather than distributed throughout the lumbar region. The thoracic kyphosis is usually maintained in extension, and may often continue into the lumbar spine as far as the hyperextended segment. A visible, dominant skin crease is usually observable at the hypermobile segment.

Excessive anterior translation of the pelvis. This again creates increased localized translational segmental stresses, producing relative 'shearing' between segments. The thoracic kyphosis may also be retained in this movement pattern. The long abdominals tend to be hyperactive and the lateral abdominal wall inhibited.

Protocols for restrictive dysfunction in extension

- Lumbar extension in prone (observe for localized hyperextension)
- Lumbar extension with fixation (Fig. 37.7)
- Thoracic extension with lumbar spine stabilized
- Extension over ball/roll
- Extension in standing (with facilitation)
- Hip extension in side-lying
- Hip extension in Thomas's position (Fig. 37.8)
- Knee flexion in prone (lengthening rectus femoris).

Protocols for motor control deficits in extension

- Core stabilization in four-point (previously described)
- Four-point alternate arm lifts
- Four-point alternate leg lifts
- Extension over ball/roll (eccentric abdominal work)

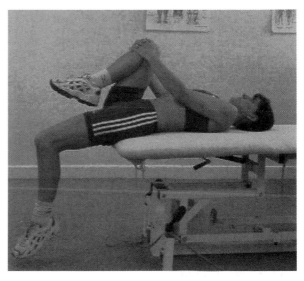

Figure 37.8 Hip extension in Thomas's position.

- Multifidus activation (Fig. 37.9)
- Hip flexion in sitting
- Supine extension (over bench)
- Abdominal holds in crook lying (Fig. 37.10)
- Posterior pelvic rotation in standing (neutral spine).

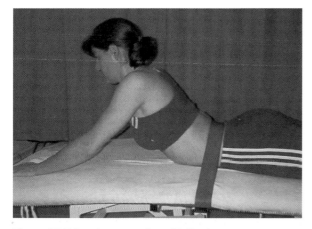

Figure 37.7 Lumbar extension with fixation.

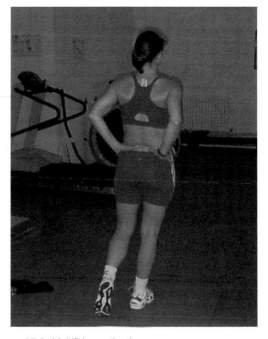

Figure 37.9 Multifidus activation.

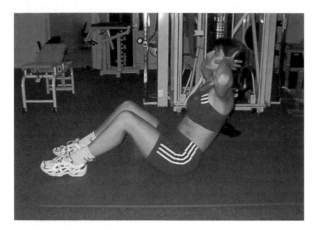

Figure 37.10 Abdominal holds in crook lying.

Rotation

Biomechanics

Rotation occurs in a transverse plane about a vertical axis. The majority of rotation occurs in the thoracic spine with relatively little available in the lumbar spine (approximately 3° per segment; Bogduk & Twomey 1987) due to the orientation of the facet joints. Rotation of the pelvis occurs about the femoral heads such that right trunk rotation produces medial rotation of the right hip and lateral rotation of the left hip. Intrapelvic rotation also occurs between the sacrum and the innominate bones. The precise coupling of movements occurring during rotation remains controversial, and appears to vary according to the degree of relative flexion or extension. The pattern is a function of the articular geometry and muscular control (Lee 1999). The dominant muscular forces are produced by the oblique abdominals because of their large cross-sectional area, fibre orientation and mechanical advantage. The fibre orientation of the paraspinals and their proximity to the axis of motion result in relatively small rotary forces. Their prime function is to generate anti-flexion moments created by the abdominals and torso (Bogduk 1994, Bogduk et al 1992).

Functionally, rotation usually occurs in combination with flexion, extension and varying degrees of side flexion. This implies that control of movement in primary planes is a necessary prerequisite for multi-plane motion, as occurs in complex patterns. Clinically, flexion/rotation mechanisms of spinal injury are very common, and, whilst acknowledging the associated high stress in these situations, rehabilitation should attempt to optimize the individual's capacity rather than promote avoidance. This is perhaps one reason why education in manual handling over several decades has not reduced the incidence of low back pain. It seems more logical to optimize the function of musculoskeletal components involved with motion, rather than attempt to eliminate movements which are part of everyday function. It is virtually impossible to undertake activities of daily living without requiring multi-plane motion (Adams & Dolan 1997). These principles must be observed in the prescription of exercise.

Movement dysfunctions

Rotation in flexion may accentuate segmental hyperflexion, particularly if sustained or repetitive (vacuuming, gardening). This is not always easily visible, but palpation of the spinous processes or manually supporting the painful segment is useful clinically. Given the frequency of these functional impairments, it represents a clinical challenge to rehabilitate these movement patterns without provocation.

Rotation in extension may produce localized segmental overstrain evidenced by skin crease and the appearance of 'kinking' at the relevant level. Again, manual facilitation is useful to assist in the diagnosis of movement dysfunction.

In either of these presentations, it is important to evaluate each of the movement components, as exercise prescription may need to address the individual components prior to incorporation into complex patterns.

Protocols for restrictive dysfunction in rotation

- Leg rotation
- Trunk rotation (Fig. 37.11)
- Side bending in standing
- Hip flexion
- Hip flexion/adduction
- Hip rotation in flexion
- Hip rotation in extension
- Thoracic rotation in sitting.

Protocols for motor control deficits in rotation

Neutral extension
- Core stabilization in four-point (previously described)
- four-point alternate arm lifts
- four-point alternate leg lifts
- Rotational trunk stability
  — in sitting

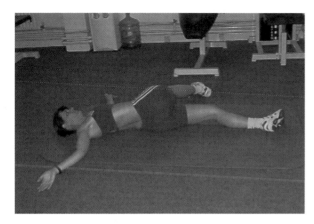

Figure 37.11 Trunk rotation.

— in bridging
— in side-lying
— bent knee fall-outs
● Hip abductors
— in side-lying
— in sitting
— in standing
● Single leg stance
— static holds
— wobble board
— pull-throughs with contralateral arm.

Flexion/rotation

● Exercise sequential rotation in varying degrees of flexion using pulleys, medicine ball, elastic tubing (Figs 37.12, 37.13).

Extension/rotation

● Exercise sequential rotation in varying degrees of extension using pulleys, medicine ball, elastic tubing (Figs 37.13, 37.14).

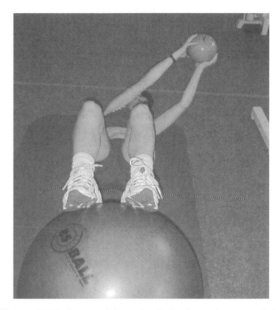

Figure 37.13 Sequential rotation in flexion using a medicine ball.

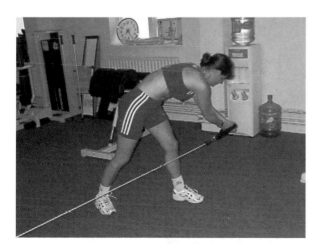

Figure 37.12 Sequential rotation in flexion using a pulley.

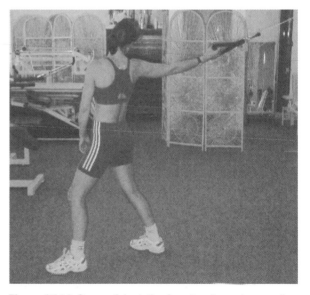

Figure 37.14 Sequential rotation in extension using a pulley.

CONCLUSIONS

Before using exercise in the management of patients with low back pain, it is necessary to consider certain factors: the objectives of the exercise, the source of symptoms, the pathological process, the nature of the mechanical dysfunction, and any contraindications to exercise. Only when these issues have been considered in detail will it be possible to construct a relevant programme of exercise specific to individual requirements.

This chapter has provided a clinical framework from which rational exercise prescription can be selected and incorporated into rehabilitation programmes specific to the clinical presentation.

REFERENCES

Adams M, Dolan P 1997 The combined function of spine, pelvis and legs when lifting with a straight back. In: Vleeming A, Mooney V, Dorman T, Snijders C, Stoeckart R (eds) Movement stability and low back pain. Churchill Livingstone, Edinburgh, p 195–205

Allison G, Kendle K, Roll S, Schupelius J, Scott Q, Panizza J 1997 The role of the diaphragm during abdominal hollowing exercises. Australian Journal of Physiotherapy 44(2): 95–102

Arnoldi C, Lempberg R, Linderholm H 1975 Interosseous hypertension and pain in the knee. Journal of Bone and Joint Surgery 57B: 360–363

Åstrand P 1987 Exercise physiology and its role in disease prevention and in rehabilitation. Archives of Physical Medicine and Rehabilitation 68: 305–309

Beimborn D, Morrissey M 1988 A review of the literature related to trunk muscle performance. Spine 13: 655

Bergmark A 1989 Stability of the lumbar spine. A study in mechanical engineering. Acta Orthopaedica Scandinavica 230(suppl): 20–24

Bogduk N 1994 The lumbar back muscles and their fascia. In: Twomey L, Taylor J (eds) Physical therapy of the low back. Churchill Livingstone, Edinburgh, p 133–138

Bogduk N, Twomey L 1987 Clinical anatomy of the lumbar spine. Churchill Livingstone, Edinburgh

Bogduk N, Twomey L 1991 Clinical anatomy of the lumbar spine, 2nd edn. Churchill Livingstone, London

Bogduk N, Macintosh J E, Pearcy M J 1992 A universal model of the lumbar back muscles in the upright position. Spine 17(8): 897–913

Butler D 1991 Mobilisation of the nervous system. Churchill Livingstone, London

Caix M, Outrequin G, Descotes B et al 1984 The muscles of the abdominal wall: a new functional approach with anatomical deductions. Anatomy Clinics 6: 101

Cohen M, Cambell J 1996 Pain treatment centres at a crossroads: a practical and conceptual reappraisal. IASP Press, Seattle

Cresswell A 1993 Response of intra-abdominal pressure and abdominal muscle activity during dynamic loading in man. European Journal of Applied Physiology 66: 315–320

Cresswell A, Thorstensson A 1989 The role of the abdominal musculature in the elevation of the intra-abdominal pressure during specific tasks. Ergonomics 32: 1237–1246

Cresswell A, Thorstensson A 1994 Changes in intra-abdominal pressure, trunk muscle activation and force during isokinetic lifting and lowering. European Journal of Applied Physiology 88: 315–321

Cresswell A, Grundstrom A, Thorstensson A 1992 Observations on intra-abdominal pressure and patterns of abdominal intra-muscular activity in man. Acta Physiologica Scandinavica 144: 409–418

Deyo R, Deihl A, Rosenthal M 1986 How many days bed rest for acute low back pain? The New England Journal of Medicine 315(17): 1064–1070

Dieppe P 1989 Why is there such poor relationship between radiographic joint damage and both symptoms and functional impairment in osteoarthritis. British Journal of Rheumatology 28: 242

Gatchel R, Turk D 1996 Psychological approaches to pain management. Guilford Press, New York

Gertzbein S D, Holtby R, Tile M, Kapasouri A, Chan K W, Cruickshank B 1984 Determination of a locus of instantaneous centres of rotation of the lumbar disc by moire fringes. Spine 9(4): 409–413

Gertzbein S D, Seligman J, Holtby R, Chan K H, Kapasouri A, Tile M, Cruickshank B 1985 Centrode patterns and segmental instability in degenerative disc disease. Spine 10(3): 257–261

Gracovetsky S, Farfan H, Helleur C 1985 The abdominal mechanism. Spine 10(4): 317–324

Hall G L, Hetzler R K, Perrin D, Weltman A 1992 Relationship of timed sit-up to isokinetic abdominal strength. Research Quarterly for Exercise and Sport 63(1): 80–84

Harding V 1998 Cognitive behavioural approach to fear and avoidance. In: Gifford L (ed) Topical issues in pain 1. CNS press, Falmouth

Hides J, Richardson C, Jull G 1996a Multifidus muscle recovery is not automatic following resolution of acute first episode low back pain. Spine 21: 2763–2769

Hides J, Richardson C, Jull G 1996b Multifidus muscle rehabilitation decreases recurrence of symptoms following first episode low back pain. Proceedings of the National Congress of the Australian Physiotherapy Association, Brisbane

Hodges P, Richardson C 1996 Inefficient muscular stabilisation of the lumbar spine associated with low back pain: a motor control evaluation of transversus abdominis. Spine 21(22): 2640–2650

Janda V 1978 Muscles, motor regulation and back problems. Plenum, New York

Janda V 1983 Muscle function testing. Butterworths, London

Janda V, Schmid H T A 1980 Muscles as a pathogenic factor in low back pain. In: Proceedings of the 4th International Conference of the International Federation of Orthopaedic Manipulative Therapists, Christchurch, New Zealand

Jull G A, Janda V 1987 Muscles and motor control in low back pain: assessment and management. Churchill Livingstone, New York

Jull G A, Richardson C A 1994 Rehabilitation of active stabilisation of the lumbar spine. In: Twomey L T, Taylor J R (eds) Physical therapy of the low back. Churchill Livingstone, New York

Jull G A, Richardson C, Toppenberg R, Comerford M, Bui B 1993 Towards a measurement of active muscle control for lumbar stabilisation. The Australian Journal of Physiotherapy 39(3): 187–193

Kendall F P, McCreary E K, Provance P G 1993 Muscles: testing and function, 4th edn. Williams and Willkins, Baltimore

Koes B A, Bouter L M, van Mameren H et al 1992a The effectiveness of manual therapy, physiotherapy, and treatment by the general practitioner for nonspecific back and neck complaints. Spine 17(1): 27–35

Koes B A, Bouter L M, van Mameren et al 1992b Randomised clinical trial of manipulative therapy and physiotherapy for persistent back and neck complaints: results of one year follow up. British Medical Journal 304: 601–604

Lee D 1999 The pelvic girdle, 2nd edn. Churchill Livingstone, Edinburgh

Lewit K 1994 The functional approach. Journal of Orthopaedic Medicine 16: 73–74

Lewit K 1999 Manipulative therapy in rehabilitation of the locomotor system, 3rd edn. Butterworth-Heinemann, Oxford

Loeser J D 1977 Low back pain. In: Bonica J J (eds) Low back pain. Raven Press, New York, p 155–162

Lund J, Stohler C, Widmer C 1993 The relationship between muscle pain and muscle activity in fibromyalgia and similar conditions. In: Vaeroy H, Mersky H (eds) Progress in fibromyalgia and myofascial pain. Elsevier, Amsterdam, p 311–328

Macintosh J E, Bogduk N 1987 The morphology of the lumbar erector spinae. Spine 12(7): 658–668

Macintosh J E, Bogduk N, Pearcy M J 1993a The effects of flexion on the geometry and actions of the lumbar errector spinae. Spine 18(7): 884–893

Macintosh J E, Pearcy M J, Bogduk N 1993b The axial torque of the lumbar back muscles; torsion strength of the back muscles. Australia and New Zealand Journal of Surgery 63(3): 205–212

Mirka G, Marras W 1993 A stochastic model of trunk muscle coactivation during trunk bending. Spine 18: 1396–1409

Newton M, Waddell G 1993 Trunk strength testing with iso-machines: part 1. Review of a decade of clinical evidence. Spine 18: 801–811

Nouwen A, Van Akkerveeken P F, Versloot J M 1987 Pattern of muscular activity during movement in patients with low back pain. Spine 12: 777

O'Sullivan P B 2000 Lumbar segmental instability: clinical presentations and specific stabilising exercises. Manual Therapy 5(1): 2–12

O'Sullivan P, Twomey L A G 1998 Altered abdominal muscle recruitment in back pain patients following specific exercise intervention. Journal of Orthopaedic and Sports Physical Therapy 27(2): 1–11

O'Sullivan P B, Twomey L, Allison G, Sinclair J, Miller K, Knox J 1997 Altered patterns of abdominal muscle activation in patients with chronic low back pain. Australian Journal of Physiotherapy 43(2): 91 98

Panjabi M 1992a The stabilising system of the spine. Part 1. Function, dysfunction, adaptation and enhancement. Journal of Spinal Disorders 5: 383–389

Panjabi M 1992b The stabilising system of the spine. Part 2. Neutral zone and stability hypothesis. Journal of Spinal Disorders 5: 390–397

Pearcy M, Portek I, Shepherd J 1984 Three-dimensional X-ray analysis of normal movement in the lumbar spine. Spine 9(3): 294–297

Potvin J R, McGill S M, Norman R W 1991 Trunk muscle and lumbar ligament contributions to dynamic lifts with varying degrees of trunk flexion. Spine 16(9): 1099–1107

Raschke U, Chaffin D 1996 Trunk and hip muscle recruitment in response to external anterior lumbosacral shear and moment loads. Clinical Biomechanics 3: 145–152

Richardson C, Toppenberg R, Jull G 1990 An initial evaluation of eight abdominal exercises for their ability to provide stabilisation for the lumbar spine. The Australian Journal of Physiotherapy 36(1): 6–11

Richardson C, Jull G, Hodges P, Hides P 1999 Therapeutic exercise for spinal segmental stabilisation in low back pain. Churchill Livingstone, Edinburgh

Sahrmann S A 1987 Muscle imbalances in the orthopaedic and neurological patient. 10th International Congress of the World Confederation of Physical Therapy, Sydney, Australia

Shekelle P, Adams A, Chassin M, Hurwitz E, Brook R 1992 Spinal manipulation for low back pain. Annals of Internal Medicine 117(7): 590–598

Sherman R, Arena J 1993 Biofeedback for assessment and treatment of low back pain. In: Basmajian J, Nyberg R (eds) Rational manual therapies. Williams & Wilkins, Baltimore, p 177–197

Shorland S 1998 Management of chronic pain following whiplash injuries. In: Gifford L (ed) Topical issues in pain 1. CNS Press, Falmouth, p 115–134

Shumway-Cook A, Wollacott M 1995 Motor control – theory and practical applications. Williams & Wilkins, Baltimore

Tesh K M, Dunn J S, Evans J H 1987 The abdominal muscles and vertebral stability. Spine 12(501): 501–508

Twomey L, Taylor J 1994 Lumbar posture, movement, and mechanics. In: Twomey L, Taylor J (eds) Physical Therapy of the low back. Churchill Livingstone, Edinburgh, p 57–91

Vaeroy H, Mersky H 1993 Progress in fibromyalgia and myofascial pain. Elsevier, Amsterdam

Vleeming A, Mooney V, Dorman T, Snijders C, Stoeckart R 1997 Movement, stability and low back pain. Churchill Livingstone, Edinburgh

Waddell G 1998 The back pain revolution. Churchill Livingstone, Edinburgh

Watson P 2000 Psychosocial predictors of outcome from low back pain. In: Gifford L (ed) Topical issues in pain 2. CNS Press, Falmouth

Witt I, Vostergaard A, Rosenklint A 1984 A comparative analysis of X-ray findings in the lumbar spine in patients with and without lumbar pain. Spine 9: 298–300

Wolf L, May P, McClure M, Parrdy W 1993 Exercise and training for spinal patients. In: Basmajian J, Nyberg R (eds) Rational manual therapies. Williams & Wilkins, Baltimore, p 177–197

Wright A 1995 Hypoalgesia post manipulation therapy: a review of a potential neurophysiological mechanism. Manual Therapy 1(1): 11–16

Zusman M 1998 Irritability. Manual Therapy 3(4): 195–202

APPENDIX: PRINCIPLES OF EXERCISE PROGRESSION

There are a number of variables which can be utilized in order to progress the degree of difficulty, including the following.

Starting position. Changing the position of the body segment relative to gravity.

Leverage. Changing the angle of limb segments relative to the axis of motion. The force generated by the centre of mass of the limb segment multiplied by the distance from the axis of motion constitutes the torque force which must be opposed by muscle activity.

Base of support. Reducing the base of support increases muscle demand. For example, progression from double leg to single leg support constitutes a significant increase in muscle force and is a necessary functional component of gait.

Range of motion. One of the basic parameters of muscle physiology is the length–tension relationship which implies that muscle force output is directly related to its length. Proper function requires muscle force output throughout the range of motion. The clinical application is the requirement to restore inner range function of lengthened muscles and outer range function of shortened muscle.

Contraction time. There is selective dysfunction of the slow-fibre, monarticular anti-gravity muscles which potentially compromises articular stability. Progression is made from improvement in muscle recruitment to sustaining holding time with progressively increasing load. This satisfies the principle of specificity in relation to postural muscle function.

Repetitions. The general principle of increased repetitions promoting endurance applies here with some modification. Because the physiological responses to postural muscle disuse is a reduction in endurance coupled with an increased contraction velocity (a shift to the right of the force–velocity curve), therapeutic exercise should aim to stimulate sustained contractions. Whilst repeated contractions will stimulate fibre endurance, the intermittent stimulation is unlikely to reinforce the optimal motor firing pattern. Therefore, a compromise solution is to utilize modest numbers of repetitions (10–15) but sustaining the holding time. This fulfils the criteria of improving endurance through prolonged muscle activation and stimulating motor recruitment patterns more specific to postural function.

Speed of contraction. In accordance with the rightward shift in the force–velocity curve, the initial focus of exercise is to promote slow, sustained contractions maintaining stable muscle activation. This can then be progressed to movements which require synergic stability and mobility functions, i.e. trunk stability with limb motion, bending backwards.

Complexity of motor activation

In conjunction with variables which increase muscle loading, progression can be made by altering the complexity of motor activation.

Static positioning. The therapist positions the body part in a desired position. This provides proprioceptive input in preparation for muscle activation.

Static positioning + hold. Muscle synergies are stimulated via the therapist rather than utilizing preferred recruitment strategies.

Active/assisted positioning. Promotes spontaneous recruitment with some facilitation and mechanical assistance.

Active positioning. Spontaneous recruitment.

Active positioning + dynamic movement. Simulates requirements of functional activities.

38

Sport and exercise in diabetes

Matthew Kiln

KEY POINTS

1. Exercise and sport are still not used as part of the standard treatment plan for diabetic patients, despite being recognized as such for over 40 years.
2. The threefold increase in premature death rate that occurs in patients with diabetes can be halved by regular exercise or sport.
3. Many of the complications of diabetes can be reduced, delayed or prevented by a reasonable level of exercise.
4. Soft tissue healing time is lengthened in diabetic patients/athletes who do not have near normoglycaemic blood glucose levels.
5. Exercise programmes should be embarked upon at a more graduated level in diabetic patients, because of the risk of silent ischaemic heart disease and possible silent myocardial infarction as a consequence of this.
6. Competitive and non-competitive athletes and their coaches need to remember that awareness of hypoglycaemia during exercise may be difficult.

INTRODUCTION

There are two types of diabetes:

- *Type 1.* This occurs generally in those under 26 years of age. Treatment requires injections of insulin. Patients are not usually overweight, the onset is usually sudden, and patients' general fitness tends to be reasonably good once they are stabilized on insulin.

- *Type 2.* This occurs in those generally over 35 years of age. The condition is controlled by diet alone, diet plus exercise, or diet, exercise and tablets; insulin injections are sometimes required as well. Patients tend to be overweight and have high levels of insulin production, but they are resistant to it. This insulin resistance is partially due to obesity, and also to lack of exercise.

Although it has been suspected since the early 1950s that exercise has had a role in helping the management of diabetes and its complications (Persson & Thoren 1980), no one has been able to come up with proof of this, or understood the reasons why. Some proof has come to light over the last 15 years. We still do not know beyond 'all reasonable doubt', but thankfully 'the balance of probabilities' suggests that regular aerobic exercise will reduce the risk of premature ischaemic heart disease and strokes in diabetic patients (Kennet & Sonlie 1979).

For these reasons, the push to incorporate exercise into diabetes care has been understandably cautious, primarily because little was known about how it could be practically done with absolute safety. In short, it cannot be. Nothing in life, including sport and diabetes can ever be done with absolute safety. Caution at the start and a gradual, controlled increase in exercise level will eliminate most risks, but not all.

In the mid-1970s I was told by probably the most eminent diabetes specialist in the world at the time, that 'it was impossible for a type 1 diabetic patient to run a marathon'. It was difficult, and it took me 2 years to work out how to do it. Since completing a marathon in the 1970s, many other diabetic patients have done so. Listening to practical experiences is often the best way to learn how to advise other patients on similar matters on which you have little practical experience. Much of the information presented in this chapter is based on the experiences of athletes and other diabetic competitors from the sports of football, rugby, hockey, athletics and sub aqua diving. (I believe the reason I was advised that it was impossible for a diabetic person to run a marathon was that this eminent professor and I were friends, and he did not want me to put myself through a training regime with unknown risks.)

MUSCULOSKELETAL SYSTEM PHYSIOLOGY IN DIABETES

When advising diabetic patients and athletes, it is important to know whether the physiology of all soft tissues, including respiration, is exactly the same as in the non-diabetic subject. In the main, the answer to this is yes (Bjorntorp & Krotkiewski 1985), but there are two areas where differences have been observed.

Muscle fibre training and development are the same in diabetic and non-diabetic patients (Persson & Thoren 1980). Therefore, from a power and endurance point of view, diabetic athletes can train on the same schedules as non-diabetic athletes, once their blood sugar level control has taken account of the exercise programme (Fig. 38.1).

In my experience, I have found that capsular injuries in diabetic athletes take approximately 50% longer to heal than those in non-diabetic athletes. Acute and

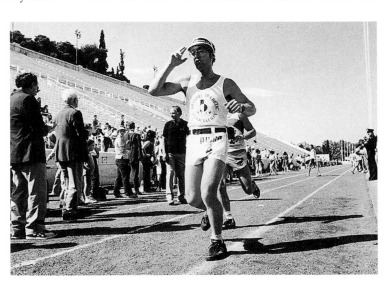

Figure 38.1 A weary diabetic finishing the Athens marathon, one of the most difficult of all. Diabetics can succeed at the most demanding sporting events.

semi-acute tendon injuries do not seem to have any lengthening in the healing process in diabetic athletes.

I have observed acute overload training myositis in diabetic athletes, which takes 7–9 days to settle but does so without any drug treatment. This, again, is 50% longer than one usually sees in non-diabetic athletes. An example of this was a weight-lifter who had suffered from diabetes for over 10 years. He markedly increased his free lift load and then developed rectus abdominis and pectoralis myositis.

The physiological explanation for these observed differences has not yet been established, but it is likely to be related to the soft tissue blood supply, or lack of it! Tendons have very little blood supply, in both diabetic and normal subjects; capsular and muscle blood supply is higher and there is more potential for differences between diabetic and non-diabetic athletes. This, however, does not explain these differences entirely.

GLUCOSE BALANCE, GLYCOGEN AND ENERGY SUPPLY

In non-diabetic subjects, insulin levels fall during and after prolonged exercise. In type 1 diabetic patients during exercise, a set insulin amount has already been injected, so exercise cannot reduce its level (Drazin & Patel 1998). In type 2 diabetic patients, the blood insulin level will not fall in response to one episode of exercise, but it will fall if exercise is on a regular, fairly frequent basis (i.e. two to three times a week) (Jun 1994).

Glucose is the initial energy source in exercise. At first, this is taken out of the blood glucose pool. It is quickly replenished from glycogen stores. Blood glucose levels in type 1 and 2 diabetic patients will fall during exercise, except when the serum insulin level is very low, when muscles cannot utilize blood glucose (insulin is required for the absorption of glucose into the cell; only then it can be metabolized). Consequently the blood glucose will rise and the patient may become ketotic. If the exercise continues without extra insulin, the athlete could rapidly develop diabetic ketoacidosis. This only happens rarely in type 1 diabetes, when the subject stops taking insulin completely prior to exercise. Occasionally, it may also occur in poorly controlled type 1 or type 2 diabetic patients (Box 38.1).

Glycogen and glucose debt

Prolonged intense exercise will produce a glycogen debt, which will often require about 100 g of glucose or its carbohydrate equivalent to replenish. This is done

> **Box 38.1** Case study: exercising with a low serum insulin in type 1 diabetes
>
> A 25-year-old male type 1 diabetic decided to go training at 18.00 h. He took his last insulin at 07.00 h. This was his standard dose, a mixture of quick-acting and medium-duration insulin. He ate a larger than usual business lunch. He was also recovering from a cold, and he felt a run would 'help to burn it off'. His blood glucose at 18.00 h was 15 mmol/L.
>
> He ran 2–3 miles, but found himself feeling more and more tired and his speed slowed. He considered that his blood sugar might be becoming a little low, so he ate three dextrose tablets that he had in his pocket. He began to feel more lethargic and took a short cut home.
>
> On arriving home, his blood sugar was 29 mmol/L and he found ketones on a urine test. He then took his evening quick-acting insulin plus two extra units. One hour later he felt a lot better.
>
> **What did he do wrong?**
>
> Firstly, it is all very well to be wise after the event, but at the time he went running he would have had very little of his morning insulin still working. This would have been all right if his blood sugar had been 'normal' when he started running, i.e. 4–7 mmol/L. Really he should not have gone training with his blood sugar starting at 15 mmol/L, or he should have given himself 1–2 units of quick-acting insulin prior to the exercise. (However, if whilst running he then decided to continue on to a long training session, i.e. 40 min plus, he would then have run this risk of becoming hypoglycaemic!) Having a cold as well would result in some insulin resistance, making this potentially dangerous scenario more likely.

by the muscles taking up this glucose and storing it as glycogen which is in preference to liver storage when exercise has been undertaken. In addition, the brain has a preferential demand for glucose of about 150 g/day. This means that the majority of carbohydrate consumed will already be 'earmarked' to replenish these muscle glycogen stores and the brain's vital supply (Bjorntorp & Krotkiewski 1985). Akin to this process, muscle and peripheral tissues all become more sensitive to insulin during and after exercise (Yamanouchik et al 1995).

This 'earmarking' of glucose is the same in diabetic and non-diabetic athletes, but in the latter the body will make the necessary adjustments itself (reducing insulin release and increasing adrenaline production) to achieve stable blood glucose levels and energy supplies. In diabetic athletes, a set amount of insulin has already been injected and self-adjustment by the body does not occur. Hence it is easy to see why type 1 diabetic patients will probably need to reduce their insulin injections by 10–20% once they start regular exercise, and type 2 diabetic patients may either improve their blood sugar levels and/or reduce their drug therapy (Grimm 1995, Kiln 1996).

WHY IS EXERCISE IMPORTANT IN DIABETES?

Primary prevention

From a public health perspective, 'sport for all' is a broad method of preventing or delaying the onset of diabetes in people at risk, as shown by Helmrich et al (1991). Those at a higher risk of type 2 diabetes should be encouraged to take up sport through their relatives with diabetes. This is particularly so for Asian at-risk patients, as they are generally at a higher risk of developing diabetes.

In the Framington study, Kennet & Sonlie (1979) clearly demonstrated that exercise resulted in an improvement in glucose tolerance. The only consequential effect of this, in practical terms, is that exercise will result in fewer of the at-risk members of the population actually developing diabetes. As yet no research has been completed to prove this point. However, I do not consider that we need lengthy, costly research to prove something that is obvious common sense and that follows from proven physiology.

Control of established diabetes

Many studies have shown an improvement in different glycaemic indices that is clearly linked to exercise. Eriksson et al (1997) demonstrated a significant reduction in HbA1c levels, and Dunstan et al (1998), after adjusting for the reduction in body mass associated with exercise, showed a significant reduction in baseline blood glucose and insulin measurements. Mosher et al (1998) confirmed, in adolescent patients with type 1 diabetes, that HbA1c levels were reduced by 0.96% with regular aerobic circuit training (in diabetes a 0.96% improvement in HbA1c is substantial).

Reducing complication rates in diabetes

Macrovascular complications

Diabetic patients generally have an increased risk of 'heart attacks' and strokes. When diabetes is associated with raised lipids, the risks escalate. My concerns are in line with a statement by Alberti (1998), who said we have a potentially 'fatal combination'. Myocardial ischaemia is by far the single highest cause of morbidity and mortality in diabetic patients, as shown by the United Kingdom Prospective Diabetes Study (UKPDS) (Turner et al 1998). It was also demonstrated in this study that when one improved blood pressure and glycaemic control, it failed to have any significant beneficial effect on the cardiovascular mortality rate in diabetic subjects. Cholesterol reduction with drugs and diet helps to reduce cardiovasular risk factors, but exercise is more generally available and probably of greater benefit. This is demonstrated well by the British Regional Heart Study (conducted on 7735 men). This study can be divided into two subsections: in the first part Shaper and Wannamethee (1991) found a 50% reduced risk of stroke; in the second part Wannamethee and Shaper (1992) demonstrated a 60% reduced risk of heart attack in those men undertaking moderate exercise.

These studies and an overall review of all such studies use whole population data, and consequently the levels found for the reduction in risk of strokes and 'heart attacks' may not be strictly accurate for diabetic patients. However, as diabetic men are at an increased risk from both, the reduction of risk from strokes and heart attacks is likely to be even higher.

Microvascular complications

The incidence of proliferative diabetic retinopathy was found by Cruickshanks et al (1992) to be reduced in diabetic women who previously and currently took part in physical activity. In diabetic men, however, there was no reduction in the incidence of proliferative diabetic retinopathy.

Diabetic nephropathy should, in theory, also be reduced by exercise, as an effect of the improvement in HbA1c brought about by exercise. As yet no research has been completed to confirm this logical assumption.

Other health benefits

Other health benefits accruing from exercise include psychological well-being, a reduction in the risk of osteoporosis, and weight loss or reduced body fat ratio. These benefits apply to the population as a whole, but are just as important to patients suffering from diabetes.

Many of the other benefits of exercise are social or psychological (Martinsen 1990), and they are often overlooked or are not easy to quantify with research, e.g. self-esteem enhancement, perceptions of mastery, and the benefit of social interaction with other people, which is important in combating feelings of isolation or alienation.

MECHANISMS INVOLVED IN THE PROTECTIVE EFFECT OF EXERCISE

As the causes of diabetes and its complications are multifactorial, the mechanisms involved in the protective effect of exercise are not clear-cut and are often interlinked. Each mechanism will be considered separately.

Fibrinolysis

Van Loon et al (1992) found that the potential for exercise to activate the fibrinolytic system remains intact in diabetic patients. Long-distance running slows the progression of atherosclerosis by stimulating fibrinolysis. This effect on fibrinolysis would also tend to reduce the severity, and consequently the morbidity, following an acute ischaemic event.

Cholesterol levels

High density lipoprotein (HDL) cholesterol levels have been shown to be raised with exercise in many research studies (Goldberg & Elliot 1987). Low-density lipoprotein (LDL) cholesterol levels, on the other hand, have been found to be lowered by exercise. Although data are inconsistent, this has generally been confirmed.

Blood pressure lowering

It is difficult to know whether this should be included as a mechanism or an effect of exercise (Duncan et al 1985). Either way, lowering blood pressure through exercise slows the rate of progression and delays the end-point of macrovascular diabetic complications.

RISKS OF EXERCISE

Hypoglycaemia. This occurs as a result of increasing insulin absorption rate and carbohydrate metabolism. It may occur up to 24 h after the exercise event.

Diminished awareness of hypoglycaemia. This occurs particularly with human insulin in some patients. A switch to animal insulin has helped many of these patients. Also, athletes may confuse the symptoms of hypoglycaemia with the usual effects of exercise, i.e. hot, sweaty, tiredness and a rapid heartbeat (Kiln 1997).

Ketoacidosis. This may be accelerated in patients with poorly controlled diabetes (Persson & Thoren 1980).

Acute myocardial infarction. This is a risk particularly if too much is attempted when the person is unfit.

Exacerbation of established microalbuminuria. Athletes need to ask their doctor to monitor this carefully initially, if it is established.

Special precautions

● The presence of autonomic neuropathy may make the pulse rate an unreliable measure of exercise intensity.

● Patients with peripheral neuropathy will have to be extremely careful with their sports footwear, as they will be at an increased risk of foot ulcers, corns, blisters etc. Any blisters/corns occurring may also be at increased risk of infection. Advice from a chiropodist is recommended.

● Unstable diabetes must be corrected by the athlete and/or the nurse specialist/doctor prior to an exercise programme.

● Exercise training must be started very slowly in patients over 40, remembering the unlikely possibility of silent myocardial infarction (Tunstall-Pedoe 1991).

ADVISING A PERSON WITH DIABETES PLANNING TO TAKE UP EXERCISE

Start the patient off slowly, with graduated walking.

Check if the patient is at particular risk from exercise. If so, you may want to request an opinion from a secondary care physician, as you may not feel confident or competent to assess this risk. This is a crucial point; indeed, it is perhaps the most important point of this chapter: **anyone advising or proposing to train diabetic athletes must know and realize the limits of their knowledge and expertise. Never give advice in areas that you are unsure about. If you do not know something then say so and advise the client where the information may be obtained** (see 'useful address' at the end of the chapter).

It is advisable for all clients with diabetes who wish to take up exercise to check that this is acceptable with their GP or hospital specialist, especially if they are over 35 years old. In clients for whom there are no real concerns, I would advise that they can start on any sports training programme that is 20–30% more moderate in the early stages than for other non-diabetic subjects. Such programmes are available at many established leisure centres and are sometimes prescribed on subsidy by local GPs. Here the patient will have a trainer who is experienced in sports science and who will be able to work out a suitable exercise programme. This is why it is important that doctors do not refer any patient who presents a real or perceived risk from undertaking exercise.

If, as a GP, you are asked whether or not a diabetic client can take up aerobic exercise, the answer will be easy if the patient is slim, has normal blood pressure, good diabetic control, normal cholesterol and serum lipid levels, and no family history of ischaemic heart disease. However, life is never as simple as that. If you are not sure, ask for help or advice. Even the hospital specialist may not be able to give a confident answer as to whether it is relatively safe for a middle-aged, overweight patient to take up aerobic exercise. The patient may have to be referred to a cardiologist to perform treadmill exercise ECG testing, which in itself can present a few risks and occasionally give false-positive or false-negative results.

If possible, the patient should measure blood sugar before and 30 min following exercise. Keep a record of this and also of the distance walked or run, and the amount of carbohydrate eaten before and during the run. Also record the time of the last tablet or injection of insulin and any adjustments in the amounts (Table 38.1; for a fuller explanation, see Kiln 1996).

From these data, one can gradually calculate the amount of carbohydrate consumed per mile. After doing this for quite a few exercise periods, the athlete will then be able to start doing the calculations to predict how much carbohydrate an exercise session will consume.

Club, elite and serious athletes

One assumes that serious athletes will have coped well with moderate exercise levels. If they have not undertaken a recording method of exercise and carbohydrate, then they should do so (Table 38.1). As this table is expanded, it can be used to slowly work out by how much the insulin and other drug dosages can be reduced on days when a fair amount of exercise is to be taken, i.e. in excess of 1 h. A 25% or greater reduction in insulin dosage is not uncommon (see Table 38.2 and Kiln 1996). The dosage of sulphonylurea drugs can often be reduced or stopped on such days.

Team games

The amount of exercise that will be required in team games is unpredictable, especially matches (Fig. 38.2 and Boxes 38.2 and 38.3). It is therefore sensible for

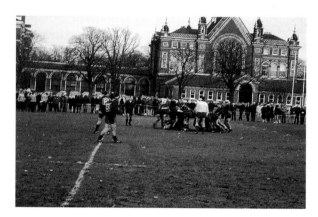

Figure 38.2 In team games the carbohydrate consumed depends largely on the quality of the opposition, particularly the opponent the diabetic athlete is marking.

Table 38.1 Chart showing how to record the details of each run. Patients can then calculate roughly how much carbohydrate they will consume on future runs. The same principle can be used for any sport

Time taken to do exercise (min)	Mile split[a] (min)	Distance (miles)	Carbohydrate eaten (g)	Blood sugars (start, finish)	Exercise type	Carbohydrate consumed per mile (g)
16	15.4	1.1	0	9.0, 8.2	Walk	5
34	12.2	2.8	12	11.0, 9.0	Walk	8
110	8.2	13.5	80	9.0, 6.5	Run	8.8
50	7.1	7.0	85	4.5, 5.0	Run	11.0
40	7.8	5.1	55	3.0, 4.0	Run	9.4

[a] Mile split is the time taken to run each mile.

Table 38.1 Recording of more advanced training and insulin dosage reduction

Time taken to do run (min)	Mile split[a] (min)	Distance of run (miles)	Carbohydrate eaten (g)	Blood sugars (start, finish)	Insulin dosage reduction	Carbohydrate consumed per mile (g)
85	8.5	10	84	8.0, 6.0	No	8.4
110	7.3	15	104	6.0, 4.0	8 → 6 units	6.9
140	7.8	18	142	10.0, 4.0	No	7.9
150	8.3	18	117	13.0, 2.0	8 → 6 units	6.5

The above runs were in the morning, so the quick-acting insulin is reduced

220	8.4	26.2	36	4.0, 4.0	8 → 2 units	1.4
225	8.6	26.2	78	4.0, 1.5[a]	8 → 2 units	3.0
204	7.7	26.2	31	7.0, 4.0	8 → 2 units	1.2

The above marathons were in the morning, so the quick-acting insulin is reduced.
A reduced amount of medium-length insulin is not taken until after the marathon, and then with a top-up dosage of quick-acting insulin. One needs to do this, otherwise the blood sugar climbs rapidly once exercise has ceased.

240	9.2	26.2	0	10, 20.0	14 → 3 units	?

This marathon was a 16.30 h start. The usual dose of quick-acting insulin was taken in the morning, the medium-length insulin was reduced (too much).
Late afternoon is not a good time to run a marathon. It was the first international marathon ever held in Moscow.

[a] This was the only marathon this athlete ran whilst on human insulin.

Box 38.2 Case study: unpredictable carbohydrate metabolism during a hockey match

A club hockey player did not reduce her morning insulin as she was playing a match in the afternoon. She ate 30–40 g of extra mixed carbohydrate in the changing room just before the game (a fruit snack bar and a piece of bread). She played in the centre-half position and, as the centre-forward she was marking was very mobile, she continually had to chase. She ate a further 40 g of carbohydrate at half-time, but towards the end of the second half she started failing to mark her opponent, and ended up tackling any player anywhere on the pitch. When she came off, her friends sensibly encouraged her to eat some of the dextrose tablets she was carrying in her pocket.

Her blood glucose test was 2.0 mmol/L. The amount of carbohydrate a diabetic hockey, soccer or rugby player will use up in a match is largely dependent upon how good and how active the opposition is. And of course you will not find this out until the match is well underway.

Box 38.3 Case study: hypoglycaemia during a rugby match

In an inter-school rugby cup semi-final, a boy with type 1 diabetes followed his usual regime of not reducing his insulin and eating three chocolate crispy bars while changing for the match, i.e. approximately 90 g of carbohydrate. He always felt a little bloated at the start of the game, but after 10 min this always seemed to go.

He was fine in the game, but at the end of full time, the score was Millfield 20, Kings-Weston 20. The match was close and all-involving, and hence he did not think to have any additional carbohydrate before extra time started. In the second half of the extra time period, he was staggering all over the pitch. He was helped off and half carried to the pavilion, where the coach decided it was not concussion but hypoglycaemia. He soon recovered, once given Glucose Gel, but it was too late for him to resume playing. Try and think of the unpredictable!

---

athletes to lower their insulin only slightly, i.e. 10–15%. They should use the morning quick-acting insulin if the match is to take place in the morning, and the morning medium-duration insulin if the match is in the afternoon.

Lowering the insulin or oral diabetic drug dosage too much before a match or event may be counter-productive, because it may result in an elevated blood sugar at the commencement of exercise, which can affect performance due to the slight lethargy it may induce.

CONCLUSIONS

1. Regular exercise, at a reasonable level, is one of the most beneficial aspects in diabetes care. This is primarily because of a reduction in the number of macrovascular complications. Patients do not need to participate in formalized sport to get useful exercise. They can walk more, avoiding using the car for short trips, and they can use the stairs, where possible, rather than the lift or escalator.

2. There are two difficulties in advising active regular sport for patients with diabetes: the first has to do with the patient finding the time to undertake regular exercise (not limited to diabetic patients!), and the second has to do with the cardiovascular risks of starting an exercise programme too quickly.

3. Advising elite diabetic athletes is a little easier than advising those starting to exercise from scratch.

4. When a diabetic person takes up exercise, caution is required to unsure that a balance is achieved between exercise, medication and carbohydrate. Each patient will have unique requirements and will need to build a log of previous exercise and carbohydrate requirements.

5. Remember the importance of being cautious when starting a diabetic patient on exercise, and give warnings appropriately. If you feel you do not know enough on this topic to give advice, ask for help. Following this common sense approach, you will not go far wrong and will help to prevent a number of diabetic patients from developing complications, possibly even preventing several premature deaths.

REFERENCES

Alberti K G M M 1998 Lipids and diabetes: a fatal combination? Diabetic Medicine 15: 359

Bjorntorp P, Krotkiewski M 1985 Exercise treatment in diabetes mellitus. Acta Medica Scandinavica 217(suppl): 3–7

Cruickshanks K J, Moss S E, Klein R, Klein B E 1992 Physical activity and proliferative retinopathy with diabetes before age 30 yr. Diabetes Care 15(10): 1267–1272

Draznin M B, Patel D R 1998 Diabetes mellitus and sports. Adolescent Medicine 9(3): 457–465

Duncan J J, Farr J E, Upton S J, Hagan R D, Oglesby M E, Blair S N 1985 The effects of aerobic exercise on plasma catecholamines and blood pressure in patients with mild hypertension. Journal of the American Medical Association 254: 2609–2613

Dunstan D W, Puddey I B, Beilin L J, Burke V, Morton A R, Stanton K G 1998 Effects of a short-term circuit weight training program on glycaemic control in NIDDM. Diabetes Research and Clinical Practice 40(1): 53–61

Erikson J, Taimela S, Erikson K, Pariainen S, Peltonen J, Kujala U 1997 Resistance training in the treatment of non-insulin-dependent diabetes mellitus. International Journal of Sports Medicine 18(4): 242–246

Goldberg L, Elliot D L 1987 The effect of exercise on lipid metabolism in men and women. Sports Medicine 4: 307–321

Grimm J J 1995 Sports and diabetes. Schweiz Rundsch Med Practice 84(35): 939–943

Helmrich S P, Ragland D R, Leung R W, Pathfinder R S 1991 Physical activity and reduced occurrence of non-insulin-dependent diabetes. New England Journal of Medicine 325: 147–152

Jun J Y 1994 The effects of programmed jogging on metabolism and cardiopulmonary function of type 2 diabetic patients. Kanhohak Tamgu 3(1): 19–42

Kennet W B, Sonlie P 1979 The Framington Study. Some health benefits of physical activity. Archives of Internal Medicine 139: 857–861

Kiln M R 1996 Advice on long distance running for diabetics. IDDT, PO Box 294, Northampton NN1 4XS

Kiln M R 1997 Exercise and sport in diabetes. Diabetes in Primary Care Group (now PCD UK), BDA, 10 Queen Anne St, London W1M 0BD

Martinsen E W 1990 Physical fitness, anxiety and depression. British Journal of Hospital Medicine 43: 194–199

Mosher P E, Nash M S, Perry A C, LaPerriere A R, Goldberg R B 1998 Aerobic circuit exercise training: effect on adolescents with well controlled insulin-dependent diabetes mellitus. Archives of Physical Medicine and Rehabilitation 79(6): 652–657

Persson B, Thoren C 1980 Prolonged exercise in adolescent boys with juvenile diabetes mellitus. Acta Paediatrica Scandinavica 283(suppl): 62–69

Shaper A G, Wannamethee G 1991 Physical activity and ischaemic heart disease in middle aged man. British Heart Journal 66: 384–394

Tunstall Pedoe D 1991 The London Marathon, medical aspects for the first 10 yrs. A report to the London Sports Medicine Institute, Charterhouse Sq, London EC1M 6BQ

Turner R C, Mills H, Neil H A W, Stratton I M, Manley S E, Matthews D R et al for the United Kingdom Prospective Diabetes Study Group 1998 Risk factors for coronary artery disease in non-insulin dependent diabetes mellitus. British Medical Journal 316: 823–828

Van Loon B J, Heere L P, Kluft C, Briet E, Dooijewaard G, Meinders A E 1992 Fibrinolytic system during long-distance running in IDDM patients and in health subjects. Diabetes Care 15(8): 991–996

Wannamethee G, Shaper A G 1992 Physical activity and stroke in British middle aged men. British Medical Journal 304: 597–601

Yamanouchik K, Shinozaki T, Chikada K et al 1995 Daily walking combined with diet therapy is a useful means for obese NIDDM patients not only to reduce body weight but also to improve insulin sensitivity. Diabetes Care 18(6): 775–778

FURTHER READING

Berg K E 1996 The diabetic's guide to health and fitness. Life Enhancement Publications, Human Kinetics, Champaign, IL

USEFUL ADDRESS

The International Diabetes Athletes Association (UK)
24 Eden Drive
Sedgefield
Cleveland TS21 3DX
England, UK

39

The physiology of walking performance in peripheral arterial disease

Simon Green   Christopher Askew

KEY POINTS

1. Peripheral arterial disease (PAD) is a debilitating atherosclerotic disease which can lead to intermittent claudication in the lower limbs, and consequently pain in response to walking.
2. Intermittent claudication most often follows a benign course, but the symptoms of atherosclerosis are associated with a substantial increase in overall mortality.
3. The physical and social constraints of intermittent claudication often constitute a serious and underrated problem for patients. Central to these constraints is the intolerance to common forms of exercise, such as walking.
4. In people with chronic diseases such as PAD, the design of effective therapies, such as physical activity, depends upon an understanding of the physiology of walking intolerance.

INTRODUCTION

Peripheral arterial disease (PAD) is a debilitating atherosclerotic disease that leads to stenosis and occlusion of the peripheral arteries and restricts the arterial circulation to the limbs. Intermittent claudication is the hallmark of atherosclerosis in large arteries of the lower extremities, and pain in response to walking is the result of an inadequacy of regional blood flow to meet metabolic demands of the exercising muscle. The reported frequency of intermittent claudication varies in different studies from approximately 2% in subjects aged 45–55 years to up 10–20% of individuals over the age of 60 years (Donovan 1994, Kannel et al 1970). Intermittent claudication most often follows a benign course, leading to critical leg ischaemia or amputation in less than 20% of patients within the first decade (Jelnes et al 1986), but the symptoms of atherosclerosis are associated with a substantial increase in overall mortality, and the physical and social constraints of the disease often constitute a serious and underrated problem for patients. Central to these constraints is the intolerance to common forms of exercise, such as walking.

Within the last decade, there have been several reviews on exercise in PAD that have focused on either physiological aspects of exercise performance (Brass & Hiatt 1994, Green & Mehlsen 1999) or rehabilitation through the use of exercise training (e.g. Barnard 1994, Gardner & Poehlman 1995, Regensteiner & Hiatt 1995). Relatively few reviews, however, have focused on the underlying physiology and pathophysiology of PAD and its contribution to walking intolerance (Brass & Hiatt 1994, Green & Mehlsen 1999). In people with chronic disease, such as PAD, the design of effective therapies, such as physical activity, depends upon an understanding of the physiology of walking intolerance. In a recent review we focused on the influence of the circulation on exercise performance in PAD (Green & Mehlsen 1999). The present review complements this focus on the physiology of performance in PAD to consider mainly phenomena occurring within skeletal muscle that contribute to walking intolerance. Methodological effects on walking performance are also important for interpreting the physiological contributions to walking performance and have been discussed elsewhere (Green & Mehlsen 1999, Hiatt et al 1995).

A CONCEPTUAL MODEL OF WALKING PERFORMANCE AND PHYSIOLOGY

Figure 39.1 illustrates a simple conceptual model of walking performance and its underlying physiology. Like quantitative, mathematical models of performance (Olds et al 1993, Peronnet & Thibault 1989), the qualitative model in the figure views performance from an energetic perspective. Walking performance in people with PAD has usually been assessed as either the total distance walked (m) or the period spent walking (s). Since most test protocols have used a gra-

dient beyond zero, the external mechanical work done during such walking tests is work done in displacing the body's mass in the vertical direction (i.e. vertical work). The expression of this vertical work done as performance is modified by the individual's body mass (Fig. 39.1), since this latter variable is not usually considered in assessing performance. The consequence is that, if performance is similar between two people, a heavier person will have done more mechanical work, something which has rarely been considered (Green & Mehlsen 1999). The external work done is the product of the external mechanical power, which is a function of the body mass, treadmill speed and gradient, and the time over which this power is sustained. As shown in Figure 39.1, the mechanical power generated at any moment is established by the rates of aerobic ($E_{aerobic}$) and anaerobic ($E_{anaerobic}$) metabolism and the efficiency with which this chemical energy is transduced into mechanical power (η_{mech}). Amongst other things, such as fibre type recruitment, mechanical efficiency (η_{mech}) is influenced by walking technique (i.e. gait) which, in turn, is subject to learning how to walk on a motorized treadmill. At a given mechanical power, $E_{anaerobic}$ will be inversely related to the extent to which $E_{aerobic}$ meets the energy requirements of walking. Given that the capacity for anaerobic metabolism ($E_{anaerobic}$) is limited, the time over which a mechanical power, and thus performance, can be sustained will depend inversely on the rate at which this limited energy source is used. The extent to which $E_{aerobic}$ meets the energy requirements during the early period of exercise depends on its kinetic response and is often expressed as the time constant of $\dot{V}O_2$ ($E_{aer}\tau$).

Consequently, walking performance depends on aerobic metabolism and the extent to which it meets the energy requirements, mechanical efficiency, anaerobic capacity and body mass. Some of the physiological phenomena stated in Figure 39.1 that underpin the energetic characteristics will be discussed in this chapter. Since the functional capacity of the leg muscles, particularly triceps surae, is usually most affected in PAD, walking performance and its energetic characteristics are ultimately limited by physiological phenomena occurring in one or both legs.

Walking performance

Walking performance, whether expressed in units of time or distance, has two main dimensions: pain-free and maximal performance. Although maximal

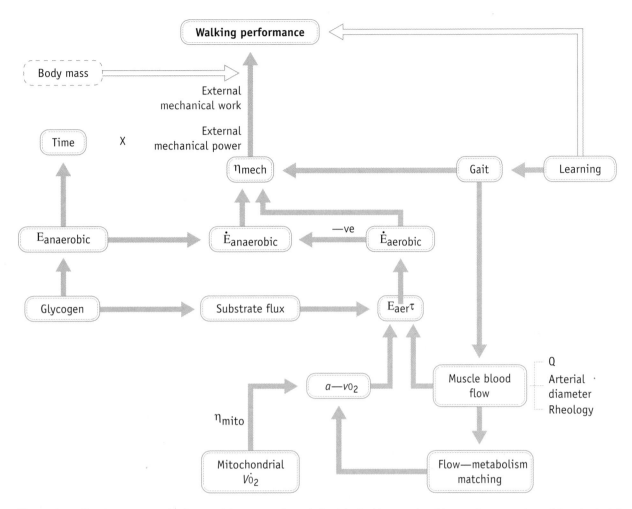

Figure 39.1 Simple, conceptual schema of the energetic and physiological bases of walking performance in peripheral arterial disease.

performance is the focus of Figure 39.1, pain-free walking performance is highly relevant to the comfort associated with walking for people with PAD. On average, the maximum time spent on walking tests is several minutes and, for incremental protocols, usually ranges between 6 and 11 min (Barker et al 1998, Hiatt et al 1988, Womack et al 1997). This performance is ~40–50% of that observed in healthy, age-matched controls (Regensteiner et al 1993). For incremental protocols, the time to the onset of muscle pain lies, on average, between 2 and 4 min or ~30–50% of maximum time (Askew et al 1997, Hiatt et al 1988, Womack et al 1997). Thus, the majority of walking performed on treadmill tests occurs in the presence of pain.

Mechanical efficiency

Mechanical efficiency (η_{mech}) is the ratio of mechanical power to energy expenditure. Mechanical efficiency during walking is more commonly measured as walking economy, which is the $\dot{V}_{O_2}$ at a given walking speed. Improvements in walking economy (i.e. η_{mech} in Fig. 39.1) increase performance (Olds et al 1993, Peronnet & Thibault 1989). There are no comparative data on walking economy for patients and controls. However, short-term training can improve both walking economy and performance in PAD (Hiatt et al 1990, 1994, Womack et al 1997). For example, a 20% increase in walking economy observed after 6 weeks of training occurred in the presence of a 55% increase in walking performance and no change in peak $\dot{V}O_2$ (Hiatt et al 1990). Although it is not possible to accurately quantify the contribution of this change in economy to walking performance, these data illustrate that a major cause of the increase in walking performance during the initial periods of training is probably an improved η_{mech}. Some of the underlying mechanisms of training-induced improvements in walking economy have been discussed by others (Green & Mehlsen 1999, Hiatt et al 1990, Womack et al 1997).

AEROBIC METABOLISM ($E_{aerobic}$)

The duration a given mechanical power output can be sustained for depends on the extent to which $E_{aerobic}$ can meet the energy requirements (Fig. 39.1). Since the capacity for anaerobic ATP synthesis is very limited, sustaining mechanical power outputs for longer than ~30–60 s depends critically on increasing $E_{aerobic}$, or $\dot{V}O_2$, rapidly and to peak values that meet the energy requirements. An impairment in these responses will increase the contribution of $E_{anaerobic}$ to energy expenditure, reduce the time it takes to maximize anaerobic ATP synthesis and ultimately fail to sustain the required power output.

Considerable attention has been given to the importance of the limitation in peak $\dot{V}O_2$ to performance in PAD, which is ~50% of that seen in older, healthy adults (Regensteiner et al 1993). In contrast, there has been very little focus on $\dot{V}O_2$ kinetics despite the fact that an increase in $\dot{V}O_2$ kinetics, independent of increases in peak $\dot{V}O_2$, can improve exercise performance considerably (Olds et al 1993). Recent evidence, however, suggests that the rate of increase in $\dot{V}O_2$ (i.e. $E_{aerobic}\tau$ in Fig. 39.1) is slowed in PAD (Bauer et al 1999). Given that these impaired 'whole body' responses are primarily limited by phenomena local to the exercising legs, then the limitation to whole body $\dot{V}O_2$ is presumably localized to the exercising leg muscles and, in particular, triceps surae. Explaining impairments in both $\dot{V}O_2$ kinetics and peak $\dot{V}O_2$ and their alleviation through training focuses attention on leg muscle $\dot{V}O_2$ and its determinants, leg muscle blood flow and the arterial–venous O_2 difference (i.e. $a–vO_{2\,diff}$) (Fig. 39.1). Leg muscle blood flow has been discussed in a companion review (Green & Mehlsen 1999) and will not be addressed here.

AEROBIC METABOLISM AND $a–vO_2$ DIFFERENCE (O_2 EXTRACTION)

There is no evidence that either the temporal increase in, or peak value of, O_2 extraction across active skeletal muscle during exercise is impaired in PAD. Prior to training, the peak level of O_2 extraction, as represented by femoral venous PO_2, during exercise by the calf or thigh is relatively higher in PAD than in 'controls' (Lundgren et al 1988, Pernow et al 1975, Sorlie & Myhre 1978, Zetterquist 1970). Following exercise training, the femoral venous PO_2 during maximal walking is further reduced in PAD (Sorlie & Myhre 1978, Zetterquist 1970). As shown elsewhere (Green & Mehlsen 1999), this training effect could increase calf muscle $\dot{V}O_2$ by ~9%, and perhaps performance by a slightly larger extent.

Differences in either the kinetics or peak values of O_2 extraction might be attributed, in part, to differences in mitochondrial $\dot{V}O_2$ (Fig. 39.1). It has long been argued that muscle 'oxidative capacity' adapts to PAD (Bylund-Fellenius et al 1981, Jansson et al 1988, Lundgren et al 1989). This argument is based on evidence of higher than normal activities for citrate synthase (Bylund et al 1976, Bylund-Fellenius et al 1981, Hiatt et al 1996, Jansson et al 1988, Lundgren et al 1989) and cytochrome oxidase (Bylund et al 1976, Bylund-Fellenius et al 1981, Lundgren et al 1989), although this is not always observed (Clyne et al 1985, Henriksson et al 1980). It is also based on the finding of a lower muscle lactate/pyruvate ratio at a given muscle PO_2, and it was suggested that this would enable patients to maintain a higher oxidative rate at a given muscle PO_2 (Bylund-Fellenius et al 1981). The importance of muscle oxidative capacity to exercise performance in PAD is reflected in evidence that cytochrome oxidase activity was positively related to walking performance, and that the training responses of these two variables were also positively related (Lundgren et al 1989). We have recently shown that the peak rate of ATP synthesis of mitochondria isolated from muscle samples taken from the gastrocnemius medialis muscle is positively related to pain-free walking time in PAD (Hou et al 1999). Therefore, muscle mitochondrial function appears to be important to walking performance in PAD and its response to training.

In contrast to adaptive changes in muscle oxidative metabolism, there is evidence of impaired mitochondrial metabolism in PAD (Brevetti et al 1988, Hands et al 1986, Hiatt et al 1992, 1996, Kemp et al 1993). Using ^{1}H magnetic resonance spectroscopy to study gastrocnemius metabolism immediately following calf exercise, Kemp et al (1993) revealed, relative to normal responses, a reduced and 'right-shifted' relationship between maximal mitochondrial ATP synthesis and [ADP]. This is similar to that observed in mitochondrial myopathy (Kemp et al 1993), but different to skeletal muscle dysfunction in other cardiovascular diseases, such as coronary heart failure, that might be due simply to the loss of mitochondria (Kemp et al 1993, Magnusson et al 1996). We have also found that differences in muscle mitochondrial function between people with PAD are not due to differences in mitochondrial volume, but rather due to functional changes inherent in mitochondria (Hou et al 1999). These data suggest that functional impairments in skeletal muscle mitochondria might occur and contribute to the walking intolerance in PAD.

The nature of such an impairment and its contribution to walking intolerance are not clear. As illustrated in Figure 39.1, in addition to blood flow, 'substrate flux' is an important determinant of the kinetic response of $\dot{V}o_2$. The primary substrate for aerobic metabolism is acetyl-CoA, which, in turn, is mainly supplied through glycolysis and beta-oxidation. Using both a dog and human exercise model characterized by reduced muscle blood flow, Timmons et al (1996, 1998) showed that increasing the availability of acetyl groups and, thus, acetyl-CoA in skeletal muscle prior to exercise increases the rate of oxidative phosphorylation during the initial period of exercise. Thus, flux through the tricarboxylate (TCA) cycle can be limited by acetyl-CoA supply, even under conditions of low blood and O_2 supply. TCA flux can also be impaired by low levels of TCA intermediates caused by reduced anapleurosis (Sahlin et al 1990). Testable hypotheses are that a lower than normal TCA flux occurs during the initial periods of exercise and contributes to the slowed $\dot{V}o_2$ kinetics in PAD, and that training improves TCA flux, $\dot{V}o_2$ kinetics and walking performance.

When acetyl-CoA supply exceeds its oxidation through the TCA cycle, the accumulation of acetyl-CoA is buffered by carnitine, resulting in the formation of acetylcarnitine. Short-chain acylcarnitines, of which acetylcarnitine is one type, are higher than normal in PAD skeletal muscle and inversely correlate with walking performance (Hiatt et al 1992). Plasma acetylcarnitine levels are also higher and decrease during walking in people with PAD who perform worse than their counterparts with lower acetylcarnitine levels and which increase with exercise (Brevetti et al 1996). Walking training reduced muscle short-chain acylcarnitine levels, and the reduction was correlated with the improvement in walking performance (Hiatt et al 1996). As yet, the likely mechanisms underpinning these effects have not been suggested. Acetyl-CoA is in equilibrium with acetylcarnitine and inhibits pyruvate dehydrogenase (PDH) activity. Consequently, during the initial period of exercise when PDH activity is still

less than maximal, TCA flux, and thus muscle $\dot{V}o_2$, might be lower in people with higher muscle acetylcarnitine (and acetyl-CoA) due to an impaired supply of acetyl-CoA. This would help to explain the relationships between muscle short-chain acylcarnitine and performance (Hiatt et al 1992, 1996), which would be mediated by difference in $\dot{V}o_2$ kinetics, as well as the findings of Brevetti et al (1996) since a net use, rather than formation, of acetylcarnitine in poor performers reflects a relatively slower production of acetyl-CoA from fat or carbohydrate oxidation and compensatory use of acetyl groups from acetylcarnitine.

Lactate accumulation and release from PAD skeletal muscle during exercise occurs when pyruvate production exceeds its utilization. In response to exercise, PAD muscle usually releases more lactate to the circulation (Lundgren et al 1988, Rexroth et al 1989), presumably because it accumulates more, although there is no direct evidence of this (Bylund-Fellenius et al 1981). In fact, in more severely affected limbs of claudicants, muscle lactate may not accumulate significantly during maximal walking (Hiatt et al 1992), and in people with 'mild' claudication, the muscle pH response to similar, fatiguing exercise was not different from that of healthy controls despite the considerably worse exercise performance (Hands et al 1986). These latter data raise the possibility that, relative to TCA flux, glycolysis is not always accelerated during ischaemic exercise in PAD muscle. Even during short-term ischaemic exercise, PAD muscle oxidizes very little carbohydrate despite extracting relatively more O_2 from the circulation (Lundgren et al 1988), an abnormal response. Given that calf muscle glycogen levels can be lower in PAD muscle (Pastoris et al 1996) and that carbohydrate oxidation is reduced in the glycogen depleted state (Putman et al 1993), it is tempting to suggest that the aforementioned reduced supply of acetyl-CoA might, in some people with PAD, also be due to low glycogen levels and glycogenolysis. Increasing muscle glycogen content in PAD skeletal muscle has also improved exercise performance (Dahllof et al 1975), which demonstrates that glycogen content can limit exercise performance, presumably by limiting substrate flux and, to some extent, the aerobic synthesis of ATP.

The possibility of metabolic impairments in PAD skeletal muscle might appear to be at odds with the higher than normal O_2 extraction during exercise, since the latter appears to suggest that the muscle's capacity to use and extract O_2 from the circulation is not impaired. However, there are possible explanations for the relatively high O_2 extraction which do not necessarily favour improved muscle performance.

First, the lower RQ and the higher rate of oxidation of ketone bodies (Lundgren et al 1988) increase the O_2 cost of ATP synthesis and contribute to a decrease in muscle, and perhaps, walking economy. Second, O_2 extraction will increase as capillary flow decreases and erythrocyte transit time increases. Although there are no reasonable estimates for erythrocyte transit times through muscle capillaries during human exercise, it is likely that when perfusion pressure is very low, such as occurs in PAD (Angelides et al 1978), these transit times will be greater and O_2 extraction will be higher. This effect increases the risk of hypoxia in regions of muscle fibres at the distal ends of capillaries where blood Po_2 is very low. It is unlikely that the higher O_2 extraction is due to improved matching of perfusion with metabolism (Fig. 39.1), given the presence of endothelial dysfunction in PAD and reduced arterial flow to working muscles, both of which would tend to reduce perfusion–metabolism matching (Green & Mehlsen 1999).

O_2 extraction also depends upon the morphology of capillaries and their density in skeletal muscle, as well as the rheological properties of blood (Fig. 39.1). Their importance to aerobic metabolism, walking performance and training responses has been discussed elsewhere (Green & Mehlsen 1999).

ANAEROBIC METABOLISM

Anaerobic ATP synthesis during exercise occurs almost entirely through PCr hydrolysis and lactate production. In healthy humans, the capacity for anaerobic ATP synthesis ($E_{anaerobic}$, Fig. 39.1) can be maximized within ~1–2 min of high-intensity exercise and, depending on the type of exercise, can be as high as 300–400 mmol ATP/kg dry weight (Bangsbo et al 1990, Spriet et al 1987). During maximal activity over this duration, anaerobic metabolism contributes ~30–50% to total ATP synthesis (Medbø et al 1988, Withers et al 1991) and progressively decreases as a function of exercise so that it would contribute ~5–15% to exercise lasting 10 min. Therefore, although anaerobic metabolism during walking or its relative contribution to energy expenditure has not been determined in PAD, it is not likely to contribute to ATP synthesis by any more than 15%. Nevertheless, and as shown in Figure 39.1, $E_{anaerobic}$ is potentially important as it helps to sustain performance when $E_{aerobic}$ cannot meet the energy requirements of walking.

The anaerobic potential of muscle, which is often equated with anaerobic capacity, can be defined by its level of anaerobic fuels (i.e. PCr and glycogen), enzyme activities and buffer value (Green 1994). PAD muscle consists of similar (Bylund-Fellenius et al 1981, Henriksson et al 1980, Hiatt et al 1996, Jansson et al 1988, Lundgren et al 1989, Regensteiner et al 1993) or even higher (Bylund et al 1976, Clyne et al 1985, Henriksson et al 1980) glycolytic enzyme activities, which suggests that the anaerobic potential of skeletal muscle, relative to its size, is not reduced in PAD. In contrast, muscle glycogen and PCr can be less than normal in PAD (Bylund-Fellenius et al 1981, Pastoris et al 1996). Using data on muscle PCr hydrolysis and lactate accumulation during maximal calf exercise of ~2.5 min (Bylund-Fellenius et al 1981), anaerobic ATP synthesis in PAD muscle was only 40% of that calculated for control muscle (60 vs. 150 mmol ATP/kg dry muscle). The apparent mismatch between anaerobic potential and anaerobic ATP synthesis suggests that the anaerobic potential of PAD skeletal muscle is not expressed (as anaerobic ATP) to the same extent as healthy muscle. This might be related to the relatively low PCr and glycogen levels. Approximately 80% of the calculated difference in anaerobic ATP synthesis was due to lactate production, which suggests that reduced glycogenolysis due to reasons previously given (see 'Aerobic metabolism' and 'a–vo_2 difference') may primarily explain the lower anaerobic capacity of PAD muscle. The relatively low anaerobic capacity might also be explained by a lower lactate efflux (relative to lactate production) and impaired [H^+] regulation due to poor blood flow (Green 1994), and/or a reduced activation of skeletal muscle.

Regardless of the reasons, the lower anaerobic ATP yield would help to explain the lower than normal calf capacity to sustain short-term exercise in PAD (Bylund-Fellenius et al 1981, Gerdle et al 1986) and contribute to some extent to the walking impairment in PAD. Whether or not this can increase with training and contribute to the improvement in walking performance has not been tested.

MUSCLE MORPHOLOGY AND HISTOLOGY

The cross-sectional area (CSA) of triceps surae is slightly lower (5%) in diseased compared with non-symptomatic PAD limbs, with the latter being similar to healthy control values (Regensteiner et al 1993). That atrophy worsens in more severe PAD is confirmed in autopsy material, where a lower CSA was observed in PAD muscle that was entirely attributed to the lower CSA (by 40%) of gastrocnemius, rather than soleus (Hedberg et al 1989).

Some studies have reported that the distribution of type I and type II fibres in either gastrocnemius or tibialis anterior is similar in PAD compared with controls (Clyne et al 1982, Henriksson et al 1980) or asymptomatic limbs (Henriksson et al 1980, Jansson et al 1988, Sjostrom et al 1980). In more severe PAD, however, gastrocnemius is composed of relatively more type I and fewer type II fibres than controls (Clyne et al 1982, Hedberg et al 1989, Makitie & Teravainen 1977). In gastrocnemius, the CSA occupied by type II fibres is lower in ischaemic limbs compared with asymptomatic or healthy control limbs (Clyne et al 1982, Regensteiner et al 1993). This is due to both the reduced type II fibre area (Clyne et al 1982, Makitie & Teravainen 1977, Regensteiner et al 1993), which might be specific to type IIb muscle (Hammarsten et al 1980), and type II fibre loss (Hedberg et al 1989). This fibre loss is more extensive in severe PAD (Clyne et al 1982) and can result in amputation (Hedberg et al 1989).

That walking performance in PAD is fuelled primarily by aerobic metabolism suggests that the recruitment of fatigue-resistant type I or type IIa fibres is crucial to performance. This has been confirmed by the positive relationship between the proportion of type I fibres in the ischaemic limb (i.e. tibialis anterior muscle) and walking performance (Sjostrom et al 1980). On the basis of this evidence, Sjostrom et al (1980) suggested that ischaemic muscle invokes 'selective metabolic exploitation' to maximize walking performance in the presence of PAD. This assumes that a relatively more fatigue-resistant muscle, as reflected in the relative increase in type I area, is created out of either the selective death (Hedberg et al 1989) or, perhaps in less severe PAD (Hammarsten et al 1980), transformation of type II fibres.

This view should be contrasted with the loss of calf strength associated with calf and type II fibre atrophy in PAD (Regensteiner et al 1993). It should also be tempered by the evidence that type I fibre area might also be reduced in PAD (Clyne et al 1982, 1985, Henriksson et al 1980) and that type I fibre loss occurs, at least when the disease is severe (Hedberg et al 1989). Regardless of its aetiology, the end result would be a reduced peak $E_{aerobic}$, $E_{anaerobic}$ (Fig. 39.1) and muscle capacity for sustained work (Gerdle et al 1986). When the endurance capacity of lower limb muscles, such as triceps surae, is reduced in the absence of reductions in body weight, the load imposed on such muscle during weight-bearing exercise, relative to its capacity to sustain the load, is increased. This would reduce the time the load can be sustained for (Hillestad 1963), and in this way, walking performance could be progressively reduced.

CONCLUSIONS

1. As illustrated using a conceptual model of walking performance and physiology, walking intolerance in PAD has a multifaceted aetiology.
2. While the reduced leg blood flow is a primary manifestation of PAD and a contributor to walking intolerance, both morphological and biochemical changes in skeletal muscle also contribute to walking intolerance.
3. Although it is not known whether walking economy is impaired in PAD, it does improve with training and could be a major contributor to the training-induced improvement in walking performance.
4. Peak aerobic power and $\dot{V}_{O_2}$ kinetics are reduced in PAD, probably a result of both the impaired leg blood flow and substrate flux in skeletal muscle.
5. The impaired substrate flux could also account for the lower anaerobic capacity in PAD skeletal muscle.
6. This variety in physiological impairment means that potentially a number of different therapies can be designed to help improve walking performance in PAD.

REFERENCES

Angelides N, Nicolaides A, Needham T, Dudley H 1978 The mechanism of calf claudication: studies of simultaneous clearance of $^{99}Tc^m$ from the calf and thigh. British Journal of Surgery 65: 204–209

Askew C, Green S, Walken P J, Codd C 1997 The reproducibility and stability of walking and cycling capacity in people with intermittent claudication. ANZ Angiology Conference, Brisbane, Australia, 1997

Bangsbo J, Gollnick P D, Graham T E, Juel C, Kiens B, Mizuno M, Saltin B 1990 Anaerobic energy production and O_2 deficit-debt relationship during exhaustive exercise in humans. Journal of Physiology (Lond.) 422: 539–559

Barker G, Green S, Askew C, Walker P W 1998 Effect of propionyl-L-carnitine supplementation on exercise performance in peripheral arterial disease. Third Annual Conference of the European College of Sports Science, Manchester

Barnard R J 1994 Physical activity, fitness, and claudication. In: Bouchard C, Shephard R J, Stephens T (eds) Physical activity, fitness, and health. Human Kinetics, Champaign, IL, p 622–632

Bauer T A, Regensteiner J G, Brass E P, Hiatt W R 1999 Oxygen uptake kinetics during exercise are slowed in patients with peripheral arterial disease. Journal of Applied Physiology 87: 809–816

Brass E P, Hiatt W R 1994 Carnitine metabolism during exercise. Life Sciences 54: 1383–1393

Brevetti G, Chiariello M, Ferulano G et al 1988 Increases in walking distance in patients with peripheral vascular disease treated with L-carnitine: a double-blind, cross-over study. Circulation 77: 767–773

Brevetti G, di Lisa F, Perna S, Menabo R, Barbato R, Martone V D, Siliprandi N 1996 Carnitine-related alterations in patients with intermittent claudication. Circulation 93: 1685–1689

Bylund A-C, Hammarsten J, Holm J, Schersten T 1976 Enzyme activities in skeletal muscles from patients with peripheral arterial insufficiency. European Journal of Clinical Investigation 6: 425–429

Bylund-Fellenius P, Walker M, Elander A, Holm S, Schersten T 1981 Energy metabolism in relation to oxygen partial pressure in human skeletal muscle during exercise. Biochemistry Journal 200: 247–255

Clyne C A C, Weller R O, Bradley W G, Silber D I, O'Donnell T F, Callow A D 1982 Ultrastructural and capillary adaptation of gastrocnemius muscle to occlusive peripheral vascular disease. Surgery 92: 434–440

Clyne C A C, Mears H, Weller R O, O'Donnell T F 1985 Calf muscle adaptation to peripheral vascular disease. Cardiovascular Research 19: 507–512

Dahllof A-G, Holm J, Kral J, Schersten T 1975 The relationship between glycogen content of leg muscles and working capacity in patients with intermittent claudication. Acta Chirurgica Scandinavica 141: 329–332

Donovan J 1994 Australia's Health 1994. Australian Government Publishing Service, Canberra, p 322

Gardner A W, Poehlman E T 1995 Exercise rehabilitation programs for the treatment of claudication pain. Journal of the American Medical Association 274: 975–980

Gerdle B, Hedberg B, Angquist K-A, Fugl-Meyer A R 1986 Isokinetic strength and endurance in peripheral arterial insufficiency with intermittent claudication. Scandinavian Journal of Rehabilitation and Medicine 18: 9–15

Green S 1994 A definition and systems view of anaerobic capacity. European Journal of Applied Physiology 69: 168–173

Green S, Mehlsen J 1999 Peripheral arterial disease. In: Saltin B, Boushel R, Secher N, Mitchell J (eds) Exercise and the circulation in health and disease. Human Kinetics, Champaign, IL

Hammarsten J, Bylund-Fellenius A-C, Holm J, Schersten T, Krotkiewski M 1980 Capillary supply and muscle fibre types in patients with intermittent claudication: relationships between morphology and metabolism. European Journal of Clinical Investigation 10: 301–305

Hands L J, Bore P J, Galloway G, Morris P J, Radda G K 1986 Muscle metabolism in patients with peripheral vascular disease investigated by ^{31}P nuclear magnetic resonance spectroscopy. Clinical Science 41: 283–290

Hedberg B, Angquist K-A, Henriksson-Larsen K, Sjostrom M 1989 Fibre loss and distribution in skeletal muscle from patients with severe peripheral arterial insufficiency. European Journal of Vascular Surgery 3: 315–322

Henriksson J, Nygaard E, Andersson J, Eklof B 1980 Enzyme activities, fibre types and capillarization in calf muscles of patients with intermittent claudication. Scandinavian Journal of Clinical and Laboratory Investigation 40: 361–369

Hiatt W R, Hirsch A T, Regensteiner J G, Brass E P 1995 Clinical trials for claudication. Assessment of exercise performance, functional status, and clinical end points. Circulation 92: 614–621

Hiatt W R, Nawaz D, Regensteiner J G, Hossack K F 1988 The evaluation of exercise performance in patients with peripheral vascular disease. Journal of Cardiopulmonary Rehabilitation 12: 525–532

Hiatt W R, Regensteiner J G, Hargarten M E, Wolfel E, Brass E P 1990 Benefit of exercise conditioning for patients with peripheral arterial disease. Circulation 81: 602–609

Hiatt W R, Wolfel E E, Meier R H, Regensteiner J G, Brass E P 1992 Skeletal muscle carnitine metabolism in patients with unilateral peripheral arterial disease. Journal of Applied Physiology 73: 346–353

Hiatt W R, Wolfel E E, Meier R H, Regensteiner J G 1994 Superiority of treadmill walking exercise versus strength training for patients with peripheral arterial disease. Implications for the mechanism of the training response. Circulation 90: 1866–1874

Hiatt W R, Regensteiner J G, Wolfel E E, Carry M R, Brass E P 1996 Effect of exercise training on skeletal muscle histology and metabolism in peripheral arterial disease. Journal of Applied Physiology 81: 780–788

Hillestad L K 1963 The peripheral blood flow in intermittent claudication. IV. Significance of the claudication distance. Acta Medica Scandinavica 173: 467–478

Hou X-Y, Green S, Askew C, Walker P W 1999 Mitochondrial function, blood flow and walking performance in peripheral arterial disease. The Fifth IOC World Congress of Sports Science, Sydney

Jannson E, Johansson J, Sylven C, Kaijser L 1988 Calf muscle adaptation in intermittent claudication. Side-differences in muscle metabolic characteristics in patients with unilateral arterial disease. Clinical Physiology 8: 17–29

Jelnes R, Cnudsting O, Jensen K H, Bokgaard N, Tonnesen K H, Schroder T 1986 Fate in intermittent claudication. Outcome and risk factors. British Medical Journal 293: 1137

Kannel W B, Skinner J J, Schwartz M J, Shurtleff D 1970 Intermittent claudication. Incidence in the Framingham study. Circulation 41: 875

Kemp G J, Taylor D J, Thompson C H, Hands L J, Rajagopalan B, Styles P, Radda G K 1993 Quantitative analysis by 31P magnetic resonance spectroscopy of abnormal mitochondrial oxidation in skeletal muscle during recovery from exercise. NMR in Biomedicine 6: 302–310

Lundgren F, Bennegard K, Elander A, Lundholm K, Schersten T, Bylund-Fellenius A-C 1988 Substrate exchange in human limb muscle during exercise at reduced blood flow. American Journal of Physiology 255: H1156–1164

Lundgren F, Dahllof A-G, Schersten T, Bylund-Fellenius A-C 1989 Muscle enzyme adaptation in patients with peripheral arterial insufficiency: spontaneous adaptation, effect of different treatments and consequences on walking performance. Clinical Science 77: 485–493

Magnusson G, Kaijser L, Rong H, Isberg B, Sylvens C, Saltin B 1996 Exercise capacity in heart failure patients: relative importance of heart and skeletal muscle. Clinical Physiology 16: 183–195

Makitie J, Teravainen H 1977 Histochemical changes in striated muscle in patients with intermittent claudication. Archives in Pathological and Laboratory Medicine 101: 658–663

Medbø J I, Mohn A C, Tabata I, Bahr R, Vaage O, Sejersted O H 1988 Anaerobic capacity determined by maximal accumulated O_2 deficit. Journal of Applied Physiology 64: 50–60

Olds T S, Norton K I, Craig N P 1993 Mathematical model of cycling performance. Journal of Applied Physiology 75: 730–737

Pastoris O, Panella L, Foppa P et al 1996 Instrumental and metabolic evaluation of patients affected by peripheral arterial occlusive disease (PAOD) following surgical revascularisation surgery. Giornale Italiano di Medicina del Lavoro 18: 41–49

Pernow B, Saltin B, Wahren J, Cronestrand R, Ekestrom S 1975 Leg blood flow and muscle metabolism in occlusive arterial disease of the leg before and after reconstructive surgery. Clinical Science and Molecular Medicine 49: 265–275

Peronnet F, Thibault G 1989 Mathematical analysis of running performance and world running records. Journal of Applied Physiology 67: 453–455

Putman C, Spriet L, Hultman E et al 1993 Pyruvate dehydrogenase activity and acetyl group accumulation during exercise after different diets. American Journal of Physiology 265: E752–760

Regensteiner J G, Hiatt W R 1995 Exercise rehabilitation for patients with peripheral arterial disease. Exercise and Sports Sciences Reviews 23: 1–24

Regensteiner J G, Wolfel E E, Brass E P et al 1993 Chronic changes in skeletal muscle histology and function in peripheral arterial disease. Circulation 87: 413–421

Rexroth W, Hageloch W, Isgro F, Koeth T, Manzl G, Weicker H 1989 Influence of peripheral arterial occlusive disease on muscular metabolism. Klinische Wochenschrift 67: 576–582

Sahlin K, Katz A, Broberg S 1990 Tricarboxylic acid cycle intermediates in human muscle during prolonged exercise. American Journal of Physiology 259: C834–841

Sjostrom M, Angquist K-A, Rais O 1980 Intermittent claudication and muscle fiber fine structure: correlation between clinical and morphological data. Ultrastructural Pathology 1: 309–326

Sorlie D, Myhre K 1978 Effects of physical training in intermittent claudication. Scandinavian Journal of Clinical and Laboratory Investigation 38: 217–222

Spriet L L, Soderlund K, Bergstrom M, Hultman E 1987 Anaerobic energy release in skeletal muscle during electrical stimulation in men. Journal of Applied Physiology 62: 611–615

Timmons J, Gustafsson T, Sundberg E, Jansson E, Greenhaff P 1998 Substrate availability limits human skeletal muscle oxidative ATP regeneration at the onset of exercise. Journal of Clinical Investigation 101: 79–85

Timmons J, Poucher S, Constantin-Teodosiu D, Worrall V, Macdonald I, Greenhaff P 1996 Metabolic response of canine gracilis muscle during contraction with partial ischaemia. American Journal of Physiology 270: E400–406

Withers R T, Sherman W M, Clark D G, Esselbach P C, Nolan S R, Mackay M H, Brinkman M 1991 Muscle metabolism during 30, 60 and 90 s of maximal cycling on an air-braked ergometer. European Journal of Applied Physiology and Occupational Physiology 63: 354–362

Womack C, Sieminski D J, Katzel L I, Yataco A, Gardner A 1997 Improved walking economy in patients with peripheral arterial disease. Medicine and Science in Sports and Exercise 29: 1286–1290

Zetterquist S 1970 The effect of active training on the nutritive blood flow in exercising ischemic legs. Scandinavian Journal of Clinical and Laboratory Investigation 25: 101–111

40

Anabolic steroid use in adolescents

Pirkko Korkia

KEY POINTS

1. American and Canadian studies of anabolic-androgenic steroid (AS) use among adolescents suggest that substantial numbers may be taking them. Information from the UK is lacking although some studies suggest that one in three adult users start AS use in their teens.
2. The major reasons for taking AS among young people involve improved sports performance and appearance.
3. The risks of their use are thought to be much the same for both adolescents and adults, apart from the possibility of growth arrest in adolescents and, generally, their greater sensitivity to the drug effects.
4. There are no studies on the effects of self-administered AS use among adolescents, and therefore little is known about the long-term effects and their severity.
5. Attitudes and risk-taking behaviour can be used to predict AS use among adolescents.
6. Early adolescence may be a critical time to prevent AS use, because normal adolescent growth and maturation might be incorrectly thought of as AS-assisted improvement in size and performance.

INTRODUCTION

In the USA and Canada, sizeable proportions of the young are reported either to have taken anabolic-androgenic steroids (AS) or to be at risk of taking them in the future. Currently, only data from one British survey, from a small town in Scotland, are available, but interviews with adult users in the UK indicate that AS use often starts in the teenage years.

The American Association of Pediatrics (AAP) has unequivocally condemned the use of AS because of the toxic side-effects, because it constitutes cheating in sport and because AS users put others at risk of becoming users. This is because young athletes who do not want to take AS are forced either to live with the fact that others may have an unfair advantage, or to join in and accept the attendant risks of side-effects. It clearly is unfair that young athletes should even have to consider such a choice. In the current economic climate in sport, with the financial and personal advantages brought by sporting success, it is not surprising that young athletes are tempted to resort to banned performance-enhancing agents such as AS. Much adolescent AS use, however, appears to be associated with the 'body culture' rather than competitive sport, and such peer pressure appears to be influential. Previous studies suggest that adolescents who begin to use AS at an early age often continue to use several types of AS for extended periods of time. They tend to show behaviour, perceptions and opinions that are consistent with habituation. For these reasons alone, prevention of AS use is important.

Although much media attention has been directed at AS use in recent years, it is not a new phenomenon among adolescents: the USA, as long ago as 1959, a Texan physician was rumoured to have administered Dianabol to a high school football team for an entire season (Yesalis et al 1993). In the 1960s, a secret study was undertaken on steroid use by a high school football team who were allegedly given AS by the team physician working with a pharmaceutical company (Gilbert 1969). Sadly, coaches, parents, older athletes and doctors were found to be involved in abetting the use of these drugs. Results from intervention trials among high-risk adolescent athletes suggest that school-based prevention programmes can be successful in deterring AS use.

WHAT ARE ANABOLIC-ANDROGENIC STEROIDS?

Anabolic steroids are derivatives of the male hormone testosterone. They have two main actions: anabolic (tissue-building) and androgenic (male-producing).

Young adults and adolescents use them to improve muscle mass, strength and sporting performance. They have four main postulated mechanisms of action. One of these is improved protein synthesis, which results in increased muscle mass. They are anti-catabolic, allowing the user to train at a greater intensity for longer and with shorter rest periods between bouts of training. They appear to stimulate the central nervous system, thereby increasing motivation, confidence and perceived energy levels, and they seem to delay the sense of fatigue. AS are also known to have a powerful placebo effect. Due to their anti-catabolic actions, AS can be viewed as useful in almost any sport where training and competition tend to be limited by 'overtraining' and injury. Although their effectiveness is still somewhat debated, there is good evidence to show that they do improve muscle mass and size. Less is known about their anti-catabolic and stimulatory effects in sports persons.

Anabolic steroids are commonly taken in tablet form and by injection. They are mostly taken in cycles of 5–8 weeks on, followed by 5–8 weeks off. It is common to take two or more AS and other drugs at the same time. Other drugs taken together with AS are intended either to enhance their effects or to prevent side-effects. Much of the information on the relative effectiveness of the various drug-taking regimes employed by users is based on trial and error.

PREVALENCE OF AS USE AMONG THE YOUNG

The first nationwide study of AS use among adolescents was published in the USA (Buckley et al 1988). The study found that of the 3403 questionnaire respondents, 6.6% of 12th grade high school pupils had taken AS, and that the user group tended to be older (>19 years) than non-users. Based on their studies, the researchers suggested that there might be between 250 000 and 500 000 adolescents in the USA taking AS. Other studies following this publication have found the prevalence of AS use to be between 1.9 and 11%, with about 1% of girls taking them (Table 40.1). In some cases, AS use started as early as the age of 8. Apparently, the numbers of teenage girls taking AS in the USA is on the increase, while male use has stabilized (Yesalis et al 1997). Research by the Canadian Centre for Drug-Free Sport (CCDS) in 1994 showed that 2.8% of the 16 000 11- to 18-year-olds had taken AS (Melia 1994). Some 83 000 of the 3 million young Canadians are estimated to be taking them. The single UK study by Williamson (1993) found that 4.4% of technical college students in the west coast of Scotland

Table 40.1 Summary of studies of the prevalence of AS use among adolescents

Authors	No. of responses	AS used (%)	Reasons for taking AS	Age at first use (years)
Buckley et al (1988), USA	3403 (M)	6.6	47% ↑ sports performance, 27% ↑ appearance, 17% due to peer pressure	14.8 (average start age)
Johnson et al (1989), USA	853 (M)	11.1	64% strength, 50% size, 27% appearance, 10% because friends used	–
Terney & McLain (1990), USA	2113	6.5, 2.5 (M,F)	5.5% of athletes, 2.4% of non-athletes. Highest use among football players and wrestlers	–
Adlaf & Smart (1992), Canada	3892	2.1, 0.2 (M,F: in past yr)	Not specified, but users participated – significantly more in weight-lifting and bodybuilding than non-users	–
Komoroski & Rickert (1992), USA	1492	7.6, 1.5 (M,F)	64% ↑ strength, 48% ↑ size, 44% ↑ appearance, 17% peer pressure	14.8 (average start age)
Gaa et al (1994), USA	3047	35, 0.9 (M,F)	22% ↑ performance 16% ↑ appearance, 14% injury prevention	10 or younger
Tanner et al (1995), USA	6930	4, 1.3 (M,F)	In athletes: 50% to ↑ performance, 16% ↑ appearance, 10% peer pressure In non-athletes: 49% ↑ appearance	8 (youngest)
Melia (1994), Canada	16 000	7, 2 (M,F)	50% ↑ performance, 46% ↑ appearance	11

M, males; F, females.

admitted prior use of AS. Some information can be obtained from less specific surveys; for example, Korkia & Stimson (1993) reported that, of 1310 male respondents in their survey of 21 gyms, 75 were 18 years or younger, and six (8%) of these admitted having taken AS. Of the 110 AS users interviewed for the same study, 10 were between 17 and 19 years of age. Lenehan et al (1996) later surveyed the north-west of England and found that, of the 1105 respondents from 43 gymnasia, 26.7% (258 of 967) of the men and 4% (5 of 125) of the women were currently using AS; the youngest user was 16 years of age. They estimated that 1 in 50 of the 25- to 29-year-olds in the north-west of England are taking AS. More importantly, of the 386 AS users Lenehan et al (1996) also interviewed, 1 in 3 said that they had started taking AS in their teens. Very few teenage AS users have been reported in UK surveys, and it is possible that this has remained a hidden problem as teenagers are not accessed through surveys of the gymnasia.

WHY DO YOUNG PEOPLE TAKE AS?

In the UK, unlike the USA, sports scholarships generally play no role in attracting youngsters to experiment and use performance-enhancing aids. The reasons for,

and prevalence of, use of such aids among the young are therefore likely to be different from those in the USA and elsewhere. Studies of UK youth populations have suggested that improved appearance/physique and improvement in sporting performance were the most common reasons for taking AS (Williamson 1993). Data from Korkia & Stimson's (1993) study on five 17- to 18-year-olds revealed that increased strength (4), muscle mass (3) and sports performance (3) were the reasons for taking AS. Reasons for weight training included improved condition (4), appearance (3) and self-esteem (3). Larger-scale investigations in the USA and Canada show similar trends. Table 40.1. summarizes previous studies, including information on the prevalence, reasons for use and the age at which AS were first tried. Adult and adolescent users tend to cite similar reasons for AS use (Korkia & Stimson 1993, Lenehan et al 1996).

Body-building competitions are largely perceived to be the pastime of adults, but competition categories for the under-18s/teens exist both in the USA and in UK. Although the number of youngsters taking part in such competitions in UK is likely to be small, those who do will inevitably be exposed to a variety of growth agents and other drugs used with them. Gaa et al (1994) drew attention to the fact that school athletes often train with weights in an unsupervised situation, thus exposing themselves to dealers and AS. Like adults, teenagers tend to feel that AS can benefit performance. Unlike in adults, improvement is not necessarily the result of training and drug use alone, but may reflect the nature of the growth process itself and the surge in circulating testosterone levels. The use of AS among high school athletes is now considered to be a major national problem in the USA (Goldberg et al 1996). Peer pressure and pressure at school to 'win at all cost' are in part responsible for this. Sadly, substantial numbers of AS users in US studies have reported that teachers and coaches actively encourage their use. It is not surprising to find relatively high levels of use with these types of pressures, especially when coupled with easy access to the drugs.

KNOWLEDGE ABOUT AS

Studies investigating the knowledge of and attitudes towards the risks of AS use among adolescents generally indicate a lack of critical knowledge or denial about the effects of these drugs and healthy alternatives, such as optimal nutrition and physical training. Tanner et al (1995) found that non-AS users recognized more of the health risks than did users, although they postulated that this could be due to denial on the part of the users. Goldberg et al (1996) reported critical knowledge deficits about AS effects among those who were associated with a greater intent to use AS in the future. A survey of 3353 students in high schools in Denver discovered that 60% did not realize that liver disease is a potential risk, about 30% failed to identify heart disease and growth arrest, and about 20% were unable to identify risks of addiction, aggressiveness, cancer and breast enlargement in males (Tanner et al 1995). Interestingly, a considerable number of students thought that AS can be used to increase height (Johnson et al 1989, Tanner et al 1995), and such beliefs may provide a temptation to experiment with them. As in most other studies, Komoroski & Rickert (1992) reported that in the majority of cases, AS are bought on the 'black market' and the suppliers provide an important source of information about them, thus compromising the advice offered. Overlooking health risks, real or perceived, tends to be consistent with other adolescent drug use behaviour.

PATTERNS OF USE

Little is known about actual patterns and practices of self-administering AS use among adolescents.

Table 40.2 AS cycle of an 18-year-old (Korkia & Stimson 1993)

Drug taken	Dose (mg/week)	Period taken (weeks)
Dianabol (methandrostenolone)	175	10
Deca Durabolin (nandrolone decanoate)	100	10
Anavar (oxandrolone)	70	10
Tamoxifen (anti-oestrogen)	70	6

Table 40.3 Self-reported side-effects of AS use in five 17- to 18-year-olds (Korkia & Stimson 1993)

Observations (no.)	Side-effect reported
5	Acne
4	Increased appetite
3	Testicular atrophy
3	Nose bleeds
3	Deepening of voice
2	Water retention
2	Increased body hair
1	Baldness
1	Gynaecomastia
1	Reproductive problems

Examples from a UK government report (Korkia & Stimson 1993) include an 18-year-old taking 175 mg of Dianabol (methandrostenolone, oral) per week for 8 weeks, a 17-year-old taking 250 mg of testosterone (unspecified, injected) for 6 weeks and an 18-year-old taking Deca-Durabolin (nandrolone decanoate, injected) 800 mg/week for 8 weeks. All took only one preparation during the specified cycle. Table 40.2 details the last cycle described by another 18-year-old, and Table 40.3 shows the side-effects reported by the five young users interviewed by Korkia & Stimson (1993). Much of this information suggests that AS use may be similar in the young and adults. The young are also at risk of involuntary under- or overdosing through the use of black market preparations, often of dubious quality and composition.

RISKS INVOLVED IN AS USE
Adverse effects on health

Short-term studies of the adverse effects of AS on adults have shown a transitory effect on a variety of health indices involving the cardiovascular system, liver, reproductive system, musculoskeletal system, skin, hair, immune system, endocrine system and the

---

> **Box 40.1** Adverse health effects associated with AS use
>
> - *Cosmetic effects* – acne, changes in facial, body and scalp hair patterns, deepening of voice, development of breast tissue in men and clitoral enlargement in women
> - *Cardiovascular effects* – derangement of plasma lipids (↓HDL and ↑LDL levels), cardiomyopathy, stroke and elevated blood pressure
> - *Liver toxicity* – liver function abnormalities, cholestatic jaundice and peliosis hepatitis
> - *Liver tumours* – appear to promote, rather than initiate, tumour development
> - *Infertility* – lowered sperm production and abnormalities in sperm in men; cessation of menstruation in women

psyche (Box 40.1) (see Korkia 1998a,b for a review). Isolated cases where AS use has been strongly associated with death and serious illness have been a major cause for concern (Capasso 1994, Huie 1994). Reports of Eastern European athletes who were given AS and other drugs throughout their career have been sad, illustrating the potential for harm especially when use starts at a relatively early age. Yesalis et al (1989) have emphasized that stunted growth, suppressed sperm production and increased risk of injury with chronic use could be particularly relevant in adolescents (see Box 40.2 for an index of suspicion that a young athlete may be using AS). The possibility of transmission of blood-borne viruses (especially HIV, hepatitis B and C) has also been raised: Buckley et al (1988) reported that 38% of high school users injected AS, and DuRant et al (1993) found that 25% of the users they investigated had shared needles. At present, few case studies and no long-term studies of health-associated risks of AS use have been carried out in adolescents. Similar to

> **Box 40.2** Index of suspicion of AS use
>
> - A sudden and dramatic weight gain and/or oedema
> - Breast tissue development or sexual dysfunction in males
> - Virilism, especially acne and growth of facial hair in women or prepubertal males
> - Mood swings, ranging from euphoria to aggression and depression
> - Signs of liver dysfunction
> - Increased curiosity about or advanced knowledge of AS

adults, individual responses and reactions to AS are likely to vary a great deal, depending on the type and dose of drug taken.

Surveys of physicians have provided additional information about side-effects. Salva & Bacon (1991) attempted to gather information about the adverse effects of AS in the young by surveying physicians and paediatricians in Texas. Of the 517 respondents, 55% reported having been asked about AS during the past 5 years; 261 physicians reported 1682 enquiries, 60% of which were made by high school boys and 26% by their parents. Less than 1% were made by non-whites. The majority were interested in AS for psychosocial reasons. Although the questionnaire did not ask about side-effects, several physicians volunteered laboratory findings and their own observations. Aggressive behaviour was reported most frequently, followed by sudden large increases in weight, hypertension, acne, elevated values of liver function tests, striate, impotence and testicular atrophy. The types of adverse effects reported by physicians are similar to those commonly observed in adult users.

Growth delay

Stunted growth is a commonly cited side-effect of AS use, although little hard evidence for this exists, perhaps because it is almost impossible to verify with any certainty. The risk of growth arrest continues until bone growth is completed. On average, this occurs by the age of 16 in girls and 18–20 in boys. Studies investigating the delay of growth and puberty provide some information about the potential harm of AS use. Early studies (Sobel et al 1956) suggested that androgen therapy stimulates skeletal maturation more than linear growth, resulting in accelerated closure of the epiphyses in the long bones and shorter than predicted stature. Later studies have generally disagreed, and have concluded that short-term low-dose androgen therapy would not compromise final predicted height (Albanese et al 1994, Bayley et al 1957, Richman & Kirch 1988, Stanhope et al 1988). Accelerated epiphyseal closure has been attributed to the dose and potency of the androgen and to children between the ages of 5.5 and 10. It appears that those with more advanced skeletal maturation fare better with treatment than those with younger skeletal maturation levels (Jackson et al 1973).

Generally, growth delay studies have involved only one drug, low doses (commonly between 2.5 mg/day and 0.25 mg/kg per day) and they have been of short duration, quite unlike self-administered AS use. The true impact of growth agents on bone arrest are therefore yet to be examined. Growth delay studies have also investigated the possible delay in the progression of puberty by the suppression of physiological increase of gonadotrophins (required for the maturation of testicles and the secretion of testosterone) with contradictory results. Generally, adverse health effects in growth delay trials have been minimal and have included virilization with high doses, moderate increase in appetite resulting in some weight gain, and the development of breast tissue with 5–20 mg weekly methyltestosterone treatment. In the absence of significant adverse short-term changes observed in these studies, the need for an assessment of the possibility of delayed side-effects has been raised (Richman & Kirch 1988). Lack of significant adverse effects in clinical trials cannot be used to justify the safe use of AS, because of the fact that they have used low dosages, a single drug and a relatively short period of administration.

Psychological effects

Box 40.3 lists psychological effects commonly associated with AS use. Little is known about any specific psychological effects, or their intensity, in adolescents. Responses from the limited sample of teenage users interviewed by Korkia & Stimson (1993) suggest that, as a group, young people are likely to experience similar symptoms as adult users: aggressive feelings were reported more often when on AS than when off them; sex drive and confidence were also boosted.

It is reasonable to expect that in young people, as in adults, perceived benefits such as increased levels of confidence, feelings of well-being and increased libido may motivate continued use. Yesalis et al (1989) drew

---

Box 40.4 Postulated mechanisms for dependence on AS

Positive reinforcement
I   Brain reward system (as with opiates)
II   ↑ Arousal
     ↑ Confidence
     ↑ Pain tolerance
     ↓ Feeling of fatigue
     Ability to exert ↑ levels of effort
     Peer admiration

Negative reinforcement
Avoidance of depression
Avoidance of withdrawal symptoms
↓ Muscle mass
↓ Social rewards
Avoidance of feeling not big enough

---

attention to the issue of habituation of young people to AS. They found that those who had done more cycles and who started taking AS at a younger age were more likely to exhibit behaviours, perceptions and opinions consistent with habituation. Early intervention is therefore important if first-time AS use and habituation at an early age are to be prevented. Box 40.4 shows ways in which AS may cause dependence in users.

PREDICTING AS USE

Typical signs of AS use are shown in Box 40.2. One or more of these signs in an adolescent should raise the parents', coach's or doctor's level of suspicion. One of the first, and perhaps most important, indications of AS use in boys is that they become obsessive or compulsive about their activity, and as a result there is a sudden and unexpected increase in weight; additionally, their face may become puffy. In girls, acne and facial hair development tend to be the first telltale signs. In applying preventive strategies and early intervention in AS use, the ability to predict the likelihood of future use may be helpful (Box 40.5). This can be done, to some degree, by examining attitudes to and beliefs about the use.

Attitudes

Melia's (1994) study showed that AS use was more likely to occur with increasing level of competition in school sports. Similarly, Terney & McLain (1990) found that 10.3% of students would use AS if this would help

---

Box 40.3 Psychological effects associated with AS use

- Feeling more powerful and confident (grandiose thoughts)
- Changes in sex drive
- Mood changes
- Irritability
- Aggression
- Impulsiveness
- Euphoria
- Depression
- Paranoia
- Dependence
- Others – insomnia, difficulty with concentration

Box 40.5 Predicting AS use in adolescents – what to look for

Attitudes
- Winning and cheating
- Value of doing one's best
- Behaviour of friends
- Negative beliefs about sport

Risk-taking
- Use of other drugs
- Tobacco smoking
- Not using condoms during sex
- Drink driving
- No helmet when motor-biking
- Not wearing a seat belt

Other
- Satisfaction with body image
- Musculature
- Belief that AS improve health
- Knowing other users

---

them in high school sports, highlighting the importance of winning among the young. Melia (1994) suggested that attitudinal data can be used as a strong predictor of AS use in young people. For instance, students' attitudes towards winning and cheating, the value they place on doing their best and the behaviour of their friends can serve as indicators. He found that among students with the greatest number of negative beliefs about sport, including drug use in sport, 69% were AS users, while AS use among those who held no such views was non-existent. Not surprisingly, Buckley et al (1988) also found that users thought AS have a legitimate place in sport.

Risk-taking behaviour

DuRant et al (1993) and Goldberg et al (1996) also investigated ways of predicting AS use among adolescents. Generally, the more frequently the adolescents studied used AS, the more likely they were also to use one or more other drugs. AS use appears to be associated with other high-risk behaviours, and also to be part of a 'risk-taking syndrome' rather than an isolated behaviour. Students with higher intent to use AS also showed greater hostility, impulsivity and 'win-at-all-costs' attitude. It is interesting, for example, that in the study by Goldberg et al (1996), economic, academic and physical measures did not differ between those with high or low future intent to use AS. Whether AS use is the cause of other high-risk behaviours or whether these are linked with psychosocial factors

(genetic, social environment, personality) remains to be investigated. Box 40.5 describes risk-taking behaviours that are associated with the use of AS in adolescents.

STRATEGIES FOR PREVENTION

The reasons for getting into AS use and strategies for preventing their use among young people involve complex issues. The development and study of effective intervention strategies are important, as indicators of dependence on AS has been reported among teenagers. It is known that proneness to health-compromising behaviours, such as drug use, is related to the interaction between a teenager's personality, environment and other related behaviours.

Knowledge of the reasons why young people get into taking drugs, common characteristics of users and their general knowledge of drugs of abuse may be used to develop strategies for preventing or stopping the use of AS. Previous media attempts to limit alcohol and tobacco use have improved knowledge, but not behaviour or attitudes of recipients (US Department of Health and Human Services 1990), and some have been associated with an increase in use. The argument has been put forward that educational strategies and counselling have a minimal effect on attitudes of the young, as there tends to be little logic involved in their decision-making processes. Difficulty in changing attitudes and behaviour in this group may therefore be great.

Evidence for the effectiveness of education programmes emphasizing alternatives to AS, such as properly structured strength training regimes and optimal nutrition, in reducing the likelihood of future AS use has been fairly promising (Bents et al 1990, Goldberg et al 1996). In Canada, the realization that 40% of the children surveyed were likely to be at moderate risk, and 13% at high risk, for taking AS led to the adoption of a wide and vigorous prevention programme, including education at an early age (junior school). Programmes aiming at preventing AS use have employed various strategies, some of which are outlined in Box 40.6. The Adolescents Training and Learning to Avoid Steroids (ATLAS) Prevention Programme is an excellent example (Goldberg et al 1996). Reis et al (1994) have highlighted the power of the media in influencing adolescents, and especially targeting teenage non-users. Their studies show that beliefs, attitudes and behaviour can be influenced by media campaigns. The role of drugs in the present youth culture, the role of self-esteem and body image,

---

Box 40.6 Arguments to use to deter adolescents from AS use

- Explain the effectiveness of optimal training and diet, especially at an adolescent's stage of development
- Increase in body size does not necessarily correspond to improvement in strength or performance
- Risk of injury (especially ligament/tendon injury) through rapid growth of muscle bulk and overly intensive training
- Harmful effects on health, some of which may appear years later

---

and the media images young people generally aspire to should be examined when planning preventive strategies. There is a need for life-skills education for decision-making and health promotion – not just drugs education and information, as this will not influence behaviour. For example, Elliot & Goldberg (1996) highlight the fact that students with a higher intent to use AS may feel much less able to turn down an offer; they basically lack refusal skills. Also, parental influence not to use drugs is important for a higher intent to use AS. Some suggest that early adolescents may be the most susceptible to persuasive advertising.

CONCLUSIONS

The use of AS among adolescents is not a new issue, as evidence regarding their use in the improvement of sporting performance, at times abetted by ambitious adults, can be traced to the late 1950s. Wild rumours have persisted, and testimonials of state-supported use by Eastern block athletes, who were unaware of it at the time, have emerged in recent years. The high prevalence of AS use found among young people, especially in the USA but also in Canadian studies, is worrying, as youth trends tend to be set in these countries. The data and trends of use available from most other countries are less comprehensive. Studies of adult users suggest that the use of AS starts in the teenage years. Because much of AS use takes place outside organized sports, drug testing programmes are not a deterrent. Other alternatives are education and legislation. Punitive legislation tends to drive users and dealers underground, often making the situation more dangerous for the user (e.g. because of drugs of dubious origin and content, and lack of medical involvement). Relatively successful education strategies aiming to deter AS use have been described in the literature. It seems that such programmes ought to be implemented at a young age, and they should be designed not only to provide information but also to change attitudes. For this to succeed, campaigners must understand youth culture, prevailing peer and media pressures, and the aspirations of young people. Additional harm reduction would also include better training for the medical profession in understanding the drug-taking culture and how to recognize those who might be taking AS. Educational strategies should be arranged by sporting bodies and schools together. It should not be forgotten, however, that drugs known for their harmful side-effects and addiction potential, such as alcohol and tobacco, among others, are far more widely used than AS in all parts of the world.

REFERENCES

Adalf E H, Smart R G 1992 Characteristics of steroid users in an adolescent school population. Journal of Alcohol and Drug Education 38(1): 43–49

Albanese A, Kewley G D, Long A, Pearl K N, Robins D G, Stanhope R 1994 Oral treatment for constitutional delay of growth and puberty in boys: a randomised trial of an anabolic steroid or testosterone undecanoate. Archives of Disease in Childhood 71: 315–317

Bayley N, Gordan G S, Lisser H 1957 Long-term experiences with mathyltestosterone as a growth stimulant in short immature boys. Pediatric Clinics of North America 4: 819–825

Bents R, Young J, Bosworth E, Boyea S, Elliott D, Goldberg L 1990 An effective education program alters attitudes toward anabolic steroids in high school athletes. Medicine and Science in Sports and Exercise 20 (suppl): 64

Buckley W E, Yesalis C E, Friedl K E, Anderson W A, Streit A L, Wright J E 1988 Estimated prevalence of anabolic steroid use among male high school seniors. Journal of American Medical Association 260(23): 3441–3445

Capasso A 1994 Peliosis hepatis in a young adult bodybuilder. Medicine and Science in Sport and Exercise 26(1): 2–4

DuRant R H, Rickert V I, Ashworth C S, Newman C, Slavens G 1993 Use of multiple drugs among adolescents who use anabolic steroids. New England Journal of Medicine 328: 922–926

Elliot D, Goldberg L 1996 Intervention and prevention of steroid use in adolescents. American Journal of Sports Medicine 24(6): S46–47

Gaa G L, Griffith E H, Cahill B R, Tuttle L D 1994 Prevalence of anabolic steroid use among Illinois high school students. Journal of Athletic Training 29(3): 216–222

Gilbert B 1969 Drugs in sport: part 2. Something extra on the ball. Sports Illustrated June 30: 30–35

Goldberg L, Elliot D, Clarke G N et al 1996 The Adolescent Training and Learning to Avoid Steroids (ATLAS) prevention program. Archives of Pediatric and Adolescent Medicine 150: 713–721

Huie M J 1994 An acute myocardial infarction occurring in anabolic steroid user. Medicine and Science in Sport and Exercise 26(4): 408–413

Jackson S T, Rallison M L, Buntin W H, Johnson S B, Flynn R R 1973 Use of oxandrolone for growth stimulation in children. American Journal of Diseases in Childhood 126: 481–484

Johnson M D, Jay M S, Shoup B, Rickert V I 1989 Anabolic steroid use by male adolescents. Pediatrics 83: 921–924

Komoroski E M, Rickert VI 1992 Adolescent body image and attitudes to anabolic steroid use. American Journal of Diseases in Childhood 146: 823–828

Korkia P 1998a Adverse effects of anabolic-androgenic steroids: a review. Journal of Substance Misuse 3: 34–41

Korkia P 1998b Psychological effects of anabolic steroid use: a review. Journal of Substance Misuse 3: 106–113

Korkia P K, Stimson G V 1993 Anabolic steroid use in Great Britain: an exploratory investigation. The Centre for Research on Drugs and Health Behaviour. Final report for the Department of Health, the Welsh Office and the Chief Scientist Office, Scottish Home and Health Department. HMSO, London

Lenehan P, Bellis M, McVeigh J 1996 A study of anabolic steroid use in the North West of England. Journal of Performance Enhancing Drugs 1(2): 57–70

Melia P 1994 Sports for all! But is it suitable for children? International Journal of Drugs Policy 5(1): 34–39

Reis E C, Duggan A K, Adger H, DeAngelis C 1994 The impact of anti-drug advertising. Archives of Pediatric and Adolescent Medicine 148: 1262–1268

Richman R A, Kirch L R 1988 Testosterone treatment in adolescent boys with constitutional delay in growth and development. New England Journal of Medicine 319: 1563–1567

Salva P S, Bacon G E 1991 Anabolic steroids: interest among parents and nonathletes. Southern Medical Journal 84(5): 552–556

Sobel E H, Raymond S, Quinn K V, Talbot N B 1956 The use of methyltestosterone to stimulate growth relative influence on skeletal maturation and linear growth. Journal of Clinical Endocrinology and Metabolism 16: 241–248

Stanhope R, Buchanan C R, Fenn G C, Preece M A 1988 Double blind placebo controlled trial of low dose oxandrolone in the treatment of boys with constitutional delay in growth and puberty. Archives of Disease in Children 144: 99–103

Tanner S M, Miller D W, Alongi C 1995 Anabolic steroid use by adolescents: prevalence, motives, and knowledge of risks. Clinical Journal of Sport Medicine 5(2): 108–115

Terney R, McLain L G 1990 The use of anabolic steroids in high school students. American Journal of Diseases in Children 144: 99–103

US Department of Health and Human Services 1990 Seventh special report to the US Congress on Alcohol and Health. National Institute of Alcohol Abuse and Alcoholism, Rockville, MD, DHHS pub No ADM-90-1656

Vaughan R, Walter H, Gladis M 1991 Steroid use among adolescents – another look. AIDS 5: 112–113

Williamson D 1993 Anabolic steroid use among students at a British College of Technology. British Journal of Sports Medicine 27: 200–201

Yesalis C E, Barsukiewicz C K, Kopstein A N, Bahrke M S 1997 Trends in anabolic-androgenic steroid use among adolescents. Archives of Adolescent Medicine 151: 1197–1206

Yesalis C E, Courson S P, Wright J 1993 History of anabolic steroid use in sport and exercise. In: Yesalis C E (ed) Anabolic steroids in sport and exercise. Human Kinetics, Champaign, IL, p 35–47

Yesalis C, Wright J, Lombardo J 1989 Anabolic-androgenic steroids: a synthesis of existing data and recommendations for future research. Clinician and Sportsmedicine 1: 109–134

41

Exercise in subjects with haematological disorders

Henry G. Watson   Michael Greaves

KEY POINTS

- Tissue oxygen delivery is affected by both the concentration and kinetics of haemoglobin.
- Sickle cell trait and poor athletic condition may predispose to sudden exertional death, which may be seen following extreme exertion and exhaustion in adverse environmental conditions.
- At very high haemoglobin levels, increased blood viscosity may offset the increased oxygen-carrying capacity.
- Choice of sports for patients with congenital or acquired bleeding disorders should be based on enjoyment, with some consideration for avoiding serious injury.
- Rapid control of bleeding and early physiotherapy assessment form the basis of appropriate management of haemarthrosis in haemophilia.
- The availability of exercise bikes and light weights in in-patient settings may improve the physical and psychological well-being of patients with haematological malignancy.

INTRODUCTION

Many highly prevalent and treatable disorders of the blood and bone marrow adversely influence exercise capacity or place the affected individual at risk during competitive sport. Examples are iron deficiency, the commonest cause of anaemia, and bleeding disorders.

In this chapter, the more common and clinically relevant conditions are described, in the context of exercise and sport.

ANAEMIAS

Anaemia is defined as a haemoglobin concentration more than 2 standard deviations below the healthy population mean (less than approximately 12 g/dL in adult females and 14 g/dL in adult males). Clearly, the haemoglobin concentration is a major determinant of the oxygen-carrying capacity of the blood, and therefore of oxygen delivery to all tissues and organs, including the heart and skeletal muscles. The oxygen dissociation characteristics of abnormal haemoglobins also influence oxygen delivery. For example, those in which the oxygen dissociation curve is moved to the right, such as sickle haemoglobin, result in improved oxygen release to the tissues, which may partially compensate for the reduced haemoglobin concentration. In contrast, athletic performance may be enhanced by an increased haemoglobin concentration. Thus, although the optimal haematocrit for tissue oxygenation at rest appears to be around 35%, a supranormal haemoglobin concentration and haematocrit have been demonstrated to improve aerobic capacity.

There is some evidence that highly trained individuals may develop a so-called 'sports anaemia'. This does not represent a true anaemia, as the body total red cell mass is normal or increased, the reduced peripheral blood haematocrit and haemoglobin concentration being due to an accompanying and proportionately greater increase in plasma volume. This is analogous to the physiological 'anaemia' of pregnancy, where the increased red cell mass allows an increased oxygen-carrying capacity to support the needs of the fetus. The adjustment to plasma volume is necessary to fill an increased vascular capacity and may also allow improved heat dissipation. If unappreciated, the phenomenon of sports anaemia may therefore lead to misdiagnosis and inappropriate treatment.

Iron deficiency

Adequate iron is essential for synthesis of haem and some muscle enzymes. However, because excess iron accumulation leads to tissue damage, and there is no physiological mechanism for iron excretion, intestinal iron absorption is normally carefully regulated. Around 10% of dietary iron is absorbed in the jejunum, and this proportion may rise to a maximum of around only 30% in response to tissue iron deficiency. An average Western diet contains 6 mg of iron/1000 kcal, but only a small proportion of this is in an available form. Red meat and fortified cereals are the principal sources of iron. The daily iron requirement in an adult is 1 mg, needed to replace incidental losses. Females require an additional 1 mg/day because of menstrual losses. Iron metabolism is therefore finely balanced in the healthy subject, and any chronic additional loss of blood or consumption of an iron-poor diet inevitably leads to tissue iron depletion. Iron stores (which amount to 3 g, mostly in the form of haemoglobin) become depleted, haem synthesis is then compromised, and microcytic haemopoiesis and, ultimately, progressive anaemia ensue. Whether the stage of tissue iron depletion alone impairs athletic performance is unclear, but there is no doubt that iron deficiency anaemia is a correctable cause of impaired performance.

From the above considerations, it is not surprising that iron deficiency is common in women of childbearing age. The situation may be exacerbated in athletes through dietary faddism, particularly in sports where weight restriction is a consideration. The oligo- or amenorrhoea associated with intensive training may, however, act as a counterbalancing influence. Increased gastrointestinal iron loss, probably as blood, has been described in distance runners, and this would further stress iron balance, as would haemoglobinuria which is occasionally described ('march haemoglobinuria').

Iron deficiency anaemia should be considered in an athlete in whom there is an unexplained and persistent loss of endurance capacity. This is particularly relevant in females and in those who adopt a vegetarian diet. The adolescent growth spurt can also stress tissue iron stores, especially in boys. In evaluating a patient with anaemia, a full blood count should be performed and the serum ferritin assayed. Iron supplements, preferably oral ferrous sulphate 200 mg t.d.s., should be prescribed for the treatment of iron deficiency anaemia. The supplement should be continued for a sufficient duration to fully correct iron stores, typically for 3 months after the haemoglobin concentration has reached a normal value. Parenteral iron is rarely indicated. If there is gastrointestinal intolerance, this frequently responds to a change of iron formulation, e.g. to ferrous fumarate or a slow-release preparation. Tissue iron depletion without anaemia, detected as a subnormal serum ferritin concentration, should be managed in the same way. There is, though, no indication for long-term oral iron supplementation in the absence of demonstrable iron deficiency.

Consideration should be given to the cause of the iron deficiency. Attention to diet may be necessary. Gastrointestinal investigations to seek a source of blood loss may be indicated in males and non-menstruating females.

Other acquired anaemias, such as those due to vitamin B_{12} and folic acid deficiency, and the haemolytic anaemias may affect the trained individual and must be investigated and managed in the usual manner.

Sickle haemoglobin disorders

Sufferers from sickle cell anaemia are homozygous for haemoglobin S (SS). In such patients, a point mutation in the beta-globin gene results in substitution of valine for glutamic acid in the beta chain of haemoglobin. Deoxyhaemoglobin S undergoes intracellular aggregation and polymerization, with an altered erythrocyte configuration and the development of the classical sickle shape. A clinically similar disorder results from co-inheritance of a haemoglobin S gene and beta-thalassaemia (sickle cell beta-thalassaemia), and a related, but clinically less severe, condition results from double heterozygosity for haemoglobin S and a different point mutation in the beta-globin gene – haemoglobin C (haemoglobin SC disease).

In sickle cell trait there is heterozygosity for haemoglobin S (AS). The distribution of the haemoglobin S gene throughout the world parallels that of falciparum malaria, and the disease is therefore one of dark-skinned races. For example, 8% of American blacks have the sickle cell trait.

Sickle cell disease and sickle cell beta-thalassaemia are serious disorders manifesting as a chronic anaemia in which the clinical history is punctuated by episodes of painful crisis due to a sudden increase in the proportion of irreversibly sickled cells within the circulation. These cause vaso-occlusion, resulting in tissue ischaemia and infarction accompanied by extreme pain (most commonly bone pain), prostration and, frequently, fever. There may be progressive pulmonary dysfunction due to vessel occlusion and recurrent infections; cardiomegaly due to high-output anaemic stress, pulmonary hypertension and, possibly, myocardial ischaemia; and neurological impairment, including ischaemic stroke. There is splenomegaly during childhood, but hyposplenism develops by adult life due to recurrent splenic infarction. Other manifestations include chronic leg ulcers, retinopathy and pigment gallstones. Death may occur during acute crisis, particularly in the form known as acute chest

syndrome, in which a vicious circle of pulmonary vaso-occlusion, hypoxia, further sickling and vessel obstruction occurs. Longevity is reduced overall, and death in middle age is common. The clinical phenotype is, however, extremely variable, ranging from frequent crises with stroke and death in childhood to a largely asymptomatic state with only an occasional painful crisis. In haemoglobin SC disease, the anaemia is less severe, painful crises are infrequent, and splenomegaly often persists in adult life.

From the above description it is clear that subjects with sickle cell disease have compromised exercise capacity. However, involvement in some sporting activities is not precluded. Furthermore, unsurprisingly, the condition potentially carries a considerable psychological burden, and adoption of as normal a lifestyle as possible is clearly desirable. Situations which increase the risk of hypoxia must be avoided, including very vigorous exertion. Dehydration and exposure to low environmental temperatures can potentially induce an acute sickle crisis, as can intercurrent infection. Close attention to fluid replacement and use of clothing appropriate to the prevailing conditions are essential. Some pursuits are clearly contraindicated, including high-altitude activities and scuba diving. Sufferers from sickle cell disease can travel safely in pressurized aircraft, but should be advised to maintain good hydration and not to embark if there is any current symptom of acute sickle crisis or infection, or a recent acute episode, e.g. within the previous 7 days.

Subjects with sickle cell disease rapidly learn to recognize symptoms of acute crisis, and any new symptom must be assessed rapidly and treatment instituted. Painful crisis represents an acute medical emergency, which demands administration of adequate analgesia, often employing narcotics, intravenous hydration, oxygen and nursing in a warm environment. Infection should be vigorously sought and treated. The hyposplenic state increases the risk of overwhelming bacterial infection.

General anaesthesia is well tolerated provided that intra- and postoperative hypoxia are avoided. Where there is a particular concern regarding the ability to sustain adequate oxygenation, preoperative exchange transfusion should be considered. Procedures in which a 'bloodless field' is achieved through use of a tourniquet are contraindicated.

In sickle cell trait, the full blood count is normal. There is no anaemia and sickled erythrocytes are not present. The condition is usually subclinical, but there are important exceptions. Haematuria is the most common complication, occurring in up to 1% of subjects with sickle cell trait and is presumably due to renal medullary microinfarction. Renal concentrating ability is usually impaired in sickle cell trait (Reeves et al 1984), although this is not generally associated with clinical symptoms. Splenic infarction and cerebrovascular events have been reported to occur at high altitude. A well conducted general anaesthetic is safe, but local hypoxia must be avoided and, therefore, prolonged use of a tourniquet is contraindicated.

Of particular concern are reports of sudden death during vigorous exercise in subjects with the sickle cell trait (Kark et al 1987). Most cases have occurred in the context of military basic training, during which soldiers with the trait have been estimated to carry a 40-fold increased risk of sudden exertional death. It has not been reported in soldiers beyond basic training, which implies that extreme exertion against a low background level of physical conditioning may be a factor. The complication has also been reported in athletes, both during pre-season training and in competition. Sudden exertional death is characterized by rhabdomyolysis, hyperthermia and cardiac arrhythmias. Extreme exertion and exhaustion in adverse environmental conditions, especially altitude and heat, in a deconditioned individual with sickle cell trait appear to be precipitating factors. The defect in renal concentrating ability may contribute, through exacerbation of dehydration. It is hypothesized that hyperlactataemia with acidosis, dehydration, hypoxia and hyperthermia trigger a sickle cell crisis, disseminated intravascular coagulation, myoglobinuria and acute renal failure.

Whatever the pathogenesis of sudden exertional death in sickle cell trait, it is clear that identification of those at risk, adoption of a staged programme of physical fitness training and avoidance of high-risk environmental conditions should be the basis for the development of a preventive strategy.

Other congenital anaemias

Hereditary spherocytosis

Among Caucasians, this is the most prevalent inherited haemolytic anaemia. It is dominantly inherited and characterized by abnormal red cell morphology, with prominent spherocytes and chronic haemolysis. Hereditary spherocytosis is genotypically and phenotypically heterogeneous, but in the majority of instances symptoms are mild, with only modest anaemia and a variable degree of jaundice. There is splenomegaly and, therefore, an increased risk of traumatic splenic rupture during contact sports and following collisions and falls. In severely symptomatic individuals, splenectomy is an effective therapeutic strategy. The lifelong increased susceptibility to overwhelming bacterial infection and the increased risk from malaria infection must be borne in mind in any splenectomized or hyposplenic individual.

Thalassaemia

Thalassaemia major is a life-threatening disorder with severe anaemia requiring lifelong blood transfusion. In the heterozygote (beta-thalassaemia trait) the haemoglobin concentration is normal. There is, though, marked red cell microcytosis, giving the potential for diagnostic confusion, as the blood picture resembles iron deficiency. However, the red cell count is unusually high. Iron stores are normal and supplementation is not indicated. The condition should be considered when a microcytic blood picture is detected in a subject of Mediterranean or Asian origin. Alpha-thalassaemia trait also results in microcytosis and is a very occasional disorder among Caucasian races.

POLYCYTHAEMIA

Polycythaemia (an abnormally high red cell and haemoglobin concentration and haematocrit) is the result of a restricted plasma volume or increased red cell mass. Low plasma volume is a particular feature in sedentary, overweight males (spurious polycythaemia). An increase in the total red cell mass (true polycythaemia) occurs in the myeloproliferative disorder of bone marrow known as polycythaemia rubra vera, and occasionally as a secondary phenomenon in association with solid tumours. True polycythaemia, however, is most frequently an adaptive response to chronic hypoxia. In clinical practice, this is seen principally in patients with chronic pulmonary disease with alveolar hypoventilation and in congenital heart disease with venous–arterial shunting.

Training at altitude is thought to improve endurance at sea level. This is unlikely to be entirely through enhanced oxygen-carrying capacity due to induced polycythaemia, as the time spent at, and the level of, altitude is frequently insufficient to have a major effect on haemopoiesis, making any advantage on return to sea level relatively short-lived. However, a rare form of familial polycythaemia has been implicated in the outstanding achievements of a three-time Olympic champion long distance skier (Roush 1995), and an increased haemoglobin concentration achieved through transfusion of autologous predonated erythrocytes has been convincingly shown to improve both maximal oxygen uptake and endurance performance (Brien & Simon 1987, Sawka et al 1987) and has been practised as a form of doping in sport. More recently, there has been a move toward achieving the same ends through parenteral administration of recombinant human eythropoietin. This haemopoietic hormone is easily obtainable as it has licensed clinical applications, primarily the management of the anaemia of chronic renal failure. When administered intravenously or subcutaneously thrice weekly over a period of several weeks, usually with parenteral iron, there is an increase in the red cell mass, haemoglobin concentration and haematocrit which persists whilst the drug administration continues. 'Blood doping' was added to the International Olympic Committee's list of prohibited methods in 1985, after several United States cyclists admitted to having used such practices at the Olympics. However, recombinant erythropoietin cannot be reliably detected by currently available gas liquid chromatography/mass spectrometry analysis of urine, and testing of blood has not yet been widely introduced.

Although polycythaemia is accompanied by an improved oxygen-carrying capacity of the blood, the red cell concentration is also the major determinant of blood viscosity. It is therefore clear that, above a certain red cell concentration, compromised microvascular perfusion may more than offset any increase in oxygen delivery arising from the increase in haemoglobin concentration. This may explain reports, from continental Europe, of sudden death in a large number of competitive cyclists who were believed to be using erythropoietin as a performance-enhancing drug. Haematocrit levels in excess of 65% have been achieved. The combination of extreme polycythaemia and dehydration is likely to be particularly dangerous, with a risk of cardiac and cerebral hypoperfusion and ischaemia.

The possibility of the presence of polycythaemia, and the need for urgent rehydration, should be considered in the management of collapse following severe exertion in competition or training. Hyperviscosity due to induced polycythaemia could also complicate the management of acute sports injuries which require surgery under general anaesthesia.

CONGENITAL BLEEDING DISORDERS

The cardinal feature of the inherited coagulation factor deficiencies is excessive or even unprovoked bleeding.

The most common manifestations of the X-linked conditions haemophilia A and B, which are due to deficiencies of factors VIII and IX, respectively, are soft tissue bleeding, muscular haematoma and haemarthrosis. Haemophilia A and B provide the bulk of significant work in haemophilia centres. However, other autosomally inherited coagulation factor deficiencies may also be complicated by haemarthrosis and muscular haematoma, although these are less prominent features of this group of disorders. In haemophilia A and B, the severity of the bleeding diathesis is determined by the residual level of activity of the deficient clotting factor. Severely affected individuals with less than 2% activity will bleed spontaneously, while in moderately affected (2–5%) and mildly affected (5–30%) patients, bleeding is almost always provoked by trauma or surgery. The severity of the bleeding diathesis in the other inherited factor deficiencies is less predictable, but in general, individuals with lower levels of measurable activity will be more likely to bleed.

It is only as a result of the development, in the last 30 years, of efficacious therapeutic factor VIII and IX concentrates that we are able to discuss the participation of severely affected haemophiliacs in many sporting activities. In the 1930s in western Europe, the mean age at death in severely affected haemophiliacs was 7.8 years, with only 18% of babies surviving for 3 years (Ikkala et al 1982). The introduction of efficacious factor VIII and IX concentrates prevented premature death from bleeding, and with the increased availability of material, the introduction of home treatment resulted in a significant reduction in hospital admissions and days off work or school through sickness, allowing haemophiliacs to participate more fully in employment and leisure activities. The ongoing improvement in the quality, safety and quantity of replacement therapy and advances in the management of bleeding episodes and haemophilic arthropathy have resulted in further improvement in the quality and diversity of life for haemophiliacs and their families, and this includes participation in a greater range of sporting activities.

Sporting activities in haemophilia

Choice of sports

Parents of children with congenital bleeding disorders and their physicians may spend a lot of time agonizing about the appropriate sports and pastimes for their youngster. It can be difficult to advise parents in these matters as there is little published evidence regarding the benefits and caveats of individual sports. There are, however, three main considerations worth bearing in mind:

- encouragement of muscle strength and tone
- avoidance of unacceptable injury
- enjoyment.

Muscle strength and tone. There is little doubt that muscle strength significantly contributes to improved joint health. The overall integrity of the major synovial joints depends on the stabilizing effects of capsules, ligaments and muscle. Muscle weakness, which results from disuse, often arises as a result of the reflex inhibition of muscle contraction following joint injury. In this way, the vicious cycle of haemarthrosis, muscle inhibition and wasting resulting in reduction of joint support and increased risk of further bleeding is embarked upon. Small studies have demonstrated a reduction in frequency of haemarthrosis in haemophiliacs following programmes of exercise to improve muscle strength.

Avoidance of unacceptable injury. There is little published evidence about the benefit of combat sports like judo, karate and the other martial arts, boxing and wrestling. However, whilst it is possible that severely affected haemophiliac children might enjoy and benefit from these activities, there can be little doubt that, in sports aiming to induce submission or knock-out, these children are at a significantly increased risk of sustaining severe injury when compared with individuals without a bleeding diathesis.

Clearly, the type and severity of a congenital bleeding diathesis along with previous medical history and musculoskeletal health of an individual need to be considered when embarking on new sporting activities. Similarly, the risks involved in the sport and the appreciation of these by the individual require consideration. Activities which repeatedly provoke bleeding on a regular basis, especially in the same muscles or joint, should be investigated. Faults in technique, apparatus and footwear and protective clothing, if identified, should be addressed. Persistence of significant joint bleeding or other injury may result in abandoning or modifying the activity.

How are doctors most likely to advise haemophilic patients about sporting activities? A 1995 World Federation of Hemophilia survey of sports recommended for haemophiliacs by their treaters showed a high degree of concordance of opinion as to which sports were most appropriate for severely affected haemophiliacs. Of 69 sports surveyed, 10 were recommended by more than 93% of haemophilia treaters who responded (Jones 1996). While it is relatively easy to recommend certain sports, it is more difficult to advise against a sport which has been chosen by a child. In the absence of reliable data only a common sense approach can be adopted. It is clear, however, that even sports perceived as exceedingly dangerous can be performed by children with severe haemophilia, with the appropriate preparation and supervision. One of the authors has participated in rock climbing and abseiling with severely affected boys without observing significant injury.

Enjoyment. There is significant evidence to suggest that sport and exercise are beneficial for children with haemophilia, but two things must be remembered: firstly, similar objectives can be achieved by many different forms of sport and exercise; and secondly, for a child to persist with a sport or activity, it must be fun. Several studies have confirmed that compliance with exercise programmes that are boring and mundane is very poor (Greenan-Fowler et al 1987, Greene & Strickler 1983). In the study of Greenan-Fowler et al, poor compliance to exercise (50% at 1 week) was altered by praise, prizes and a high level of encouragement. This study emphasized the role of peer pressure, the input of a friendly adult, and the importance of an element of competition as well as fun in sporting activities for this group.

Prevention of injury

Factors considered in the previous section, including the appropriateness of a sport given a child's age, diagnosis, disease severity, clinical and musculoskeletal state and capacity for judgement, are clearly important in preventing children from participating in a sport that is unsuitable for them.

Several other factors require attention in order to reduce the risk of injury:

- Appropriate training with good attention to development of technique.
- Use of suitable footwear and other protective clothing. Haemophilic children should all wear shock-absorbing material such as sorbothane in their shoes to reduce the impact of heel strike on the ankles and knees.
- Participants in sports should be encouraged to undertake warm-up and warm-down routines.
- Where appropriate, suitable supervision should be available.
- Prophylaxis with appropriate coagulation factor concentrate is not a prerequisite for all sport, and is

certainly not required for many non-contact activities. There are no controlled trials to evaluate the use of coagulation factor concentrates in the prevention of sports injury, but, again, it seems to be common sense to use concentrate prophylactically before sports which are physically demanding, involve a lot of impact on joints, or involve a lot of body contact.

Management of injury

The general principles of treatment of sports injuries in haemophiliacs should be the same as in non-haemophiliacs. There are, however, several features of injury in haemophiliacs that do require special attention and that are worth particular mention.

Immediate management of nearly all musculoskeletal sports injuries is similar. Local ice-pack application reduces pain, muscle spasm and possibly bleeding. Fifteen minute applications 1- to 2-hourly are recommended, paying attention to preventing damage to the skin from the ice-packs. Compression by firm crepe bandaging and elevation of the affected limb in the first 24 h post injury all help to limit inflammation. Temporary immobilization of the injured joint or muscle may be beneficial or even unavoidable. However, periods of immobilization should be kept to an absolute minimum, and rapid return to activity encouraged as detailed below.

Initial assessment. Often, the need for coagulation factor replacement or other therapy to raise coagulation factor levels will be rapidly made by individuals or their parents. In this situation, for haemarthrosis or muscle haematoma, sufficient replacement to raise the plasma level to around 30% activity should be given as soon as possible. Schools and sports clubs attended by haemophiliacs have often been briefed about the appropriate management of injured subjects, and additionally individuals with congenital bleeding disorders in the UK carry cards detailing the nature and severity of their disorder along with emergency medical contact numbers. Individuals with very serious injuries (e.g. to the head) should be given replacement therapy as soon as possible and transferred to the nearest accident and emergency unit.

More often than not, haemophiliacs with musculoskeletal injuries will attend their local haemophilia centre, where appropriate assessment, investigation (e.g. radiology), attention to haemostasis, and early involvement of other specialists, such as orthopaedic surgeons and physiotherapists, will all be arranged.

Haemophiliacs travelling abroad should take time before departure to refer to the WFH publication *Passport* to identify the closest haemophilia centre to their holiday resort. They should of course carry with them adequate amounts of coagulation factor concentrate (to allow treatment without exposure to new products), stored under appropriate conditions. Where possible, a letter of introduction from their local haemophilia centre should be arranged.

Local haemostasis. Open wounds in individuals with bleeding disorders resulting from trauma should be treated appropriately with regard to prevention of infection. Local cleaning, debridement and removal of foreign bodies are performed as they would be in normal individuals. Attention should be paid to state of immunity against tetanus. Several materials, such as thrombin, fibrin sealant and topical adrenaline, may be considered for use, especially in those individuals with anti-factor VIII antibodies. In most situations, these are however, unsatisfactory, and recourse to systemic replacement therapy is required. It is worth noting that in previously untreated patients (PUPS) or recipients of recombinant material only, use of topical thrombin or fibrin sealant represents a first exposure to plasma-derived blood products. Such an exposure would defeat the purpose of using recombinant material and is therefore inappropriate. Wound clips, Steri-Strips and sutures should be used as required.

The majority of haemophiliacs over the age of 12 years will have been infected with the persistent hepatitis viruses B and C – some, in addition, will be infected with HIV. There is no documented transmission of any viral infection by recombinant material to date. Individuals frequently treating haemophiliacs should be vaccinated against hepatitis B virus and should follow standard procedures to avoid parenteral transmission of viruses when treating open wounds in any haemophiliac.

Coagulation factor replacement. For the majority of sports injuries in persons with congenital coagulation factor deficiencies a single treatment to raise the deficient factor to around 30% will be sufficient to stop the bleeding. More severe injuries, often with clear visible signs of large muscular haematoma or haemarthrosis, may require treatment for longer periods, ranging from 48 h to 10 days. Psoas muscle bleeding is notoriously problematic and must be treated to complete resolution to prevent re-bleeding, which is common and may be complicated by femoral nerve compression with devastating consequences. Fractures and their manipulation may require prolonged coagulation factor replacement. Closed immobilized fractures require treatment for 3–5 days or longer if there is concern about the development of a compartment syndrome.

When it is likely that more than 48 h of therapy will be required, continuous infusion therapy is now the treatment of choice of many haemophilia treaters. The likely benefits include improved haemostasis and reduced overall concentrate use when compared with bolus therapy.

Where it is available and of proven safety, replacement should be with a high purity single factor concentrate, either plasma-derived or recombinant. Individuals with factor II or X deficiency should be treated with a virus-inactivated prothrombin complex concentrate (PCC). Attention should be paid to the possible consequences of treatment in patients with concomitant liver disease or disseminated intravascular coagulation. Factor V deficient patients should be treated with single donor virus-inactivated plasma (VIP). Factor XI concentrates are available but there is concern about activation of coagulation in association with their use and VIP should certainly be considered in individuals with a pre-existing prothrombotic state or significant arterial disease. Individuals with von Willebrand's disease may respond to treatment with DDAVP which increases VIII:c and vWF levels approximately three- to fourfold, probably by inducing release from endothelial cells. DDAVP may be given intravenously or by the intranasal route and is associated with minimal side-effects in adults, but is subject to the effect of tachyphylaxis, which limits the number of successive days on which treatment can be given. DDAVP is contraindicated in individuals with myocardial ischaemia and those with type 2B von Willebrand's disease, and does not produce haemostasis in individuals with severe haemophilia or type 3 von Willebrand's disease.

Inhibitory antibodies to coagulation factors are most commonly seen in haemophilia A patients, but may occasionally arise in other congenital bleeding disorders. Treatment with materials which activate the tenase complex by alternate means, e.g. FEIBA or rVIIa, or alternatively non-human factor VIII, may be used to stop bleeding. In all of the above situations, expert haemophilia advice should ideally be sought.

Physiotherapy. Early physiotherapy assessment and appropriately timed introduction of treatment are integral to the management of joint and muscle bleeding in haemophilia. Following haemarthrosis, the emphasis is very much on avoiding prolonged immobilization. Haemarthrosis is complicated by reflex inhibition of surrounding muscle groups, which together with voluntary immobilization results in muscle wasting and loss of joint support. If the stability of the joint is affected, this may result in an increased likelihood of further joint bleeding and the development of a vicious cycle resulting in the evolution of a target joint, chronic synovitis and haemophilic arthropathy. Management of significant muscle haematoma depends on the appropriate timing of active mobilization of the affected muscle, with attention being paid to the prevention of damaging re-bleeding.

In haemophiliacs who have sustained significant repeated joint and muscle bleeds, it is almost certain that damage to proprioceptive function will have been sustained. A strong emphasis on proprioceptive training and addressing problems of chronic muscle imbalance has recently emerged in physiotherapy practice.

HAEMATOLOGICAL MALIGNANCY

We tend to encourage exercise and sport in our patients with haematological malignancies. We find, anecdotally, that it often improves both physical and psychological well-being. A few points merit a mention:

- We discuss pastimes and sport with patients on an individual basis.
- Patients with Hickman lines are advised to avoid swimming. If involved in other sports, we encourage patients to carefully tape the line securely to the body.
- Patients with profound thrombocytopenia are discouraged from sports in which they are likely to sustain head trauma. Cycle helmets and protective clothing (e.g. knee and elbow pads) are encouraged where it is deemed appropriate.
- Patients are discouraged from activities which regularly induce bleeding.
- Weight-bearing and gentle exercise are encouraged in patients with skeletal disease such as myeloma.
- Patients receiving high-dose chemo-radiotherapy are encouraged to exercise during their in-patient stay when they feel up to it. Static cycling and the use of light weights are encouraged.

THROMBOCYTOPENIA

Significant thrombocytopenia may arise as a feature of many haematological conditions and their management. The clinical presentation of thrombocytopenia depends to a degree on its severity and possibly the speed of its onset. Patients with significant thrombocytopenia ($<100 \times 10^9/L$) may present with easy bruising, epistaxis or gum bleeding, but more often than not will be completely asymptomatic. Spontaneous bleeding in an otherwise healthy individual with thrombocytopenia is unusual at a count of $>20 \times 10^9/L$.

In advising parents of children with idiopathic thrombocytopenic purpura (ITP), it is known that the incidence of fatal intracranial haemorrhage in childhood ITP is around 1 in 10 000 and that fatal haemorrhage is positively correlated to head injury.

ANTICOAGULANT THERAPY

Anticoagulant therapy is widely practised. For long-term thromboprophylaxis, low-dose aspirin is used in subjects with known arterial disease. It acts through inhibition of the platelet cyclo-oxygenase enzyme required for normal platelet aggregation. Aspirin is well tolerated and safe, gastrointestinal intolerance and haemorrhage being the principal side-effects. Aspirin produces only a mild systemic haemostatic defect. The skin bleeding time is marginally prolonged and there may be an increased tendency to bruise.

In relation to sport and exercise, warfarin anticoagulant therapy is of greater importance, as it induces a clinically very significant coagulopathy with an associated risk of haemorrhage. Warfarin may be indicated for the treatment of disease in subjects capable of sporting activity. It is the treatment of choice for thromboprophylaxis after an episode of venous thromboembolism. Although an active lifestyle and low adiposity reduce the risk of venous thrombosis, it is a condition which not uncommonly affects young adults, including sportsmen and women. An Olympic medallist rower and a national representative distance runner are among sufferers of venous thrombosis known to the authors. The acute thrombotic event – deep vein thrombosis and/or pulmonary embolism – usually arises through the interaction of inherited and acquired prothrombotic influences. The former constitute a group of disorders known as familial thrombophilia, which includes a common point mutation in the gene for coagulation factor V, known as factor V Leiden. This is of particular importance, as around 4% of Caucasians are heterozygous for this gene and have a risk of venous thrombosis which is some sevenfold greater than that of the unaffected population. The condition is clinically silent until the first episode of venous thrombosis, which frequently occurs between the ages of 20 and 50 years. Acquired factors which predispose to venous thromboembolism include tissue trauma and the postoperative state, and use of the combined oral contraceptive. The latter increases risk around fourfold, but interacts in a multiplicative fashion with factor V Leiden, resulting in a relative risk for venous thrombosis which is approximately 40 times greater than baseline.

Warfarin is also widely used to reduce the risk of embolic stroke in patients with mechanical heart valve prostheses, and in subjects with chronic atrial fibrillation who have evidence of cardiac or arterial disease. Atrial fibrillation occurs with increased prevalence in middle-aged males who indulge in regular vigorous exercise compared with a sedentary control population (Karjalainen et al 1988). In this situation, the arrhythmia occurs in the absence of evidence of underlying cardiovascular disease and therefore fulfils the criteria for the diagnosis of 'lone atrial fibrillation'. Fortunately, the embolic risk in lone atrial fibrillation is not considered to be sufficient to warrant warfarin therapy.

Warfarin acts through inhibition of vitamin K, which is necessary for the complete synthesis of clotting factors II, VII, IX and X in the liver. The degree of prolongation of the prothrombin time is used to determine optimal dosage. The result is standardized, as the International Normalized Ratio (INR), in order to achieve conformity. For most indications, a target INR of 2.5, with an optimal range of 2.0–3.0, is desirable. This recommendation is based on the exponential increase in risk of haemorrhage associated with a rising INR above 4.0, and the increased thrombotic risk at levels below 2.0.

There is a risk of fatal haemorrhage, principally intracranial bleeding, of 0.25% per annum in a subject receiving warfarin. Up to a third of these bleeds occur at a time when the INR falls within the recommended therapeutic range, the remainder occurring at times of overanticoagulation. These statistics indicate the very real hazards associated with oral anticoagulant therapy. Despite this, exercise, and even competitive sport, is not absolutely contraindicated, but some sporting activities are hazardous in this situation and should be discouraged. This includes contact sports and any other activity where head trauma is a risk, e.g. high diving. The use of protective headgear is essential where permissible, and in any case should be worn during recreational exercise such as cycling, canoeing and equestrian activities. Careful counselling at the induction of warfarin therapy is mandatory in order to explore the level of risk, and the duration of warfarin exposure must be kept to a safe minimum. Occasionally, alternative antithrombotic strategies may be appropriate. Use of self-administered once-daily low-molecular-weight heparin prophylaxis, instead of warfarin, could be considered in the management of venous thromboembolism in subjects who wish to continue their involvement in high-risk sports. The relative efficacy of such an approach is, however, unknown. An increased bleeding risk is not excluded, and long-term administration of heparin has been associated with symptomatic osteoporosis.

It is essential to consider the well-known potential for hazardous drug interactions when prescribing for the patient on warfarin therapy. Of particular relevance are the non-steroidal anti-inflammatory agents, many of which can cause a further increase in the INR and also, potentially, gastrointestinal haemorrhage. Whenever possible, a drug which is least likely to interact should be selected and the INR carefully monitored after its introduction and withdrawal.

Intramuscular injections carry the risk of haematoma formation in the warfarin-treated subject and should be avoided whenever possible. Many surgical procedures can be carried out safely when the INR is 2.0 or less, but neurosurgical and ophthalmological operations usually demand normal haemostasis.

Where haemorrhage occurs in an individual receiving warfarin, management depends on the nature and severity of the bleed and the level of the INR. Discontinuation of warfarin will result in a gradual fall of the INR to 1.0 over 4–5 days. Where a more rapid correction is required, this can be achieved over 6–8 h by the slow intravenous injection of 2 mg of vitamin K. When bleeding is life-threatening, complete and immediate normalization of coagulation can only be guaranteed by infusion of a concentrate of factors II, IX and X, preferably given under the guidance of a haematology specialist. Administration of fresh frozen plasma is insufficient (Makris et al 1997). Vitamin K should also be given, in order to achieve lasting correction of coagulation. This potentially life-saving therapy with factor concentrate and vitamin K would clearly be appropriate in a warfarin-anticoagulated subject with head trauma and neurological deterioration.

CONCLUSIONS

The central role of haemoglobin in ensuring tissue oxygenation, and other factors which affect oxygen delivery such as haemoglobin dissociation kinetics and blood rheological factors have resulted in the in-depth study of haematological variables in relation to sports and exercise. Unfortunately, competitive athletes have applied this knowledge in an unacceptable fashion to gain a performance advantage.

The possibility that anaemia is contributing to reduced athletic performance should always be considered, especially in females. Specialist medical practitioners who are aware of the particular requirements of individuals undertaking vigorous exercise should perform the detection, investigation and treatment of anaemia in athletes.

Appropriate advice on sport and exercise activities may be requested by different groups of patients with haematological disorders. We have attempted to summarize general principles, but acknowledge that there is little published evidence relating to sport or exercise in these disorders. As such, an appreciation of the physiology and pathology of these conditions should be borne in mind, and advice, based on this knowledge and common sense, offered.

REFERENCES

Brien A J, Simon T L 1987 The effects of red blood cell infusion on 10-K race time. Journal of the American Medical Association 257: 2761–2765

Greenan-Fowler E, Powell C, Varni J W 1987 Behavioral treatment of adherence to therapeutic exercise by children with haemophilia. Archives of Physical Medicine and Rehabilitation 68: 846–849

Greene W B, Strickler E M 1983 A modified isokinetic strengthening program for patients with severe hemophilia. Developmental Medicine and Child Neurology 25: 189–196

Ikkala E, Helske T, Myllyia G, Nevanlinna H R, Pitkanen P, Rasvi C 1982 Changes in the life expectancy of patients with severe haemophilia in Finland in 1930–79. British Journal of Haematology 52: 7–12

Jones P 1996 Living with haemophilia, 4th edn. Oxford University Press, Oxford

Karjalainen J, Kujala U M, Kaprio J, Sarna S, Viitasalo M 1988 Lone atrial fibrillation in vigorously exercising middle aged men: case-control study. British Medical Journal 316: 1784–1785

Kark J A, Posey D M, Schumacher A R, Ruehle C V 1987 Sickle cell trait as a risk factor for sudden death in physical training. New England Journal of Medicine 317: 781

Makris M, Phillips W S, Greaves M, Kitchen S, Rosendaal F R, Preston F E 1987 Emergency oral anticoagulant reversal: the necessity for prothrombin complex concentrates. Thrombosis Haemostasis 77: 477–480

Reeves J D, Lubin B, Embury S H 1984 Renal complications of sickle cell trait are related to the percent of HbS. Blood 64(suppl 118): 5

Roush W 1995 An 'off switch' for red blood cells. Science 268: 27–28

Sawka M N, Young A J, Muza S R, Gonzalez R R, Pandolf K B 1987 Erythrocyte infusion and maximal aerobic power. Journal of the American Medical Association 257: 1496–1499

42

Problems with sport surgery in HIV-positive patients

G. Schweitzer   L. Schlebusch

KEY POINTS

1. HIV (human immunodeficiency virus) spreads from one person to another by a number of means, including, among others, sexual transmission, the intermingling of blood and needlestick infection.
2. The virus attacks the immune system of the body, leaving the individual vulnerable to infection and malignancy. Progression to full-blown AIDS may take several years.
3. HIV-infected sportspersons often show a similar psychological response to their infection as that shown by athletes in the face of injury. Of course, there are additional factors to contend with in the HIV-infected individual.
4. The stress response to discovery of HIV infection will affect both psychological and physical functioning.
5. The management of HIV-positive patients should be considered from a multidisciplinary perspective, especially in view of the potential psychological and neuropsychological complications.

INTRODUCTION

HIV (human immunodeficiency virus) infection is caused by a retrovirus. HIV spreads from one individual to another by heterosexual and homosexual intercourse, by blood transfusion, by administration of blood products, across the placenta in pregnant women, by needlestick infection, in the milk of lactating women, and by shared needles among drug addicts.

Cannon (1992) stated that the virus invades the body, frequently mutates, and, by attacking the immune system, leaves the individual vulnerable to infection and malignancy. Progression from HIV infection to full-blown AIDS may take several years, and is not at present completely understood. It is known that the virus enters cells and replicates. When the virus enters CD4 helper T lymphocytes, the RNA genome of the virus is transcribed into a DNA copy which integrates into the cellular chromosome. Thereafter, the virus exists in a latent or productive state. In the latent state, little RNA or protein is made and no virions are produced. Later, modulation into viral replication can occur with cell death. Viral titres are highest during the initial and terminal stages of HIV infection. Time between the initial HIV infection and clinical manifestations of AIDS can be as long as 10 years, although the usual time is about 6–8 weeks. The latter time is known as the window period and is very important when dealing with sportspersons. The patient may initially be negative, and may be in this window period. Thus repeated ELISA and Western blot tests may be necessary for several years if infection with HIV is suspected.

Luck et al (1996) stated that as long as the CD4 count remains at greater than 200, the risk of opportunistic infection is about the same as that in a normal person. If it drops below 200, however, opportunistic infection, and infection with the more common pathogens, may occur. They also recommended that elective surgery should not be performed on patients with a CD4 count less than 200 or a serum albumin less than 25 g/L. We agree with these recommendations.

An injured athlete typically goes through psychological phases similar to those described for patients facing death, i.e. disbelief, denial, isolation, anger, bargaining, depression, acceptance and resignation, whilst remaining hopeful (Rotella 1982). This situation can be worsened in the case of an HIV-positive patient, who typically responds with shock, anger, guilt, anxiety, depression and obsessive-compulsive behaviour, such as persistent probing for explanations, a relentless search for improved treatment or new diagnostic evidence, and a preoccupation with physical decline (Christie 1990). At the same time, athletes have different perceptions of injury, ranging from seeing it as a disaster, to perceiving it as an opportunity to be excused from strenuous training, as a good excuse for poor performance, or as an opportunity to show courage.

Injured athletes often wonder what their chances of recovery are, remaining hopeful whilst being faced with the prospect of preparing themselves for an end to participating in sport. This occurs in HIV-infected individuals. Should there be an end to a patient's sports career, this may, as for other injured athletes, precipitate an 'identity crisis', with concomitant dysfunctional thinking and potential psychopathology, including anxiety and depression (Rotella 1988).

Stress is a critical psychosocial factor in performance, and the role of stress in disease and immune suppression has been extensively documented in the literature (Kaplan & Sadock 1995, Schlebusch 1990, 2000). Not only can the demands of competitive participation in sport be stressful, but sports injuries can also be very stressful and emotionally devastating, and much has been written about this, and the appropriate psychological treatment (Yukelson & Murphy 1993). The same would apply to HIV-infected sportspersons. Clearly the situation can be exacerbated considerably if HIV infection forms a part of the equation, and the different and complex variables will interact with each other. This can be overwhelming for the patient. A central issue is the patient's stress response, which affects both psychological and physical functioning.

An important factor is the sportsperson's ability to cope with training demands and competition, and to maintain a balanced personal life. Sports people who follow intense training schedules and who strive to maintain a balance between their training, work, marriage and social life are exposed to a great deal of stress, with increased risk for further injury or disease (Yukelson & Murphy 1993). Apart from endocrinological and autonomic effects, stress can impact negatively on the patient's thought processes and psychological status. This can be aggravated by HIV infection. It has been suggested that with an increase in stress levels, the visual fields of a patient narrow, resulting in the patient overlooking relevant cues in the environment, and thus further increasing the possibility of an injury (Williams et al 1991).

As HIV attacks the immune system, it follows the increased stress levels produced by injury, and knowledge of being HIV-positive can further reduce a patient's ability to cope with the various psychological and physical concomitants.

In addition, HIV is a neurotropic virus which may affect the neurons of the occipital cortex, thus further narrowing the visual fields.

We practise in a community where HIV infection is endemic and epidemic. Halpern & Preston (1994) reported that raised intracranial pressure and focal neurological deficits, together with autoimmune dysfunction, are anaesthetic problems found in HIV-infected individuals. Our anaesthetists take this into account when we operate.

Patients with HIV infection who are immunocompromised are subject to several disorders of the central nervous system (CNS). Many patients present with a constellation of cognitive, motor and behavioural changes characteristic of subcortical dementia (Van Gorp & Cummings 1995). Psychomotor slowing, difficulty in concentrating, poor retrieval of information, problems with mood and affect, and visuospatial skills are often the initial features in HIV-infected individuals, and this of course would also apply to sportsmen and sportswomen. The presentation is consistent with early involvement of the thalamus and basal ganglia. It has been argued that the predilection for subcortical and limbic structures suggests that psychological disorders may be partly attributed to psychological underpinning.

Given this, and in view of our experience, the biological, psychological and social variables in HIV-positive patients should be holistically considered from a multidisciplinary point of view, as has been emphasized before (Schlebusch & Cassidy 1995). This is especially so in view of the potential psychological and neuropsychological complications in these patients (Grant & Atkinson 1995, Schlebusch et al 1998).

In December 1997, *The Lancet* commented:

The global HIV epidemic is far worse than previously thought, with about one in every 100 adults aged 15–49 infected. And surprisingly, for a disease that continually reflects social inequalities, the situation has improved in several industrialised nations, while the developing world now bears more than 90% of the world's HIV/AIDS burden. (Morris 1997)

INCIDENCE

The incidence of HIV infection varies according to the geographical area, and this has an important bearing on the incidence of infection in sportspersons. The highest incidence is in individuals aged between 15 and 40 (Lachman 1997), and of course this is the age group that actively participates in sport. The highest incidence in the world is in sub-Saharan Africa. In Central and East Africa, the incidence is reported to be 60–70% of the population. The latest figures available to us from King Edward VIII Hospital, Durban of attendees at the antenatal clinic, is more than 30% (A Smith, Department of Virology, University of Natal, South Africa, personal communication, 1998). This is the largest teaching hospital in the region. An incidence of

25% or more is also reported from similar antenatal clinics in the North-Western Province of South Africa.

In North America, the figures vary depending on the community. Sloan et al (1995), writing from a grade 1 trauma centre at the Cook County Hospital in Chicago, found the incidence at their institution to be 12–21% in critically injured patients who needed shock resuscitation. Similarly, McAuliffe et al (1997), reporting figures from an urban level 1 trauma centre in Miami, Florida, stated that 9.1% of major trauma patients and 19.4% of all adult patients admitted with infections were seropositive for HIV. However, their survey was performed prior to 1991 when their series was first published.

The majority of infected individuals are in the childbearing age group: 15–40 years.

If we take into account the latest available figures from the Province of KwaZulu Natal and the North Western Province of South Africa, it is highly likely that the sexual partners of HIV-positive pregnant women are also HIV-positive. It is very likely that the male sexual partners of HIV-positive pregnant women play competitive sport, as this is a common recreational activity in this age group. Thus it is very likely that they will present with injuries sustained whilst playing sport. It is highly significant that a special facility has recently opened in Richards Bay, a harbour city north of Durban, to deal specifically with HIV-related problems.

Ching et al (1996), writing from the Hand Clinic at Johannesburg hospital, have stated that the majority of HIV patients are asymptomatic and do not present to medical practitioners either inside or outside the hospitals. We suspect that the majority of HIV-infected sportsmen and sportswomen in South Africa fall into this category. The professional requirements for many contemporary sports participants are such that these people are geographically highly mobile and may be at risk of infection in foreign centres. We are seeing this in South Africa.

By far the most popular contact sport in South Africa is soccer. This sport is played nearly all year round by all races and all age groups. Young men in particular, and to a lesser extent young women, participate in this sport. Based on the available figures given above, five or six players in each soccer club could be HIV-positive. This would present a major problem to the club doctor. The problem would be both ethical and administrative. Some clubs place pressure on the club doctor to reveal which players are HIV-positive, and this could result in a player being asked to leave. One of us (GS) acted as a club doctor to a professional soccer club. He refused to perform routine HIV tests on all players on ethical and legal grounds. Only one player was tested for HIV during the doctor's tenure at the club, and this will be discussed later in the chapter.

The incidence of HIV-positive individuals among sportspersons in South Africa is not known. Anecdotal information is that some professional soccer clubs in South Africa which import players from abroad perform routine HIV tests on these individuals. HIV-positive players are not employed by these clubs and are returned to their home countries. The information about the players and clubs is a closely kept secret, but rumours abound.

The club doctor must exercise constant vigilance in South Africa because of the high incidence of HIV-positive individuals in the community.

In this country there are stringent ethical regulations regarding testing for HIV. The patient must be very carefully counselled before blood is taken for testing, and again when the results of tests become available.

As most sports training sessions take place in the early evening, and most sports events take place in the early evenings or at weekends, trained AIDS counsellors are not always available in the acute situation. Language may be a problem, as in South Africa there are 11 official languages. Usually the club doctor is English-speaking, and errors in interpretation and translation may arise if the patient or the interpreter is not fluent in English.

Another problem which crops up from time to time is that patients are aware of their HIV-positive status, or of the status of their sexual partners or their children, but conceal this from the club doctor who examines them for sports injury.

CLINICAL PRESENTATION

This is well documented in standard texts, and will be mentioned in this chapter only briefly.

The vast majority of men and women who participate in sport are healthy individuals. It must be remembered that these patients may be in the window period of their HIV infection. Many sportsmen and women also lead very active social and sex lives.

Neither of the authors has, to the best of his knowledge, treated an HIV-positive sportsperson or a person with full-blown AIDS. One of us has treated a patient whose child was HIV-positive, so it is very likely that the father was also HIV-positive.

The only patient treated with a sexually transmitted disease (STD) was a player who presented with gonococcal urethritis. This player had unprotected, casual sexual contact whilst playing an away match in Johannesburg and presented with a urethral infection. The ELISA and Western blot tests for HIV were negative. It is not known whether the player was in a window phase of HIV infection. Shortly after consulting the club doctor, the player was dismissed by the club for disciplinary reasons which were not associated with his STD. Attempts to trace the player were unsuccessful.

PREVENTION OF HIV INFECTION IN A SPORTS CLUB

As at the present time there is no effective cure for HIV infection, the emphasis must be on prevention. With this in view, one of us (GS) has, at the beginning of each soccer season, talked to the players in his club about HIV infection. The players were advised to practise monogamy, to use condoms and to avoid casual, unprotected sexual contact. Each time a new player joined the club during the course of the soccer season, he was given similar advice.

A controversial topic at present is whether HIV infection can be spread from bleeding wounds on the sports field. This is especially so in body contact sports such as boxing, wrestling, judo, karate, soccer and rugby. In South Africa, rugby and soccer players with bleeding wounds are obliged to leave the sports field, and have their wounds bandaged before resuming play. What is not certain is what happens when the blood seeps through the bandages. Although adequate provision was made for disposal of bloodstained bandages in the author's sports club, it is not known what provisions were made by other clubs.

TREATMENT

The majority of doctors involved in sports medicine in South Africa are general practitioners. Some of these individuals have additional sports medicine qualifications from the University of Cape Town. Several orthopaedic surgeons and other specialists are also involved at local, regional and national levels.

To the best of our knowledge, there are no guidelines at present for the treatment of sports injuries in HIV-positive individuals. The opinions expressed in this chapter are based on a review of the current literature and on our own experience and practice of sports medicine.

In our opinion, some modification is essential in the management of individuals suspected of HIV infections who are injured on the sports field.

Paiemont et al (1994), in a paper on postoperative infections in asymptomatic HIV-positive orthopaedic trauma patients, stated that the infection rates are high in seropositive individuals. These authors went as far as· to say that asymptomatic seropositive individuals are at higher risk of postoperative orthopaedic infections. More recently, McAuliffe et al (1997), from the University of Miami, Florida, found that patients with AIDS were significantly more likely to present with spontaneous onset of infection in the absence of a penetrating injury than those patients who are HIV-seropositive but asymptomatic. What is significant in their series is that the risk factors they list include intravenous drug use as the commonest: 46 of their 90 patients were intravenous drug users, while three were listed as having acquired HIV infection by heterosexual contact; 20 patients, however, were listed as uncertain, so it cannot be said with certainty how they acquired the HIV infection.

Our policy is to act on the safe side. Where a patient needs to undergo a major reconstructive procedure, e.g. the knee ligaments, we would carefully counsel the patient to have an HIV test. If the HIV test came back positive we would again counsel the patient and suggest that a conservative approach be performed rather than a major operative procedure. More recently it has been stated that the presence of a CD4 lymphocyte count of less than 200 would preclude elective reconstructive surgery. The same would apply to an albumin count of less than 25 g/L.

Our reason for adopting this approach is that in addition to the higher risk of infection, the life expectancy of HIV-infected individuals is unpredictable. Surgery places further stress on the already compromised immune system, which may be overwhelmed, resulting in opportunistic and non-opportunistic infections.

The drug management of an HIV-infected sportsperson falls outside the scope of the average club doctor, and this includes ourselves. In this type of case, consultation should be sought with a person with a particular interest and expertise in HIV infection, usually an immunologist, physician or dermatologist.

The club doctor's duty, in our opinion, is to provide objective and systematic assessment of the patient's physical, psychological and neurocognitive status, to assist with the differential diagnosis (Schlebusch et al 1998). Very often the psychopathology, notably depressive and anxiety states, becomes evident at this stage of diagnosis of HIV infection. However, these patients may (and often do) have psychological and neurological difficulties which are secondary to their primary HIV infection. Furthermore, any psychological sequelae which could be associated with other physical problems, e.g. diabetes mellitus, have to be considered.

In addition, common sequelae of HIV infection can contribute to behavioural reactions, and these can mimic cognitive changes seen in anoxia resulting from head injury, chest injury or adult respiratory distress syndrome. HIV enters the CNS and both dementia and delirious states can result from CNS infection. CNS neoplasms and abnormalities caused by systemic disorders, together with endocrinopathies, as well as adverse CNS reactions to drugs, can occur (Kaplan & Sadock 1995). Differential diagnosis in this instance is important for both management (delirium should always precipitate a medical work-up of an HIV-infected patient to assess the underlying CNS-related process) and prognosis.

An evaluation should be made of the impact of the sports injury on behaviour, i.e. an assessment of deficits in function that are causally related to a head injury sustained in sport. Clinically, neuropsychiatric complications occur in at least 50% of HIV-infected patients (Kaplan & Sadock 1995), and neuropsychological symptoms may be the first sign of the disease in about 10–30% of such cases (Kaplan & Sadock 1995, Lezak 1995). Damage to the brain can occur as a result of HIV infection involving brain cells, or indirectly from pressure or mass lesions, tumours or infectious processes resulting from a deteriorating immune system (Lezak 1995).

In our community, cryptococcosis is a relatively common infection of the CNS in HIV-positive patients. Further, the often subtle neuropsychological sequelae of a mild head injury, i.e. headaches, dizziness, concentration and memory problems, fatigue, irritability, anxiety and depression, may easily be misattributed to causes other than the brain injury (Schlebusch et al 1998). The presence of a pre-existing condition such as substance abuse, psychiatric illness, CNS damage due to previous head injury or infection can influence the impact and serve to exacerbate any real damage due to the head injury (McCaffrey & Lynch 1995). The most common substance abused in our community is cannabis, which is locally known as 'dagga'. It may be of interest in passing that the dagga available in our community contains the highest concentration of d-tetrahydrocannabinol in the world. In our practice we frequently encounter cannabis-related substance disorders. Although one of us (GS) has previously treated patients with dagga withdrawal symptoms following major trauma, to the best of our knowledge neither of us has seen this problem following a sports injury.

Recommendations regarding treatment options/decisions and management should consider the findings of the neuropsychological assessment. Such an assessment can also give information on the behaviour of patients in hospital, and on their neurocognitive ability (Schlebusch et al 1998). Another important issue is the patient's ability to understand explanations and instructions, i.e. comprehension (La Marche & Boll 1955). It is also of significance in the assessment of the patient's ability to comply with treatment (La Marche & Boll 1955), to perform activities of daily living, and to live independently, if such is the case (Long & Kibby 1995, McCaffrey & Lynch 1995). Neuropsychological assessment will also give information as to which patients will benefit from specific interventions and rehabilitation (Long & Kibby 1995). It also facilitates the generation of a medical climate that is patient-orientated and psychologically minded. Moreover, it takes cognizance of the effect of the hospital environment on the patient's reactions, and meets the needs of the staff as mental health facilitators, by providing practical suggestions for management (Schlebusch 1983).

There is, in addition, a need to address both the pre-morbid psychological disorders and the onset of new ones, which may complicate diagnosis and the patient's response to treatment. It is important not to make the error of ascribing any psychological disorders to variables that are unrelated to the HIV infection, and to consider any iatrogenic phenomena. The treatment can be both psychological and pharmacological, and the patient should be informed of the neuropsychological findings and be taught coping measures. It is important to stress that the patient's safety is a priority. Research has shown that patients with advanced HIV disease have a 30-fold increased risk of suicidal behaviour when compared with seronegative individuals (Grant & Atkinson 1995).

Some of the principles (Rotella 1988) that are applied to the management of an injury are also applicable in the case of the HIV-positive athlete with an injury. The patient should be encouraged to adopt a rational, self-enhancing, rather than a self-defeating, perspective. Although the problem might be untimely and inconvenient, leading to emotional difficulties, it is not appropriate to deny the situation. The patient's 'self-talk' can, to a large extent, determine the behavioural response. Coping skills can be learnt to control dysfunctional thoughts. As for other injuries, the patient should be able to distinguish between 'trying your hardest and doing your best' (Rotella 1988). A significant attitudinal change might be required if the patient

is to accept the change in health status. The development of trust between the patient and the treatment team, as well as the coach, is critical. The key issue is to act in the best interests of the athlete. Adequate family and social support systems tend to reduce the effects of stress in these cases (Schlebusch & Cassidy 1995). This would also apply to HIV-positive athletes.

CONCLUSIONS

The management of the injured HIV-infected sportsperson is a multidisciplinary one. Psychological assessment and support are vital. A social worker, if possible, and the family must be involved. The role of the medical practitioner is to educate members of sports teams about HIV problems, to diagnose the injury and the infection, and to tailor the treatment appropriately to the patient's needs.

REFERENCES

Cannon W 1992 AIDS and arthroscopic surgery. Arthroscopy 8: 279–286

Ching V, Ritz M, Song C, de Aguir G, Mohanlal P 1996 Human immunodeficiency virus infection in an emergency hand service. Journal of Hand Surgery 21-A: 696–699

Christie G 1990 Applications of clinical health psychology to sexually transmitted diseases (specifically AIDS). In: Schlebusch L (ed) Clinical health psychology. A behavioural medicine perspective. Southern Book Publishers, Johannesburg, ch 17

Grant I, Atkinson J 1995 Psychiatric aspects of acquired immunodeficiency syndrome. In: Kaplan H, Sadock B (eds) Comprehensive textbook of psychiatry, 6th edn. William and Wilkins, Baltimore, vol 2, ch 29.2

Halpern S, Preston R 1994 HIV infection in the parturient. International Anaesthesiology Clinics 32(2): 11–30

Kaplan H, Sadock B (eds) 1995 Comprehensive text book of psychiatry, 6th edn. Williams and Wilkins, Baltimore

Lachman S 1997 Heterosexual HIV/AIDS as a global problem: towards 2000. An updated guide for all medicine practitioners and health care workers. Pharmaceutical Society of South Africa, Johannesburg

La Marche J, Boll T 1995 The neuropsychological evaluation of organ transplant patients: a review. Advances in Medical Psychotherapy 8: 79–100

Lezak M 1995 Neuropsychological assessment, 3rd edn. Oxford University Press, New York.

Long C, Kibby M 1995 Ecological of neuropsychological tests: a look at neuropsychology's past and the impact that ecological issues may have on its future. Advances in Medical Psychotherapy 8: 59–78

Luck J, Logan L, Benson D, Glasser D 1996 Human immunodeficiency virus infection: complications and outcome of orthopaedic surgery. Journal of American Academy of Orthopaedic Surgeons 4: 297–304

McAuliffe J, Seltzer D, Hornicek F 1997 Upper extremity infections in patients sero-positive for human immunodeficiency virus. Journal of Hand Surgery 22-A: 1084–1089

McCaffrey R J, Lynch J K 1995 Issues in forensic clinical neuropsychology. Advances in Medical Psychotherapy 8: 35–46

Morris K 1997 HIV epidemic could number 40 million by year 2000. The Lancet 350: 1683

Paiemont G, Hymes R, La Douceur M I, Gosselin R, Green H 1994 Post-operative infections in asymptomatic HIV – sero-positive orthopaedic trauma patients. Journal of Trauma 37: 545–551

Rotella R 1982 Psychological care of the injured athlete. In: Kulund D (ed) The injured athlete, 2nd edn. J B Lippincott, Philadelphia, ch 5

Schlebusch L 1983 Consultation – liaison clinical psychology in modern hospital general practice. South African Medical Journal 64: 781–786

Schlebusch L 1990 Clinical health psychology. A behavioural medicine perspective. Southern Book Publishers, Johannesburg

Schlebusch L 2000 Mind shift. Stress management and your health. University of Natal Press, Pietermaritzburg

Schlebusch L, Cassidy M 1995 Stress, social support and biopsychosocial dynamics in HIV/AIDS. South African Journal of Psychology 25: 27–30

Schlebusch L, Schweitzer G, Bosch B 1998 Psychological considerations in the management of the HIV-infected patient with polytrauma. A case presentation. In: Schlebuch L (ed) South Africa beyond transition. Psychological well-being. Psychological Society of South Africa, Pretoria, ch 56

Sloan E P, McGill B A, Zalenski R et al 1995 Human immunodeficiency virus and hepatitis B virus seroprevalence in an urban trauma population. Journal of Trauma 38: 736–741

Van Gorp W, Cummings J 1995 Neuropsychiatric aspects of infectious diseases. In Kaplan H T, Sadock B J (eds) Comprehensive textbook of psychiatry, 6th edn. Williams and Wilkins, Baltimore, ch 2

Williams J, Tonyman P, Anderson M 1991 Effects of stress, stressors and coping resources on anxiety and peripheral narrowing. Journal of Applied Sports Psychology 3: 126–141

Yukelson D, Murphy S 1993 Psychological considerations in injury prevention. In Renstrom P (ed) Sports injuries. Basic principles of prevention and care. Blackwell Scientific Publications, Oxford, ch 25

43

Biomechanical problems of the lower limb – the key to overuse injury?

Simon J. Bartold

KEY POINTS

1. The foot transmits enormous loads from the body to the ground as a part of everyday life, and is the structure which provides stability for all the more proximal segments.
2. The integrity of the foot is fundamental to mobility in humans.
3. Any disturbance in normal foot function will cause inefficiency, fatigue and overuse injury.
4. Faulty lower limb biomechanics contribute to the vast array of overuse injuries seen in sport.
5. Biomechanics is at the centre of very complex and sophisticated research. As this continues to expand, new and improved techniques are always arising to manage injury in the athlete.

INTRODUCTION

The foot is arguably the most remarkably engineered structure in the human body. It is required to accept enormous loads as a part of everyday life, and is the structure upon which all segments above are dependent for stability. Any disturbance in normal foot function will have repercussions for the weight-bearing athlete, as this disturbance must be compensated at another level, causing inefficiency, fatigue and overuse. The integrity of the foot is fundamental to the human capacity for mobility. Human locomotion is often described as a series of falls linked together, but always on the brink of catastrophe. Failure of the foot in the realm of human motion and gait is likely to tip us further toward 'the brink of catastrophe'.

For most of us, normal, pain-free foot function is taken for granted. Despite the tremendous loads and delicate, precise function of the foot, a lifetime of functional locomotion is expected. What can we expect, however, when normal lower limb biomechanics are interrupted and especially when the increased stress of sport is considered? How much do faulty lower limb biomechanics contribute to the myriad overuse injuries seen by sports medicine practitioners? The very term 'biomechanics' has expanded in recent times and is now the centrepiece of very complex and sophisticated research. Our understanding of the structures subjected to abnormal biomechanical loads now includes not just tendon, ligament, joint and bone, but neural and biochemical pathways. The boundaries are rapidly expanding, and with this expansion comes new and improved techniques to wage the battle against injury in the athlete.

THE BIOMECHANICS OF LOWER LIMB INJURY

The science of the biomechanics of human movement is an extremely complex topic that is not within the scope of this chapter. It is, however, important to address the basic features of injury with a biomechanical basis.

Whilst our understanding of the sequential nature of human gait and fundamental segmental skeletal arrangement is essentially clarified, it is important to note that considerable controversy exists in relation to exact biomechanical measurement and analysis. This is an area of intense scientific scrutiny and increasingly sophisticated research. For the purpose of this book we shall limit the discussion to a summary of closed kinetic chain (i.e. weight-bearing) analysis of the foot and lower limb, as this is the injury-producing state.

General principles

In any discussion of human biomechanics it is necessary to revisit the concept of the cardinal body planes, as they provide the framework for all future joint and segmental position references. The cardinal body planes are the frontal, sagittal and transverse planes (Fig. 43.1):

- sagittal plane – divides the body into left and right halves
- transverse plane – divides the body into superior and inferior halves
- frontal plane – divides the body into anterior and posterior halves.

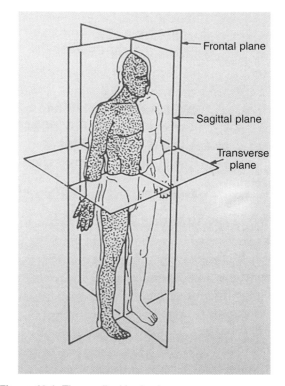

Figure 43.1 The cardinal body planes.

JOINTS

Of the numerous joints in the foot, we shall discuss three which play a major role in biomechanical function: the ankle, the subtalar joint and the midtarsal joint.

The ankle joint

The ankle or talocrural joint joins the leg to the foot and is the articulation between the tibia and fibula to the trochlear surface of the talus. The ankle joint itself may be regarded as a hinge joint, with motion restricted to almost pure dorsiflexion and plantarflexion in the sagittal plane. This motion is determined by the joint axis which lies approximately 8° from the transverse plane (or 82° from the sagittal plane) and 20–30° from the frontal plane (Valmassey 1993) (Fig. 43.2) (Author's note: It is very important when considering any discussion of a joint axis in the foot that theoretical models only can be put forward. This is due to the extreme complexity of accurately measuring a joint axis either *in vivo* or *in vitro*. Whilst research techniques have improved considerably in recent

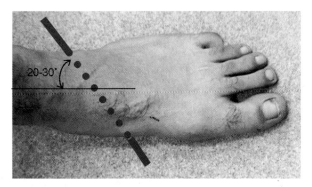

Figure 43.2 The ankle joint axis lies 20–30° from the frontal plane.

times, reliability of measurement is still not good enough to establish absolute joint axial values. All measurements quoted in this text should therefore only be considered as the most up-to-date approximations at this time.)

The ankle joint axis moves during plantarflexion and dorsiflexion, deviating plantarmedially with plantarflexion, and plantarlaterally with dorsiflexion (Hicks 1954b, Lundberg et al 1989).

The lateral collateral ligaments and the medial collateral ligament, or deltoid ligament, establish the ligamentous integrity of the ankle joint, and these structures limit and stabilize the range of motion at the ankle joint. The range of motion required for normal locomotion is variously quoted in the literature, but it is generally agreed that between 5° and 10° of dorsiflexion at the ankle is required for the leg to pass forward on the foot during the propulsive phase of gait (Bartold & Taylor 1993). Unlike the knee, the ankle joint has no major surrounding stabilizing muscles. All muscles acting to move the foot at the ankle joint arise in the leg, and so the ankle joint is susceptible to injury in the frontal plane (i.e. inversion/eversion).

The subtalar joint

The subtalar joint is the articulation with the calcaneus located immediately below the talus, created by three articular facets – anterior, middle and posterior – located on the inferior surface of the talus and the superior surface of the calcaneus (Brukner 1987).

The subtalar joint is often regarded as the most important joint in the foot because of its ability to convert transverse rotations of the leg into a smooth forward progression of gait. It is occasionally referred to as a 'torque converter' joint and is the keystone of the ankle joint complex. It is also suggested that most compensa-

tion to biomechanical malalignment will take place at the level of the subtalar joint. Motion at the subtalar joint is triplanar, i.e. non-weight-bearing, the foot abducts,' dorsiflexes and everts with pronation. Conversely the foot adducts, plantarflexes and inverts with supination. Closed kinetic chain, or weight-bearing, changes this situation in that once the calcaneus contacts the ground, it can move in the frontal plane only (i.e. inversion/eversion), due to ground reaction forces. Therefore, during closed kinetic chain, when the foot pronates, the calcaneus everts while the talus adducts and plantarflexes. During supination, the calcaneus inverts, with abduction and dorsiflexion of the talus.

Subtalar joint axis

The axis of the subtalar joint runs from posterior, plantar and lateral, to anterior, dorsal and medial. The angulation of the axis has been variously reported as 42° average inclination from the transverse plane and 16° average inclination medially from the sagittal plane (Manter 1941) (Fig. 43.3) and 23° deviation from the sagittal plane medially and 42° deviation from the

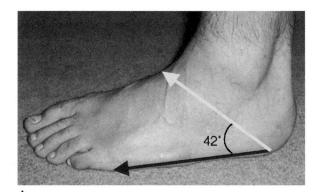

A

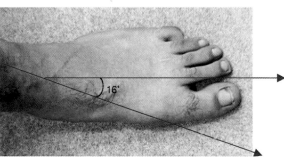

B

Figure 43.3 The subtalar joint axis deviates approximately 42° from the transverse plane (A) and 16° from the sagittal plane (B).

transverse plane (Mann & Inman 1964). Wide variations in these measurements have been reported and there is considerable variation in the deviation of the axes from both sagittal and transverse planes (Englesberg & Andrews 1987). Individual variation in the deviation of the axes has a profound effect on subtalar joint range of motion in a specific direction. This in turn influences compensation patterns in the biomechanically unsound lower limb.

The midtarsal joint

The midtarsal joint is sometimes called the transtarsal joint, and comprises the combined articulations of the talonavicular joint and the calcaneocuboid joint. It represents the functional articulation between the rearfoot and the midfoot. These articulations have been described anatomically as plane or gliding joints which function as a single unit (Karpanji 1970). The midtarsal joint is complicated by the fact that it has two joint axes, a longitudinal axis and an oblique axis, which act independently of each other. Although this statement is hotly debated, especially given the findings of Lundberg & Svensson (1988) and van Langelaan (1983), it is arguably the most practical working model.

Motion about the longitudinal axis is primarily in the frontal plane (inversion/eversion) due to the close anatomical alignment of the axis to the sagittal and transverse planes. Motion about the oblique axis occurs primarily in the sagittal (dorsiflexion/plantarflexion) and transverse (adduction/abduction) planes. This is due to the positioning of the axes at near to 50° from both transverse and sagittal planes. An important concept is the linking and interdependability of midtarsal joint function with subtalar joint function. The range of the midtarsal joint is dependent upon subtalar joint position. A pronated subtalar joint increases midtarsal joint motion, whilst a supinated subtalar joint decreases midtarsal joint motion. Our current understanding is that the midtarsal joint plays an important role in the compensation of many biomechanical anomalies, and failure of correct midtarsal joint function may be an important feature of many lower limb biomechanical problems (Bartold 1998).

BASIC BIOMECHANICS

In gait, the foot acts in a predictable and synchronous manner. Any interruption of the normal sequential events in gait may play an important role in lower limb injury generation. Whilst the ankle joint allows the leg to pass over the foot in gait, the subtalar and midtarsal joints are responsible for allowing key lower limb movements in sport.

The gait cycle

During gait, the foot must be able to fulfil the following obligations:

- It must contribute to the shock-absorbing mechanism.
- It must be able to adapt to unevenness in the terrain.
- It must allow normal transverse rotation of the lower limb.
- It must convert to a rigid lever for effective forward propulsion.

So that gait is simplified and the complex function of the foot is better understood, we divide the gait cycle into two phases, with the foot expected to fulfil its function strictly within these guidelines. One complete gait cycle is described by heel strike of the foot until the next heel strike of the same foot. The phases of the gait cycle are as follows:

- *Swing phase.* This relates to the time the foot is non-weight-bearing and has little influence on lower limb injury. However, it is important in that the swing phase of gait determines foot position immediately prior to weight-bearing.
- *Stance phase.* This phase describes weight-bearing and is divided into three periods (Fig. 43.4):
  — contact
  — midstance
  — propulsion.

Contact period

The contact period lasts for approximately 25% of the stance phase of gait and begins immediately the foot strikes the ground, i.e. 'heel contact'. At this time, the foot should be slightly inverted with activity of tibialis anterior, and should immediately begin to pronate at the subtalar joint. This contact period pronation allows the foot to absorb the impact of heel strike and fulfil its role as a shock absorber. This initial contact period pronation is driven above by knee flexion, which occurs immediately after heel strike. Subtalar joint pronation also allows for the foot to adapt to variations in terrain. Subtalar joint pronation continues up until the forefoot begins to bear weight, known as forefoot loading, and this marks the end of the contact period

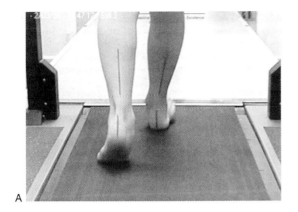

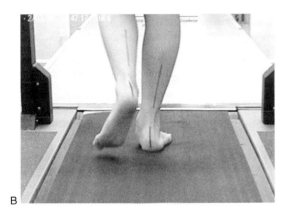

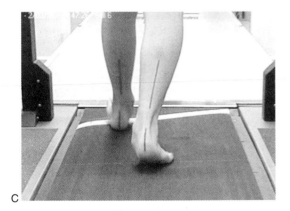

Figure 43.4 The gait cycle showing the three periods of the stance phase of gait. These photographs demonstrate an abnormal gait pattern with substantial abnormal subtalar and midtarsal joint pronation. A: Contact. B: Midstance. C: Propulsion. Note the pronated position of the subtalar and midtarsal joints at a time when they should be supinated. This is likely to alter normal muscle action and timing significantly, and may be an important contributing factor in injury.

and the beginning of the midstance period of the stance phase of gait.

Midstance

By the time the forefoot is finally weight-bearing, the foot should have finished pronating. Any apparent pronation beyond this point in the gait cycle indicates severe abnormal foot function. This amplifies the great importance of accurate gait analysis in the assessment of overuse injury. The quality of gait is of vital importance and it is imperative the sports medicine practitioner is able to correctly interpret any interruption of the normal gait cycle.

The midstance period finishes at approximately the 65% mark of the stance phase, and is identified by the event known as heel lift, which marks the beginning of the propulsive period of the stance phase of gait.

Propulsion

For effective propulsion to occur, the foot must act as an efficient lever and therefore must be 'locked'. The forefoot can only act as a rigid lever if the subtalar joint is supinated. This supinated position of the subtalar joint pronates the midtarsal joint by way of ground reaction forces and reduces the available midtarsal joint motion, thereby producing a stable forefoot platform suitable for effective forward propulsion. The end of the propulsive period, and therefore the stance phase of gait, is marked by toe-off, which during a normal walking gait cycle corresponds to forefoot loading on the opposite foot. It is essential to understand the basic nature of lower limb biomechanics. It is not so much a question of how much pronation or supination, but when it occurs. It is also important to accept that foot function has a significant effect higher up the limb. Because of the articulation of the talus within the ankle mortise, pronation is inextricably linked to internal rotation of the tibia. Because of these rotational changes, abnormal pronation or supination can often be major contributors to injury in the lower limb. The remainder of the chapter will explore one of the most common lower limb injuries in sport, plantar fasciitis, and how faulty biomechanics may contribute.

PLANTAR FASCIITIS

This is by far the most common sports injury presenting to the office of the sports podiatrist. This debilitating injury has the potential to severely restrict, or even prohibit, the athlete from normal training or competition.

However, with correct history, medical work-up and definitive diagnosis, plantar fasciitis is one of the most responsive of all sports injuries to treatment.

History

Plantar fasciitis presents in a most characteristic manner, and the diagnosis *clinically* is often made within the first few minutes of history-taking. Typically plantar fasciitis is:

- *Insidious*. The onset is gradual and worsens over a period of time, often weeks or even months. Eventually the pain degenerates to a stage where the patient is compelled to seek treatment. Plantar fasciitis is occasionally acute in onset, but this is invariably preceded by some traumatic incident. Interestingly, if the history is complete enough, the examining practitioner will often elicit a report of injury to the general region of the plantar fascia at the time the pain first started. An example of this would be catching the heel on the edge of a footpath whilst crossing the road. At the time this does not cause pain, but at a microscopic level it may be enough to cause separation of the cross-linking structure of the collagen fibres of the plantar fascia and precipitate a symptomatic, chronic condition.
- *Painful in the morning on rising from rest*. The patient will report pain, severe on first weight-bearing in the morning or on rising after a prolonged period of rest (e.g. after a long car journey). This pain will inevitably improve after a short period of walking. Likewise, the pain is worst at the commencement of sporting activity and improves after a period of 'warm-up'. The pain is, however, likely to worsen after cessation of sport. The basis of this pain after rest is presumed to be due to the accumulation of inflammatory by-products which impinge on nerve endings when compressed during weight-bearing (Bartold 1998). This pain, i.e. morning and rise from rest pain, is one of the most reliable and characteristic features diagnostically for plantar fasciitis.
- *Localized over the medial slip of the origin of the fascia*. Plantar fasciitis is usually a very well localized condition and this assists greatly in making the diagnosis. It is relatively uncommon for pain to be spread over a more diffuse area, but there may be poorly defined pain in the mid-substance of the fascia or even spreading up the medial and lateral aspects of the calcaneus.

Anatomy

The plantar fascia is perhaps more correctly called the *plantar aponeurosis*, and lies superficial to the muscles of the plantar surface of the foot. The plantar fascia has a thick and strong central part which covers the central muscle of the first layer, *flexor digitorum brevis*, and is immediately deep to the superficial fascia of the plantar surface. It is attached proximally to the calcaneus at the anterior calcaneal tubercle, the site of the muscle attachments, while distally it blends with the skin at the creases at the bases of the digits and also sends five slips, one to each toe. Each of these splits into two, which pass deeply, one on each side of the flexor tendons of that toe, and finally fuse with the *deep transverse metatarsal ligaments*.

This anatomical arrangement is integral to the pathogenesis of plantar fasciitis. Also of great importance anatomically are the perifascial structures, most notably the subcalcaneal bursa and the medial tibial branch of the posterior tibial nerve (Fig. 43.5). Both these structures may be involved in what is seen as the general symptom complex of plantar fasciitis, especially in the more chronic cases.

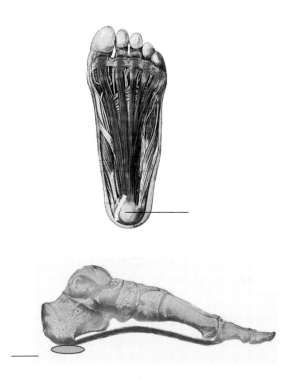

Figure 43.5 The perifascial structures. The anatomy of the plantar fascia. The broad, fan-shaped fascia provides important support to the medial longitudinal arch of the foot.

Biomechanics of the plantar fascia

The plantar fascia has two main functions, both of which are essential to the normal functioning of the foot.

Firstly, it maintains the integrity of the medial longitudinal arch of the foot. Rupture of the plantar fascia severely compromises the arch structure of the foot and may lead to a profoundly flat foot. This, however, is dependent upon the site of rupture, and in fact surgical sectioning of the plantar fascia near its origin may have little effect on the arch profile.

Secondly, because of its manner of insertion into the medial aspect of the calcaneus, the plantar fascia has a vital role in the resupination of the foot during the propulsive period of the stance phase of gait. This is achieved through what is known as the windlass function of the hallux (Hicks 1954). This so-called windlass function describes the tightening of the plantar fascia on dorsiflexion of the hallux. During the propulsive period of the stance phase of gait, the heel has left the ground and the hallux is therefore in a dorsiflexed position. This tightens the plantar fascia and, through its more medial insertion, exerts an inversion influence on the calcaneus and thereby supinates the subtalar joint in closed kinetic chain (Fig. 43.6). Recent research has confirmed this phenomenon, and demonstrates that the peak loading force in the plantar fascia occurs during the propulsive period of the stance phase of gait (Scott & Winter 1990).

Specific abnormal foot types may subject the plantar fascia to increased strain. Prolonged abnormal subtalar pronation has long been implicated in the pathogenesis of plantar fasciitis (Clement et al 1981, Kibler et al 1991, Meissner & Pittala 1988, Warren & Jones 1987). Kogler et al (1996) demonstrated *in vitro* that strain in the plantar fascia was measurably reduced in nine cadaver specimens when a lateral forefoot wedge was introduced and load applied. Bartold (1998) confirmed that pain scores were significantly reduced with taping and lateral forefoot wedging in a study of 55 plantar fasciitis patients. Both studies indicate the relative biomechanical contribution to the injury and suggest that altering the midtarsal joint moment may have a significant strain-reducing effect on the plantar fascia.

Physical examination

- *Local tenderness*. Pain will usually be localized over a small area near the origin of the fascia at the proximal insertion into the anterior tubercle of the calcaneus. The pain response to palpation over this small area involves considerable apprehension, and evasive action may be taken by the patient to avoid further investigation (Fig. 43.7)!
- Commonly there will be *pain over the midline of the plantar surface* of the calcaneus, which may be either diffuse or localized in nature. This pain may characteristically be seen in patients with weight-bearing occupations (nurses, storemen etc.), and probably represents some inflammation of the subcalcaneal bursa (Fig. 43.8).

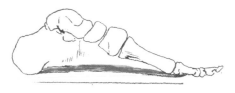

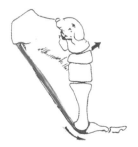

Figure 43.6 Diagrammatic representation of the windlass mechanism demonstrating how the plantar fascia tightens during the propulsive period, assisting with resupination of the subtalar joint and conversion of the foot from mobile adapter to rigid lever.

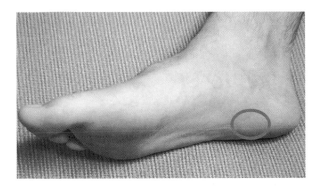

Figure 43.7 The classic site for palpation of local tenderness with plantar fasciitis.

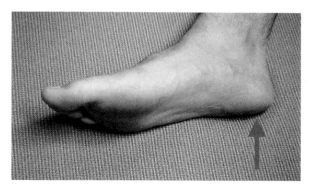

Figure 43.8 Typical site for location of pain from a subcalcaneal bursa. Note that this is more proximal to the site of pain of plantar fascia origin.

- There is often *diffuse tenderness* up the medial or lateral aspect of the calcaneus, which is typical of the more severe inflammatory processes. This needs to be differentiated from calcaneal stress fracture or referred pain from the subtalar joint (Fig. 43.9).
- *Positive windlass manoeuvre*, i.e. pain with passive dorsiflexion of the hallux thereby loading the plantar fascia. This positive windlass test is often quoted in the texts, but in reality is seen in only a tiny percentage of cases, and then only the most severe. A positive windlass response may indicate rupture of a significant proportion of the fascia (Fig. 43.10).
- *No swelling*. Swelling with plantar fasciitis is relatively rare and usually reserved to the most severe cases or an acute fascial injury. The presence of swelling, however, can be an important diagnostic clue and may indicate other injury such as fracture, muscle injury or rupture to the fascia.

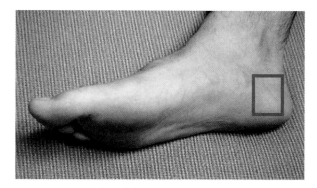

Figure 43.9 Pain is commonly palpated over the medial or lateral body of the calcaneus. This pain must be differentiated from a calcaneal stress fracture.

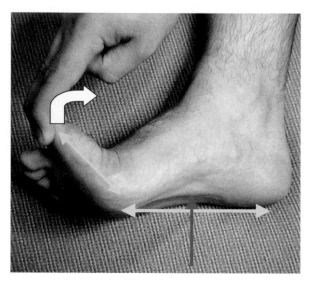

Figure 43.10 Demonstration of the windlass manoeuvre in which the hallux is dorsiflexed to tighten the plantar fascia. Increased tension in the plantar fascia is clearly demonstrated by the arrow.

- *Nodular change to the fascia* is a very common finding and represents fascial granulomata formed as the result of repeated fascial injury which has healed with scarring. These granulomata can become quite large (the size of a golf ball is not uncommon), and therefore very uncomfortable during weight-bearing. If these lesions cannot be accommodated with the appropriate orthotic device, surgical intervention is appropriate.
- *Pain with passive talocrural joint dorsiflexion*. Because of the intimate anatomical relationship between the plantar fascia and the triceps surae, dorsiflexion at the ankle joint will commonly elicit pain. Stretching of a tight posterior group is mandatory in the rehabilitation of plantar fasciitis (Fig. 43.11).

Radiographic evaluation

Plain radiographs are used routinely in the medical community to screen for the so-called 'spurs' often associated with plantar fasciitis (Fig. 43.11). This practice is not only of limited value clinically, but in fact may cloud the issue, especially in the mind of the patient. A calcaneal spur, as visualized on a standard lateral radiograph of the foot, is in fact a shelf of friable, non-cancellous bone, extending the full width of the plantar fascia, but most commonly insinuated in the origin of flexor digitorum brevis (Baxter & Thigpen

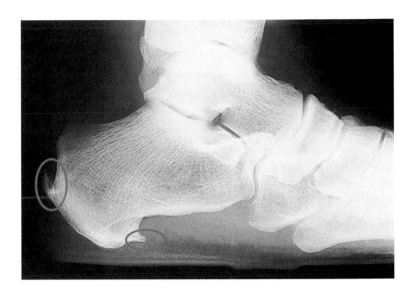

Figure 43.11 Large plantar and posterior calcaneal 'spurs'. These lesions are often asymptomatic and discovered only during investigation for other, unrelated entities.

1984). It probably represents an attempt by the body to provide a support shelf for the injured fascia, rather than the formation of a true traction spur secondary to enthesopathy. Plain radiographs and other investigative radiology studies such as isotopic bone scan, CT scan, ultrasound studies and MRI should only be utilized when there is suspicion of fascial disruption or malignancy/infective process.

Differential diagnosis

As with any sporting injury, making an accurate diagnosis is of utmost importance. This is particularly highlighted when one considers that some of the more serious systemic diseases and tumours can present as simple overuse injuries such as plantar fasciitis. The practitioner must therefore always take the most complete history and listen to the patient for the clues that may indicate a more sinister diagnosis. The following are some of the diagnoses that may result in heel pain:

- complete rupture of the plantar fascia
- subcalcaneal bursitis
- medial calcaneal nerve entrapment
- ruptured fat pad
- Sever's disease
- tarsal tunnel syndrome
- calcaneal stress fracture
- seronegative arthropathy, e.g. ankylosing spondylitis, Reiter's syndrome, psoriatic arthritis, irritable bowel syndrome

- diffuse connective tissue disease including seropositive arthropathy (rheumatoid arthritis)
  — Behçet's syndrome
  — systemic lupus erythematosus
  — necrotizing vasculitis and other vasculopathies
  — Sjögren's syndrome
  — Marie–Strumpel disease
- tumour.

Management

The immediate treatment for plantar fasciitis is as with all overuse injuries, i.e. rest, ice, compression, elevation and medication to reduce inflammation and control pain. The specific management involves a review of the following:

- *Training techniques* – with specific reference to those drills that may have contributed to the injury, e.g. hill running, running on non-supporting surfaces such as sand, stair climbing, bounding, sudden increases in training or sudden changes to training routine.
- *Shoes* – a very large and complex area, especially given the increased sophistication of current athletic footwear. The onus is on the sports medicine practitioner to be aware of the specific requirements of the different sports and the way in which a shoe can be either beneficial or detrimental. Specific recommendations should be made for the individual needs of the athlete (Fig. 43.12).

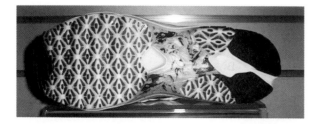

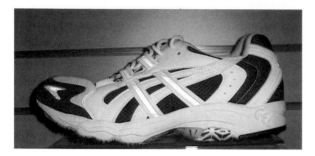

Figure 43.12 The complexities of modern athletic footwear means the sports medicine practitioner must be aware of the technical features of each shoe.

- *Stretching* – especially of the triceps surae, but ability to assess and address all tight structures is essential. **Note**: it is particularly important to be able to identify and treat tight neural structures in overuse injury (Fig. 43.13).

- *Taping* – modified low-dye/moccasin taping is particularly helpful in the early management of plantar fasciitis (Fig. 43.14).
- *Modalities* – may be beneficial in the reduction of inflammation associated with plantar fasciitis.
- *Cross-fibre friction* – this is an especially useful technique in this condition and is easily taught to the patient as an ongoing home management treatment.
- *Subtalar joint mobilization* – important in the presence of reduced subtalar joint mobility.
- *Orthoses* – these are arguably the most important treatment modality for plantar fasciitis of a biomechanical origin. Many authors have cited prolonged abnormal pronation as an important factor in the pathogenesis of the condition (Kwong et al 1988). Management should revolve around control of the abnormal foot position, with particular attention to the midtarsal joint. This joint must be maintained in a maximally pronated position to reduce the strain in the plantar fascia (Bartold 1998, Kogler et al 1996).
- *Surgery* – good results can be achieved with sectioning of the plantar fascia near its origin and decompression of the medial calcaneal branch of the posterior tibial nerve where appropriate. Surgery should, however, only be considered when other conservative measures have failed.

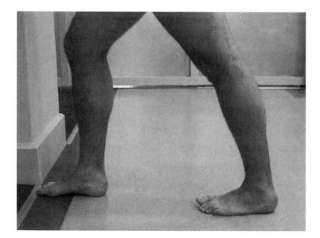

Figure 43.13 Stretching, particularly for tight triceps surae, is an important part of the management of plantar fasciitis. Note: this patient has a very tight gastrocnemius muscle and is compensating this deficiency by allowing the knee to move into recurvatum.

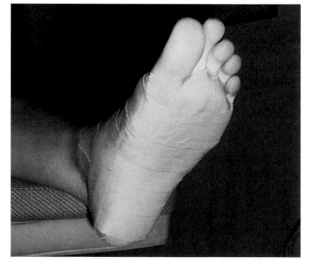

Figure 43.14 Strapping for plantar fasciitis.

CONCLUSIONS

An understanding of the biomechanical basis of overuse injury is essential for any practitioner working in the field of sports medicine. Nowhere is this more evident than in an injury such as plantar fasciitis. Future research must focus on patterns of compensation for biomechanical abnormalities and methods of accommodation for these anomalies once identified, e.g.:

- the role of the midtarsal joint in both the generation and treatment of the condition
- the role of dynamic and passive arch support
- improved accuracy of joint axial measurement
- improved dynamic gait analysis in relation to injury production.

REFERENCES

Barnett C H 1952 The axis of rotation of the ankle joint in man. Its influence upon the form of the talus and the mobility of the fibula. Anatomy 86: 1–8

Bartold S J 1998 The biomechanics of plantar fascial injury: calcaneal inversion does not reduce plantar fascial strain. Proceedings of the 18th Australian Podiatry Conference, Australian Podiatry Association, Melbourne.

Bartold S J, Taylor G 1993 Common foot and ankle problems in sport: their assessment, management and prevention. Australian Sports Medicine Federation, Canberra

Baxter D E, Pfeffer G B 1987 Chronic heel pain – treatment rationale. Orthopedic Clinics of North America 20(4): 563–568

Baxter D E, Thigpen C M 1984 Heel pain – operative results. Foot Ankle 5: 16–25

Brukner J 1987 Variations in the human subtalar joint. Journal of Orthopedic Sports Physical Therapy 8: 489–494

Clement D B, Taunton J E, Smart G W 1981 A survey of overuse injuries. Physician and Sportsmedicine 9: 47–58

Englesberg J R, Andrews J G 1987 Kinematic analysis of the talocalcaneal/talocrural joint during running support. Medicine and Science in Sport and Exercise 3: 275–284

Hicks J H 1954a The mechanics of the foot I. The plantar aponeurosis and the arch. Journal of Anatomy 88: 25–30

Hicks J H 1954b The mechanics of the foot II. The plantar aponeurosis and the arch. Journal of Anatomy 88: 345–357

Karpanji I A 1970 The physiology of the joints: lower limb, vol 2. Churchill Livingstone, Edinburgh

Kibler W B, Goldberg C, Chandler T C 1991 Functional biomechanics in running athletes with plantar fasciitis. American Journal of Sports Medicine 19(1): 66–71

Kogler G F, Solomonidis S E, Paul J P 1996 Biomechanics of longitudinal arch support mechanisms in foot orthoses and their effect on plantar aponeurosis strain. Clinical Biomechanics 11(5): 243–252

Kwong P K, Kay D, Voner R T, White M W 1988 Plantar fascia mechanics and pathomechanics of treatment. Clinical Sports Medicine 7(1): 119–126

Lundberg A, Svenssen D 1988 The axis of rotation of the talo-calcaneal and talo-navicular joints. In: Lundberg A (ed) Patterns of motion of the ankle/foot complex. Karolinska Institute, Gotab, Stockholm

Lundberg A, Svensson D, Nemeth G, Selvik G 1989 The axis of rotation of the ankle joint. Journal of Bone and Joint Surgery (Br) 71: 94–99

Mann R A, Inman V T 1964 Phasic activity of intrinsic muscles of the foot. Journal of Bone and Joint Surgery (Am) 46: 469

Manter J T 1941 Movements of the subtalar and transtarsal joints. The Anatomical Record 80(4): 397–410

Meissier S P, Pittala K A 1988 Etiological factors associated with selected running injuries. Medicine and Science in Sports and Exercise 20(5): 501–505

Scott S H, Winter D A 1990 Internal forces at chronic running injury sites. Medicine and Science in Sports and Exercise 22(3): 357–369

Valmassy R L 1996 Clinical biomechanics of the lower extremities. Mosby, St Louis

van Langelaan E J 1983 A kinematic analysis of the tarsal joints. Acta Orthopaedica Scandinavica 54(suppl): 204

Warren B L, Jones G J 1987 Predicting plantar fasciitis in runners. Medicine and Science in Sports and Exercise 19(1): 71–73

44

Sports for children with physical disabilities

A. D. J. Webborn

KEY POINTS

1. In recent decades, there have been increasing efforts to enable people with disabilities to enjoy the benefits of regular physical activity.
2. The choice of sport for a child with disabilities will be influenced by various factors, including, *inter alia*, the child's preference, the sport's characteristics, the child's medical condition and cognitive and social skills, and the availability of facilities.
3. There are relatively few absolute contraindications to participation, but risks relating to, for example, a concomitant cardiac condition or altered thermoregulation should be properly considered.
4. Sports for people with disabilities have developed in relation to particular groups of disability, e.g. spinal cord lesions, visual impairment, cerebral palsy and amputees, and there is also a group for those not falling into any particular category, termed 'les autres'.
5. With the continued advances in sport for children with disabilities, and in particular the competitiveness of the environment, physicians have a duty of care to protect young athletes from exploitation.

INTRODUCTION

The potential benefits in medical terms of regular and appropriate physical activity are now well established. The risks of a sedentary lifestyle are also well recognized (Blair et al 1995), and the last few decades have seen increasing efforts to enable people with disabilities to enjoy these benefits too. For most people, their first introduction to organized sport is in childhood, often through their school, and for many years children with disabilities have been denied this opportunity. Sport plays a major part in society today, with particular regard to social integration, and exclusion of people with disabilities from aspects of society in general are reflected in the history of exclusion from sport. The reasons for this are many and often cultural and include:

- Parental overprotection – the concept that a child with a disability is too frail to participate (Nixon 1988)
- Medical overprotection – medical restrictions may have been placed on children because of a lack of understanding (Peck & McKeag 1994). If in doubt, doctors seem to advise against anything that might involve some risk
- Reluctance to integrate children with disabilities in able-bodied sport in school
- A lack of organized sport programmes for children with disabilities
- Absence of appropriate and accessible sport facilities and coaches with appropriate training.

TERMINOLOGY

Prior to embarking on any discussion of sport for children with disabilities, it is useful to consider the current terminology in use. Terms such as 'handicapped', 'retarded' and 'incapacitated' are avoided. The emphasis is on the positive attributes of the person and a 'people first' approach is used, e.g. 'people with special needs', 'people with learning difficulties'. Handicap derives from a person being 'cap in hand' – begging. Similarly, with reference to sports, terms to be avoided are 'handicapped sport' or 'disabled sport'. Sport itself cannot be disabled. Disability sport is the adopted term for sport that has been designed for or specifically practised by athletes with disabilities. It may seem a small point but it is important that both coaches and athletes are comfortable with the terminology used so as not to cause offence.

Although there are potential health gains from appropriate levels of physical activity for children with disabilities, we should also consider the social and psychological benefits of involving these children in sport (Brown 1982). This may be within the confines of disability sport or in integration with sport for non-disabled. Each can improve self-efficacy and self-worth. Allowing children with disabilities to compete and achieve in a sporting environment provides fulfilment. The benefits must be also seen in the light of the risks of continued inactivity and its effects on bone density, muscle strength and cardiovascular risk factors.

CHOOSING A SPORT

For those who are considering offering children with disabilities the potential benefits of sport, there are certain issues to address, including, for example, 'What are you aiming to achieve?'. If the aim is primarily for physical health benefits for a disease process then one has to consider the difference between exercise and sport. These terms are often incorrectly used interchangeably. Sport is not always exercise, and vice-versa. Sport implies competition and the physiological demands are determined by the sport, e.g. wheelchair sprint racing (anaerobic) versus wheelchair road racing (aerobic) versus pistol shooting (skill). Sport may also involve trauma, which will be particularly undesirable in some conditions. Alternatively, the focus may be on socialization and building self-esteem. While the ability to achieve one of these aims is not necessarily exclusive of the others, it is helpful to consider one's goals. Not all sports need to be organized or competitive.

The choice of sport will be influenced by various factors, including:

- The personal preference of the child – an emphasis on fun, enjoyment and taking part in a sport that stimulates and interests the child is important for continued participation
- The characteristics of the sport – physiological demands, collision potential, team or individual, coordination requirements
- The medical condition – beneficial and detrimental aspects
- Problems associated with the condition – although motor dysfunction may initially appear to be the major limitation to participation, there may be, for example, an associated cardiac condition to consider
- The cognitive ability and social skills of the child – ability to follow rules and interact with others
- Availability of facilities

- Availability of appropriate coaching and support staff (lifting and handling)
- Equipment availability and cost – as disability sport has evolved, so has the technology. At elite level, wheelchairs are designed particularly for the sport in question and are not used for activities of daily living. Wheelchair racing has derived much influence from cycling technology. Specialist chairs are available for sports such as tennis, rugby and basketball. While it is not necessary to have sport-specific chairs for initial participation, it does become a consideration as children develop their interest and feel more limited by their equipment.

Sports can be classified based upon their aerobic intensity, potential for trauma and demands for coordination. Exercise intensity may be monitored satisfactorily by rating of perceived exertion (Ward et al 1995). Examples of categorizations of sport are shown in Table 44.1.

RISKS OF PARTICIPATION

Although this chapter aims to highlight the positive aspects of sport for children with disabilities, it would be inappropriate not to consider the potential risks. In general terms there are relatively few absolute contraindications to participation, and for any child or adult, able-bodied or not, the general principles of training apply. Training is an adaptation response to gradual and progressive overload governed by the duration, intensity, frequency and mode of activity. If the principles of training are applied, then the risk of adverse effects are minimized and improvements in cardiovascular fitness can be made in a variety of disabilities (O'Connell & Barnhart 1995).

Sudden death in sport

Sudden deaths that occur during sport or exercise participation are rare but catastrophic events that may occur regardless of age or health status. Sudden deaths associated with vigorous exercise or sports participation in children are invariably related to cardiac conditions, except perhaps for incidents related to seizures in water or other dangerous situations. Examples are:

- hypertrophic obstructive cardiomyopathy
- anomalous coronary vessels
- aortic dissection associated with Marfan's syndrome
- arrhythmias
- aortic stenosis
- septal defects and right-to-left shunts.

For children with a disability, it requires greater awareness from their physician of conditions that may have associated cardiac disease. For example, it is estimated that 50% of children with trisomy 21 (Down's syndrome) will have some congenital cardiac defect and this will require evaluation if strenuous participation is intended. Exercise intensity is an important consideration in sport selection where cardiac anomalies may be present. Physicians should not exclude children from appropriate levels of activity on the basis of possible cardiac disease without good evidence (Bergman & Stamm 1967).

Environmental issues

Children are more vulnerable than adults to extremes of temperature due to an increased surface area to body weight ratio. They will lose heat more rapidly in a cold environment, and conversely gain heat more rapidly in a hot environment. Sweating rates in children are less

Table 44.1 Examples of sports' collision potential, aerobic intensity and coordination needs (American Academy of Pediatrics 1982)

	Collision/contact potential	Aerobic intensity	Coordination
High	Judo Basketball Alpine skiing	Athletics Nordic skiing Swimming	Basketball Shooting Archery
Moderate ('limited' for collision/contact potential)	Athletics Volleyball Nordic skiing	Equestrain Table tennis Judo	Volleyball Goalball Soccer
Low ('none' for collision/contact potential)	Archery Table tennis Shooting	Archery Boccia Bowling	Power lifting Athletics – track Boccia

than in adults, and as a result children have a reduced capacity for heat loss in a hot environment. The relatively lower blood volume of a child makes dehydration more likely. Children with disabilities have additional risks with temperature regulation, as follows:

- Neurological disorders, e.g. spinal cord injury. There is a reduction in functioning peripheral receptors and the heat loss mechanisms below the level of the lesion are impaired. In general terms, the higher the level of the spinal cord lesion, the greater the problems of temperature control appear to be.
- Some children will need assistance with their daily living needs and need to be able to access appropriate fluids. This may be as a result of physical or visual impairment. An increased awareness and training of coaching and support staff are necessary.
- The effects of dehydration may also increase the possibility of epileptic seizures. The incidence of epilepsy in disabled sportsmen is higher than the average population. Ten per cent of the Great Britain swimming team for the European Championships in 1995 had some form of epilepsy.
- Muscle tone in children with cerebral palsy may be affected with excessive exposure to heat and have detrimental effects on performance.
- Bilateral amputees have less surface area to sweat and lose heat.
- Children with a learning disability will require particular guidance and supervision regarding fluid intake and hydration.
- In cold environments, children require appropriate clothing and headgear with adequate wind-proofing. Circulatory disorders associated with their disability may make them more susceptible to cold injury.

Trauma

Most sports involve some risk of injury, but particular sports have higher associations than others. They may be contact sports such as football or sports where there is the risk of collision injuries occurring, such as skiing or cycling. Children with congenital heart disease may be at increased risk of dysrhythmias from blunt trauma to the chest, and subcutaneous pacemakers or cerebrospinal fluid (CSF) shunts also may be susceptible to trauma. Bone mineral density may be reduced by the nature of the condition, e.g. osteogenesis imperfecta, or secondary to immobilization, e.g. in paraplegia, and the risk of spontaneous fracture or fracture with minimal trauma exists. The risk of atlantoaxial instability in patients with Down's syndrome remains

an issue of contention, with the relaxation of recommendations in more recent guidelines still being a matter of debate (Pueschel 1998).

Overuse injuries

Children with disabilities participating in sport are no less susceptible to overuse injuries than their able-bodied counterparts and the risk factors are the same:

- sudden increases in training volume
- biomechanical factors – more prevalent and often more pronounced in children with disabilities
- growth – osteochondritides, avulsion and growth plate injuries
- technical factors – probably more prevalent with coordination difficulties
- poor flexibility – muscle contractures.

THE GROUPING OF CHILDREN BY DISABILITY

In reality, people with disabilities can take part in virtually every sport available, including high-risk sports such as mountain climbing, sub-aqua diving and skiing. Historically, sports for people with disabilities have developed in relation to particular disabled groups, and for the purposes of this text, it is easier to consider these disability groups and the medical problems they face individually. These groups also represent the elite level that children may go on to (see 'elite disability sport') and are as follows:

- spinal cord lesions – congenital (spina bifida) or acquired (injury or disease)
- visual impairment
- cerebral palsy
- amputees
- 'les autres' (or 'the others') – a term used for people with certain disabilities that do not fit into another category, e.g. muscular dystrophy, multiple sclerosis
- children with learning difficulties, including The Special Olympics (discussed further in Ch. 45).

Spinal cord lesions

The motor loss that occurs following spinal cord injury is the most obvious to the uninitiated and reflects the level of the spinal cord lesion. This may involve all limbs (quadriplegia) or both legs (paraplegia), and may be a complete or incomplete paresis. In terms of sport performance for a child, this is probably the major determining factor, but from the medical point of view it is the sensory and autonomic losses that are more important. The level of the motor loss will determine whether there is any loss of intercostal muscle function, which will be reflected in reduced ventilatory capacity. It will also influence postural stability, and bracing may be required for some sports. Paralympic sports for athletes with spinal cord lesions include archery, equestrian events, lawn bowls, tennis, athletics, fencing, power lifting, basketball, shooting, yachting, swimming, quad rugby and table tennis.

Sensory loss

The sensory loss that accompanies the motor loss at the same level has important implications for a child taking part in sport. Skin pressure areas occur commonly in people with spinal cord injuries, and increased pressure and shear forces from sports activities may increase the risk of skin ulceration. Because pain is not appreciated at the cortical level, prolonged sitting in a sports chair, designed for performance rather than comfort, may increase the risk of tissue damage. It is unlikely to be detected unless exaggerated local spinal cord reflexes give warning signs of nociception with increased muscle tone or possibly autonomic dysreflexia (see later). Careful inspection of chairs for sharp edges etc. should be carried out along with skin inspection after activity.

Autonomic loss

Bowels and bladder. Dysfunction of the autonomic nervous system following spinal cord injury leads to impaired function of bladder and bowels, with loss of control. Children with spinal cord lesions may manage their urinary function with condom and leg bag drainage (with or without reflex activity), indwelling catheter or intermittent self-catheterization. Sports activities increase the risk of 'failure' of the urinary collecting system through leakage or increased intra-abdominal pressure, causing inappropriate voiding or soiling. Children may be embarrassed about their urinary or bowel function, particularly if participating with able-bodied children. Urine leakage is a potential risk and supervising staff should be aware of the potential problems and help to reassure children. It may be given as a reason for non-participation.

Children with a neurological bladder are at risk of recurrent urinary tract infection and renal calculi. It is important that dehydration does not occur as this not only impairs sport performance and risks heat illness, but is also likely to aggravate renal calculi and infection.

Thermal regulation. The problems associated with thermal regulation and spinal cord injury have been alluded to in the section on environmental issues. In spinal cord-injured child, there is:

- Peripheral receptor mechanism function loss – causing inability to detect temperature change.
- Loss of autonomic control on the sweating effector mechanism (Guttman et al 1958) – there is a basal sweat rate below the level of the lesion which is unaffected by ambient temperature or activity. In tetraplegics, in particular, there is an increased sweat rate above the level of the lesion which may be of the order of a sixfold increase (Petrofsky 1992). This may lead to sweat dripping off and being ineffective in heat loss.
- Loss of control of the ability to vasoconstrict or vasodilate the peripheral vasculature appropriately.
- A different thermoregulatory set point – this is a variable function of the ambient temperature and makes appropriate thermoregulation problematic (Attia & Engel 1983, Downey et al 1973).

It is important to ensure that children with spinal cord injuries take the necessary preventive measures for exercise in the heat (Webborn 1996), with reductions in duration and intensity of exercise while offering regular drinking opportunities and the usual methods of cooling (e.g. hat, fan, appropriate clothing).

In a cold environment, the muscles of a child with a spinal cord lesion will not shiver, and the skin responses are not appropriate and increase the rate of heat loss. Appropriate protective clothing should be worn, including wind protection, and the extremities should be checked for cold injury.

Cardiovascular. Children with a spinal cord lesion above the level of T1 will have an absence of sympathetic cardiac innervation, producing a depressed maximal heart rate. The level is determined by the intrinsic sinoatrial activity and is usually between 110 and 130 beats/min (Hoffman 1986). This reduction in heart rate reserve and also in stroke volume accounts for a reduced cardiac output. These factors are related to the reduced catecholamine response and decreased preload from reduced peripheral vascular tone.

Autonomic dysreflexia. This phenomenon occurs in spinal cord lesions of T6 and above and is triggered by nociceptive input below the level of the lesion. Sensory impulses enter the cord below the lesion, and the sympathetic nervous system responds to local spinal reflexes with an excessive discharge which is uncorrected. There is an inappropriate response of noradrenaline output that produces hypertension, sweating, skin blotching and headache. The usual causes are blockage of a urinary catheter, constipation, urinary calculi, anal fissure or ingrowing toenail. In the hospital setting, this has been reported to produce severe hypertension, cerebral haemorrhage, fits and deaths, and as such is treated as a medical emergency with management aimed at removing the nociceptive stimulus and reducing the blood pressure with sublingual nifedipine if required.

Recently, there have been reports of athletes with a quadriplegia intentionally inducing the dysreflexic state to achieve performance enhancement. This technique is known as 'boosting', and has been achieved by clamping the catheter to cause bladder distension, tightening leg straps, twisting/sitting on the scrotum or prolonged sitting in the racing chair. The noradrenaline response is reported to enhance exercise performance by achieving a greater response from the sympathectomized heart. Rating of perceived exertion is reduced for a given exercise intensity and improvements are seen in treadmill exercise capability. Moreover, increases in simulated race times of 9.7% in the 'boosted' state have been seen (Burnham et al 1994). Although there have been no serious reported consequences from use in the 'athletic situation', possibly as a result of increased cardiovascular fitness in the trained athlete compared with the hospitalized patient, for reasons of safety it is a practice not to be encouraged and it has been deemed a banned method of doping by the International Paralympic Committee.

Musculoskeletal injuries. Data on the true incidence and type of injury in people with spinal cord lesions are limited and are often self-reported diagnoses (Bloomquist 1986, Ferrara & Davis 1990). Data on children are even more elusive. However, the sort of injuries typically seen include chronic and overuse symptoms in the cervical and thoracic spines and the shoulder. The shoulder, in particular, is reported to be a major source of pain, but the author's personal experience at the Atlanta Paralympic Games with the Great Britain team found that a larger proportion of complaints of shoulder pain were attributable to the cervical spine and not the shoulder. Traumatic injuries to the forearm, hand and fingers are common. As in any sport, prevention should address warm-up, attention to technique, equipment, flexibility and appropriate conditioning and cool-down.

Spina bifida

Spina bifida is a congenital disorder involving faulty closure of the neural tube. Children with spina bifida are sometimes equated with children with a spinal cord lesion, but the clinical presentation may vary from no visible abnormality to a child who has a quadraparesis and severe learning difficulties. Hydrocephalus is common, with cerebrospinal fluid (CSF) shunting required. The shunt should be protected from trauma in at-risk sports. An abnormality of the hindbrain, the Arnold–Chiari malformation, is not uncommonly present. There is downward displacement of the brain stem into the cervical spine, and this may become symptomatic with neck pain and motor or sensory neurological changes or respiratory impairment. Sports that place the cervical spine at risk should therefore be avoided.

Depending on the level of the motor loss, children may be ambulant or require a wheelchair for activity. Those who are ambulant have relatively few limitations in sport. Those with higher lesions are more prone to significant scoliosis, which may require bracing or spinal fusion. Contractures are common, and stretching and flexibility should be an important part of the exercise programme. The principles of bowel and bladder function described above may also apply, as does the sensory loss.

Visually impaired

Visual impairment can range from complete blindness to partial-sightedness, combining loss of visual acuity and field loss. Children with visual impairment have the opportunity to take part in many sports. They may be aided by guides or callers, who call directions, or alternatively by adaptations such as a sound-emitting ball or a tandem cycle with a sighted pilot rider. In swimming, an assistant taps the head or shoulder with a soft-ended pole to indicate the pool end to enable turning and finishing. Adaptations can be made to rifles to give an audible tone when on target.

The main problems for visually impaired children taking part in sport relate to falls and collisions causing injury. Assistants may help the visually impaired by offering an arm as a guide, which the child can then hold onto to be led, rather than grasping the child's arm and leading him or her.

Cerebral palsy

Cerebral palsy is a non-progressive cerebral impairment that occurs before, during or shortly after birth. There are three primary motor disorders that characterize the condition:

- Spasticity – there is marked increase in muscle tone, with weakness, poor movement and posture.

The tone is a variable parameter dependent upon environmental factors, fatigue and emotion.

- Choreoathetosis – uncontrolled jerky movements, due to involvement of the basal ganglia, which are more noticeable during slow movement.
- Ataxia – this presents as poor balance and coordination as a result of cerebellar involvement.

Hypotonic cerebral palsy is far less common. Although the more obvious limitations to sport for children stem from the motor dysfunction, there are several other commonly associated disorders which should be considered in sport selection, including:

- epilepsy
- visual defects
- deafness
- intellectual impairment
- perceptual deficits.

At the elite level, half of the competitors will compete in a wheelchair while the others are ambulant. The energy cost for ambulation, however, is high in cerebral palsy. For children in wheelchairs, the positioning of the body is crucial. Because of the extensor pattern of the spasticity, the hips extend and place the body in a poor pushing position. Securing the legs in place with the knees flexed greater than 90° and higher than the hips may help.

Previously, there has been controversy over the benefit of strength training in people with cerebral palsy, with its effect on muscle tone. However, benefits have been seen in adolescents (McCubbin & Shasby 1985) and elite-level athletes. Flexibility is a key component in an exercise programme in maintaining range of motion in the presence of spasticity. Stretching may involve assisted techniques such as proprioceptive muscular facilitation methods, but care should be applied in handling the limbs which may increase tone. Care should be taken to avoid pain. In some children, stretching may result in reduced performance by reducing motor tone, on which the child is dependent for stability or function. Stretching for flexibility may best be performed in these children after the performance in the warm-down period.

Amputees

Children with an amputation may participate in sport either with a prosthesis (e.g. sprinting, cycling) or without (e.g. high jump, swimming), or may compete in a wheelchair (e.g. basketball). It may be an upper or lower limb amputation, but lower limb amputations are more common. The potential benefits of sports par-

ticipation relate to the general benefits of exercise and improving musculature and circulation in the residual limb. This is not without risk to the residual limb from the effects of friction and compression when the prosthesis is used. This can result in skin abrasions and infection and musculoskeletal injury. The fit of the prosthesis is important for athletic performance, and is a fine balance between overcompression of the residual limb and slipping of a loose prosthesis on a sweaty residual limb. The fit will require continual adjustment because of growth and muscle adaptations to training. The alignment of the prosthesis is also an important consideration in injury prevention and may be altered by repetitive forceful impacts in running. The biomechanical effects of the 'short leg' on the prosthetic side, to allow easier ground clearance, may contribute to musculoskeletal disorders in the normal limb or low back. Impact loading is also a concern for the residual limb, with increased ground reaction forces that may lead to degenerative change in joints higher in the kinetic chain. Technological advances in prosthetic design may reduce this loading. The 'Flex-foot' design offers greater impact absorption while storing energy to facilitate propulsion, but is not without a cost implication for a child who requires a sports prosthesis as well as a prosthesis for daily use (see Figs 44.1 and 44.2).

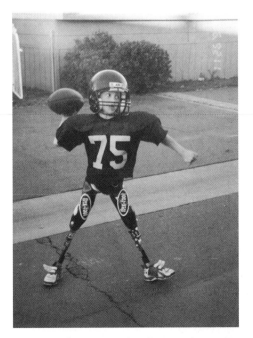

Figure 44.1 A child wearing 'Flex-foot' prostheses. By courtesy of Ossur/Flex-Foot Inc, Aliso Viejo, California. This illustration also appears on the cover of this book.

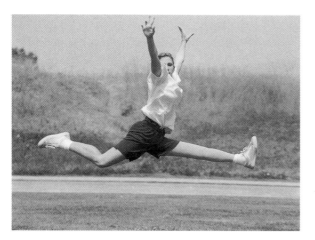

Figure 44.2 A young girl with a left-leg 'Flex-foot' prosthesis. By courtesy of Ossur/Flex-Foot Inc, Aliso Viejo, California.

'Les autres'

Somehow it seems more acceptable to describe those people with disabilities that do not fit into another category as 'the others' by translating the term into French – *les autres*. As sport for people with disabilities has expanded, so people outside the traditional disability groups have become involved, but by their nature they are fewer in number. Examples include the muscular dystrophies, multiple sclerosis, short stature, limb deficiencies, ankylosis, arthrodesis or arthritis of major joints.

It is beyond the scope of this chapter to describe each of these in detail, but the principles described previously apply in a similar way. Common sense application of general guidelines and a medical dictionary for the rare syndromes are probably the major requirements!

ELITE DISABILITY SPORT

Sports for people with disabilities have developed over the last century from minor sports clubs for a few conditions to the staging of the Paralympic Games, which is now the second largest sporting event, in terms of numbers of competitors, after the Olympics. Sport organizations for people with disabilities date back to the 1800s and include sports clubs for the deaf in Germany and a documented amputee race in Newmarket, England, in 1880 (Fallon 1995). However, the main impetus in advancing sport for disabled people is credited to Sir Ludwig Guttman of the spinal injuries centre at Stoke Mandeville. In 1944, Guttman started introducing sport as a stimulus for rehabilitation in servicemen injured in World War II. Wheelchair sports were developed and included table tennis, archery and basketball. This led to the first Stoke Mandeville games in 1948, with 16 competitors. This progressed to more than 3500 competitors at the Atlanta Paralympic Games with six major disability groups. As the size and prestige of the games has progressed, the emphasis has changed for some coaches, from encouraging of children with disabilities to take an interest in sport, to identifying talented children with the potential to win medals at major competition. The age of competitors in the Paralympic games is declining, with some competitors aged 15 and 16 years in the Great Britain Atlanta Paralympic team. The Paralympic sports best represent those sports most orientated towards people with disabilities and those with historical and technological development. It is therefore likely that children will gravitate towards these sports where organizations best represent their interests and the coaching structures are in place (Box 44.1).

Some of the sports are disability-specific, e.g. judo and goalball for the visually impaired, boccia for cerebral palsy and rugby for tetraplegics. In sports such as athletics, competitors will compete in events against athletes with similar disabilities, whilst in sports such as swimming, athletes with different physical disabilities will compete against each other, classified according to the severity of disability. A swimmer with cerebral palsy may compete alongside a swimmer with limb deformities and one with a spinal cord injury. The classification system for each sport is beyond the scope of this article, but it attempts to produce fair competition among the disability groups and may include functional assessment of sport performance as well as objective assessment by medical examination. Needless to say, it can be an area of great contention, as the change of classification group can mean the difference between being world champion and not even making the team.

Box 44.1 Sports of the 1996 Paralympic Games

- Archery
- Athletics
- Basketball
- Boccia
- Cycling
- Equestrian
- Fencing
- Football
- Goalball
- Judo
- Lawn bowls
- Power lifting
- Shooting
- Swimming
- Table tennis
- Tennis
- Volleyball
- Yachting
- Quad rugby

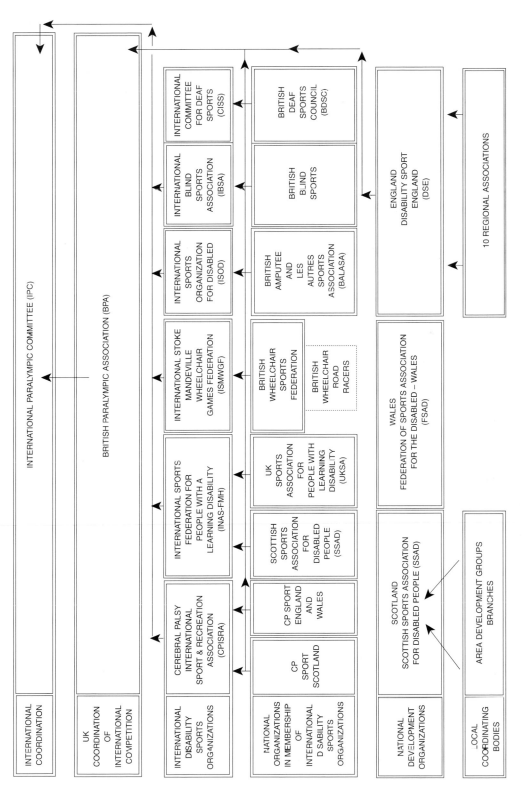

Figure 44.3 The structure of sport for people with disabilities.

ORGANIZATION

On an international level, there are a number of disability- and sport-specific organizations representing the international interests of athletes. At a national level it can be even more confusing. An example of the structure of the national disability sports movement in the United Kingdom is shown in Figure 44.3 and is not for the faint-hearted.

As sport for people with disabilities develops, it is hoped that this will simplify. However, the debate regarding integration into versus segregation from able-bodied sport continues (Downs 1995). Demonstration events of disability sport do occur at the Olympic and Commonwealth Games.

CONCLUSIONS

The potential for children with disabilities to perform in sport in general and in elite sport is increasing. The medical limitations to activity are few, but physicians also have a duty of care to protect young athletes in a competitive environment from exploitation. There are still many political issues surrounding sport and disability, both between disability groups and regarding integration into or segregation from able-bodied sport. For the physician, the duty of care is to aid the provision of safe sport which provides health benefits and raises self-esteem through enjoyable participation.

REFERENCES

American Academy of Pediatrics 1982 Recommendations for participation in competitive sports. Pediatrics 81: 737–739

Attia M, Engel P 1983 Thermoregulatory set point in patients with spinal cord injuries (spinal man). Paraplegia 21(4): 233–248

Bergman A B, Stamm S J 1967 The morbidity of cardiac nondisease in school children. New England Journal of Medicine 276(18): 1008–1013

Blair S N, Kohl H W 3rd, Barlow C E, Paffenbarger R S Jr, Gibbons L W, Macera C A 1995 Changes in physical fitness and all-cause mortality. A prospective study of healthy and unhealthy men. Journal of the American Medical Association 273: 1093–1098

Bloomquist L E 1986 Injuries to athletes with physical disabilities: prevention implications. Physician & Sports Medicine 14(9): 96–105

Brown R S 1982 Exercise and mental health in the pediatric population. Clinics in Sports Medicine 1: 515–527

Burnham R, Wheeler G, Bhambini Y, Belenger M, Eriksson P, Steadward R 1994 Intentional induction of autonomic dysreflexia among quadriplegic athletes for performance enhancement: efficacy, safety, and mechanism of action. Clinical Journal of Sports Medicine 4: 1–10

Downey J A, Huckaba C E, Myers S J, Darling R C 1973 Thermoregulation in the spinal man. Journal of Applied Physiology 34(6): 790–794

Downs P 1995 Willing and able: an introduction to inclusive practices. Australian Sports Commission, Canberra

Fallon K E 1995 The disabled athlete. In: Bloomfield J, Fricker P A, Fitch K D (eds) Science and medicine in sport. Blackwell Science, Carlton, p 550–551

Ferrara M, Davis R 1990 Injuries to elite wheelchair athletes. Paraplegia 4: 24–37

Guttman, L, Silver J R, Wyndham 1958 Thermoregulation in spinal man. Journal of Physiology 406–419

Hoffman M D 1986 Cardiorespiratory fitness and training in quadriplegics and paraplegics. Sports Medicine 3: 312–330

McCubbin J A, Shasby G B 1985 Effects of isokinetic exercise on adolescents with cerebral palsy. Adapted Physical Activity Quarterly 2: 56–64

Nixon H L 1988 Getting over the worry hurdle: parental encouragement and the sports involvement of visually impaired children and youths. Adapted Physical Activity Quarterly 5: 29–43

O'Connell D G, Barnhart R 1995 Improvement in wheelchair propulsion in pediatric wheelchair users through resistance training: a pilot study. Archives of Physical Medicine and Rehabilitation 76: 368–372

Peck D M, McKeag D B 1994 Athletes with disabilities; removing medical barriers. Physician & Sports Medicine 22(4): 59–62

Petrofsky J S 1992 Thermoregulatory stress during rest and exercise in heat in patients with a spinal cord injury. European Journal of Applied Physiology & Occupational Physiology 64: 503–507

Pueschel S M 1998 Should children with Down syndrome be screened for atlantoaxial instability? Archives of Pediatric & Adolescent Medicine 152(2): 123–125

Ward D S, Bar Or O, Longmuir P, Smith K 1995 Use of rating of perceived exertion (RPE) to prescribe exercise intensity for wheelchair-bound children and adults. Pediatric Exercise Science 7: 94–102

Webborn A D J 1996 Heat-related problems for the Paralympic Games, Atlanta 1996. British Journal of Therapy & Rehabilitation 3: 429–436

45

Sport for children with intellectual disabilities

Carolyn C. O'Brien

KEY POINTS

1. A major barrier to physical participation of children with an intellectual disability is the negative attitude of teachers, parents and coaches towards their involvement in sport.
2. Intellectually disabled children have delays in their developmental milestones, fundamental movement skills and motor performance skills which hinder them from interacting physically at a similar skill level as their peers. Some, e.g. those with Down's syndrome, also have physiological differences from their normally developing peers.
3. Intervention programmes for intellectually disabled children should progress from sensory and perceptual-motor programmes in early childhood to skill-based learning and fitness activities in middle childhood.
4. Children with an intellectual disability need to be taught physical skills in a different way to their normally developing peers, e.g. they require much repetition.
5. People conducting physical activity sessions for children who are intellectually disabled must have a good knowledge of their physical, learning and developmental differences.

INTRODUCTION

Sport and physical activity are important for children's health, growth, and physical and social development (Shepard 1995). In children with an intellectual disability, sport not only improves health-related factors such as obesity and cardiovascular risk factors, but also helps overcome poor self-esteem, loneliness, depression, poor motor skills, low physical fitness and lack of social contacts, especially in adolescence and adulthood.

Intellectual disability occurs in about 3% of the population, and has a varied aetiology, including brain damage from trauma, infection such as cytomegalovirus, rubella and meningitis, metabolic disorders including phenylketonuria, galactosaemia and hypothyroidism, and noxious substances such as alcohol. Chromosome disorders which affect brain development, including Down's syndrome and fragile X syndrome, account for up to 10% of the intellectually disabled population. Some other causes of intellectual disability may be low birthweight or prematurity, hydrocephalus and microcephaly. Although the primary disability is intellectual, many of these children may have other disabilities, such as cerebral palsy, spina bifida, congenital heart defects, hearing and visual impairment, and behaviour dysfunction caused by autism or Asperger's syndrome (Eichstaedt & Lavay 1992, Sherrill 1998).

People in Australia are regarded as intellectually disabled if they are more than two standard deviations below the norm on standardized intelligence tests. Account is also taken of their communication and life skills. In the UK these people are classified as having learning difficulties. In the USA and Canada, the same people are classified as being mentally retarded (Eichstaedt & Lavay 1992, Sherrill 1998).

Sport for children with an intellectual disability is important, but special support services should be available in the school and the community. The presence of these services makes it easier to address the attitudinal, biological and participation barriers that these children need to overcome to participate in sporting activities of a highly competitive nature or in physical activity for recreation and leisure.

ATTITUDE BARRIERS

A negative attitude is one of the greatest barriers that intellectually disabled children need to overcome before they can successfully participate in sport or physical activity. The attitude barrier may be negative feelings by the disabled person, parents, other children in the class or community setting, health professionals, physical education teachers or coaches.

In comparison with the rest of the population, people with a disability are less likely to participate in regular sport or physical activity. This has resulted in what has been called the disabled or sick child syndrome. Children with this syndrome are socially withdrawn, have poor physical fitness and low motor ability. The origins of this syndrome are largely due to low societal expectations of what disabled children can achieve. These negative expectations often result in overprotection of disabled children by parents, teachers and health professionals (Marley 1997).

Unfortunately, a negative attitude towards disabled children participating in sport deprives them of the positive outcomes derived from regular physical activity. These positive outcomes include an improvement in mood state, physical fitness, self-concept and self-esteem. Increased physical activity participation has also been shown to improve social acceptance, so that people with a disability gain an increased perception of themselves as worthwhile (Hutzler & Bar-Eli 1993). A major thrust in recent years has been the inclusion of people with a disability in a less restrictive environment. The philosophy behind current inclusion policy is that a positive attitude towards disabled children is fostered by interaction between these children and their normally developing peers. The theoretical assumption is that non-disabled children will develop positive attitudes towards peers with a disability, provided the inclusion setting is based on equal status and common goals. On the other hand, negative attitudes are likely to occur in non-disabled peers if the inclusion programme is not appropriate for them.

Tripp et al (1995) found evidence that contradicted this general philosophy in children aged 9 to 12 years old. They found that children in an integrated physical education setting had more negative attitudes towards their disabled peers than children who had physical education in segregated settings. An important finding that needs to be addressed by those advocating inclusion policy is that competition in an inclusive setting caused frustration between the children and more negative attitudes towards children with a disability. Additional findings from this study were that girls tended to have a more favourable attitude than boys to peers with a disability. Overall, the positive attitude of children without a disability towards those with a disability decreased according to the type of disability – the most favourable attitudes were towards children with a physical disability, followed by those with an intellectual disability, and then those with a behavioural disorder.

Another study investigated the effect of academic learning and positive experiences of future physical education teachers and advanced undergraduate physical education teachers. The undergraduate physical education teachers who had academic preparation and positive experiences in working with children and people with disabilities felt more competent in their role of including disabled children in their classes (Rizzo & Kirkendall 1995).

It is apparent, therefore, that a way to overcome negative attitudes towards participation in sport by disabled people is to educate parents and teachers about the importance of health-related benefits derived from sport and physical activity. In addition, trainee physical education teachers should learn about disabilities as well as having the opportunity to work in programmes that foster positive attitudes towards participation in sport by people with a disability.

Teachers or coaches working with intellectually disabled people in sport and physical activity settings need to know about motor development delay and early intervention strategies; the reasons for poor motor performance and methods of improving the skills of these children; and the structural, physiological and learning dysfunction in people with an intellectual disability. All these factors need to be taken into account, as they may interfere with the opportunity for people with a disability to increase physical fitness as well as improving their performance at an elite level. These biological barriers include different physiological responses, anatomical anomalies, and neuromuscular and learning dysfunction, all of which hinder successful participation by intellectually disabled people in sport and physical activity.

BIOLOGICAL BARRIERS

Delayed motor development in intellectually disabled children

Children with intellectual disability, including those with Down's syndrome, have deficits in all phases of motor development. Intellectually disabled children without Down's syndrome are delayed in their development of postural reflexes, and many have abnormalities in muscle tone, poor body awareness and slower reaction times for their age. Children with Down's syndrome also have persistent delays in reflex development, and very low muscle tone, abnormally high joint laxity, perceptual deficiencies in postural, auditory

and visual areas, and marked memory deficits in storage and retrieval of information (O'Brien & Hayes 1995). These delays and differences mean that most of the developmental milestones of these children, including sitting, crawling and walking, are delayed. Consequently, these children are delayed in their acquisition of the fundamental movement patterns of running, jumping, throwing and catching, and acquire more advanced movement skills later. This delay implies that intellectually disabled children will have fundamental motor skills well below their age norms, and this alone will preclude normal social and physical interaction (O'Brien & Hayes 1995).

In addition to delayed motor development, O'Brien & Hayes (1995) found that intellectually disabled children with and without Down's syndrome had delays in motor performance as measured by the following items from the Bruininks–Oseretsky test of motor proficiency: running speed and agility, dynamic and static balance, bilateral coordination, and throwing and catching a ball. Overall, the results from 6-year-old children suggested that there was no significant difference between children who were clumsy (developmental coordination disorder) and those who had intellectual disability and Down's syndrome, but these three groups of children were below age norms. At 10 years of age, however, there was a significant difference in motor performance, and the clumsy children had a better performance than the two intellectually disabled groups (O'Brien & Hayes 1995).

Moreover, a longitudinal study conducted on the motor performance of children with Down's syndrome aged from 10 to 16 years showed that they continued to improve on subtests of the Bruininks–Oseretsky test of motor proficiency. The rate of improvement was slower after 12 years of age, and by 16 years they had a much lower level of motor performance than normally developing age peers. It was also found that the lowest scoring items in terms of the age norms was in the balance tasks (Jobling 1998), confirming the weakness in this area of motor control that has been frequently reported in the literature.

Physiological responses in people with an intellectual disability and Down's syndrome

In addition to motor delay and differences, intellectually disabled people and those with Down's syndrome are physiologically different from the normal population. Young adults with an intellectual disability have such low levels of cardiorespiratory fitness that their values are similar to those of middle-aged people or post-myocardial infarction patients. Nevertheless, some adults do show normal cardiovascular responses to training. Furthermore, there does not appear to be any physiological reason why people without Down's syndrome or any secondary disabilities do not have normal physiological function. Nevertheless, the finding of such low levels of fitness must have serious implications for the health of these people as well as their ability to participate in competitive sport (Fernhall et al 1996).

Other research has shown that people with Down's syndrome have impaired brain glucose utilization, thyroid hormonal deficiency, heart and blood vessel abnormalities, pulmonary hypoplasia, narrowed aorta, and small nasal and oral cavities. These physiological differences compromise their cardiovascular fitness, which is lower than those people with intellectual disability without any secondary disabilities (Eberhard et al 1989, 1991, Fernhall et al 1996).

Until recently, little was known about the physiological response of children with Down's syndrome to maximal exercise exertion. In regard to exercise response, current research has demonstrated that, as well as their lower aerobic capacity on maximal exertion, these children have irregular rises in blood pressure and a lower increase in heart rate than their normally developing peers. Examination of blood parameters of Down's syndrome children after intense maximal exercise has suggested that they have similar biochemical changes, even though they have different endocrine responses (Eberhard 1989).

These studies on cardiovascular responses raise the question as to whether individuals with Down's syndrome have physiological limitations to increasing their cardiovascular capacity with intense exercise. If this is true, then people who have Down's syndrome will have lower levels of physical fitness, which may contribute to their known higher risk than the rest of the population of developing coronary heart disease, secondary diabetes, obesity and hypertension in middle age. Furthermore, there is a paucity of research into the cardiovascular responses of children with Down's syndrome to physical activity and sport, and without this information it is difficult to design programmes to reduce common health risks with increased age.

Structural impairment in children with Down's syndrome

Although children with Down's syndrome derive many benefits from participation in regular physical activity and sport, certain precautions must be taken to ensure their safety. Common serious health problems of these children should be identified, particularly cardiac abnormalities and atlantoaxial instability, which has been estimated to occur in 10–40% of children with Down's syndrome (Cremers et al 1993).

Atlantoaxial instability is caused by laxity of the transverse atlantal ligaments. In these children, there is a risk that, during sport, spinal compression or dislocation may occur at the atlantoaxial joint if the neck is in extreme flexion or extension. The consequence of spinal compression or dislocation can be loss of co-ordination and generalized muscular weakness, or there may be more severe outcomes such as diplegia, hemiplegia or torticollis. Medical opinion is divided, however, about the actual risk to children with Down's syndrome who have a 4 mm or greater distance between the posterior rim of the anterior arch of the atlas and the axis. The conservative opinion is that all high-risk sports, such as diving, gymnastics and football, are contraindicated. According to other medical authorities, there is little increased risk to these children, so they should not be restricted in the sports in which they wish to participate. Indeed, the small increased risk is outweighed by the health benefits derived through regular participation in physical activity and sport, especially as the gap between the atlas and axis usually decreases with age (Cremers et al 1993).

Neuromuscular impairment in children with cerebral palsy

Intellectual disability occurs frequently in people with cerebral palsy, especially spasticity, in which it has been estimated that 70% of patients have some form of intellectual disability (Sherrill 1998). The consequences of sport participation in children with cerebral palsy are far-reaching.

People with cerebral palsy, whether they have spasticity, athetosis, ataxia or a mixed condition, all have similarities as well as distinct differences in their condition and in the parts of their bodies that are affected. Similar symptoms across all types of cerebral palsy are abnormalities of muscle tone, persistence of more primitive brain reflexes, marked coordination difficulties, and abnormalities in perceptual processing. Even mildly affected children with spastic cerebral palsy have reduced anaerobic power in the arms and legs. This finding may be due to muscle fibre changes, as they have more slow fibres, probably because a lesion in the upper motor neurons causes atrophy of fast fibres in the antigravity muscles in children with spasticity (Parker et al 1992).

Another finding from electromyographic (EMG) research has shown that people with cerebral palsy have major difficulties in descending motor commands, including reflex control and muscle contractions. These recent observations have led to the hypothesis that the brain lesion resulting in cerebral palsy causes processing abnormalities in sensori-motor information, and hence the construct of faulty models of motor functioning. Because of this developmental difference in children with cerebral palsy, it is doubtful, even with extensive intervention, that these children are able to learn adaptable patterns of movement with appropriate temporal sequencing (Parker et al 1993).

Due to abnormal voluntary control of movement, persistent reflexes and poor muscle control, most children with cerebral palsy who are capable of self-initiated ambulation have abnormal gait patterns. The abnormalities in walking have been extensively researched in children, but there is a paucity of research in abnormal running patterns and the effect this has on elite running performance. The limited number of studies in this area have shown that self-ambulatory elite athletes with cerebral palsy have abnormalities in their running pattern, including a shortened stride length, asymmetry in distance and phasing of their steps, and a longer airborne phase on their affected side. Frequency of steps, on the dysfunctional side, or if both sides are affected equally, is higher for the same velocity than that of able-bodied runners. These abnormalities in gait result in a much higher energy cost than for able-bodied people, which means that they fatigue more easily. This is compounded by the fact that most people with cerebral palsy have low aerobic work capacity (Pope et al 1993).

Structuring the learning environment for intellectually disabled children

It is more difficult for children and adults with an intellectual disability to learn complex skills than it is for normally developing people. The cognitive limitations of these children both in learning new skills and in participating in a sport environment must be acknowledged even in those children with a mild intellectual disability. Many children with an intellectual disability have attention problems, so they become easily distracted by irrelevant stimuli. One way of overcoming this problem when trying to teach them a new skill is to limit the amount of distracting stimuli. These include noise, excessive movement and colour. It is also important to gain their attention by using something that is new to them, something that is very brightly coloured or is a surprise (Sherrill 1998, Thomas 1984).

Children with intellectual disability have problems with short-term memory. One way of overcoming this in sport is to teach them strategies to cope with the complexity of the games situation. It must be remembered, however, that these children may not transfer the taught strategy from one situation to a slightly different one, and that they usually do not develop their own strategies (Thomas 1984). Teachers and coaches should break a sport or physical skill down into smaller units of information for the child to learn. They must also give children with an intellectual disability a large number of rehearsals in a particular task until the task is well learnt (Thomas 1984). A new skill may be taught by modelling the activity, encouraging the children to image what they are trying to remember, or talking themselves through what they are to do. Children should receive positive reinforcement when they succeed in a task. Verbal praise is a good reinforcement.

In summary, biological barriers to participation must be taken into account when sport and physical activity options are presented to the child with an intellectual disability. Some traditional sports may be contraindicated in children with Down's syndrome because they may have atlantoaxial instability, cardiac abnormalities, hearing and visual impairment. Other children with an intellectual disability may also have cerebral palsy or spina bifida, and many of them have epileptic seizures. Finally, structuring the optimum learning environment is an important aspect of teaching these children sports skills.

The final barrier to be discussed is the mode of participation in sport. This will be called the participation barrier.

PARTICIPATION BARRIER

Finding the correct placement in sport and physical activity for intellectually disabled children is equally as important as overcoming the attitudinal and biological barriers to their participation in sport. Much of the recent discussion on this aspect of participation in sport and physical activity has been centred around inclusion. Inclusion in the USA is mandated by law, but this is not the case in other countries such as Australia. This means that inclusion practices might be slower, but it also means that the reasons for inclusion can be carefully evaluated.

Before intellectually disabled children are included in sport and physical activity, teachers, parents and health professionals should ask the following questions. Why is it important to try to include these children? What strategies can be used to make the physical activity beneficial to the intellectually disabled child and non-disabled peers? Would either groups of children learn better in a more segregated environment?

The answers to these questions are complex. For example, if the disabled child is placed in a normal sport or physical activity session, the environment is more stimulating. As a consequence, the disabled child will be exposed to age-appropriate social skills and behaviours, as well as experiencing age-appropriate activities. Moreover, even non-disabled children need different types of instruction. This means that, provided modifications can be made easily, it is better to include the disabled child within normal school and community activities (Block 1994). Any accommodation to the activity, however, must allow the person with the disability and non-disabled peers to participate successfully, without making the activity meaningless or more dangerous (Block 1994).

People in charge of the inclusion activity must have an understanding of the particular disability and its implications in the sport or physical activity setting. They must also have knowledge of specific activities that might be suitable for children with a particular disability. For example, if Down's syndrome children are being taught, the people conducting the session should know which children have atlantoaxial instability, to ensure that these children avoid all activities that place pressure on the neck when hyperextended or flexed. In another example, swimming is a suitable activity for children with cerebral palsy, but extra personnel are needed to ensure that help is available if any children have an epileptic seizure.

Resource implications would include the number of extra people needed to assist the disabled child and the teacher to make the learning experience beneficial to all the children participating in the session. Other resource requirements may include lighter balls and bats, or modified equipment, games or rules. The teacher may be able to include some children successfully by allocating peer tutors to assist the child. If this is the case, there needs to be a number of peer tutors to assist each child so that the tutors can participate in all the activities.

Decisions also need to be made about whether the intellectually disabled child has skills at a similar level to the other children participating in the sport or physical activity. This is because acceptance of the child within that setting mainly depends on whether the child has similar sports skills to the other children in the group, especially if the activity is highly competitive.

It must be remembered that the primary aim of sport and physical activity for children with an intellectual disability is that the programme for these children must improve their participation rate, their physical skills and physical fitness. It is assumed that improvement in these three areas will increase the social acceptance and feelings of competency of these children, so that they can participate in sport and physical activity in school and the community.

Finally, successful sport and physical activity programmes for intellectually disabled children must provide for a continuum of physical experiences, from leisure and recreation to participation in elite competition like the Special Olympics, which is discussed below.

Special Olympics

The Special Olympics is founded on the belief that people with mental retardation can, with proper instruction and encouragement, learn, enjoy and benefit from participation in individual and team sports, adapted as necessary to meet the needs of those with special mental and physical limitations (Eichstaedt & Lavay 1992, p. 387).

The Special Olympics originated in the USA, where summer day camps for intellectually disabled children and adults were sponsored by the Kennedy family between 1963 and 1968. In 1968, the first International Special Olympics were held in Chicago. In the same year, Special Olympics International was formed as a non-profit charitable organization. In 1977, the Winter Special Olympics was established, in addition to the Summer Olympics (Eichstaedt & Lavay 1992). Since its inception, the Special Olympics organization has set up training programmes throughout the USA, so that anyone aged over 8 years with an IQ of 80 or below, with or without other disabilities, can participate in events that are ability-, gender- and age-appropriate. In 1989, motor active training programmes were set up by the Special Olympics for people with a severe intellectual disability who could not take part in the Special Olympics or the training programmes for these events.

Paralympic Games

In 1992, another important milestone occurred in Barcelona, when athletes with an intellectual disability competed for the first time in the Paralympic Games (Doll-Tepper 1994). By being included in the Paralympics, people with an intellectual disability now have the full spectrum of opportunity in sport, recreation and leisure. It places the responsibility on professionals assisting intellectually disabled children to ensure they have the proper foundation in motor development and sport skills to enable them to take advantage of the opportunities that are now available to them.

CONCLUSIONS

1. Negative attitudes towards participation in sport and physical activity by intellectually disabled children may not necessarily be overcome by placing them in the least restrictive environment. Some studies have shown that an inclusion policy may foster more negative attitudes than when these children participate in a segregated setting. Negative attitudes occur in competitive activities and in situations where the intellectually disabled child does not have the equivalent skill levels of the other children. It has to be assumed, therefore, that inclusion in these situations will not be beneficial to the child with an intellectual disability, who may derive more benefit from non-inclusion settings. It must be remembered that many people without a disability enjoy playing sport against people of their own gender, which is in fact a segregated setting!

2. Children with an intellectual disability with and without Down's syndrome have many delays and differences in their motor development, physiological responses to maximum exercise, anatomical anomalies and learning impairment, in comparison with their normally developing peers. Children with intellectual disabilities and Down's syndrome have delayed motor development partly due to persistent primitive reflexes and delayed postural responses. Consequently, they have delayed developmental milestones and fundamental movement patterns that make it difficult for them to have normal play interactions with other children. In middle childhood through adolescence they have lower motor performance scores on age-referenced motor performance tests, which disadvantages them in regular sports and physical activity settings.

3. Children with Down's syndrome also have different physiological responses to maximal exercise. They have a lower aerobic capacity, irregular rises in blood pressure, and a lower increase in heart rate than children without Down's syndrome. Many children with Down's syndrome also have anatomical differences such as heart defects and atlantoaxial instability, which may mean that certain sports and activities should not be attempted. Intellectually disabled children without Down's syndrome or any secondary disabilities also have lower motor performance and fitness scores than their normally developing peers. In most cases, there is no apparent reason for these low scores, so they may reflect lack of play, games and sports opportunities for these children.

4. Infants and young children with an intellectual disability, whatever its origin, should participate in sensorimotor programmes. Once they have acquired basic fundamental movement patterns they should participate in activities that improve limb coordination, balance, strength and locomotor and manipulative skills. In middle childhood, the emphasis should initially be on elementary games and sport skills. In addition, unless contraindicated, children with an intellectual disability should participate in fitness activities at a submaximal level. Children who have a higher standard in sport skills and fitness levels should be encouraged to train and compete with their normally developing peers. Physical leisure and recreational skills should also be taught to all children with an intellectual disability so that they can remain physically active and maintain social contacts throughout life.

5. The learning environment for intellectually disabled children should reduce distracting stimuli because of attentional problems in these children. Their attention to relevant stimuli can be enhanced by novel and

brightly coloured stimuli. Because of their memory deficits, particularly in short-term memory, the task to be learned should be broken down into small units and repeated until it is well learned. Children with intellectual disabilities should be taught strategies such as imaging or talking themselves through the task in order to learn skills and remember what they should do when playing games and sports. Appropriate actions and tactics will also have to be well rehearsed, as these children do not generalize readily from one situation to another. Frequent positive reinforcement also enhances learning.

6. Personnel conducting the sport or physical activity session must have a thorough knowledge of the disability and what precautions need to be taken to enable these children to participate successfully and safely with other children. Additional resource implications for participation in sport and physical activity might include more personnel as well as modifications to the rules of the game and/or the equipment. Any decisions about including an intellectually disabled child in regular sport or physical activity should depend on the skill level of that child and the competitiveness of the activity. Decisions about optimal placement in sport and physical activity must take into account whether it will improve their participation rate, physical skills, physical fitness and social interactions. Opportunities should also be provided to allow these children to participate in physical leisure and recreational activities.

7. Athletes with an intellectual disability should be able to receive coaching and experience competition in individual and team sports that are adapted to meet their special needs. The Special Olympics organization meets these needs very well in the USA, but its role in other countries may be met by other organizations at the community and interstate level. The Special Olympics International does provide an international competition for many intellectually disabled athletes from around the world. The competition caters for summer and winter sports at an individual and team level that are ability-, age- and gender-specific. Elite athletes with an intellectual disability have been included in the Paralympics since 1992. This means that intellectually disabled people should now have the opportunity to participate in sport from a recreational to an elite level.

REFERENCES

Block M E 1994 Including students with disabilities in regular physical education. Paul H Brookes, Baltimore

Cremers M J G, Bol E, de Roos F, van Gijn J 1993 Risk of sports activities in children with Down's syndrome and atlantoaxial instability. Lancet 342: 511–514

Doll-Tepper G 1994 Adapted physical education programs for mentally retarded children. In Yabe K, Kusano K, Nakata H (eds) Adapted physical activity. Springer-Verlag, Tokyo, p 20–25

Eberhard Y, Eterradossi J, Rapacchi B 1989 Physical aptitudes to exertion in children with Down's syndrome. Journal of Mental Deficiency Research 33: 167–174

Eberhard Y, Eterradossi J, Therminarias A 1991 Biochemical changes and catecholamine responses in Down's syndrome adolescents in relation to incremental maximal exercise. Journal of Mental Deficiency Research 35: 140–146

Eichstaedt C B, Lavay B W 1992 Physical activity for individuals with mental retardation. Human Kinetics, Champaign, IL

Fernhall B, Pitetti K H, Rimmer J H et al 1996 Cardiorespiratory capacity of individuals with mental retardation including Down syndrome. Medicine and Science in Sports and Exercise 28(3): 366–371

Hutzler Y, Bar-Eli M 1993 Psychological benefits of sports for the disabled people: A review. Scandinavian Journal of Medicine and Science in Sports 3: 217–228

Jobling A 1998 Motor development in school-aged children with Down syndrome: a longitudinal perspective. International Journal of Disability, Development and Education 45(3): 283–291

Marley W P 1997 The disability syndrome and the instinctive wisdom of the body. Palaestra 26–29

O'Brien C, Hayes A 1995 Normal and impaired motor development: theory into practice. Chapman & Hall, London

Parker D F, Carriere L, Hebestreit H, Bar-Or O 1992 Anaerobic endurance and peak muscle power in children with cerebral palsy. American Journal of Diseases in Children 146: 1069–1073

Parker D F, Carriere L, Hebestreit H, Salsberg A, Bar-Or O 1993 Muscle performance and gross motor function of children with spastic cerebral palsy. Developmental Medicine and Child Neurology 35: 17–23

Pope C, Sherrill C, Wilkerson J, Pyfer J 1993 Biomechanical variables in sprint running of athletes with cerebral palsy. Adapted Physical Activity Quarterly 10: 226–254

Rizzo T L, Kirkendall D R 1995 Teaching students with mild disabilities: what effects attitudes of future physical educators. Adapted Physical Activity Quarterly 12: 205–216

Sherrill C 1998 Adapted physical activity, recreation and sport. WCB/McGraw-Hill, Boston

Shepard R J 1995 Physical activity, health and well being at different life stages. Research Quarterly for Exercise and Sport 66(4): 298–302

Thomas J R 1984 Motor development during childhood and adolescence. Burgess, Minneapolis

Tripp A, French R, Sherrill C 1995 Contact theory and attitudes of children in physical education programs towards peers with disabilities. Adapted Physical Activity 12: 323–332

Index